Essentials of
Human Nutrition

Essentials of
Human Nutrition

Fourth Edition

Edited By

Jim Mann
Professor of Human Nutrition and Medicine, University of Otago,
New Zealand

A. Stewart Truswell
Emeritus Professor of Human Nutrition, University of Sydney, Australia

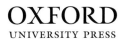

OXFORD
UNIVERSITY PRESS

OXFORD
UNIVERSITY PRESS

Great Clarendon Street, Oxford OX2 6DP

Oxford University Press is a department of the University of Oxford.
It furthers the University's objective of excellence in research, scholarship,
and education by publishing worldwide in

Oxford New York

Auckland Cape Town Dar es Salaam Hong Kong Karachi
Kuala Lumpur Madrid Melbourne Mexico City Nairobi
New Delhi Shanghai Taipei Toronto

With offices in

Argentina Austria Brazil Chile Czech Republic France Greece
Guatemala Hungary Italy Japan Poland Portugal Singapore
South Korea Switzerland Thailand Turkey Ukraine Vietnam

Oxford is a registered trade mark of Oxford University Press
in the UK and in certain other countries

Published in the United States
by Oxford University Press Inc., New York

© Oxford University Press 2012

British Library Cataloguing in Publication Data

Data available

Library of Congress Cataloging in Publication Data

Library of Congress Control Number: 2011939854

Typeset by Techset Composition Ltd, Salisbury, UK
Printed in Great Britain
on acid-free paper by
Ashford Colour Press Ltd, Gosport, Hampshire

ISBN 978-0-19-956634-1

10 9 8 7 6 5 4 3 2

Preface

Several excellent textbooks of human nutrition are available. We have attempted to produce a book that differs from most of them by asking our contributors to describe what they regard as those aspects of their topics that are essential to the understanding and practice of human nutrition. Most of the authors are international authorities on the subjects on which they have written and all are very experienced teachers.

We were initially reluctant to accept the offer of the publishers to produce yet another textbook of human nutrition. We were persuaded to do so because we felt there was a need for a book that described the essential information required by students embarking on a University course in human nutrition, and by those in training in the health and food science professions, where the importance of nutrition is being increasingly recognized. Many of our clinical colleagues in medicine, dentistry, nursing and physiotherapy, and school teachers, provided strong encouragement for this project, since they too required a simple reference volume, having themselves received little formal training in nutrition. An increasingly informed public expects its health providers to have knowledge of one of the most important determinants of individual and public health. Health professionals and food scientists need to be able to disentangle scientifically established nutrition principles from the morass of misinformation available in the public domain. The book may also be of value to those in the fitness industry, and, last but not least, individual members of the public who have sufficient knowledge of biology and chemistry and who wish to be informed of the essentials of human nutrition. The book is not intended to be a detailed reference volume and each chapter contains further reading for those wishing to extend the information provided in the text.

We have tried to emphasize that nutritional science encompasses a spectrum of disciplines and involves the use of many methodologies. In the past, the major advances in nutrition were made at the level of organs and organisms, many from studies of experimental animals. Most present advances have been at the population level and, even more recently, at the molecular level. The discovery that dietary alteration can modify gene expression suggests that what we eat has even more profound implications than had previously been believed. These disciplines now need to be integrated at the human level to promote the practical application of nutritional science in metabolic, clinical, and public health nutrition.

This medium-sized textbook has become popular, especially in universities in Europe and the Southern Hemisphere. Human nutrition science continues to evolve since our third edition in 2007 and thus Oxford University Press asked us to prepare this fourth edition.

Seventeen new writers have joined the authorship of the book. Most are very well-known nutritional scientists. Six of the 42 chapters are completely rewritten and all the others have been revised and updated. Professor John Milner and Dr Young Kim, have written a new chapter on 'Genes, nutrition, and disease risk,'

Professor Tim Lang and Dr Helen Crawley have written a new chapter entitled 'Nutrition, the environment, and sustainable diets', and case studies have been included in four of the chapters. In a few chapters, potentially controversial views regarding the implementation of nutrition interventions have been expressed. These are not necessarily the views of the editors.

We are very grateful to our chapter writers for their expert and well-described material—and also for their tolerance of our editing of what they wrote. We have been somewhat interventionist in our attempt to keep the writing simple and readable and the different chapters fairly consistent. We thought it important not to let 'essentials' get wordy, long, heavy, and costly.

Although we two editors live and work in separate countries, it has been an enjoyable and creative task to work together, with the help of many e-mails and teleconferences.

We hope that readers will find our book useful in their study of human nutrition. For those who would like more detail, each chapter has a list of suggestions for further reading. These references are not comprehensive but selected, and most of them should be accessible.

We have arranged to participate in an Editors' Forum via OUP's Online Resource Centre. Twice a year we will send notes on new developments in the whole area of human nutrition. In addition, we would welcome comments from students, lecturers, or general readers.

Prof. Jim Mann, jim.mann@otago.ac.nz
Prof. Stewart Truswell, stewart.truswell@sydney.edu.au

New to this edition

- Six chapters entirely rewritten, all others revised and updated.
- New chapters: 'Genes, nutrition, and disease risk' and 'Nutrition, the environment, and sustainable diets'.
- Enhanced coverage of the B vitamins and obesity.
- Several new case studies.

To see topical and scientifically robust updates on nutrition associated with this textbook and web links to many of the journal articles in the Further Reading sections, please see the dedicated Online Resource Centre at www.oxfordtextbooks.co.uk/orc/mann4e/.

Acknowledgements

The editors are very pleased that so many leading nutrition scientists have been prepared to contribute and have tolerated our editing. Our knowledge of nutrition has been moulded by many discussions with many colleagues over several years. Lesley Day has been the main editorial assistant for the book in Otago. She assisted with the revision of many of the chapters following the editorial process and ensured the standardized format required by the publishers. She has also been responsible for obtaining permissions to reproduce original material from other sources. We are grateful to her for playing a crucial role in the production of the book.

Marianne Alexander was Professor Truswell's secretary in Sydney for the first three editions and since early 2010, he has been assisted by Theodora Sideratou. Elizabeth Gray, editorial assistant for the first two editions, provided support for the third and fourth editions. For this edition, Gordon Hargreaves carried out the drawing and preparation of figures as required.

Contents

*deceased

Part 3 Nutrition-related disorders

*deceased

Part 7 Changing food habits

Part 8 Applications

Abbreviations

AA	arachidonic acid
AAS	atomic absorption spectrophotometry
ACE	angiotensin-converting enzyme
ACP	acyl carrier protein
ADH	alcohol dehydrogenase; antidiuretic hormone
ADI	acceptable daily intake
AGP	α1-acid glycoprotein
AGRP	agouti-related proteins
AI	adequate intake
AIDS	acquired immunodeficiency syndrome
ALDH	aldehyde dehydrogenases
AN	anorexia nervosa
AOAC	Association of Official Analytical Chemists
APC	adenomatous polyposis coli
ARE	antioxidant response element
ATP	adenosine triphosphate
BMD	bone mineral density
BMI	body mass index
BMR	basal metabolic rate
BN	bulimia nervosa
BSE	bovine spongiform encephalopathy
BST	bovine somatotrophin
CAP	Common Agricultural Policy
CBT	cognitive behavioural therapy
CHD	coronary heart disease
CCK	cholecystokinin
CoA	co-enzyme A
COMA	Committee on Medical Aspects of Food Policy
COX2	cyclooxygenase 2
CPAP	continuous positive airways pressure
CRP	C-reactive protein
CSA	childhood sexual abuse
CT	computerized tomography
CVD	cardiovascular disease
DASH	Dietary Approaches to Stop Hypertension
DE	digestible energy
DEXA	dual energy X-ray absorptiometry
DFEs	dietary folate equivalents
DGGs	dietary goals and guidelines
DHA	docosahexaenoic acid
DIT	diet-induced thermogenesis
DLW	doubly labelled water
DP	degree of polymerization
DRI	dietary reference intakes
DRV	dietary reference values
DV	daily value
EAR	estimated average requirement

EASD	European Association for the Study of Diabetes
ECF	extracellular fluid
EDNOS	eating disorder not otherwise specified
EFA	essential fatty acids
EFSA	European Food Safety Authority
EGRA	erythrocyte glutathione reductase activity
EPA	eicosapentaenoic acid
FAD	flavin adenine dinucleotide
FAO	Food and Agriculture Organization
FDA	Food and Drug Administration
FEP	free erythrocyte protoporphyrin
FFM	fat-free mass
FFQ	food frequency questionnaires
FG	fasting glucose
FIVE	familial isolated vitamin E deficiency
FMN	flavin mononucleotide
FSA	Food Standards Agency
FSANZ	Food Standards of Australia and New Zealand
GABA	γ-amino butyric acid
GE	gross energy
GFR	glomerular filtration rate
GI	glycaemic index
GL	glycaemic load
GLC	gas–liquid chromatography
GM	genetically modified
GPx	glutathione peroxidase
GRAS	generally regarded as safe
GST	glutathione S-transferase
GTP	guanosine triphosphate
HAART	highly active antiretroviral therapy
HACCP	hazard analysis of critical control points
HCP	haem carrier protein
HDAC	histone deacetylase
HDL	high-density lipoprotein
HERP	human exposure/rodent potency index
HG	hyperemesis gravidarum
HIV	human immunodeficiency virus
HPLC	high-performance liquid chromatography
ICF	intracellular fluid
ICCIDD	International Council for the Control of Iodine Deficiency Disorders
IDA	iron deficiency anaemia
IDD	iodine-deficiency disorders
IDDM	insulin-dependent diabetes
IF	intrinsic factor
IFG	impaired fasting glucose
IGF	insulin-like growth factor
IGT	impaired glucose tolerance
IHD	ischaemic heart disease
IL	interleukin
IOTF	International Obesity Taskforce
IPT	interpersonal psychotherapy

IRBP	interstitial retinoid binding protein
IRP	iron-responsive protein
IU	international units
JEFCA	joint expert committee on food additives
KKP	key kitchen person
LBM	lean body mass
LBW	low birth weight
LCP	long-chain ω-3 polyunsaturated
LDL	low-density lipoprotein
ME	metabolizable energy
MPOD	macular pigment optical density
MRDR	modified relative dose–response
MSG	monosodium glutamate
MTHFR	methylene tetrahydrofolate reductase
MUAC	mid-upper arm circumference
MUFA	monounsaturated fatty avids
MZ	meso-zeaxanthin
NAD	nicotinamide-adenine-dinucleotide
NADP	nicotinamide-adenine-dinucleotide phosphate
NASH	non-alcoholic steatohepatitis
NDO	non-digestible oligosaccharides
NE	niacin equivalents
NIDDM	non-insulin-dependent diabetes
NMES	non-milk extrinsic sugar
NOEL	no observed effect level
NPRQ	non-protein respiratory quotient
NPY	neuropeptide Y
NRV	nutrient reference values
NSP	non-starch polysaccharide
NTD	neural tube defects
p.p.m.	parts per million
PAF	platelet-activating agent
PAL	physical activity level
PBM	peak bone mass
PCB	polychlorinated biphenyls
PCV	packed cell volume
PEM	protein-energy malnutrition
PIVKA	protein induced by vitamin K absence
PLP	pyridoxal 5′-phosphate
PPAR	peroxisome proliferator-activated receptor
PTH	parathyroid hormone
PUFA	polyunsaturated fatty acids
PVC	polyvinyl chloride
PYY	peptide YY
RBP	retinol binding protein
RDA	recommended dietary allowance
RDI	recommended dietary intake
RDS	rapidly digestible starch
RE	retinol equivalents
RES	reticuloendothelial system
RMR	resting metabolic rate

RNI	recommended nutrient intake
RS	resistant starch
SCFA	short-chain fatty acids
SHP	starch hydrolysis product
SNP	single-nucleotide polymorphisms
SNRI	selective norepinephrine reuptake inhibitor
SSRI	selective serotonin reuptake inhibitor
TBW	total body water
TEE	total energy expenditure
TfR	transferrin receptor
THF	tetrahydrofolatereductase
TIBC	total iron binding capacity
TNF	tumour necrosis factor
TPP	thiamin pyrophosphate
TTR	transthyretin
UDP	uridine diphosphate
UIL	upper intake level
UNAIDS	United Nations Programme on HIV/AIDS
USI	universal salt iodization
UV	ultraviolet
vCJD	variant Creutzfeldt–Jakob disease
VDR	vitamin D receptor
VLCD	very-low-calorie diets
VLDL	very-low-density lipoprotein
WHO	World Health Organization

Contributors

Margaret Allman-Farinelli, PhD, MPhilPH, Dip Nutr Diet
Associate Professor
Human Nutrition Unit
Building G08
University of Sydney
NSW 2006
Australia

Annie S. Anderson, BSc, PhD, SRD
Professor and Director for Centre for Public Health
Nutrition Research
Ninewells Hospital & Medical School
University of Dundee
Dundee, DD1 9SY
Scotland, UK

Vishal Avinashi, MD, MPhil
Research Fellow
Division Gastroenterology,
Hepatology and Nutrition
The Hospital for Sick Children
555 University Avenue
Toronto, Ontario
Canada

Katrine Baghurst, PhD
Nutrition Consultant
82, Cave Avenue
Bridgewater, 5155
South Australia

Kim Bell-Anderson, PhD
Human Nutrition Unit
Building G08
University of Sydney
NSW 2006
Australia

Sheila Bingham*, BSc, MA, PhD
Deputy Director
MRC Dunn Human Nutrition Unit
Welcome Trust/MRC Building
Hills Road
Cambridge, CB2 2DH
UK

Louise M. Burke, PhD, Grad Dip Diet, FACSM
Head of Department of Sports Nutrition
Australian Institute of Sport
Bruce
ACT 2617
Australia

*deceased

Alexandra Chisholm, PhD
Senior Lecturer/Research Dietitian
Department of Human Nutrition
University of Otago
Dunedin
New Zealand

Helen Crawley, PhD
Reader in Nutritional Policy
Centre for Food Policy
City University London
Northampton Square
London, EC1V 0HB
UK

John Cummings, MB, ChB, MSc, MA, FRCP (Lond), FRCP (Edin)
Professor of Experimental Gastroenterology
Department of Pathology and Neuroscience
Ninewells Hospital and Medical School
Dundee, DD1 9SY
UK

Lisette CPGM de Groot, MSc, PhD
Professor of Nutrition and Ageing
Division of Human Nutrition
Wageningen University
Bomenweg 2
Wageningen
The Netherlands

Zoltán H. Endre, MB BS, BSc(Med), PhD, FRACP
Professor and Head of Department of Nephrology
Prince of Wales Hospital Sydney
NSW 2031
Australia and
Professor of Medicine
University of Otago
Christchurch Campus
New Zealand

Lawrence Eyres, PhD
ECG Consultant to the Food Industry
127 Point Wells Road
Point Wells
Auckland 0986
New Zealand

Meika Foster, BA, LLB (Hons), BSc(Hons)
Nutrition Researcher
Human Nutrition Unit
Building G08
University of Sydney
NSW 2006
Australia

Ailsa Goulding, PhD, FACN
Professorial Fellow
Department of Medicine
Otago Medical School
University of Otago
Dunedin
New Zealand

Andrea Grant, MSc
Assistant Research Fellow
Department of Medical and Surgical Sciences
University of Otago
Dunedin
New Zealand

Trish Griffiths, BSc, Dip Nutr Diet, MPH, Grad Dip Comm M
Manager, Nutrition Services
Bread Research Institute Australia
North Ryde
NSW 2113
Australia

Ohood Hakim, BSc (Hons), MSc
PhD Research Fellow
Nutrition and Metabolism Department
University of Surrey
Guildford, GU2 7XH
UK

Anne-Louise Heath, BA (Hons), BSc (Hons), PhD
Senior Lecturer
Department of Human Nutrition
University of Otago
Dunedin
New Zealand

Caroline Horwath, PhD
Senior Lecturer in Human Nutrition
University of Otago
Dunedin
New Zealand

Alan A. Jackson, CBE, MA, MD, FRCP, MRCPCH
Professor of Human Nutrition
University of Southampton
Southampton General Hospital
Tremona Road
Southampton, SP16 6YD
UK

W. Philip T. James, CBE, MD, DSc, FRCP (Edin), FRSE
Professor
Chairman, International Obesity Task Force
231 North Gower Street
London, NW1 2 NR
UK

Martijn B. Katan, PhD
Professor of Nutrition
Institute of Health Sciences
VrijeUniversiteit Amsterdam
De Boelelaan 1085
1081 HV
Amsterdam

Young Sook Kim, PhD
Nutritional Research Group
Division of Cancer Prevention
National Cancer Institute
National Institute of Health
6130 Executive Boulevard
Executive Plaza, Room 3156
Rockville, MD 20892
USA

Tim Lang, PhD
Professor of Food Policy
Centre for Food Policy
City University, London
Northampton Square
London, EC1V 0HB
UK

Susan A. Lanham-New, BA, MSc, PhD, RPH Nutr
Professor of Nutrition
Head, Nutrition and Metabolism Department
University of Surrey
Guildford, GU2 7XH
UK

Anita S. Lawrence, M. MedSci, PhD
Nutrition Manager
Dairy Australia
60, City Road
Southbank
Victoria 3006
Australia

Helen M. Leach, MA (Hons), PhD, FRSNZ
Emeritus Professor in Anthropology
Department of Anthropology
University of Otago
Dunedin
New Zealand

Claus Leitzmann, BSc, MSc, PhD
Professor of Human Nutrition
Institut für Ernährungswissenschaft
Justus-Liebig Universität Giessen
Wilhelmstraße 20
Germany

Philippa Lyons-Wall, PhD, Dip Nutr Diet
Lecturer in Nutrition and Dietetics
School of Public Health
Queensland University of Technology
Victoria Park Road
Queensland, 4059
Australia

A. Patrick MacPhail, MB, BCh, PhD, FCP(SA), FRCP
Professor Emeritus
Department of Medicine
University of the Witwatersrand
Helen Joseph Hospital
Perth Road, West Dene, 2092
Johannesburg
South Africa

Jim I. Mann, CNZM, MA, DM, PhD, FRACP, FRSNZ
Professor in Human Nutrition and Medicine
Department of Human Nutrition
University of Otago
Dunedin
New Zealand

Jennifer McMahon, MBE, FN, PhD, MBA
Department of Human Nutrition
University of Otago
Dunedin
New Zealand

John A. Milner, PhD
Chief of Nutritional Research Group
Division of Cancer Prevention
National Cancer Institute
National Institute of Health
6130 Executive Boulevard
Executive Plaza, North Suite 3164
Rockville, MD 20892
USA

Yasmin Mossavar-Rahmani, PhD, RD
Associate Professor
Division of Health Promotion & Nutrition Research
Department of Epidemiology and Population Health
Albert Einstein College of Medicine of Yeshiva University
Bronx, NY
USA

M. Alain Mourey, MSc
Nutritionist
Economic Security Unit
International Committee of the Red Cross
19, Ave de la Paix
1202 Geneva
Switzerland

Winsome R. Parnell, BHSc, MSc, PhD, NZRD
Associate Professor in Human Nutrition
Department of Human Nutrition
University of Otago
Dunedin
New Zealand

Robert Peveler, BM BCh, MA, DPhil, FRCPsych
Professor of Liaison Psychiatry
Clinical Neurosciences Division
University of Southampton

Andrew M. Prentice, PhD
Professor of International Nutrition
London School of Hygiene & Tropical Medicine
Keppel Street
London, WC1E 7HT
UK

Neville Rigby
Independent Consultant
Convenor of the International Obesity Forum

James Robinson*, MD, ScD, FRACP, FRSNZ
Emeritus Professor in Physiology
Department of Physiology
Otago Medical School
Dunedin
New Zealand

Stephan Rössner, MD, PhD
Professor Emeritus
Director of Obesity Unit M73
Karolinska University Hospital
Huddinge
SE-141 86
Stockholm
Sweden

Samir Samman, PhD
Associate Professor
Human Nutrition Unit
Building G08
University of Sydney
Sydney, NSW 2006
Australia

Donna Secker, MSc, PhD, RD
Clinical Dietitian
The Hospital for Sick Children
555, University Avenue
Toronto, Ontario
Canada

*deceased

C. Murray Skeaff, PhD
Professor in Human Nutrition
Department of Human Nutrition
University of Otago
Dunedin
New Zealand

Sheila Skeaff, PhD
Senior Lecturer
Department of Human Nutrition
University of Otago
Dunedin
New Zealand

Ross C. Smith, MD, BS, FRACS
Associate Professor of Surgery
University Department of Surgery
Royal North Shore Hospital
St Leonards
NSW 2065
Australia

Rachael Taylor, BSc (Hons), PhD
Associate Professor
Edgar National Centre for Diabetes and
Obesity Research
Department of Medicine
University of Otago
Dunedin
New Zealand

Christine D. Thomson, MHSc, PhD
Emeritus Professor in Human Nutrition
Department of Human Nutrition
University of Otago
Dunedin
New Zealand

David I. Thurnham, PhD
Emeritus Professor of Human Nutrition
Northern Ireland Centre for Food and Health
University of Ulster
Cromore Road
Coleraine, BT52 1SWA
UK

**Stewart Truswell, AO, MD, DSc,
FRCP, FFPH, FIUNS**
Emeritus Professor of Human Nutrition
School of Molecular Bioscience
Building G08
University of Sydney
NSW 2006
Australia

Hannah Turner, BSc, DClinPsych
Clinical Psychologist
University of Southampton Mental
Health Clinical Group
Royal South Hants Hospital
Southampton, SO14 0YG
UK

Wija A. van Staveren, MSc, PhD, RD
Emeritus Professor
Nutrition and Gerontology
Division of Human Nutrition
Wageningen University
Wageningen
The Netherlands

Bernard Venn, PhD
Senior Lecturer
Department of Human Nutrition
University of Otago
Dunedin
New Zealand

H.H. (Esté) Vorster, DSc
Professor and Director of Research
Faculty of Health Sciences
North-West University
Potchefstroom, 2520
South Africa

Bernhard Watzl, PhD
Adjunct Professor of Human Nutrition
Max Rubner-Institut
Federal Research Centre for Nutrition and Food
Haid-und-Neu-Straße 9
736131 Karlsruhe
Germany

Peter Williams, PhD, Dip Nutr Diet, MHP, FDAA
Associate Professor in Nutrition and Dietetics
School of Health Sciences
University of Wollongong
NSW 2522
Australia

Martin Wiseman, MB, BS, FRCP, FRCPath
Medical & Scientific Adviser
World Cancer Research Fund International
19, Harley Street
London, W1 9QJ
UK and
Visiting Professor in Human Nutrition
Institute of Human Nutrition
University of Southampton
Southampton
UK

Stanley H. Zlotkin, MD, PhD, FRCPC
Professor
Department of Gastroenterology and Nutrition
The Hospital for Sick Children
555, University Avenue
Toronto, Ontario
Canada

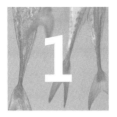

Introduction

Stewart Truswell and Jim Mann

1.1 Definition

This book is about what we consider the essentials of human nutrition.

The science of human nutrition deals with all the effects on people of any component found in food. This starts with the physiological and biochemical processes involved in nourishment—how substances in food provide energy or are converted into body tissues—and the diseases that result from insufficiency or excess of essential nutrients (malnutrition). The role of food components in the development of chronic degenerative diseases, like coronary heart disease, cancer, dental caries, and so on, are major targets of research activity nowadays. The scope of nutrition extends to any effect of food on human function: fetal health and development, resistance to infection, mental function, and athletic performance. There is growing interaction between nutritional science and molecular biology, which may help to explain the action of food components at the cellular level and the diversity of human biochemical responses.

Nutrition is also about why people choose to eat the foods they do, even if they have been advised that doing so may be unhealthy. The study of food habits thus overlaps with the social sciences of psychology, anthropology, sociology, and economics. Dietetics and community nutrition are the application of nutritional knowledge to promote health and wellbeing. Dietitians advise people how to modify what they eat in order to maintain or restore optimum health and to help in the treatment of disease. People expect to enjoy eating the foods that promote these things; and the production, preparation, and distribution of foods provides many people with employment.

A healthy diet means different things to different people. Those concerned with children's nutrition—parents, teachers, and paediatricians—aim to promote healthy growth and development. For adults in affluent communities, nutrition research has become focused on attaining optimal health and 'preventing' (which mostly means 'delaying') chronic degenerative diseases of complex causation, especially obesity (Chapter 17), cardiovascular diseases (Chapter 21), cancer (Chapter 22), and diabetes (Chapter 23). These chronic diseases have also become major causes of ill health and premature death in many developing countries (Chapter 18), where they may coexist with malnutrition (Chapter 19) and even periods of famine (Chapter 19).

Apart from behavioural and sociological aspects of eating there are two broad groups of questions in human nutrition, with appropriate methods for answering them:

First, what are the essential nutrients, the substances that are needed in the diet for normal function of the human body? How do they work in the body and from which foods can we obtain each of them? Many of the answers to these questions have been established.

Second, can we delay or even prevent the chronic degenerative diseases by modifying what we usually eat? These diseases, like coronary heart disease, have multiple causes, so nutrition can only be expected to make a contribution—causative or protective. The answers to these questions are at best provisional; much still has to be disentangled and confirmed.

1.2 Essential nutrients

Essential nutrients have been defined as chemical substances found in food that cannot be synthesized at all or in sufficient amounts in the body, and are necessary for life, growth, and tissue repair. Water is the most important nutrient for survival. By the end of the nineteenth century the essential amino acids in proteins had been mostly identified, as well as the major inorganic nutrients such as calcium, potassium, iodine, and iron.

The period 1890–1940 saw the discovery of 13 vitamins, organic compounds that are essential in small amounts. Each discovery was quite different; several involve fascinating stories. The research methods have comprised observations in poorly nourished humans, animal experiments, chemical fractionation of foods, biochemical research with tissues in the laboratory, and human trials.

Animal experiments played major roles in discovering which fraction of a curative diet was the missing essential food factor and how this fraction functions biochemically inside the body. The white laboratory rat is widely used, but it is not suitable for experimental deficiency of all nutrients; the right animal model has to be found. Lind demonstrated as early as 1747, in a controlled trial on board *HMS Salisbury*, that scurvy could be cured by a few oranges and lemons, but progress towards identifying *vitamin C* had to wait until 1907 when the guinea-pig was found to be susceptible to an illness like scurvy. Rats and other laboratory animals do not become ill on a diet lacking fruit and vegetables; they make their own vitamin C in the liver from glucose.

For *thiamin* (vitamin B_1) deficiency, birds provide good experimental models. The first step in the discovery of this vitamin was the chance observation in 1890 by Eijkman in Java (while looking for what was expected to be a bacterial cause of beri-beri) that chickens became ill with polyneuritis on a diet of cooked polished rice but stayed well if they were fed cheap unhusked rice. Human trials in Java, Malaysia, and the Philippines showed that beri-beri could be prevented or cured with rice bran (or 'polish'). A bird that is unusually sensitive to thiamin deficiency, a type of rice bird, was used by Dutch workers in Java to test the different fractions in rice bran. The anti-beri-beri vitamin was first isolated in crystalline form in 1926. It took another 10 years of work before two teams of chemists in the USA and Germany were able to synthesize vitamin B_1, which was given the chemical name thiamin.

To find the cause of *pellagra*, which was endemic among the rural poor in the south-eastern states of the USA at the beginning of this century, Goldberger gave restricted maize diets to healthy volunteers, some of whom developed early signs of the disease. But the missing substance, niacin, could not be identified until there was an animal model—in this case 'black tongue' in dogs.

In the 1920s, linoleic and linolenic acids were identified as essential fatty acids. Then came the development of analytical techniques for determining micro amounts of trace elements in foods and tissues. In this way the other group of essential micronutrients emerged, the trace elements copper, zinc, manganese, selenium, molybdenum, fluoride, and chromium.

There is an additional group of food components such as dietary fibre and some carotenoids that are not considered to be essential but which are important for maintenance of health and possibly also for reducing the risk of chronic disease.

1.3 Relation of diet to chronic diseases

More recent is the realization that environmental factors, including dietary factors, are of importance in many of the chronic degenerative diseases that are major causes of ill health and death in affluent societies. The nutritional component of these is more difficult to study than with classical nutritional deficiency diseases because chronic diseases have multiple causes and take years to develop. It may be a 'risk factor' rather than a direct cause, but for some of these diseases there is sufficient evidence to show that dietary change can appreciably reduce the risk of developing the condition. The scientific methods for investigating chronic diseases, their causes, and treatment and prevention differ from those used for studying adequacy of nutrient intakes.

Often the first clue to the association between a food or nutrient and a disease comes from observing striking differences in incidence of that disease between countries (or groups within a country); these differences correlate with differences in intake of dietary components. Sometimes dietary changes over time in a single country have been found to coincide with changes in disease rates. Such observations give rise to hypotheses (theories) about possible diet–disease links rather than proof of causation because many potential causative factors may change in parallel with dietary change and it is very difficult to disentangle the separate effects.

Animal experiments, because they are usually short term, are not as useful for investigating diet and chronic diseases and can be misleading. More information has come, and continues to come, from well-designed (human) *epidemiological* studies that record the relationship between dietary intake, or variables known to be related to diet, and the chronic disease under question. Studies can either investigate subjects after diagnosis of the disease (retrospective studies) or before diagnosis (prospective studies).

Retrospective or *case–control studies* are quicker and less expensive to carry out, but are less reliable than prospective studies. A series of people who have been diagnosed with cancer of the large bowel, for example, will be asked what they usually eat, or what they ate before they became ill. These are the 'cases'. They are compared with at least an equal number of 'controls' who are people without bowel cancer but of the same age and gender and, if possible, social conditions. Weaknesses of the method include: the possibility that the disease may affect food habits; that the cases cannot recall their diet accurately before the cancer really started; that the controls may have some other disease (known or latent) that affects their dietary habits; and that food intakes are recorded by cases and controls in a different way (bias).

Prospective or *cohort studies* avoid the biases involved in asking people to recall past eating habits. Information about food intake and other characteristics are collected well before onset of the disease. Large numbers of people must be interviewed and examined; they must be of an age at which bowel cancer (for example) starts to be fairly common (in the middle aged) and in a population that has a fairly high rate of this disease. The healthy cohort thus examined and recorded is then followed up for 5 years or more. Eventually, a proportion will be diagnosed with bowel cancer and the original dietary details of those who develop cancer can be compared with the diets of the majority who have not developed the disease. Usually a number of dietary and other environmental factors are found to be more (or less) frequent in those who develop the disease. These, then, are apparent risk factors, or protective factors. But they are not necessarily the operative factors. Fruit consumption may appear to be protective but perhaps in this cohort, smokers eat less fruit and smoking may be more directly related. This 'confounding' must be analysed, in effect, by analysing the data to see the relationship of fruit to the disease at different levels of smoking.

Prospective studies usually provide stronger evidence of a diet–disease association than case–control studies, and where several prospective studies produce similar findings from different parts of the world this is impressive evidence of association (positive or negative), but it is still not final proof of causation. If an association is deemed not due to bias or confounding, is qualitatively strong, biologically credible, follows a plausible time sequence, and especially if there is evidence of a dose–response relationship, it is likely that the association is causal. However, there are some negative issues with regard to cohort studies. The prospective follow-up of large numbers of people (usually thousands or tens of thousands) is a complicated and costly exercise. Furthermore, assessing dietary intake at one point in time may not provide a true reflection of usual intake. It is also conceivable that a dietary factor operating before the study has started, perhaps even in childhood, may be responsible for promoting a disease.

Definitive proof that a dietary characteristic is a direct causative or protective factor requires one or more *randomized controlled prevention trials.* These involve either the addition of a nutrient or other food component as a supplement to those in the experimental group, and a placebo (dummy) capsule or tablet taken by the control group, or the prescription of a dietary regimen to the experimental group while the controls continue to follow their usual diet. Disease (and death) outcomes in the two groups are compared. Such trials have the advantage of being able to prove causality as well as the potential cost–benefit of the dietary change. However, they are costly to carry out because, as with prospective studies, it is usually necessary to study large numbers of people over a prolonged period of time. Quite often a single trial or a single prospective study does not in itself produce a definitive answer, but by combining the results of all completed investigations in a *meta-analysis,* more meaningful answers are obtained. For example, a much clearer picture has emerged regarding the role of dietary factors in the aetiology of coronary heart disease from meta-analyses of prospective studies or clinical trials.

In addition to epidemiological studies and trials, much research involving the role of diet in chronic degenerative disease has centred around the effects of diet on modifying risk factors rather than the disease itself. For many chronic diseases there are biochemical markers of risk. High plasma cholesterol, for example, is an important risk factor for coronary heart disease. Innumerable studies have examined the role of different nutrients and foods on plasma cholesterol or other risk factors. Such studies are cheaper and easier to undertake than epidemiological studies and randomized controlled trials with disease outcome because far fewer people can be studied over a relatively short period of time. They have helped to find which foods lower cholesterol and so should help protect against coronary heart disease. It is this information that has formed the basis of the public health messages that have undoubtedly contributed to the decline in the incidence of coronary disease in most affluent societies over the past 40 years.

Several international organizations, including the World Health Organization (WHO) and the World Cancer Research Fund (WCRF), have attempted to establish clear guidelines regarding the degree of confidence that can be placed on observed associations between dietary factors and chronic diseases. Using the approach developed by WCRF, an association is described as 'convincingly causal' when randomized controlled trials show that modifying the factor can influence disease outcome, or when several cohort (prospective) studies show consistent associations that cannot be explained by chance or confounding.

For an association to be regarded as convincing there should also be confirmatory evidence from experimental studies in humans or animals, and there should be a biological gradient or dose-response between the degree or level of exposure to the dietary factor and the disease risk—meaning the greater the exposure to the food or nutrient, the greater the risk. Associations may be defined as 'probably causal' if several cohort and/or case-control studies consistently demonstrate biologically plausible associations that cannot be explained by chance, bias or confounding. *'Convincing'* and *'probable'* associations are regarded as sufficient to warrant recommendations for dietary change, but those based on lesser degrees of evidence are not.

This approach was until recently also used by the WHO. However, more recently WHO and some other national and international organizations have espoused the GRADE (The Grading of Recommendations, Assessment, Development, and Evaluation) approach to guideline development. The system was developed for clinical practice and relies heavily on randomized controlled trials (RCT), an essential prerequisite for grading the evidence as being of high or moderate quality, a requirement for '*strong*' recommendations. Observational studies can generally only generate '*weak*' recommendations. Given that in nutrition RCTs with clinical endpoints are few and far between and that most nutrition authorities would agree that decisions regarding strength of association and recommendations should be made on the totality of evidence, not just RCTs, it will be interesting to see whether this evidence-based approach proves to be appropriate for nutrition recommendations. All would agree that we should be sure of our ground before we advise individuals or populations to change a diet to which they are accustomed. Food habits have strong cultural values.

1.4 Tools of the trade

As with any other science or profession, nutrition has its own specialized techniques and technical terms. Those that are frequently used in research and professional work are introduced here. They are described in more detail further on in the book.

1.4.1 Measuring food and drink intake

Which foods (and drinks) does a person or a group of people usually eat (and drink) and how many grams of each per day? Unless the subject is confined within a special research facility under constant observation the answer can never be 100% accurate. Information about food intake is subjective and depends on memory; people do not always notice, or know, the exact description of the foods they are given to eat (especially in mixed dishes). When asked to record what they eat they may alter their diet. People do not eat the same every day so it is difficult to obtain a profile of their usual diet.

The different techniques used are described in Chapter 30. One set of methods estimates the amounts of food produced and sold in a whole country and divides these by the estimated population. This is 'food disappearance' or food moving into consumption. Obviously, some of this food is wasted and some is eaten by tourists and pets. The main value of the data is for following national trends and for seeing if people appear to be eating too little or too much of some foods.

Other methods capture the particular foods and amounts of them that individuals say they actually ate. These methods rely either on the subjects' memories or on asking them to write down everything they eat or drink for (usually) several days.

1.4.2 Food composition tables (see Chapter 29)

Ideally, food tables would contain all the usual foods eaten in a country and give average numbers for the calories (food energy), the major essential nutrients, and other important food components (e.g. dietary fibre) of each food, measured by chemical analysis. In many smaller, less affluent countries there is no complete set of food composition data, so 'borrowed' data are used from one of the 'big' Western countries (e.g. the UK, USA, or Germany). Food tables are used to calculate people's nutrient intakes from their food intake estimates. Most food tables are also available as computer software, which greatly speeds up the computations (for 20 subjects × 4 days × 80 foods or drinks × 35 nutrients, that is 224 000 computations).

1.4.3 Dietary reference values and guidelines (see Chapter 37)

Computer software packages for dietary analyses generate printouts that show what a subject or groups of individuals have eaten in terms of nutrients. This does not mean anything unless comparison is made with normative dietary reference values. Two sets are used, but they differ somewhat from country to country. For essential nutrients (protein, vitamins, minerals) the reference is in a table of *recommended nutrient intakes* (*dietary reference intakes* in the USA). For some nutrients that are not essential but which may be related to disease risk (e.g. saturated fat, which is related to risk of coronary heart disease), advice regarding intake is in recommendations called *dietary guidelines.*

1.4.4 Biomarkers: biochemical tests

If an individual (or group) is found to eat less than the recommended intake of nutrient 'A' then they may not have any features of 'A' deficiency. The food intake may have been under-reported or only temporarily less than usual, and there are large body stores for some nutrients. Some people may have lower requirements than average. On the other hand, individuals can suffer deficiency of nutrient 'A' despite an acceptable intake if they have an unusually high requirement, perhaps because of increased losses from disease. For many nutrients, biochemical tests using blood or urine are available to help estimate the amount of the nutrient functioning inside the body (see Chapter 31). Furthermore, *biomarkers* provide a more objective and often more economical method for estimating intake of some food components (e.g. urinary sodium for salt) than food intake measurement, and they can also be used to check the reliability of subject histories or records of food intake.

1.4.5 Human studies and trials

Most of the detailed knowledge in human nutrition comes from a range of different types of human experiments. They may last from hours to years and may include just a few subjects or thousands of subjects. The following are examples:

- *Absorption studies*: Some nutrients are poorly absorbed, and absorption of nutrients is better from some foods than from others. Many studies have been done to measure *bioavailability*—that is, the percentage of the nutrient intake that is available to be used inside the body. After a test meal, the increase in some nutrients can be measured in blood or other samples. Isotopes may be needed to label the nutrient.

- *Metabolic studies*: The diet is usually changed in one way only, and the result is measured in a change in blood or excreta (urine and/or faeces). One type is the *balance experiment*. This may measure, for example, the intake of calcium and its excretion in urine and faeces. Because of the minor variability of urine production and the major variability of defecation these measurements have to be made for a metabolic period of several days every time any dietary change is made.

- Another example is the effect of a controlled (usually single) change of diet on blood plasma cholesterol, a risk factor for coronary heart disease (see Chapter 21). Such an effect is known to take 10–14 days if it is going to appear and the experiment should include control periods before and after the dietary change being examined.

Interpreting the results of such studies is a complex matter. There is individual variation in the way people absorb and metabolize nutrients (Box 1.1). There is also the possibility that changes observed over a short time period may not persist indefinitely because humans may adapt to dietary change. Furthermore, when one component is added or

---

BOX 1.1 Nutrition and genes

- Some nutrients can affect expression of some genes, for example, some forms of vitamin A, retinoic acids, affect transcription of genes for cellular differentiation (Chapter 12). Likewise 1,25-dihydroxy-vitamin D switches on the gene for calcium transport—and possibly other genes (Chapter 15).

- Second, variants of some genes (polymorphism) affect the function of some nutrients. Examples include alcohol metabolism (Chapter 7), haemochromatosis (Chapter 10), folate metabolism (Chapter 13), familial hypercholesterolaemia (Chapter 21), lipoprotein apo-E types (Chapter 21), genes and cancer (Chapter 22), lactase insufficiency (Chapter 25), and phenylketonuria (Chapter 25).

- Third, in some of the plants that provide our food, a gene from another species has been inserted or an endogenous gene has been inactivated to produce a crop that is easier to grow (e.g. genetically modified maize) or has an improved nutritional profile (e.g. Golden rice) (Chapter 27). Some nutrition research departments are now giving priority to *nutrigenomics*, the application of genomics technologies in nutrition sciences and food technology.

---

removed from the diet there are usually consequential changes to the rest of the diet, as some other food is put in its place. An apparent effect of removing one food may at least in part be due to the action of its replacement or to the energy deficit that results if it is not replaced. Before recommending dietary change it is imperative that nutritionists consider not only the role of individual nutrients as determinants of health and disease, but also diet as a whole and the complex dynamics of dietary change, in order to ensure that overall benefit will accrue from any changes that are made.

Further Reading

1. **Mann, J.I.** (2010) Evidence-based nutrition: Does it differ from evidence-based medicine? *Ann Med*, **42**, 475–86.
2. **Truswell, A.S.** (2001) Levels and kinds of evidence for public health nutrition. *Lancet*, **357**, 1061–2.

Useful Websites

 To see topical and scientifically robust updates on nutrition associated with this textbook and web links to many of the journals in the Further Reading sections, please see the dedicated Online Resource Centre at **http://www.oxfordtextbooks.co.uk/orc/mann4e/**

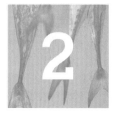

2 Genes, nutrition, and disease risk

Young Sook Kim and John A. Milner

Dietary habits are intimately linked with establishing every aspect of human growth, development, and resistance to disease. Thus, eating behaviour represents the most relevant lifelong environmental factor that can influence the duration and quality of life. Today, multiple nutrition strategies are touted for their likelihood of preventing or delaying the onset of disease, and optimizing performance. However, it is clear that not all individuals respond identically to dietary change. Assessing who will benefit more or be placed at risk because of their eating habits or dietary change represents a major scientific challenge, yet holds promise to markedly influence strategies for health promotion and disease prevention (Davis *et al.*, 2010). At least part of this variation in response relates to individual differences in genetic and epigenetic phenotypes, which influences the absorption, digestion, metabolism, excretion, and site of action of bioactive food components. Both variations in DNA sequence and epigenetic-modified chromatin structure regulate genetic activity and thus are the two major mechanisms influencing gene expression. Deciphering how these mechanisms combine to coregulate transcription should assist in explaining individual responses to food and its components.

While public health approaches will remain the major strategies for implementing nutrition messages aimed at chronic disease prevention, personalized approaches may facilitate compliance in the context of prevention and disease management. The vast majority of individuals are not average in their likes, dislikes, behaviours, or metabolism. Such personalized approaches will build on the recognition that 'one size does not fit all' when applied to diet or to genetics. Technologies which identify subpopulations who are likely to benefit most from dietary change or who are especially at high risk because of dietary intake are likely to be cost effective.

2.1 Genomic technologies and their interpretation

2.1.1 Definitions of terms

Nutrigenetics investigates an individual's genetic predisposition to respond to dietary components.

Single-nucleotide polymorphisms (SNPs) are single-base mutations in genes and are considered the most common and important interindividual genetic difference at the sequence level. SNPs can occur in both exons and introns, i.e. in coding and non-coding DNA regions, and some, but not all, have important functional consequences. Functional SNPs are common genetic variations which occur relatively frequently in the human genome (Sachidanandam *et al.*, 2000). Variation in genes also occurs as a result of additions, deletions, and translocations. These genetic variants contribute to beneficial and detrimental variations in biological responses to dietary components. The eventual outcome in terms of biological response may depend upon the interaction of a number of different gene effects. Plausible mechanism(s) as to how polymorphic genes interact with nutrients and thereby influence diseases, including cancer, cardiovascular disease (CVD), and hypertension, are briefly discussed below.

Nutrigenomics is a collective term that includes nutrigenetics, epigenomics, and transcriptomics (Fig. 2.1 and Box 2.1). Thus, it builds on a wealth of

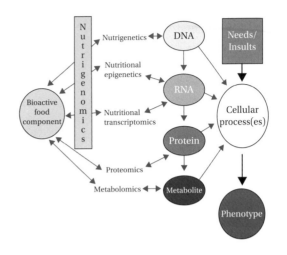

Fig. 2.1 Interactions between diet and genetics in determining overall phenotype. Knowledge about the interactions of food components with the various 'omics' will help define the most appropriate nutritional pre-emptive strategies for promoting growth, development, and disease prevention.

BOX 2.1 Terms used when describing the relationships between genes, nutrition, and disease risk

Nutrigenomics

The study of the effects of foods and their constituents on gene expression. Collectively it helps explain variation in food preferences, digestion, absorption, metabolism, excretion, and the ability of food components to influence biological processes.

Nutrigenetics

The study of individual genetic disposition that predetermines the response to food components.

SNPs (Single nucleotide polymorphisms)

The most common gene change (single-base) which sometimes leads to changes in protein formation or activity.

Transcriptomics

The study of the expression of genes that are being actively transcribed from DNA to RNA at any given time.

Epigenetics

The study of changes in genetic expression by mechanisms other than the DNA sequence. Epigenetic programming involves DNA methylation, histone modifications, and small regulatory RNAs.

(Continued)

BOX 2.1 Terms used when describing the relationships between genes, nutrition, and disease risk (*Continued*)

Proteomics

The study of proteins in terms of structure and functions including their activities, localization, modifications, and inter/intrainteractions with endogenous/exogenous cellular compounds.

Metabolomics

The systematic study of small-molecular-weight substances in cells, tissues, and/or whole organisms as influenced by multiple factors including genetics, diet, lifestyle, and drugs.

Microbiome

The total and functionality of microbial cells that interact with the environment and can influence health and disease risk.

scientific underpinning of human genetic/genomics to define variations in food preferences, digestion, absorption, metabolism, excretion, and the needs for nutrients/bioactive food components (in isolation or in combination) for biological processes. Nutrigenomics is complemented by proteomics, metabolomics, the microbiome, and other 'omic' technologies. Collectively, each 'omic' technology assists with the detection of genetically distinct responders and non-responders to particular diets or individual ingredients. It should also be noted that the overall response to bioactive food components may also be determined by a variety of insults that occur in humans, including overindulgence of calories, free radical generation, environmental contaminants, and bacteria (both beneficial and harmful) and viruses.

2.1.2 Interpreting genomic datasets

Despite the power of the profiling using 'omic' technologies, the interpretation of the resulting datasets is exceedingly complex, if not mind-boggling. Fig. 2.2 provides insights into how diet can influence cellular messages which then influence metabolic pathways that have functional consequences in terms of networks that influence the entire organism. It is clear that this information highway has two lanes such that nutrient supply influences networks and networks set the tone for

needs. Unfortunately, at present much of the available data describing the interrelationships is best described as guilt-by-association. However, there is a growing trend towards systemic approaches which incorporate multiple technologies to the same sample to develop predictive models. Bioinformatic tools are critical for understanding the multiple dimensions that integrate diet, genomics, and the overall cellular responses. While these models are exceedingly important, controlled intervention studies in genetically defined subpopulations will be needed to truly understand their physiological relevance in influencing growth, development, and disease resistance.

2.1.3 Finding interactions between genotype and diet

To predict the response to dietary change, it is critical to gain a clear mechanistic understanding about how food components function in isolation or in combination to modulate target genes. In particular it is necessary to establish the amount and species of components and durations of exposures required to modulate target genes. A wealth of evidence demonstrating the ability of multiple bioactive food components to modify the expression and/or function of regulatory genes already exists. However, the experiments have often involved exaggerated exposures to cells in culture and thus their

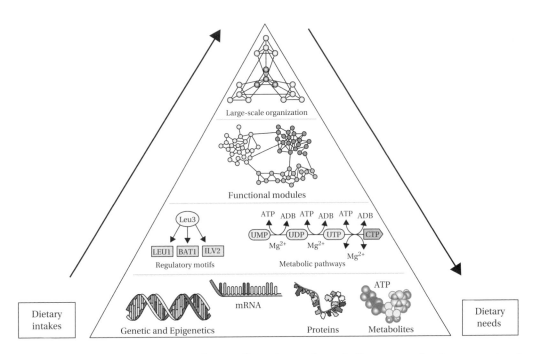

Fig. 2.2 Nutrition and genomics are an integrative science. Overall, the process is a two-way street, with intakes determining outcomes and outcomes determining needs. Bioinformatics is a critical technology that is required to evaluate the multiple dimensions that integrate diet, genomics, and overall cellular responses.

relevance to intact organisms remains uncertain. Nevertheless, there are examples, including the development of hyperplastic polyps in the colon, insulin resistance in obesity, plaque in blood vessels, and hypertension, where evidence exists that food components can have an impact. At this stage, it is unclear if response to dietary components reflects a change in one or more molecular targets and if these modulating changes influence one or more cellular processes (see Fig. 2.3). For example, in the colon, the formation of malignant polyps on colonic mucosa can be related to a number of factors, including regulatory genes such as the adenomatous polyposis coli (APC) and transforming growth factor β receptor II, inflammatory events at intestinal epithelial cells, and the influence of intestinal commensal microbes on the host's ability to uptake, metabolize, and excrete the potentially carcinogenic agents. Each of these factors, either on their own or in combination, can be markedly influenced by a variety of dietary components.

Several fundamental questions about gene–diet interactions remain to be answered. The first relates

to tissue specificity. For example, the bioavailability of active food components can vary immensely across tissues and therefore influence its ability to alter gene expression patterns. The differential tissue response has been highlighted for food items such as calcium, where evidence exists that it is a protective factor against colorectal cancer, yet may promote prostate cancer. Another issue is the similarity or inconsistency in response between normal and abnormal cells. Several studies suggest that folate may prevent the expression of aberrant genes associated with colorectal cancer yet may promote tumours once transformation has occurred. Likewise, evidence exists that antioxidants may protect normal cells from radical damage but may promote free radical generation in cancerous cells. Still another issue is when in the life cycle a dietary change brings about the greatest response. While there are limited examples about early exposures to nutrients and subsequent disease risk, one of the most frequently cited relates to the greater benefits of soy introduction earlier in life than occurs when consumed by mature women. Such timing

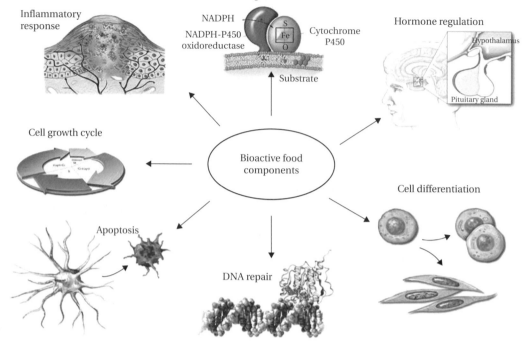

Fig. 2.3 It is critical that the genomic and diet interrelationship be put into the context of critical cellular events. These have been best characterized as they relate to cancer development, and similar types of relationship likely exist with other conditions which influence growth, development, and health. Disease conditions likely influence one or more of these processes and thus lead to detectable phenotypic changes. It remains unclear if the response to foods or food components relates to changes in one or more of these critical cellular/systemic processes.

phenomena with flavonoids suggest that flexible epigenetic rather than irreversible genetic changes may be involved. Inadequacy of the diet may also precipitate a change in health. For example, feeding a Western-style diet (characterized by a high fat intake and low calcium, vitamin D, and methyl donors) to C57Bl/6 mice for 2 years altered colon gene expression profiles, including the *APC* gene, and ultimately increased the number of tumours (Yang *et al.*, 2008).

2.2 Genetic polymorphisms influencing diet–disease relationships

Human genome sequencing during the past decade has identified about 1000 mutations responsible for human diseases and implicates multiple disease-causing genes which may be responsible for human multifactorial diseases including obesity, cardiovascular disease (CVD), and cancer. SNPs are likely to confer individuality because of their ability to influence genome plasticity and to explain gene–environment interactions, including interactions between foods and genes. Although several SNPs in key genes have been associated with chronic disorders, few of these associations have been conclusively confirmed and more definitive dietary interventions are needed to confirm the gene–nutrient interventions. Box 2.2 lists a few examples of SNP variations that have been

BOX 2.2 Genetic polymorphisms influencing diet–disease relationships. These are discussed further in the expanded version of the chapter available in the Online Resource Centre.

SNPs that influence cancer risk

Vitamin D receptor (VDR) and colon cancer

Both dietary vitamin D intake and the BsmI VDR polymorphism are correlated with the reduced colo-rectal cancer risk.

ER-β and prostate cancer

The protective effect of dietary soy may differ between the genotypes of ER-β.

Glutathione-S-transferase (GST) M1 and breast cancer

The breast-cancer preventative effects of the cruciferous vegetable component sulphoraphane is significant only in the population with GST M1 polymorphisms.

Diet genetic polymorphisms and CVD risk

APOA5

The consumption of high polyunsaturated fatty acid diet may increase CVD risk in carriers of the $-1131T > C$ allele.

APOE

Dietary saturated fat intake modifies the effects of the APOE polymorphism in determining CVD risk.

Cholesterol 7-α-hydroxylase

Polymorphism in this gene may modify triglyceride concentrations in response to a reduced-fat diet.

Polymorphic genes influencing hypertension risk

α-Adducin

The Gly460Trp type of this gene is more salt sensitive, which is associated with the increased risk for hypertension.

SNPs in aldosterone synthase and angiotensin-converting enzyme

The frequency of SNPs in the DNA of these enzymes is significantly different in salt-sensitive hypertensive patients compared with controls.

Variations in the dietary response due to gene copy numbers

Amylase activity

The AMY1 gene that encodes salivary amylase occurs in greater amounts in individuals who habitually consume increased quantities of starch.

Her2/neu

The amplification of Her2/neu gene may be predictive of the responsiveness to dietary components that target this molecule.

PI3K overexpression

The overexpression of genes in the PI3K pathway may influence the sensitivity of tumours to dietary treatment, including genistein from soy or catachins from green tea.

implicated in explaining gene–nutrient effects on disease conditions.

2.2.1 Vitamin D receptor (VDR) and colon cancer

Vitamin D is involved in the modulation of calcium and bone metabolism and a role has been suggested in cancer prevention and in promoting immuno-competence. These effects are manifested via the VDR. Polymorphisms within this gene have been extensively studied in diverse diseases including cancer, but there are inconsistencies in the literature. A recent meta-analysis supports the suggestion of an inverse association between vitamin D intake, 25-hydroxyvitamin D status, and the BsmI VDR polymorphism and rectal cancer risk when calcium intake was low (Slattery *et al.*, 2004). Furthermore, carriers of the VDR FOK I Ff or ff alleles consuming low levels of dietary calcium were at substantially increased risk for rectal cancer compared to those carrying the VDR FOK I FF genotype. This risk was reduced when individuals consumed a higher amount of calcium. Thus, the extent to which calcium might help reduce colorectal cancer is likely far greater in those with specific genetic variances. There is evidence that the ff allele is associated with reduced calcium accretion in children and thus reduced bone development. The mechanism by which exaggerated calcium brings about this protection remains to be determined. However, there is evidence that the increase in the intracellular calcium ion concentration impacts a diverse range of cell functions and gene expression patterns.

While these are interesting findings, it is clear that the VDR has many genetic polymorphisms. However, it is uncertain how these and other genetic variants influence the response to multiple food components. The considerable variability in the ability of SNPs to explain the response to vitamin D may be a result of other food components. For example, when considering the intake of calcium from dairy products, genistein from soy or resveratrol from grapes or nuts might influence the response as much as vitamin D *per se*.

2.2.2 Apolipoprotein polymorphisms and cardiovascular disease

Diet is recognized as a critical factor capable of modulating lipid metabolism and its related disorders, including CVD. Several genetic polymorphisms including APOA5 −1131T >C and apolipoprotein E have been shown to influence the interaction between dietary lipids and CVD risk.

APOA5 is an apolipoprotein that plays a key role in modulating circulating plasma triglycerides (a major risk factor for CVD). Genetic analysis of over 2000 men and women participating in the Framingham Offspring Study provided convincing evidence that the −1131T>C single-nucleotide polymorphism of APOA5 gene modulates lipoprotein particle size as well as plasma triglyceride levels (Lai *et al.*, 2006). In subjects homozygous for the −1131C allele, higher intake of polyunsaturated fatty acids (>6% of total energy) was associated with increased particle size of very-low-density lipoprotein, decreased particle size of low-density lipoprotein, and higher plasma triglyceride levels. Conversely, these changes were not present in carriers of the −1131T allele. These results suggest that for carriers of the APOA5 −1131T >C SNP, which was present in approximately 13% of the study population, a diet high in polyunsaturated fatty acids may be an important CVD risk factor.

APOE is a protein that is produced in liver and functions as a transporter of lipoproteins, fat-soluble vitamins, and cholesterol into the blood. This protein has linear relationships with both low-density lipoprotein cholesterol and coronary risk. APOE is polymorphic, with three different isoforms, APOE2, APOE3, and APOE4, that come from a single gene. APOE3 is most common and considered to be the normal isoform, whereas APOE2 is known to be associated with the slow metabolism of dietary fat and about 20% reduced risk for atherosclerosis.

Another isoform, APOE4, has been shown to be involved with increased risk for atherosclerosis and Alzheimer's disease, impaired cognitive function, and reduced neurite outgrowth. Interestingly, dietary saturated fat intake was shown to modify the effect of the APOE polymorphism in determining risk of coronary heart disease (CHD) (Bennet *et al.*, 2007). When saturated fat intake was low (<10% of energy), no statistically significant association between the APOE polymorphism and CHD risk was observed ($P = 0.682$). However, with higher intakes of saturated fat ($\geq$10%), the association between polymorphism and CHD was significant ($P = 0.005$), and the differences between E2 and E4 carriers were magnified. These results again suggest that genotypes can dramatically influence the response to dietary components and ultimately influence disease risk.

2.2.3 Polymorphic genes influencing hypertension risk

Excess salt intake is a recognized risk factor for hypertension. Dietary guidelines for Americans recommend that the majority of the US adult population, including middle-aged, senior, black, and hypertension patients should limit sodium intake to lower morbidities and mortality. These differential recommendations for varied groups, categorized in terms of age, genetic background, and disease condition, suggest that not everybody responds identically to sodium. Polymorphisms regulating the retention of water and sodium, such as those in α-adducin (Gly460Trp), angiotensin-converting enzyme (I/D), and aldosterone synthase (−344C/T), have been reported to influence the effect of salt on blood pressure via their influence on sodium homeostasis (Beeks *et al.*, 2004).

The Gly460Trp genotype of the α-adducin is associated with erythrocyte sodium transport and increases tubular sodium reabsorption and risk of hypertension. In the Ohasama Study, the Trp460 allele of α-adducin 1 was found to be linked with hypertension in young subjects with low renin activity. In addition, the −344T>C polymorphism in the promoter of the aldosterone synthase gene (CYP11B2) and the 825C>T polymorphism of the G-protein beta3 subunit gene (GNB3) are considered candidates for the genetic risk of salt-sensitive hypertension. This group of researchers compared the allele frequency of five candidate genes between Japanese and Caucasians; the results showed that the frequencies of all alleles were significantly higher in Japanese than in Caucasians. These interesting findings suggest a plausible explanation for the interracial differences in the frequency of salt-sensitive hypertension. The effects of the other polymorphisms are described in the Online Resource Centre.

2.3 Epigenetics and diet regulation

Epigenetic events alter the expression of developmental genes by adding/deleting methyl groups to/from the DNA, adding functional groups to/from histone around which DNA winds, or by the induction of non-coding microRNAs. The reversibility of these events provides yet another plausible link between dietary habits and gene expression patterns and, potentially, disease risk. Evidence continues to surface that early postnatal exposure to dietary methyl donors including folic acid, vitamin B_{12}, choline, and betaine, as well as genistein, can significantly reduce the risk of developing epigenetic-associated chronic diseases in preclinical models (Jirtle and Skinner, 2007).

Undeniably, epigenetic control mechanisms have a significant role in the regulation of embryonic development and tissue homeostasis and modulate diseases including CVD and cancer. DNA methylation status is dynamically regulated by its methylation and demethylation reactions. In animals, multiple mechanisms of active DNA demethylation have been proposed, including a deaminase-initiated and a DNA glycosylase-initiated base excision repair pathway. New information concerning the effects of various histone modifications on the establishment and maintenance of DNA methylation is broadening our understanding of the regulation of DNA methylation, but much remains to be discovered.

Histone deacetylase (HDAC) is an enzyme that removes acetyl groups from histone and thereby suppresses the expression of tumour suppressor genes, including *p21*. Evidence suggests that butyrate, which is formed in the large intestine by fermentation of dietary fibre, serves as a natural inhibitor of HDAC. Likewise, a variety of other bioactive food components, including sulphoraphane from cruciferous vegetables, diallyl disulphide from garlic, and genistein from soy, function as weak inhibitors of HDAC. Feeding these dietary HDAC inhibitors to animals and humans was correlated with a restoration of *p21* expression, which correlates with a reduction in the risks for colon and prostate cancer. While these results suggest that the HDAC inhibitory activity of specific dietary components contributes to cancer prevention, additional studies are needed to characterize gene-specific histone modifications brought about by food components. Changes in histones may also relate to other disease conditions.

The role of small non-coding RNA molecules in the regulation of gene expression is an emerging area of research. These small RNAs are thought to mediate transcriptional gene silencing, which has been shown to be correlated with changes in chromatin structure (including modulation of histone marks and DNA methylation) at specific sites in promoter regions. Interestingly, dietary methyl-deficiency-induced hepatocellular carcinoma has been characterized by prominent early changes in the expression of microRNA genes that are involved in the regulation of apoptosis, cell proliferation, cell-to-cell connections, and epithelial–mesenchymal transition. The detailed mechanisms by which diet can influence epigenetic events are discussed in the expanded version of the chapter in the Online Resource Centre.

2.4 Critical molecular targets

Dietary compounds may confer health benefits by interacting and modulating the expression and function of specific genes that are keys in various disease pathways. Relevant examples include antioxidant transcription factor nuclear factor (erythroid-derived 2)-like 2 (Nrf2), cell cycle-related apoptotic gene *p21*, and inflammation-associated enzyme cyclooxygenase 2 (COX2). The fact that multiple nutrients appear to influence the same target supports the concept that the totality of the diet rather than individual components promotes health and disease prevention. The effects of dietary factors on Nrf2 are described below. *p21*, *COX2*, and peroxisome proliferator-activated receptor (*PPAR*) are discussed in the expanded version of the chapter in the Online Resource Centre.

Nrf2 is an important transcription factor that responds to a variety of dietary antioxidants, including sulphoraphane in broccoli, n-3 fatty acids in fish, lycopene in tomatoes, and diallyl disulfide in garlic, and calorie restriction, which leads to the protection of cells from harmful oxidative damages (Fig. 2.4). In response to excess oxidative stress such as injury, inflammation, or high-fat diet consumption, specific dietary constituents release Nrf2 from its complex with an actin-binding protein, Keap 1, in the cytosol and allow it to translocate into nuclei, where it binds to a specific DNA motif called antioxidant response element (ARE), which results in the expression of phase II detoxifying enzymes, including glutathione-S-transferase and quinone reductase (Fig. 2.4). This protection programme has been well demonstrated in Nrf2-deficient mice which could not dispose of fat-generated radicals appropriately, but rather accumulated them in liver, leading to the development of fatty liver diseases (Kitteringham *et al.*, 2010). These animals were also sensitive to deficiency of methionine/choline nutrients, which resulted in abnormal lipid metabolism in liver. These results suggest that Nrf2 is critical in maintaining health in response to various stimuli by either increasing the synthesis of phase II enzymes or by regulating normal liver function.

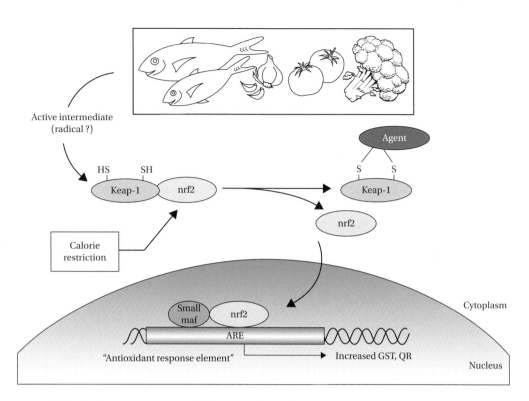

Fig. 2.4 Multiple food components can influence the nuclear transcription factor Nrf2. It remains to be determined whether excesses of one food item diminish the health benefits attributed to other potential modifiers. The effective blend of foods to optimize this process remains to be resolved. ARE, antioxidant response element; GST, glutathione S-transferase; QR, quinone reductase.

The significance of Nrf2 also comes from its fundamental role as a primary defence system in our body when it faces challenges in disease processes such as inflammation or neuroprotection in which oxidative stress has been implicated as playing a key role. Inflammatory cycles usually generate a lot of unstable oxidative radicals that could damage tissue macromolecules, including DNA and protein. Fortunately, these harmful radicals can be removed by dietary antioxidants through the nuclear transcription factor Nrf2. For example, anti-inflammatory properties of dietary flavonols, quercetin, and its metabolite isorhamnetin, shown in RAW264.7 macrophages (10 µmol/l, 24 hours), were accompanied by about a three-fold increase in a downstream target of Nrf2 that is known to antagonize chronic inflammation (Boesch-Saadatmandi *et al.*, 2011). Likewise, dietary polyphenol curcumin (100 mg/kg) found in turmeric has been shown to decrease

oxidative and cytotoxic damage that has been implicated in the pathogenesis of cerebral ischaemia, including Parkinson's disease. These results suggest that the upregulation of Nrf2 by natural dietary components could be non-toxic and promise the development of prevention strategies for inflammation and Parkinson's disease.

Summary and conclusions

It is abundantly clear that the foods and food components that are consumed interact with the human genome, either directly or indirectly. Both genetic and epigenetic events can markedly influence the response to food components. This can occur through changes in the absorption, digestion, metabolism, and excretion of the food component or by changing the activity of its molecular target. As a better understanding of genomics emerges, it will become increasingly easy to identify those who will benefit most from intervention strategies. Success will depend on: (1) the ability to identify necessary exposures (amounts and durations) for both essential and non-essential bioactive food components to bring about a desired response; (2) the predictive value of biomarkers which reflect 'effect' (molecular targets) and 'susceptibility' (nutrient–gene and nutrient–nutrient interactions); (3) effective communication to consumers about the merits of obtaining information about their personalized 'omics' values; and (4) the upholding of a bioethical framework that prevents discrimination of nutrigenomic and health data in any capacity. While there are significant challenges that must be overcome before genetic and epigenetic information for personalizing nutrition approaches can be introduced for routine use, the potential societal impact in terms of economic and health benefits are indeed enormous.

Further Reading

1. **Beeks, E., Kessels, A.G., Kroon, A.A., van der Klauw, M.M., and de Leeuw, P.W.** (2004) Genetic predisposition to salt-sensitivity: A systematic review. *J Hypertens*, **22**, 1243–9.

2. **Bennet, A.M., Di Angelantonio, E., Ye, Z., et al.** (2007) Association of apolipoprotein E genotypes with lipid levels and coronary risk. *JAMA*, *298*, 1300–11.

3. **Boesch-Saadatmandi, C., Loboda, A., Wagner, A.E., et al.** (2011) Effect of quercetin and its metabolites isorhamnetin and quercetin-3-glucuronide on inflammatory gene expression: Role of miR-155. *J Nutr Biochem*, **22**, 293–9.

4. **Davis, C.D., Emenaker, N.J., and Milner, J.A.** (2010) Cellular proliferation, apoptosis and angiogenesis: Molecular targets for nutritional preemption of cancer. *Semin Oncol*, **37**, 243–57.

5. **Jirtle, R.L., and Skinner, M.K.** (2007) Environmental epigenomics and disease susceptibility. *Nat Rev Genet*, **8**, 253–62.

6. **Kitteringham, N.R., Abdullah, A., Walsh, J., et al.** (2010) Proteomic analysis of Nrf2 deficient transgenic mice reveals cellular defence and lipid metabolism as primary Nrf2-dependent pathways in the liver. *J Proteomics*, **73**, 1612–31.

7. **Lai, C.Q., Corella, D., Demissie, S., et al.** (2006) Dietary intake of n-6 fatty acids modulates effect of apolipoprotein A5 gene on plasma fasting triglycerides, remnant lipoprotein concentrations, and lipoprotein particle size: The Framingham Heart Study. *Circulation*, **113**, 2062–70.

8. **Sachidanandam, R., Weissman, D., Schmidt, S.C., et al.** (2000) A map of human genome sequence variation containing 1.42 million single nucleotide polymorphisms. *Nature*, **409**, 928–3.

9. **Slattery, M.L., Neuhausen, S.L., Hoffman, M., et al.** (2004) Dietary calcium, vitamin D, VDR genotypes and colorectal cancer. *Int J Cancer*, **111**, 750–6.

10. **Yang, K., Kurihara, N., Fan, K., et al.** (2008) Dietary induction of colonic tumors in a mouse model of sporadic colon cancer. *Cancer Res*, **68**, 7803–10.

Useful Websites

To see topical and scientifically robust updates on nutrition associated with this textbook and web links to many of the journals in the Further Reading sections, please see the dedicated Online Resource Centre at **http://www.oxfordtextbooks.co.uk/orc/mann4e/**

Part 1

Energy and macronutrients

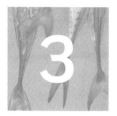

3 Carbohydrates

John Cummings and Jim Mann

Carbohydrates are stored energy. They are synthesized by plants from water and carbon dioxide using the sun's energy and have the general formula $(CH_2O)_N$. In their simplest form, glucose $(C_6H_{12}O_6)$, they are readily soluble and, after absorption from the gut, are transported in blood to the tissues where they are oxidized back to water and carbon dioxide from which process the host gains energy for cellular metabolic processes. Unlike plants, animals have limited capacity to synthesize carbohydrates but can make the disaccharide lactose and oilgosaccharides for milk and the storage carbohydrate glycogen, a branched structure of glucose molecules, found in muscle and liver. When dietary carbohydrate is not available as an energy source, and stored glycogen has been depleted, glucose can be made from lactate, glycerol, and some amino acids.

Carbohydrates are the most important source of food energy in the world, the major staples being cereals, such as rice, wheat, maize, barley, rye, oats, millet, and sorghum. Sugar is of increasing importance because the human passion for sweetness has resulted in an increase in sugar production to such an extent that it now provides more dietary energy in many countries than foods such as starchy roots, pulses, other vegetables and fruit (Fig. 3.1). Sugar cane was probably first cultivated in Papua New Guinea about 10 000 years ago and sugar beet, which can be grown in temperate climates, some 250 years ago. Carbohydrate-containing foods provide between 40% and 80% of total food energy intake, depending on culture and economic status and contribute important amounts of protein, vitamins, minerals, phytochemicals, sterols, and antioxidants to the diet.

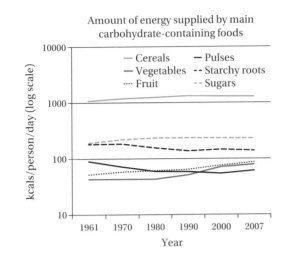

Fig. 3.1 Principal carbohydrate sources of food energy (Kcals/person/day) from major carbohydrate sources (1961–2007).

Source: FAOSTAT Food Balance Sheets 2010 (http://faostat.fao.org/site/368/default.aspx#ancor).

3.1 Classification of dietary carbohydrates

Despite being principally a source of energy, carbohydrates are a diverse group of substances that have varied chemical and physiological properties, which result in a number of important effects on health. They may be grouped or classified in different ways, but as chemistry ultimately determines function, classification according to molecular size—characterized by the degree of polymerization (DP), the type of linkage (α or non-α linked), and the individual monomers present—is the only approach that has stood the test of time (Table 3.1). This classification was recommended by the Joint FAO/WHO Expert Consultation on carbohydrates in 1997 (FAO/WHO, 1998) and endorsed at the Scientific Update in 2006 (Nishida *et al.*, 2007).

Table 3.1 The major dietary carbohydrates

Class (DP)[a]	Subgroup	Principal components
Sugars (1–2)	i Monosaccharides	Glucose, fructose, galactose
	ii Disaccharides	Sucrose, lactose, maltose, trehalose
	iii Polyols (sugar alcohols)	Sorbitol, mannitol, lactitol, xylitol, erythritol, isomalt, maltitol
Oligosaccharides (3–9) (short-chain carbohydrates)[b]	i Malto-oligosaccharides (α-glucans)	Maltodextrins
	ii Nonα-glucan oligosaccharides	Raffinose, stachyose, fructo- and galacto-oligosaccharides, polydextrose, insulin
Polysaccharides (≥10)	i Starch (α-glucans)	Amylose, amylopectin, modified starches
	ii Nonstarch polysaccharides (NSPs)	Cellulose, hemicellulose, pectin, arabinoxylans, β-glucans, glucomannans, plant gums and mucilages, hydrocolloids

[a]Degree of polymerization or number of monomeric (single-sugar) units.
[b]See IUB-IUPAC definition and Cummings *et al.* (1997).

Source: Nishida, C., Nocito, F.M., and Mann, J. (2007) Joint FAO/WHO Scientific Update on Carbohydrates in Human Nutrition. *Eur J Clin Nutr*, **61** Suppl 1, S1–137.

3.1.1 Sugars

Sugars comprise monosaccharides, disaccharides, and sugar alcohols. The three principal monosaccharides are glucose, fructose, and galactose (Fig. 3.2) and they are the building blocks of naturally occurring di-, oligo-, and polysaccharides. Free glucose and fructose occur in honey and cooked or dried fruit (invert sugar) and in small amounts in raw fruit, berries, vegetables, especially carrots, onions, swede, and turnip, and tomatoes. Corn syrup (a glucose syrup produced by the hydrolysis of corn starch) and high-fructose corn syrup (which contains glucose and fructose) are increasingly being used by the food industry. Fructose is the sweetest of all the food carbohydrates.

The principal disaccharides are sucrose (αGlc$(1 \rightarrow 2)\beta$-Fru) and lactose (β-Gal$(1 \rightarrow 4)\beta$Glc) (Fig. 3.2). Sucrose is found very widely in fruit, berries, and vegetables and can be extracted from sugar cane or beet. Lactose is the main sugar in milk. Maltose, a disaccharide derived from starch, occurs in sprouted wheat and barley. Trehalose (α-Glc$(1 \rightarrow 4)\alpha$-Glc) is found in yeast, fungi (mushrooms), and in small amounts in bread and honey. It is used by the food industry as a replacement for sucrose, where a less sweet taste is desired but with similar technological properties.

The polyols, such as sorbitol, are alcohols of glucose and other sugars. They are found naturally in some fruits and made commercially by using aldose reductase to convert the aldehyde group of the glucose molecule to the alcohol. Sorbitol is used as a replacement for sucrose in the diet of people with diabetes but confers little benefit.

3.1.2 Oligosaccharides (short-chain carbohydrates)

Oligosaccharides are compounds in which monosaccharide units are joined by glycosidic likages. Their DP is not clearly defined but, according to chemical convention, they are carbohydrates with a DP of 2–10. However, nutritionists classify the disaccharides (DP 2) as sugars. The division between oligosaccharides and polysaccharides at DP 10 is somewhat arbitrary as there is a continuum of molecular size from sugars to complex polymers of DP 100 000 or more. In reality, the division is made analytically by defining oligosaccharides as carbohydrates other than mono- and disaccharides that remain in solution in 80% (w/v) ethanol. Food oligosaccharides fall into two groups. One, the maltodextrins, which are mostly derived from starch and include maltotriose, and α-limit dextrins that have both α-1,4 and α-1,6 bonds and are on average DP 8. Maltodextrins are widely used in the food industry as sweeteners, as fat substitutes, and to modify the texture of food products. They are digested and absorbed like other α-glucans. Second are the oligosaccharides that are not α-glucans. These oligosaccharides include raffinose (α-Gal$(1 \rightarrow 6)$ α-Glc$(1 \rightarrow 2)\beta$-Fru), stachyose (($Gal)_2$ 1:6 Glu 1:2 Fru) and verbascose (($Gal)_3$ 1:6 Glu 1:2 Fru). They

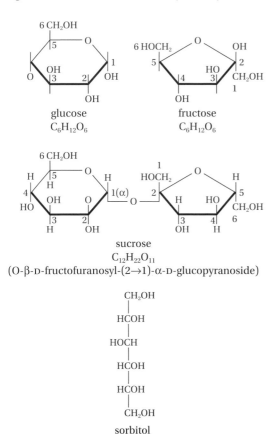

Fig. 3.2 The structure of mono- and disaccharides.

are, in effect, sucrose joined to varying numbers of galactose molecules and they are found in a variety of plant seeds such as peas, beans, and lentils. Important also in this group are inulin and fructo-oligosaccharides (α-Glc($1 \rightarrow 2$)β-Fru($2 \rightarrow 1$) β-Fru$_{(N)}$ or β-Fru($2 \rightarrow 1$)βFru$_{(N)}$). They are fructans and are the storage carbohydrates in artichokes with small amounts of the lower-molecular-weight varieties found in wheat, rye, asparagus, and members of the onion, leek, and garlic families. They may also be produced industrially. The chemical bonds linking these oligosaccharides are not α-1,4 or 1,6 glucans and, therefore, they are not susceptible to pancreatic or brush border enzyme breakdown. They have become known as 'nondigestible oligosaccharides' or NDO. Some of them, mainly the fructans and galactans, have unique properties in the gut and are known as prebiotics (see Section 3.10.5).

Milk, especially human milk, contains oligosaccharides that are predominantly galactose containing, although great diversity of structure is found. Almost all carry lactose at their reducing end and are elongated by addition of N-acetylglucosamine-linked β1–3 or β1–6 to a galactose residue, followed by further galactose with β1–3 or β1–4 bonds. Other monomers include l-fucose and sialic acid. The principal oligosaccharide in milk is lacto-N-tetraose.

Total oligosaccharides in human milk are in the range 5.0–8.0 g/L, but only trace amounts are present in cow's milk.

3.1.3 Polysaccharides

These divide into α-glucans (starch) and non-α-glucans (nonstarch polysaccharides).

Starch Starch is the storage carbohydrate found in cereals, potatoes, cassava, legumes, and bananas and consists only of glucose molecules. It occurs in a partially crystalline form in granules and comprises two polymers: amylose (DP ~ 10^3) and amylopectin (DP ~ 10^4–10^5). Most common cereal starches comprise 15–30% amylose, which is a nonbranching helical chain of glucose residues linked by α-1,4 glucosidic bonds, and 70–85% amylopectin, a high-molecular-weight, highly branched polymer containing both α-1,4 and α-1,6 linkages (Fig. 3.3). Some waxy starches (maize, rice, sorghum, barley) comprise mostly amylopectin. In animals and humans, carbohydrate is stored in liver and muscle in limited amounts as glycogen, which has a structure similar to amylopectin but is even more highly branched. The crystalline form of the amylose and amylopectin in starch granules confers on them distinct X-ray

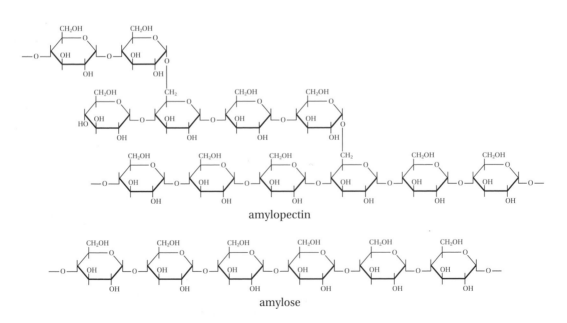

amylopectin

amylose

Fig. 3.3 The structure of amylose and amylopectin.

diffraction patterns (A, B, and C). The A type is characteristic of cereals (rice, wheat, maize) and the B type of potato, banana, and high-amylose starches, while the C type is intermediate between A and B, as found in legumes. In their native (raw) form, the B starches are resistant to digestion by pancreatic amylase. Starch, which is not digested in the small bowel, is known as 'resistant starch' (see Section 3.5.1). The crystalline structure is lost when starch is heated in water (gelatinization), thus permitting digestion to take place. Recrystallization (retrogradation) takes place to a variable extent after cooking and cooling, and is in the B form.

Modified starch Because many starches do not have the functional properties needed to impart or maintain desired qualities in food products, some have been modified, by either chemical processing or plant breeding techniques, to obtain these properties. Various processes are used to modify starch, the two most important being substitution and cross-linking. Substitution involves etherification or esterification of a relatively small number of hydroxyl groups on the glucose units of amylose and amylopectin. This reduces retrogradation, which is part of the process of staling of bread, for example. Substitution also lowers gelatinization temperature, provides freeze–thaw stability, and increases viscosity. Cross-linking involves the introduction of a limited number of linkages between the chains of amylose and amylopectin. The process reinforces the hydrogen bonding that occurs within the granule. Cross-linking increases gelatinization temperature, improves acid and heat stabilities, inhibits gel formation, and controls viscosity during processing. Techniques of plant breeding, including genetic modification, can also be used to alter the proportions of amylose and amylopectin in starchy foods. For example, high-amylose corn starch requires higher temperatures for gelatinization and is more prone to retrogradation. Varying the composition of starchy foods may alter nutritional properties, as well as conferring different functional properties.

Nonstarch polysaccharides Nonstarch polysaccharides (NSPs) are principally the polysaccharides of the plant cell wall and are the main component of dietary fibre. They comprise a mixture of many molecular forms of which cellulose, a straight-chain β-1,4-linked glucan (DP 10^3–10^6), is the most widely distributed. Because of its linear, unbranched nature, cellulose molecules are able to pack closely together in a three-dimensional lattice work, forming microfibrils. These form the basis of cellulose fibres, which are woven into the plant cell wall and give it structure. Cellulose comprises 10–30% of the NSPs in foods.

By contrast, the hemicelluloses are a diverse group of polysaccharide polymers that contain a mixture of hexose (6C) and pentose (5C) sugars, often in highly branched chains. Mostly they comprise a backbone of xylose sugars with branches of arabinose, mannose, galactose, and glucose, and have a DP of 150–200. Typical of the hemicelluloses are the arabinoxylans found in cereals. About half the hemicelluloses contain uronic acids, which are carboxylated derivatives of glucose and galactose. They are important in determining the properties of hemicelluloses, behaving as carboxylic acids, and are able to form salts with metal ions such as calcium and zinc.

Common to all cell walls are pectins, which are primarily β-1,4-D-galacturonic acid polymers, although they usually contain 10–25% other sugars such as rhamnose, galactose, and arabinose, as side chains. Some 3–11% of the uronic acids have methyl substitutions, which improve the gel-forming properties of pectin, as used in jam making. Some residues are acetylated. Calcium and magnesium salts of uronic acids are characteristic of pectins.

Chemically related to the cell wall NSPs—but not strictly cell wall components—are the plant gums and mucilages. Plant gums are sticky exudates that form at the sites of injuries to plants. They are mostly highly branched, complex uronic acid-containing polymers. Gum Arabic, named after the Arabian port from which it was originally exported to Europe, comes from the acacia tree and is one of the better-known plant gums. It is sold commercially as an adhesive and used in the food industry as a thickener and to retard sugar crystallization. Other plant gums include karaya (sterculia) and tragacanth, which are licensed food additives.

Plant mucilages are botanically very different in that they are usually mixed with the endosperm of the storage carbohydrates of seeds. Their role is to retain water and prevent desiccation. They are neutral polysaccharides like the hemicelluloses, of which guar gum, from the cluster bean, and carob gum are similar β-1,4-D-galactomannans with α-1,6-galactose single-unit side chains. Again, they are widely used in the pharmaceutical and food industries as thickeners and stabilizers in salad creams, soups, and toothpastes.

The algal polysaccharides, which include carageenan, agar, and alginate, are all NSPs extracted from seaweeds or algae. They replace cellulose in the cell wall and have gel-forming properties. Carageenan and agar are highly sulphated and the ability of carageenan to react with milk protein has led to its use in dairy products and chocolate.

Because of the nature of the chemical bonds in NSPs, they are not digested by enzymes secreted into the gut but are extensively degraded by bacteria in the lower bowel through a process known as fermentation (see Section 3.5.4).

3.2 Measurement of dietary carbohydrates

In North America, total carbohydrate in the diet has traditionally been estimated by measuring moisture, fat, protein, and ash and subtracting the sum from the total dry weight of the food. The remainder is considered to be carbohydrate 'by difference'. In Europe and Australasia, measurement is based on the sum of individual carbohydrates. The 1997 and 2006 consultations by the Food and Agriculture Organization (FAO) and the World Health Organization (WHO) use the latter approach because the figure arrived at by difference includes noncarbohydrate components (lignin, tannins, waxes, and some organic acids) and compounds the analytical errors of all the other determinations. Moreover, by difference does not allow a detailed characterization of dietary carbohydrate, which is necessary for understanding the relationship between carbohydrates and health and making claims.

A single comprehensive system to measure all the carbohydrate fractions in the diet does not exist, although one is urgently needed. Hence, food tables will often give only a figure for total carbohydrate, sugars, starch, and sometimes NSPs or fibre. What is usually missing at the present time are data on oligosaccharides and resistant starch.

After homogenization of a diet or food, and lipid extraction if necessary, free sugars (mono- and disaccharides) can be extracted into aqueous solutions and measured by gas–liquid chromatography (GLC) or high-performance liquid chromatography (HPLC). Enzymic methods also exist for individual sugars. Oligosaccharides or short-chain carbohydrates are more difficult to determine and are measured as those carbohydrates other than free sugars that are soluble in 80% ethanol and not susceptible to pancreatic amylase. Starch and maltodextrins are hydrolysed and NSPs precipitated with ethanol. Fructans are hydrolysed enzymatically and the monosaccharide constituents reduced to acid-stable alditol derivatives, while the remaining oligosaccharides are hydrolysed with sulphuric acid and measured as alditol acetates by GLC.

Starch is solubilized and then hydrolysed with a combination of amylolytic enzymes, and the increase in glucose is measured either enzymatically, colorimetrically, or by GLC. Starch can be subdivided analytically into rapidly digestible (RDS), slowly digestible (SDS), and resistant starch (RS). RDS and SDS relate to the rate of release of glucose from starch and are relevant to the concept of the glycaemic index (see Section 3.6).

After starch has been hydrolysed enzymatically, NSPs can be precipitated with 80% ethanol, hydrolysed with sulphuric acid, and the released sugars measured colorimetrically, by GLC or HPLC. Techniques exist for separate measurement of cellulose in the process. The division of NSPs (fibre) into soluble and insoluble is method (pH) dependent and is not recommended.

3.3 Other terms used to describe carbohydrates

A classification based on chemistry is necessary for a coherent and enforceable approach to measurement and labelling and to understanding the physiological and health effects of the various carbohydrates. However, chemistry does not always translate directly into physiology because each of the major classes of carbohydrate has a variety of physical properties and physiological effects. However, classification based on physiological properties alone creates a number of problems, as it requires that a single effect be considered overridingly important and used as the basis of the classification; which makes measurement difficult. This dichotomy has led to the introduction of a number of terms, chemical, physiological, and botanical, to describe various fractions and subfractions of carbohydrate.

3.3.1 Extrinsic and intrinsic sugars

Intrinsic sugars are those incorporated within the cell walls of plants, that is, they are naturally occurring and are always accompanied by other nutrients. Extrinsic sugars are those added to foods. Lactose in milk does not fall readily into either category but milk has important nutritional properties, so the term non-milk extrinsic sugar (NMES) was introduced in the UK to indicate the group of sugars other than intrinsic and milk sugars that should be identified in the diet. This terminology has not gained widespread use. The WHO/FAO Expert Consultation on *Diet, nutrition and the prevention of chronic diseases* (WHO Technical Report Series 916) in 2003 recommended the use of the term 'free sugars', which refers to all 'monosaccharides and disaccharides added to foods by the manufacturer, cook and consumer, plus sugars naturally present in honey, syrups and fruit juices.'

3.3.2 Total sugars

Analytically, it is not readily possible to distinguish in a processed food which sugars might have been added and which are naturally present in say, fruit, in that

food. Moreover, there is probably little difference physiologically between the way the body absorbs and metabolizes the sucrose present in a banana and that in a sugary drink, for example. Of course, the nutritional profile of these two foods will be very different. For labelling purposes, therefore, the category of 'total sugars' has been suggested, which includes all sugars from whatever source in a food, and is defined as all monosaccharides and disaccharides other than polyols. Other terms in use include sugars, added sugars, refined sugars, saccharose, and free sugars.

3.3.3 Complex carbohydrate

The term complex carbohydrate was first introduced in 1977 in *Dietary goals for the United States* to encourage consumption of what were considered 'healthy foods' such as wholegrain cereals, fruit, and vegetables. Subsequently, the term came to be used to distinguish between sugars and polysaccharides (Table 3.1). Complex carbohydrate has, however, never been formally defined and eventually it became equated with starch. It has not proved useful to distinguish 'healthy' food because many fruits and vegetables are low in polysaccharides and starch. Moreover, starch can have many forms, each with contrasting metabolic properties. Starch derived from most cooked starchy cereals or potatoes is almost as rapidly absorbed as many sugars. On the other hand, some starch such as that found in unripe bananas and partly milled grains and seeds is fairly resistant to digestion in the small intestine of humans and from a physiological perspective is digested and metabolized more like NSPs. The term 'complex carbohydrate', therefore, is not useful in the context of a chemically based approach to carbohydrates or in nutritional recommendations.

3.3.4 Glycaemic carbohydrate

Perhaps the most useful distinction with regard to human health is whether or not the carbohydrate does or does not directly provide glucose as an energy source for the tissues following the process of digestion and absorption in the small intestine. Carbohydrate that provides glucose for metabolism is referred to as 'glycaemic carbohydrate', whereas carbohydrate that passes to the large intestine where it is fermented is referred to as 'nonglycaemic carbohydrate'. Most mono- and disaccharides, some oligosaccharides (maltodextrins), and digestible starches may be classed as glycaemic carbohydrate. The remaining oligosaccharides, nonstarch polysaccharides and resistant starches are considered to be nonglycaemic carbohydrates. A food may contain both glycaemic and nonglycaemic carbohydrate. The extent to which carbohydrate in foods raises blood glucose concentrations compared with an equivalent amount of reference carbohydrate has also been used as a means of classifying dietary carbohydrate; it is known as the glycaemic index (see Section 3.6).

Analogous to the concept of glycaemic carbohydrate are the terms 'available and unavailable carbohydrate'. These were introduced by McCance and Lawrence in 1921 while preparing food tables for diabetic diets. Available carbohydrate was defined as 'starch and soluble sugars' and unavailable carbohydrate as 'mainly hemicellulose and fibre (cellulose)'. The terms glycaemic and nonglycaemic are probably more useful and follow on from McCance and Lawrence's original ideas.

3.3.5 Dietary fibre

There is now an internationally agreed definition of dietary fibre, which is a combination of chemistry and physiology.

Given that the main body of epidemiological and experimental data regarding health benefits of fibre derives from studies of diets based on fruit, vegetables, and wholegrain cereals, it is important to emphasize the benefits of intrinsic carbohydrates of the plant cell wall, which are characteristic of such diets (hence the first bullet point in Box 3.1).

There is experimental evidence that some carbohydrate polymers extracted from food and synthetic polymers may have physiological effects such as cholesterol lowering. However, there is a lack of long-term epidemiological evidence of health benefit, so bullet points two and three in Box 3.1 emphasize the need for 'generally accepted scientific evidence' to be accepted by 'competent authorities' before such polymers can be labelled as fibre.

The principal components of dietary fibre by any definition are the NSPs of the plant cell wall, but resistant starch also meets the criteria of the Codex

BOX 3.1 Definition of dietary fibre agreed at Codex Alimentarius in 2009

'Dietary fibre means carbohydrate polymers with ten or more monomeric units, which are not hydrolysed by the endogenous enzymes in the small intestine of humans and belong to the following categories:

- 'Edible carbohydrate polymers naturally occurring in food as consumed,
- 'carbohydrate polymers, which have been obtained form food raw material by physical, enzymatic or chemical means and which have been shown to have a physiological effect of benefit to health as demonstrated by generally accepted scientific evidence to competent authorities,
- 'synthetic carbohydrate polymers which have been shown to have a physiological effect of benefit to health as demonstrated by generally accepted scientific evidence to competent authorities'.

There are two footnotes to the definition, one of which allows countries to include oligosaccharides (DP 3–10) as fibre, which is the position taken by the European Commission, and the other which allows 'fractions of lignin and/or other compounds when associated with polysaccharides in the plant cell walls and if these compounds are quantified by the AOAC gravimetric methods'. There are no internationally agreed methods for measuring dietary fibre at present.

Source: http://www.codexalimentarius.net/web/archives.jsp?year=09, ALINORM 09/32/26 paras 27–54 and page 46.

definition. This will not be a large contributor to the overall fibre content of a food except for uncooked starch as found in banana and cooked and cooled starchy foods that are common staples in developing countries. Lignin, a plant cell-wall substance associated with NSP is not a carbohydrate, has no well-established health benefit, is very difficult to measure, and is not included in the main definition.

The terms 'soluble' and 'insoluble' fibre developed out of the early chemistry of NSPs. However, this separation is not chemically distinct, it can be changed by simply altering the pH of the extraction, and the physiological roles of soluble and insoluble NSPs in foods are not clear. Much of the early work on soluble fibre, which suggested that it had good cholesterol-lowering properties, was from studies using pure polysaccharides such as pectin, guar, psyllium, and milling fractions like oat bran. All plant cell wall/NSP complexes, as they exist in foods, contain a 'soluble' fraction and ascribing specific physiological properties to, or making dietary recommendations for distinct subfractions of NSP is not justified at present.

3.4 Availability and consumption

The major sources of carbohydrate worldwide are cereals (rice, wheat, maize, barley, oats, rye, millet, and sorghum), root crops (potatoes, cassava [manioc], yams, sweet potatoes, and taro), sugar cane and beet, pulses, vegetables, fruit, and milk products. World production of cereals, sugar cane, vegetables, and fruits has increased over the last 20–30 years (see Chapter 26). Production of root crops, pulses, and sugar beet, however, has changed little on a worldwide basis; pulse production has decreased in some Asian countries and root crop production has fallen in Europe. At first glance these data suggest that overall food production is keeping pace with population growth, which has continued in most parts of the world. Increased production, however, is due largely to improved agricultural practices, principally the increased use of fertilizers, and there has been no appreciable increase in areas under cultivation for these crops. This suggests that the steady increase in production may not be sustained in all countries. Indeed, for the continent of Africa, cereal production is already inadequate and it seems conceivable—indeed likely—that there are major problems ahead. The proportional reduction of root crops and pulses may have nutritional consequences.

Fig. 3.1 shows the kilocalories available per person per day from carbohydrate-containing foods available for consumption on a worldwide basis.

These data are lower than overall crop production statistics because much cereal production goes into animal feed (especially maize and barley) or is grown for seed, or is used in brewing and distilling (barley). In terms of agricultural production for food, in 2007 rice was the main cereal, followed by wheat, then maize. Fig. 3.1 shows clearly that cereal crops provide by far the biggest contribution to energy intake of any food—46% in 2008. Notable, however, is the steady rise in energy from sugar, which was in 1961 very similar to that obtained from starchy roots (potatoes, sweet potato, yams, etc.), while by 2008 sugar had become the second source of energy from carbohydrate, providing 231 kilocalories per person per day compared with 140 from starchy roots. Overall, including non-milk sugars, carbohydrate-containing foods provided 67% of food energy in 2008 worldwide.

Population surveys permit a broad overview of carbohydrate consumption in different parts of the world (Table 3.2). As a percentage of total energy intake, the contribution from all carbohydrates ranges from about 40% to over 80% (representing about 250–400 g carbohydrate/day) with more affluent countries such as those in North America, Europe, and Australasia at the lower end of the range, and less affluent countries at the higher end. Starch accounts for 20–50% and sugars 9–27% of

Table 3.2 Intake of carbohydrate and its components in adults in various countries since 1980

Country	Year	n	Energy (kcal)	Carbohydrate		Starch		Sugars	
				g	% energy	g	% energy	g	% energy
Malawi[a]	1997	141	1457	287	78.7	—	—	—	—
S Africa—coloured	1990	976	1981	224	45.2	147	29.7	77	15.6
China	1992	3682	2396	355	59.3	—	—	—	—
Vietnam	1988	7462	1998	407	81.5	—	—	—	—
Netherlands	1987–88	4134	2309	244	42.2	122	21.1	119	20.6
UK[b]	2001	1724	M 2313	M 275	M 47.6	M 157	M 27.3	M 118	M 20.4
			F 1632	F 203	F 49.7	F 110	F 26.9	F 88	F 21.6
Chile	1995	859	1981	287	58.0	—	—	—	—
USA	1988–91	7931	2109	244	46.3	—	—	—	—
Australia	1983	6255	2190	232	42.4	125	22.8	107	19.5
Papua New Guinea	1991	750	2628	406	61.8	349	53.1	57	8.7

[a]Gibson, R.S. (1997) Personal communication.
[b]National Diet and Nutrition Survey 2002. The Stationery Office London.

Source: **FAO/WHO** (1998) *Carbohydrates in human nutrition*. Report of a Joint FAO/WHO Expert Consultation. Paper 66. Rome, Food and Agricultural Organization, World Health Organization.

total energy, with low intakes of sugars generally associated with high total carbohydrate intakes. In Western countries 20–25% of total energy is derived from sugars, about one-third of all sugars come from naturally occurring sources (vegetables, milk, fruits, and juices) and two-thirds from added sugars, especially sucrose. In North America, a relatively high proportion of free sugars comes from corn syrup solids or high-fructose corn syrups, so that sucrose intake—but not total sugar intake—is lower than in most European countries. Trends in total carbohydrate consumption suggest a falling intake in most relatively affluent countries, reflecting a progressive decline in overall energy intake.

3.5 Digestion and absorption of carbohydrates

3.5.1 Sugars and starch (Fig. 3.4)

The mono- and disaccharides, maltodextrins, and most starches are digested and absorbed from the upper part of the small bowel. They are hydrolysed to their constituent monosaccharides before transport across the mucosa. Some carbohydrates, such as lactose in many populations, most oligosaccharides except maltodextrins, some starches, and all

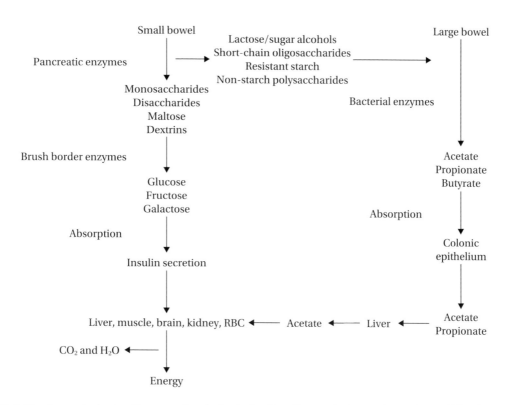

Fig. 3.4 The two principal pathways of carbohydrate digestion and absorption. RBC, red blood cells.

NSPs, resist digestion and pass into the large bowel where they are fermented (see Section 3.5.4).

Carbohydrate digestion starts in the mouth, where salivary α-amylase is secreted. However, its activity is substantially inhibited by low pH when ingested food enters the stomach and so is relatively unimportant compared with that resulting from pancreatic amylase in the small intestine. Amylase is the only active carbohydrate-digesting enzyme produced by the pancreas. α-Amylase hydrolyses the α-1,4 bonds but only those that are not at the ends of a molecule or next to α-1,6 branch points, so α-amylase produces a mixture of glucose, maltose, maltotriose, and α-limit dextrins, which are presented to the small bowel mucosa. The surface area of the small intestine is about 200 m² because it is covered with microvilli. These microvilli extend into the unstirred water-layer phase of the intestinal lumen. The microvillus layer is known as the brush border and in it are the three principal enzymes that complete digestion to monosaccharides: these are glucoamylase (α-glucosidase) and

sucrose-isomaltase, which are able to reduce the products of starch digestion to glucose monomers and sucrose to glucose and fructose, and lactase (β-galactosidase), which hydrolyses lactose to glucose and galactose. The expression of β-galactosidase is retained in the brush border after weaning in only a minority of world populations, mainly those in northern climates. In close association with these enzymes are transporters that move the monosaccharides into the portal blood. Glucose and galactose are both absorbed into the enterocyte by a process of active transport facilitated by sodium glucose cotransporters (SGLT1). Sodium is pumped from the cell to create a sodium gradient between the intestinal lumen and the interior of the cell. The resultant sodium gradient drives the cotransporter so that one molecule of sodium and one molecule of glucose or galactose are transported into the cytoplasm of the enterocyte against a concentration gradient. Glucose is pumped out of the enterocyte and into the intracellular space by glucose transporter 2 (GLUT 2). This is one of a large family of more than 12 facilitative glucose transporters that are found in tissues throughout the body, which transport d-glucose down its concentration gradient, a process described as facilitated diffusion. Fructose is taken up from the gut lumen by a similar process of facilitated transport by the glucose transporter 5 (GLUT 5), which may also be the means by which it exits the enterocyte.

Sugar alcohols such as sorbitol, mannitol, xylitol, and erythritol, have no specific transport mechanism and are absorbed by simple diffusion. At low amounts, this works well, but as the amount ingested increases, so the transport capacity of the small bowel is overwhelmed and they partly pass into the large bowel. Because of their relatively low molecular weight, they retain considerable amounts of water within the bowel, which can lead to diarrhoea after excess consumption.

Any starch that escapes the normal small bowel digestive processes is called resistant starch. As already indicated (see Section 3.2), starch may resist digestion because it is enclosed in wholegrains or is otherwise physically inaccessible (RS1), or because it is present in the B-type crystalline form (RS2) or because it has retrograded after cooking and cooling (RS3). Some modified starch (e.g. hydroxypropyl or acetylated starch) will also resist digestion (RS4). The amount of RS in the diet is not accurately known because measuring it is technically difficult. This is because almost any handling of starchy foods from diet collections (i.e. mixing with water, homogenization, freezing, or cooling) will affect RS content. Present estimates for countries with Westernized diets are in the range of 3–10 g/day. Clearly this is very diet dependent. A couple of relatively unripe bananas will readily provide 20 g RS. A biscuit made with potato flour would give 10 g. The amount of RS that escapes digestion also varies among people, partly dependent on transit time through the small bowel.

3.5.2 Oligosaccharides

Aside from the maltodextrins, which are derived from starch, the oligosaccharides are a neglected group of carbohydrates from the point of view of their nutritional value. The nature of their chemical bonds means they are not susceptible to either pancreatic or brush border hydrolysis and so they pass entirely into the large intestine. Oligosaccharides, therefore, are not glycaemic carbohydrates. The lower molecular weight species (DP 3–5) have the potential to provide an osmotic gradient in the small bowel, and if taken in large quantities (15–30 g) can cause disturbances in gut function. They are better known for their propensity to gas formation in the colon as a result of their rapid fermentation. Some of these oligosaccharides have been shown to have prebiotic properties (see Section 3.10.5)

3.5.3 Nonstarch polysaccharides (NSPs)

NSPs escape digestion in the small bowel and pass into the large bowel, where they are fermented. The reason for their resistance to digestion is partly because of their physical form and partly their chemical bonds. They are almost entirely found in plant cell walls and the chemical bonds in these molecules are not susceptible to brush border or pancreatic digestive enzymes. For example, the bonds in cellulose are principally β-1,4 in contrast to α-1,4 in starch. This minor stereochemical difference is sufficient to prevent hydrolysis by pancreatic amylase. The amount of NSPs in the diet varies (12–36 g/day), with higher amounts being characteristic of vegetarian diets or populations with high fruit and vegetable intake, such as on some Pacific islands. High NSP intake is not characteristic of diets in developing countries because rice and maize are low in NSPs and fruit and vegetables are in short supply, so intakes are in the 16–25 g/day range.

3.5.4 Fermentation

Virtually all carbohydrate that enters the large bowel is fermented by the commensal bacteria of the colon, which are present at densities of up to 10^{12}

cells/g contents. Recovery of oligosaccharides in faeces is effectively nil, while RS and NSP excretion is rarely more than 2–4 g/day when intakes are in the 20–40 g range. Only very resistant retrograded starches survive partly, the amount depending on colonic transit time, although occasional individuals are unable to digest some RS fractions. Microcrystalline cellulose may resist fermentation because of its highly condensed structure, an observation that led to the belief that cellulose was not digested in the human gut. This is because microcrystalline cellulose was used in many early experiments of cellulose digestion. However, cellulose naturally present in the cell walls of food is completely fermented unless it is in a highly lignified structure. Other polysaccharides of the plant cell wall are also readily fermented, even when given in purified forms such as pectin or guar gum. This process is facilitated by the ability of these latter substances to form gels readily accessible to the microbiota.

Microbial fermentation is an anaerobic process and produces quite different end-products from aerobic metabolism. As Fig. 3.5 shows, these include principally the short-chain fatty acids (SCFAs), acetate, propionate, and butyrate, which are the two-, three-, and four-carbon fatty acids of the same chemical series that include C12–C22 fatty acids, which are the major lipids of the diet.

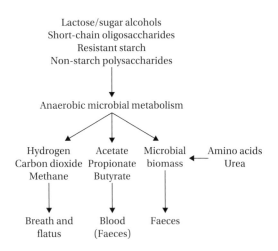

Fig. 3.5 Fermentation of carbohydrate in the large bowel.

The SCFAs are, however, much more water soluble. They are rapidly absorbed. Butyrate is the major energy source for the colonic epithelial cell, in contrast to glutamine for the small bowel and glucose for most other tissues. Butyrate also has differentiating properties in the cell, arresting cell division through its ability to regulate gene expression. This property provides a credible link between the dietary intake of fermented carbohydrates, such as NSPs, and protection against colorectal cancer.

Propionate is absorbed and passes to the liver, where it is taken up and metabolized aerobically. This molecule is not seen as having significant regulatory properties in humans, although it may moderate hepatic lipid metabolism. However, in ruminant animals, propionate is crucial to life because it is used to synthesize glucose in the liver.

Acetate is the major SCFA produced in all types of gut fermentation and the molar ratio of acetate to propionate to butyrate is around 60:20:20. Acetate is rapidly absorbed, stimulating sodium absorption, and passes to the liver and then into the blood, from where it is available as an energy source. Fasting blood acetate levels are about 50 µmol/L, rising 8–12 hours later to 100–300 µmol/L after meals containing fermentable carbohydrate. Acetate is rapidly cleared from the blood with a half-life of only a few minutes and is metabolized principally by skeletal and cardiac muscle and the brain. Acetate spares free fatty acid oxidation in humans and its absorption does not stimulate insulin release. Another precursor of blood acetate is alcohol.

Thus, fermentation is an integral part of digestion and provides energy, which is up to 70% of the available energy in equivalent monosaccharides. By convention, the energy value of oligosaccharides has been set as 2 kcal/g, and the same value could usefully be applied to RS and NSPs. The total energy provided from fermentation in the human is probably only 5% of total energy requirements, although it could be more, depending on diet.

Fermentation of amino acids, derived from protein, also occurs in the large bowel and, in addition to SCFAs, yields ammonia, amines, phenols, and sulphur compounds. Fermentation also gives rise to the gases hydrogen and carbon dioxide. Much of the hydrogen is converted to methane by bacteria, and both hydrogen and methane are excreted in breath and flatus. Gas production, especially if rapid, is one of the principal complaints of people unused to eating foods containing significant amounts of fermentable carbohydrate. Another product of fermentation is microbial biomass or microbial growth. These bacteria are excreted in faeces and this is one of the principal mechanisms of laxation by NSPs especially. Also produced from fermentation is lactate. This occurs usually during rapid fermentation of soluble carbohydrates such as oligosaccharides. Both D- and L-lactate are produced and both are absorbed. Ethyl alcohol is also produced during hind-gut fermentation, although it is more characteristic of fermentation by yeasts, as in brewing and wine making.

3.6 Glycaemic response to carbohydrate foods

Plasma glucose levels rise 5–45 minutes after any meal that contains sugars or digestible starch, and usually return to fasting levels 2–3 hours later. This rise in blood glucose is known as the glycaemic response and depends upon the rate and extent of digestion, absorption, and clearance from the plasma. The glycaemic index of a carbohydrate-containing food is defined as the incremental area under the blood glucose curve following a portion of a test food containing 50 g of carbohydrate, expressed as a percentage of the response to 50 g of carbohydrate from a standard food (either glucose or white bread) taken by the same subject. The glycaemic index (GI) of a range of carbohydrate-containing foods derived from studies in humans is shown in Table 3.3.

Table 3.3 The average glycaemic index (GI) of 62 most common carbohydrate-containing foods

	GI		GI		GI
High-carbohydrate foods		**Breakfast cereals**		**Vegetables**	
White wheat bread	75	Cornflakes	81	Potato, boiled	78
Whole wheat/whole meal bread	74	Wheat flake biscuits	69	Potato, instant mash	87
Specialty grain bread	70	Porridge, rolled oats	55	Potato, french fries	63
Unleavened wheat bread	70	Instant oat porridge	79	Carrots, boiled	39
Wheat roti	62	Rice porridge/congee	78	Sweet potato, boiled	63
Chapatti	52	Millet porridge	67	Pumpkin, boiled	64
Corn tortilla	46	Muesli	57	Plantain/green banana	55
White rice, boiled	73			Taro, boiled	53
Brown rice, boiled	68	**Fruit and fruit products**		Vegetable soup	48
Barley	28	Apple, raw	36		

Table 3.3 (*Continued*)

	GI		GI		GI
Sweet corn	49	Orange, raw	43	**Dairy products and alternatives**	
Spaghetti, white	49	Banana, raw	51	Milk, full fat	39
Spaghetti, whole meal	48	Pineapple, raw	59	Milk, skim	37
Rice noodles	53	Mango, raw	51	Ice cream	51
Udon noodles	55	Watermelon, raw	76	Yoghurt, fruit	41
Couscous	65	Dates, raw	42	Soy milk	34
		Peaches, canned	43	Rice milk	86
Snack products		Strawberry jam/jelly	49		
Chocolate	40	Apple juice	41	**Legumes**	
Popcorn	65	Orange juice	50	Chickpeas	28
Potato crisps	56			Kidney beans	24
Soft drink/soda	59	**Sugars**		Lentils	32
Rice crackers/crisps	87	Fructose	15	Soya beans	16
		Sucrose	65		
		Glucose	103		
		Honey	61		

Source: Atkinson, F.S., Foster-Powell, K., and Brand-Miller, J.C. (2008) International tables of glycemic index and glycemic load values. *Diabetes Care*, **31**, 2281–3.

GI is influenced by a number of attributes of foods (see Table 3.4). As a general rule, foods that are rich in glucose-containing sugars and rapidly digested starches, such as white bread or cornflakes, will have a relatively large glycaemic response because they are rapidly digested and absorbed. On the other hand, foods such as pulses that are rich in slowly digested and resistant starch, nonstarch polysaccharides, and oligosaccharides will have a low GI. Foods containing fructose also have a relatively low GI because fructose is metabolized and contributes very little to blood glucose. Carbohydrate-containing foods that are also high in fat and protein have a low GI because of the effects of these other components on gastric emptying.

GI is helpful when comparing foods belonging to the same group, for example different types of breads for which GI might range from relatively low (e.g. rye breads) to over 100 in the case of some white or wholemeal breads. Indices at the high or low extremes of the range are probably a true reflection of the glycaemic response and may therefore be helpful when making food choices. However, small differences in published values are probably of little relevance since most GI values are based on the study of a relatively small number of healthy individuals and there is considerable inter- and intraindividual variation in glycaemic response to carbohydrate-containing foods. Furthermore, some foods advertised as having a low GI but which have

Table 3.4 Food factors influencing glycaemic response

Amount of carbohydrate
Nature of the monosaccharide components
Glucose
Fructose
Galactose
Nature of the starch
Amylose
Amylopectin
Crystalline form A, B, or C
Starch–nutrient interaction
Resistant starch
Cooking/food processing
Degree of starch gelatinization/retrogradation
Particle size
Food form
Cellular structure
Other food components
Fat and protein
NSP (affects physical form and viscosity)

a high content of sucrose, high fructose corn syrup, and/or fat may be energy dense. So, for those wishing to restrict energy intake, GI is not necessarily a useful indicator.

The total glycaemic response to a food or meal is determined by the amount of carbohydrate consumed, the GI of each food, and the nature of the other components of the meal. A product or food may have a high GI, but if only a small quantity is consumed, the total amount of glucose available as an immediate energy source is limited. The concept of glycaemic load (GL) was introduced to quantify the overall glycaemic effect of a portion of food. GL is the product of the amount of available carbohydrate in a typical serving and the GI of the food divided by 100. While GL may be a more practical approach to determining the glycaemic response to food, this indicator is clearly dependent on GI and its pitfalls are therefore similar. The ranking of foods according to GL is in most instances similar to that for GI.

Along with the blood glucose response to carbohydrate-containing meals, there is an insulin response, which is important in the control of metabolism. It often reflects the glycaemic response but can, for some foods, be more exaggerated, so the insulin response after apple juice is much greater than that after whole apples, while the glycaemic responses are similar. The presence of fat and protein in a meal increases insulin responses.

3.7 Carbohydrate metabolism

The concentration of glucose in the blood of adults is generally controlled within the range 4.0–5.5 mmol/L. However, when a carbohydrate-containing meal is ingested, the level may temporarily rise to as high as 7.5 mmol/L and fall to as low as 3.0–3.5 mmol/L during fasting. When levels are about 10 mmol/L, such as occurs in diabetes mellitus, or even at lower levels in some people, glucose spills into the urine (glycosuria). Close regulation of blood glucose is necessary, because the brain requires a continuous supply, although it can adapt to lower levels or even use ketone bodies from fat breakdown if adaptation occurs slowly. Erythrocytes rely almost totally on glucose. Several metabolic pathways are involved in the utilization of glucose as an energy source and the maintenance of glucose homeostasis. The pathways are described in detail in textbooks of biochemistry and are summarized briefly in Fig. 3.6.

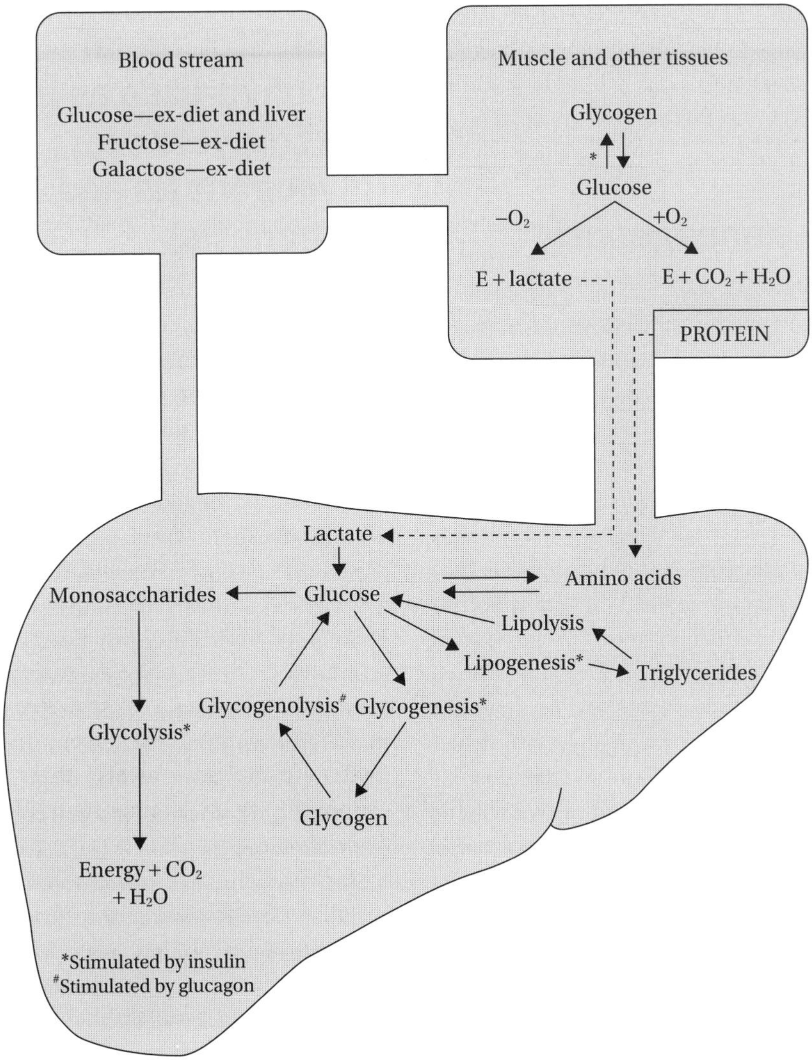

Fig. 3.6 Carbohydrate metabolism and its control.

Figure labels: Blood stream — Glucose—ex-diet and liver, Fructose—ex-diet, Galactose—ex-diet. Muscle and other tissues — Glycogen ⇌ Glucose; $-O_2$ → E + lactate; $+O_2$ → E + CO_2 + H_2O; PROTEIN. Liver: Lactate, Glucose, Amino acids, Monosaccharides, Lipolysis, Lipogenesis* → Triglycerides, Glycolysis*, Glycogenolysis#, Glycogenesis*, Glycogen, Energy + CO_2 + H_2O. *Stimulated by insulin. #Stimulated by glucagon.

3.7.1 Glycolysis

Following absorption, glucose, fructose, and galactose are transported to the liver via the hepatic portal vein. Fructose and galactose are very rapidly converted to glucose. Fructose may also enter the glycolytic pathway directly. Very low concentrations of either of these sugars can be detected in the blood immediately after ingestion.

Glycolysis (the breakdown of glucose) occurs in the cytosol of all cells and may take place in the presence (aerobic) or absence (anaerobic) of oxygen. The pathway involves the metabolism of hexoses to pyruvate. Many reactions catalysed by different enzymes are involved, but glycolysis is regulated by three enzymes that catalyse nonequilibrium reactions —namely, hexokinase (glycokinase), phosphofructokinase, and pyruvate kinase. Under aerobic conditions, pyruvate is transported into the mitochondrion and is then oxidatively decarboxylated to acetyl co-enzyme A (CoA), which enters the citric acid cycle. Under anaerobic conditions (e.g. in exercising muscles or in red blood cells), pyruvate is converted to lactate, which is transported to the liver, where glucose is reformed via the process of gluconeogenesis (see below) and again becomes available via the circulation for oxidation in the tissues. This is known as the lactic acid cycle, or the Cori cycle.

3.7.2 Gluconeogenesis

Gluconeogenesis includes all mechanisms and pathways responsible for converting noncarbohydrates to glucose. In addition to lactate, the other major substrates are the glucogenic amino acids (especially glycine, alanine, glutamate, and aspartate) and glycerol. In the liver, gluconeogenesis takes place in the cytosol, and this pathway involves the same enzymes as glycolysis except at three sites: glucose 6-phosphatase instead of hexokinase; fructose 1,6-biphosphatase instead of phosphofructokinase; and phosphoenolyruvate carboxykinase instead of pyruvate kinase.

Triglycerides of adipose tissue are continuously undergoing hydrolysis to form free glycerol, which cannot be utilized by adipose tissue and therefore diffuses out into the blood and reaches the liver, where it is first converted to fructose 1,6-biphosphate, before being converted to glucose.

Alanine is the main amino acid, which is transported from the muscle to the liver, where it may be converted to pyruvate.

3.7.3 Glycogenolysis

Glycogen represents the principal storage form of carbohydrate in animals and is present mainly in the liver and muscle. In the liver its major function is to service other tissues via formation of glucose, when dietary sugars are not immediately available as an energy source between meals or while fasting. In muscle it serves only the needs of that organ by providing an immediate source of metabolic fuel. Glycogenolysis is the pathway by which the glycogen stores are converted via glucose 1-phosphate and glucose 6-phosphate to glucose. After 12–18 hours of fasting, the liver becomes totally depleted of glycogen, whereas muscle glycogen is depleted only after exercise.

3.7.4 Storage of carbohydrates as glycogen and triglyceride (glycogenesis and lipogenesis)

Glycogen is synthesized from glucose by glycogenesis. This is not the reverse of glycogenolysis but a completely separate pathway that usually operates for several hours after a carbohydrate-containing meal, when the amount of ingested carbohydrate far exceeds energy requirements for the tissues. Glycogen stores become saturated at around 1000 g. In some animal species, carbohydrates in excess of requirements are converted to fat via the pathway of lipogenesis: triosephosphate provides the glycerol moiety of acylglycerol, and fatty acids may be synthesized from acetyl CoA ultimately derived from carbohydrate. Other than in the experimental situation of gross carbohydrate overfeeding, conversion of carbohydrate to stored lipid does not occur to any appreciable extent in humans.

Similarly, pyruvate, as well as intermediates of the citric acid cycle, provide the carbon skeletons for the synthesis of amino acids, but conversion to amino acids is an unimportant fate of ingested carbohydrate.

3.7.5 Metabolic and hormonal mechanisms for the regulation of blood glucose levels

The maintenance of stable levels of glucose in the blood is one of the most carefully regulated homeostatic mechanisms in the body (Fig. 3.6). Insulin, secreted by the β-cells of the islets of Langerhans in the pancreas, plays a central role in regulating blood glucose. About 40–50 units (15–20% of the total amount stored) are produced daily. Insulin secretion is stimulated by rising blood glucose levels as well as by amino acids, free fatty acids, ketone bodies, glucagon, and secretin. Insulin lowers blood glucose by facilitating its entrance into insulin-sensitive tissues and the liver by enhancing the activity of glucose transporters. Insulin also stimulates the storage of glucose as glycogen (glycogenesis) and enhances the metabolism of glucose via the glycolytic pathway. The action of glucagon, secreted by the α-cells of the islets of Langerhans, opposes that of insulin. Secretion occurs in response to hypoglycaemia (low blood glucose levels). Glucagon stimulates glycogenolysis by activating the enzyme phosphorylase and enhances gluconeogenesis. Hypoglycaemia also stimulates the secretion of adrenaline by the chromaffin cells of the adrenal medulla and acts by stimulating the phosphorylase and hence glycogenolysis. Thyroid hormones, glucocorticoids, and growth hormone have a smaller effect than insulin has on blood glucose, glucagon, and adrenaline in healthy individuals. Resistance to the effects of insulin occurs in diabetes and in obesity.

3.8 Recommended intakes and energy value of carbohydrates

3.8.1 Recommended intakes of carbohydrates

The minimum amount of carbohydrate required to avoid ketosis is considered to be about 50 g/day. Glucose is an essential energy source for the brain, red blood cells, and the renal medulla, the daily requirement being about 180 g/day. Approximately 130 g/day can be produced in the body from noncarbohydrate sources by gluconeogenesis, hence the amount of 50 g/day recommended intake. If this is not provided, these organs can adapt by utilizing ketones derived from fatty acid oxidation as a source of energy. A state of ketosis is undesirable because cognitive function may be impaired, and in pregnant women the fetus may be adversely affected. During pregnancy and lactation, the minimum carbohydrate required should probably be about 100 g/day.

Most people consume appreciably more than 100 g carbohydrate daily, with intakes ranging from 200 to 400 g/day (Table 3.2). The FAO/WHO Expert Consultation on carbohydrates (1998) suggested that at least 55% of total energy should be derived from carbohydrate obtained from a variety of food sources. A wide range, up to 75% of total energy, is regarded as acceptable. A significant adverse effect on health is possible with higher levels of intake because adequate amounts of protein, fat, and other essential nutrients may be excluded. A comparable range was suggested by the WHO/FAO Expert Consultation on *Diet, nutrition and the prevention of chronic diseases* (2003). The FAO/WHO Scientific Update on Carbohydrates (Nishida *et al.*, 2007) recommended a reduction of the lower limit of the acceptable range to 50%. The most recent international dietary reference values from the European Food Safety Authority (EFSA, 2010) suggest that for both adults and children, intake of total carbohydrate should range from 45–60% total energy. This recommendation is more in keeping with current dietary practices since in most western countries intake of total carbohydrate is typically below 50% of food energy. The FAO/WHO recommendations relating to free sugars suggest an intake below 10% total energy. The new EFSA reference values do not include an upper limit for sugars but potential adverse effects of excessive intakes are acknowledged. Recommendations from different countries are inconsistent, since different approaches to defining sugars are used. Food-based dietary guidelines such as that developed in South Africa (Box 3.2) may be more useful. The role of sugar in human health during the past 50–60 years is summarized in the case study (Box 3.3, p. 38).

Recommendations regarding dietary fibre also tend to vary because of lack of argument as to what

Food-based dietary guidelines:

1 Use food and drinks containing sugar sparingly and not between meals.

2 Use little or no sugar.

3 Enjoy foods that contain sugar as a treat on special occasions.

4 Try not to use sugar and sugary drinks more than four times a day and only during mealtimes.

5 Brush teeth twice a day with fluoride toothpaste.

6 Rinse the mouth after eating or drinking sweet things.

should be included as dietary fibre and how to measure it. The WHO/FAO Expert Consultation (2003) and EFSA DRVs recommend at least 25 g/day dietary fibre (20g NSP), which should be provided by wholegrain cereals, fruit, and vegetables. The recommendation is really to ensure a healthy intake of these foods, which for fruit and vegetables is five portions or 400 g a day.

3.8.2 Energy value of carbohydrates

Dietary carbohydrate has traditionally been assigned an energy value of 4 kcal/g (17 kJ/g), though when carbohydrates are expressed as monosaccharides the value of 3.75 kcal/g (15.7 kJ/g) is usually used. However, because RS and some oligosaccharides are not digested in the small intestine and the process of fermentation is less metabolically efficient than when digestion and absorption are completed in the small intestine, it is clear that these carbohydrates are providing the body with less energy. The energy value of all carbohydrate requires reassessment, but until this has been carried out, the FAO/WHO consultation recommends that the energy value of carbohydrates that reach the colon be set at 2 kcal/g (8 kJ/g).

3.9 Carbohydrates and diseases

3.9.1 Energy balance and obesity

The avoidance of obesity depends upon maintaining energy balance (see Chapters 6 and 17). However, the nature of dietary carbohydrate appears to influence energy balance. Diets rich in dietary fibre tend to be bulky, promote satiety, and reduce the risks of excessive weight gain. Furthermore, randomized controlled trials have shown the potential of such diets to promote weight loss in those who have already become overweight or obese. Conversely, a high intake of energy-dense foods, whether they be high in fats or free sugars or both, increases the risk of excessive fat accumulation. There is particular concern around the potential of a high intake of free sugars in beverages and fruit juices to contribute to the increased risk of obesity in childhood. The physiological effects of energy intake on satiation and satiety appear to differ between solid foods and fluids. High-energy beverages (invariably high in free sugars) may be less 'sensed' than comparable energy intakes from solid foods, perhaps because of reduced gastric distension and more rapid transit times. As a result, there may be a failure to adjust food intake to take into account the energy derived from beverages. This provides a major justification for recommending a restriction on intake of free sugars. The history of sugar and its potential effects on human health is summarized in the case study. There has also been recent interest in the potential of diets low or very low in total carbohydrate (e.g. Atkins-type diets) to facilitate weight loss to a greater extent than can be achieved on relatively high carbohydrate diets. However, randomized controlled trials which have continued for a year or longer suggest that, in the medium to long term, distribution of macronutrients have little influence on the magnitude of weight reduction.

3.9.2 Carbohydrates and physical performance (see Chapter 39)

A high-carbohydrate diet in the day preceding endurance-type physical activity ('carbohydrate loading') enhances physical performance, as may a high carbohydrate pre-event meal and carbohydrate supplementation in the form of beverages containing free sugars. This is presumably achieved as a result of glycogenesis and accumulation of maximum glycogen stores. Similarly, carbohydrate intake after an event can aid recovery by replenishing depleted glycogen stores. Low-intensity recreational physical activity does not require carbohydrate supplementation. Some people may consume unnecessary extra energy in this way.

3.9.3 Carbohydrate through the life cycle

During the first 6 months of life, exclusive breastfeeding is recommended by WHO, with lactose being the major source of carbohydrate and accounting for about 40% of milk energy. The concentration of lactose is tailored to the needs of the maturing neonatal and infant gut, especially while colonic microflora and pancreatic amylase production are developing. For infants fed on formulas, the carbohydrate content should be as similar as possible to breast milk. Significant spill-over of carbohydrate into the neonatal colon occurs where, in breastfed infants, a largely saccharolytic flora dominated by bifidobacteria are responsible for fermentation and salvage of energy through SCFAs and lactate absorption. Bottle-fed babies, or those who are weaned early, develop a more diverse flora, which starts to resemble that of the adult much sooner.

Preschool children can be fed the same foods as adults but, because of their rapid growth, they require a more energy-dense diet. Food should, therefore, provide more than 30% of energy from fat and less than 50% from carbohydrate. Thus, the change from breast milk, which provides more than 50% of the energy from fat, to an adult-type diet, should be gradual. The preschool years are a particularly important time to teach the avoidance of sugary drinks and puddings, increased intake of which has been shown to be associated with the onset of obesity.

Early introduction of substantial amounts of carbohydrate from a single food source is a major determinant of malnutrition in developing countries because such foods may be deficient in some essential nutrients. In more affluent countries, sometimes vegetarian and vegan children tend to be fed diets that are high in nonglycaemic carbohydrate. Thus, they too may be at risk of insufficient energy for growth, as well as nutrient deficiencies associated with a diet without meat or animal products.

Requirements for total energy and nutrients increase during pregnancy and lactation. The minimum requirement for carbohydrate is doubled to around 100 g/day, but most women achieve adequate intakes by consuming a wide variety of carbohydrate-containing foods. Particular attention to carbohydrate intake may also be appropriate for some groups of older people—as with children, a diet with excessive intakes of nonglycaemic carbohydrate may be associated with a predisposition to undernutrition as a result of inadequate intake of total energy and some essential nutrients. While many will benefit from the satiety-promoting effects of diets rich in nonstarch polysaccharides, for some an increase in sugars and rapidly digested starches may be necessary to ensure adequate energy intake.

3.9.4 Lipids and cardiovascular disease

For many adults, increasing the consumption of appropriate carbohydrate-containing foods will facilitate the reduction in saturated fatty acids that are causally linked to cardiovascular disease and increase the intake of antioxidants and other cardio-protective nutrients (see Chapter 21). High intake of wholegrain cereals and dietary fibre has been shown in prospective studies to be associated with reduced cardiovascular risk. However, high intakes of free sugars and rapidly digested starches may be associated with high triglycerides and very-low-density lipoproteins and reduced high-density lipoproteins. Large amounts of fructose or sucrose, especially when consumed in the context of relatively high fat intakes, may induce hypertriglyceridaemia. However, a high carbohydrate intake when derived from vegetables, intact fruits, and wholegrain cereals does not appear to have long-term adverse effects on the overall lipoprotein profile.

3.9.5 Blood glucose and diabetes

Wholegrain carbohydrate-containing foods rich in dietary fibre and with a low glycaemic response reduce the risk of developing type 2 diabetes. Diets high in sucrose may be associated with increased insulin resistance and, by contributing to the energy density of the diet, lead to the development of being overweight and obesity, the principal risk determinant of type 2 diabetes. Foods with a high content of dietary fibre and a low GI are associated with an improvement in glycaemic control in both type 1 and type 2 diabetes, as well as improvement in several other cardiovascular risk factors. The majority of patients with type 2 diabetes are overweight and restriction of free sugars along with other energy-dense foods will facilitate weight loss, a principal goal in the treatment of this condition, since it is almost invariably associated with improved control of blood glucose and other clinical and metabolic abnormalities associated with diabetes (see also Chapter 23).

3.9.6 Dental caries

Dental diseases are a costly burden to healthcare services, accounting for between 5% and 10% of total healthcare expenditure. Dental caries rates appear to be declining in some relatively affluent countries but prevalence is increasing in many developing countries. Dental caries has a complex aetiology. The condition occurs because of demineralization of enamel and dentine by organic acids formed by bacteria in dental plaque through the anaerobic metabolism of sugars derived from the diet.

Free sugars and readily digestible starches appear to be involved, although lactose, sugar alcohols, and oligosaccharides are less acidogenic than other carbohydrates. Dental caries occurs infrequently when the consumption of free sugars is below 15–20 kg per person per year, equivalent to a daily intake of 40–55 g per person or 6–8% of total energy intake. Frequency of consumption is particularly relevant, hence the recommendation that foods and drinks containing free sugars should be limited to a maximum of four times per day. Fluoride protects against dental caries, reducing rates by 20–40%, but it does not eliminate the condition (see Section 11.5).

3.10 Carbohydrates and gut disorders

3.10.1 Lactose malabsorption

The universal presence of lactose in milk means that all newborn mammalian species have the appropriate enzyme lactase (β1-4,galactosidase) in the brush border to deal with this sugar. However, after weaning, lactase activity declines rapidly in all species, except some human populations. These are the traditional milk-drinking people who have their ancestors in the Aryan races of the Middle East and North India. In practice this means the majority of Northern Europeans and populations deriving from them, including North American whites, and

Australian and New Zealand whites. Individuals who do not express lactase can tolerate small amounts of milk in their diet, but large amounts lead to unabsorbed lactose, which exerts an osmotic effect in the small bowel with fluid and sugar entering the large bowel. Here partial fermentation occurs and there is often rapid gas production producing abdominal pain and an osmotic diarrhoea. The use of yoghurts and other fermented milk products, as well as the use of preparations of the enzyme lactase may improve lactose tolerance. Lactose intolerance is occasionally seen in adults of European descent.

3.10.2 Other carbohydrate intolerances

There are other less frequent clinical disorders in which digestion or absorption of sugar is disturbed, resulting in sugar intolerance with consequences similar to those of lactase deficiency. Most frequently they are seen in children secondary to underlying gastrointestinal disease, especially as a result of severe gastrointestinal infections, particularly in malnourished children. They may also be congenital and, although rare, such conditions may be life-threatening in children. Three examples of these disorders are: sucrase-isomaltase deficiency, which is associated with watery diarrhoea following consumption of sucrose-containing foods; alactasia, or the total absence of lactase in infancy, which is accompanied by diarrhoea associated with milk (note the difference between this condition and lactose intolerance); and glucose-galactose malabsorption (diarrhoea from eating glucose, galactose, or lactose). The diagnosis is usually suspected on the basis of clinical observations and is confirmed by sugar tolerance tests and measurement of breath hydrogen.

3.10.3 Large bowel function and its disorders

It is in the large bowel that dietary carbohydrates come to dominate the ambient physiology. Bowel habit is determined largely by the amount of carbohydrate that enters the colon and by transit time. NSPs are the major controller of faecal bulk, with other carbohydrates, such as RS and oligosaccharides mildly laxative. NSPs from different sources have been shown to have contrasting effects on stool weight, with NSPs from wheat (particularly wheat bran) being the most potent laxative, increasing stool output by around 5 or 6 g/day per gram of NSPs fed from this source. Following close on the heels of wheat sources are NSPs from fruit and vegetables, (4 g/g of NSPs fed), after which come the gums, oats, and legumes and, probably the least laxative of the NSPs sources, pectin. The effect of NSPs on bowel habit is modified principally by gut transit time, which is an innate control of large bowel function.

The mechanism whereby fermentable carbohydrates affect bowel habit is now well established. The notion that fibre acts like an inert sponge in the colon has now been superseded because we know that NSPs are extensively metabolized by colonic bacteria. Faecal weight, therefore, increases through a variety of mechanisms that include increased bacterial biomass (Fig. 3.5), increased hydration of stool mass associated with more rapid transit time, and the presence of unmetabolized cell wall material, particularly lignified forms such as that present in bran.

It follows, because NSPs are such effective laxatives, that they have been used very widely in the management of constipation. There are many causes of constipation but the commonest one is low NSP-containing diets, often associated with a sedentary lifestyle, travel and, sometimes, therapeutic diets, such as those used for weight reduction. Other physiological causes of low stool weight are pregnancy, some phases of the menstrual cycle, and old age, where a combination of low food intake and lack of exercise are probably most important. Irritable bowel syndrome can include constipation and many drugs have constipation as a side effect. Diets high in NSPs are well established in the management of constipation. There is no universal prescription but the amount required is one that will produce a satisfactory bowel habit. The aim should be to increase the patient's NSP intake, which was likely to be around 12 g/day to 18–24 g/day. Those who fail to respond to this sort of dietary change should be carefully screened for more serious causes of the problem. Easy ways of increasing NSP intake include:

- increasing bread intake to 200 g/day and changing to 100% wholemeal;
- eating a wholegrain breakfast cereal;
- increasing fruit and vegetable intake to 400 g/day;
- eating more legumes such as beans and peas, although this may produce problems with gas due to oligosaccharide fermentation;
- using bulk laxatives such as ispagula and sterculia.

Irritable bowel syndrome (IBS) is one of the most common disorders seen in the gastroenterology clinic and has two main presenting features, namely abdominal pain and altered bowel habit. It is, however, a very diverse syndrome with no clear aetiology. While the cause is unknown, NSPs help in the management of constipation-predominant IBS. However, wheat bran is not universally beneficial in this condition, possibly because it is thought that a significant number of IBS patients are wheat-intolerant without having the diagnostic features of coeliac disease. Furthermore, changing people onto significantly increased NSP intakes leads to excess gas production and IBS patients may have a gut that is unusually sensitive to gas.

Colonic diverticular disease is another condition that benefits from carbohydrate in the diet, particularly NSPs. A diverticulum is a pouch that protrudes outwards from the wall of the bowel and is associated with hypertrophy of the muscle layers of the large intestine, particularly the sigmoid colon. Diverticular disease is very common in industrialized societies, the prevalence rising with age to about 30% of people over the age of 65. Many people with diverticula do not have symptoms, but those that do complain of lower abdominal pain and changes in bowel habit. High-NSP-containing diets were introduced in the 1960s and their use revolutionized the management of this condition. Wheat bran is thought to be more effective than other sources of NSPs or bulk laxatives, although bran is not a panacea and may aggravate gas pro-

duction, feelings of abdominal distension, and incomplete emptying of the rectum.

3.10.4 Cancer

Carbohydrates are not generally implicated either in the cause or prevention of the major cancers with the exception of colorectal cancer. In 1969, Burkitt pointed out that those countries where colorectal cancer risk was low, principally African countries, had high intakes of NSPs and large stool bulk. He suggested that lack of NSPs was the cause of large bowel cancer because it allowed slow transit time through the colon and cancer-forming chemicals to accumulate in the large bowel. We now know that there are other important contributors to colorectal cancer risk, in particular obesity, but nevertheless dietary fibre remains an important protective element of the diet. Not all epidemiological studies have shown a protective effect of fibre, probably because measuring dietary intake was not always done well and NSPs or fibre intakes were measured badly. However, in the recent European Prospective Investigation into Cancer (EPIC study) (Bingham et al., 2003), where dietary methodology and understanding of NSPs and their measurement were good, a clear inverse relationship was seen between the incidence of large bowel cancer and fibre intake. This is further discussed in Chapter 22.

3.10.5 Prebiotics

Prebiotics were defined by an FAO Technical Meeting in 2007 as 'a non-viable food component that confers a health benefit on the host associated with modulation of the microbiota.' Prebiotics alter the balance of the gut microflora to one with more bifidobacteria and lactobacilli. Bacteria from these groups are important in maintaining the gut barrier to infection, are almost entirely nonpathogenic, synthesize B vitamins, and are predominantly saccharolytic (i.e. break down carbohydrate). It is worth noting that the exclusively breastfed baby has a microflora that is very similar to this pattern. Apart from altering the balance of the flora, prebiotics are also fermented producing short-chain fatty acids.

The best-established prebiotics are fructo-oligo-saccharides, inulin, and galacto-oligosaccharides. As already noted, prebiotic oligosaccharides are relatively poor laxatives and there are few published studies of their benefits in clinical studies. However, they have been shown to reduce the risk of travel-ler's diarrhoea, and animal studies have demon-strated clear anti-inflammatory properties in the gut. Perhaps more surprisingly, prebiotic carbohy-drates increase calcium absorption and bone min-eral density in adolescents. They might well prove to be designer carbohydrates of the future.

The oligosaccharides of breast milk have long been credited with being the principal growth factor for bifidobacteria in the infant gut and thus primarily responsible for these bacteria dominat-ing the microbiota of the gut of breastfed babies. In this context, milk oligosaccharides are acting as prebiotics. Bifidobacteria can grow on milk oligo-saccharides as their sole carbon source, while lac-tobacilli may not be able to do so. The similarities between milk oligosaccharide structure and epi-thelial cell surface carbohydrates in the gut suggest that milk oligosaccharides may act as soluble receptors for gut pathogens and thus form an essential part of colonization resistance. They may also be immunomodulatory.

3.11 Other roles for carbohydrates and inborn errors of metabolism

Apart from their role in energy metabolism, carbo-hydrates are required for the synthesis of some larger complex molecules in the body, such as RNA and DNA, which use the five-carbon sugars ribose and deoxyribose produced from glucose in the pentose phosphate pathway. Also synthesized from glucose by the oxidation of uridine diphos-phate glucose is glucuronic acid, which is needed for the conjugation of sterols and foreign com-pounds like drugs to aid their water solubility and, thus, their excretion in bile and urine.

Glucose, galactose, and fructose can undergo isomerization, epimerization, and phosphorylation reactions, leading to the production of other sugars such as xylose, mannose, rhamnose, and fucose. Further transamidation leads to the formation of amino sugars such as glucosamine 6-phosphate, which can be N-acetylated to N-acetyl glucosamine, which is an important precursor for glycoprotein synthesis. Glycoproteins are proteins conjugated to sugars and are essential constituents of mucus, which covers the epithelial surfaces of the body. Other glycoproteins include plasma proteins, such as prothrombin, and immunoglobulins and peptide hormones, such as follicle-stimulating hormone. Glycoproteins also occur at all surfaces and are important in cell recognition. The surface of the human erythrocyte is covered in a complex array of polysaccharides that are responsible for the deter-mination of blood groups. In the gut, lectins (pro-teins present in foods such as beans and peas) recognize cell-surface glycoproteins and bind to them and may cause acute reactions characteristic of food intolerance.

Several different inborn errors of galactose and fructose metabolism are associated with failure to thrive and a range of serious clinical outcomes in infants if the conditions are not diagnosed. Such infants are likely to thrive if the relevant sugar (lac-tose, fructose) is withdrawn from the diet.

3.12 Future directions

There has been a considerable resurgence of inter-est in dietary carbohydrate recently with the advent of the role of GI as a means of determining optimum carbohydrate-containing foods for the maintenance

BOX 3.3 Case study

Sugar cane was first cultivated in Papua New Guinea some 10 000 years ago and sugar beet has been grown in cooler climates for the past 250 years. Production has gradually increased so that in many countries sugar is a major energy source, providing as much, if not more energy, than starchy vegetables and fruit. A desire for sweet foods, and generally widespread availability, account for this trend. The term 'sugar' is mainly used to refer to sucrose extracted from sugar cane or beet but is found in vegetables, fruit, and berries, along with small amounts of free glucose and fructose, the constituent monosaccharides of sucrose. These naturally occurring sugars which are incorporated within the cell walls of plants (sometimes referred to as intrinsic sugars) and milk sugar (lactose) are not of concern when considering potentially adverse health-related issues. However, corn syrup and high-fructose corn syrup (see 3.1.1) are increasingly used in confectionary and manufactured foods in some countries, most notably the USA. They may contribute a substantial proportion of total dietary sugar and therefore warrant consideration when examining health-related issues.

Sugar has long been regarded as a potential cause of diabetes, not surprisingly, given the body's inability to adequately handle ingested sugar and the loss of sugar in the urine; indeed, the condition was frequently referred to in lay terms as 'sugar diabetes'. In the 1950s fairly convincing evidence emerged from Sweden suggesting a strong association with dental caries that was later confirmed to be related particularly to frequency of consumption. In the 1960s and early 1970s many research publications (including a number in major international journals) appeared suggesting that sugar was not only a strong determinant of diabetes risk, but was also related to several cardiovascular risk factors (notably cholesterol, triglycerides, and blood pressure) and also clinical cardiovascular disease. The claims were based upon cross-sectional epidemiological data and trends over time and experimental studies in which the effect of feeding very large quantities of sucrose on risk factors were examined.

In contrast to these observations, more carefully controlled studies in the 1970s suggested that the epidemiological data had been misinterpreted. Studies involving isocaloric comparisons of more physiological intakes of sucrose with starches did not generally have an adverse effect on risk factors. Further reassurance regarding potential adverse health consequences of sucrose followed with a series of studies reporting no deterioration in glycaemic (blood glucose) control or lipid levels in people with diabetes when modest amounts of sucrose were incorporated into the diets of people with diabetes. It is noteworthy, though not always appreciated, that the sucrose in the experimental diets replaced relatively rapidly digested starches, that the amounts were modest, and that in all other respects the diets complied with the dietary guidelines for diabetes at the time (i.e. they were high in fibre-rich vegetables, fruits, and wholegrain cereals and low in fat, especially saturated fat). Although in reality the observations are only reassuring in the context in which the research was undertaken, this series of observations tended to allay concerns regarding adverse consequences of sugar except with regard to the link between amount and frequency of consumption and dental caries. Two exceptions to the otherwise reassuring findings did not appear to cause undue concern. Some individuals with hypertriglyceridaemia appeared to be sensitive to even fairly modest changes in sucrose intakes. They were considered to have 'sucrose-induced hypertriglyceridaemia' but the condition was believed to be relatively rare. Furthermore, free-living individuals who were asked to replace their usual dietary sucrose intake with carbohydrate foods rich in starch tended to lose weight and their triglyceride levels fell as they were unable to fully replace calories from this energy-dense source.

During the past decade or so the tide has once again started to turn. Obesity has reached epidemic proportions in many countries and the metabolic syndrome (of which hypertriglyceridaemia is frequently a feature) has been reported in around one-quarter of the adult population in some societies. While the precise role of sugars as a cause of obesity and the metabolic syndrome and in their management remains to be established, there is no doubt that excessive consumption of energy-dense foods is associated with an increased risk of obesity and that sugar, corn syrup, and high-fructose

BOX 3.3 (Continued)

corn syrup contribute to the energy density of confectionary products, snacks, and convenience foods. There is reasonably consistent evidence that high intakes of sugar-sweetened beverages increases the risk of excessive weight gain in children and emerging evidence that sugar may be associated with weight gain and some adverse metabolic effects in those with the metabolic syndrome. In the light of these observations and the increased risk of dental caries, especially associated with frequent consumption of sucrose, many sets of dietary guidelines include advice to limit intake of sugar and corn syrups. There is no universal agreement regarding the optimum upper level of intake, but more restrictive advice is recommended for those with the metabolic syndrome and for those attempting to reduce excess body fat.

The role of dietary sucrose has once again become a focus of intense interest and research.

of health and in a variety of disease states. Furthermore, the health-promoting qualities of carbohydrates that are not digested and absorbed in the small intestine are now being recognized. The prebiotic oligosaccharides, as components of functional foods, have potentially important health benefits. The extent to which sucrose and other sugars should be restricted or liberated will continue to be debated, as will the optimum contribution of total carbohydrate to the daily energy intake. Methodologies for the measurement of various dietary carbohydrates are likely to be refined, and given the advances in the field of molecular biology it seems highly likely that there will be further insights into the understanding of the molecular basis of many of the issues discussed in this chapter.

Further Reading

1. **Atkinson, F.S., Foster-Powell, K., and Brand-Miller, J.C.** (2008) International tables of glycemic index and glycemic load values. *Diabetes Care*, **31**, 2281–3.
2. **Bingham, S.A., Day, N.E., Luben, R., et al.** (2003) Dietary fibre in food and protection against colorectal cancer in the European Prospective Investigation into Cancer and Nutrition (EPIC): An observational study. *Lancet*, **361**, 1496–501.
3. **Cummings, J.H. and Macfarlane, G.T.** (1991) The control and consequences of bacterial fermentation in the human colon. *J Appl Bacteriol*, **70**, 443–59.
4. **Cummings, J.H., Beatty, E.R., Kingman, S.M., et al.** (1996) Digestion and physiological properties of resistant starch in the human large bowel. *Br J Nutr*, **75**, 733–47.
5. **Cummings, J.H., Roberfroid, M.B., and Andersson, G., et al.** (1997) A new look at dietary carbohydrate: Chemistry, physiology and health. *Eur J Clin Nutr*, **51**, 417–23.
6. **EFSA Panel on Dietetic Products, Nutrition, and Allergies (NDA)** (2010) Scientific opinion on dietary reference values for carbohydrates and dietary fibre. *EFSA J*, **8**, 1462.
7. **Englyst, H.N., Kingman, S.M., and Cummings, J.H.** (1992) Classification and measurement of nutritionally important starch fractions. *Eur J Clin Nutr*, **46**, S33–50.
8. **FAO/WHO** (1998) *Carbohydrates in human nutrition*. Report of a Joint FAO/WHO Expert Consultation. Paper 66. Rome, Food and Agricultural Organization, World Health Organization.
9. **Jenkins, D.J.A., Wolever, T.M.S., Taylor, R.H., et al.** (1981) Glycemic index of foods: A physiological basis for carbohydrate exchange. *Am J Clin Nutr*, **34**, 362–6.
10. **Macfarlane, S., Macfarlane, G.T., and Cummings, J.H.** (2006) Prebiotics in the gastrointestinal tract. *Aliment Pharmacol Ther*, **24**, 701–14.

11. **Mann, J.I. and Cummings, J.H.** (2009) Possible implications for health of the different definitions of dietary fibre. *Nutr Metab Cardiovasc Dis*, **19**, 226–9.

12. **Nishida, C., Nocito, F.M., and Mann, J.** (2007) Joint FAO/WHO Scientific Update on Carbohydrates in Human Nutrition. *Eur J Clin Nutr*, **61** Suppl 1, S1–137.

13. **WHO/FAO** (2003) *Diet, nutrition and the prevention of chronic diseases*. Report of a Joint WHO/FAO Expert Consultation. Geneva, World Health Organization.

14. **Williams, S.M., Venn, B.J., Perry T., et al.** (2008) Another approach to estimating the reliability of glycaemic index. *Br J Nutr*, **100**, 364–72.

Useful Websites

To see topical and scientifically robust updates on nutrition associated with this textbook and web links to many of the journals in the Further Reading sections, please see the dedicated Online Resource Centre at **http://www.oxfordtextbooks.co.uk/orc/mann4e/**

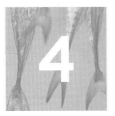

Lipids

C. Murray Skeaff and Jim Mann

Lipids are a group of compounds that dissolve in organic solvents such as petrol or chloroform, but are usually insoluble in water. The most obvious lipids in food and nutrition are edible oils, which are liquid at room temperature, and fats, which are solid at room temperature. Many people in high-income countries regard fats and oils as foods that should be avoided as far as possible because of their perceived role in the development of obesity and coronary heart disease. However, in addition to enhancing the flavour and palatability of food, lipids make an important contribution to adequate nutrition—some of them important to reduce the risk of heart disease. They are major sources of energy; some are essential nutrients because they cannot be synthesized in the body, yet they are required for a range of metabolic and physiological processes and to maintain the structural and functional integrity of all cell membranes. Lipids are also the only form in which the body can store energy for a prolonged period of time. These stored lipids in adipose tissue also serve to provide insulation, help to control body temperature, and afford some physical protection to internal organs. Lipids include the fat-soluble vitamins. Triacylglycerols, also referred to as triglycerides, make up the bulk of dietary lipid, with phospholipids and sterols making up nearly all the remainder.

4.1 Naturally occurring dietary lipids

Naturally occurring dietary lipids are derived from a wide variety of animal and plant sources, including animal adipose tissue (the visible fat on meat, lard, and suet); milk and products derived from milk fat (cream, butter, cheese, and yoghurt); vegetable seeds, nuts, oils, and products derived from them (e.g. margarines); eggs; plant leaves; and fish oil.

Many sources of dietary lipid are visible and obvious, while others are less so, for example, those found in the muscle of lean meat, avocado, nuts, and seeds, as well as those in processed or home-prepared foods such as pies, cakes, biscuits, and chocolates. In most Western countries, dietary lipid provides 30–40% of total dietary energy. In Asian

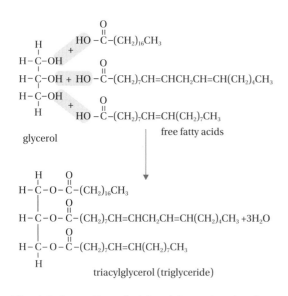

glycerol

free fatty acids

triacylglycerol (triglyceride)

Fig. 4.1 Formation of a triacylglycerol molecule.

countries and throughout the economically developing world, the proportion of energy derived from dietary lipids is usually much lower.

4.1.1 Glycerides and fatty acids

Triacylglycerols make up about 95% of dietary lipids. A triacylglycerol molecule is formed from a molecule of glycerol (a three-carbon alcohol) with three fatty acids attached (Fig. 4.1). Fatty acids consist of an even-numbered chain of carbon atoms with hydrogens attached, a methyl group at one end and a carboxylic acid group at the other (Fig. 4.2). The carbon atoms are classically numbered from the carboxyl carbon (carbon number 1). The methyl end carbon is known as the n minus (n–) or omega (ω) carbon atom. The physical and biological properties of triacylglycerols are determined by the nature of the constituent fatty acids.

Saturated fatty acids are those in which carbon–carbon bonds are fully saturated with hydrogen atoms (i.e. four hydrogens per carbon–carbon bond). When two hydrogens are absent, the carbons form double bonds with each other and monounsaturated (a single double bond) or polyunsaturated

(two or more double bonds) fatty acids result. Double bonds in polyunsaturated fatty acids are always separated by one CH_2 (methylene group). Fatty acids can be described by their common name, their chemical name, their full or simplified chemical structure, or a shorthand notation in which the first number indicates the number of carbon atoms and the second the number of double bonds (Fig. 4.2). For monounsaturated and polyunsaturated fatty acids, a third descriptor indicates the position of the first double bond relative to and including the methyl end. Inserting a double bond in a saturated fatty acid reduces its melting point. For this reason, fats (e.g. butter) containing a predominance of saturated fatty acids are usually solid at room temperature while oils (e.g. soybean oil) containing a predominance of polyunsaturated fatty acids are liquid at room temperature. The position of the unsaturated bonds in mono- and polyunsaturated fatty acids has a profound influence on their nutritional properties and health effects. The position of the first double bond relative to the methyl end indicates the 'family' to which the unsaturated fatty acid belongs. Polyunsaturated fatty acids in which the first double bond is three carbon atoms from the methyl end of the carbon chain are called n-3 or ω-3 fatty acids, and those in which the first double bond is next to the sixth carbon atom are n-6 or ω-6 fatty acids. The third important family is the n-9 or ω-9 group, in which the first double bond is next to the ninth carbon atom from the methyl end. In the body, fatty acids of one 'family' cannot be converted into those of another 'family'. Fatty acids are sometimes classified by carbon chain-length and referred to as short-chain (i.e. fewer than 8 carbons), medium-chain (8–12 carbons), long-chain (14 or more carbons), or very long-chain (22 or more) fatty acids. Almost all fatty acids have chain lengths with an even number of carbon atoms; however, there are a couple of odd-chain length fatty acids which are present in very small amounts in fats from ruminant animals. A list of the fatty acids of nutritional interest is given in Table 4.1.

A single triacylglycerol molecule may contain either three identical fatty acids or, more frequently,

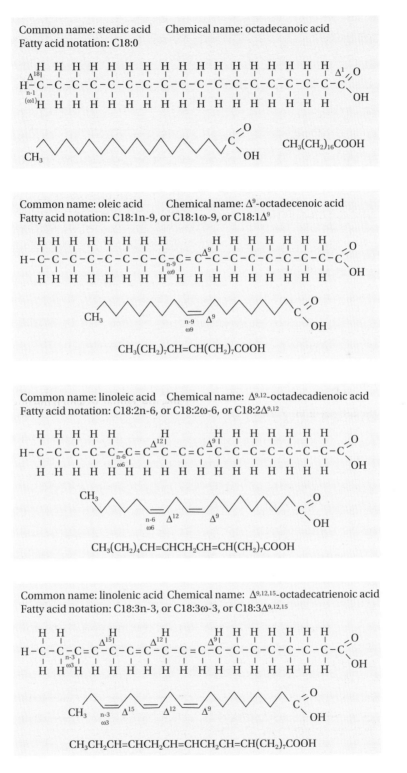

Fig. 4.2 Names and structures of some common fatty acids.

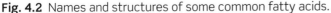

Table 4.1 Fatty acid names and occurrence

Common name	Nomenclature	Occurrence
Saturated		
Acetic	2:0	Vinegar
Butyric	4:0	Dairy fat
Caproic	6:0	Dairy fat
Caprylic	8:0	Palm kernel oil
Capric	10:0	Dairy fat, coconut oil
Lauric	12:0	Coconut oil
Myristic	14:0	Dairy fat, coconut oil
Pentadecanoic	15:0	Small amounts in fats from ruminant animals (e.g. cow)
Palmitic	16:0	Most plant and animal fats
Margaric	17:0	Very small amounts in fats from ruminant animals (e.g. cow)
Stearic	18:0	Most plant and animal fats
Arachidic	20:0	Peanuts
Behenic	22:0	Small amount in animal fats
Lignoceric	24:0	Plant cutin
Monounsaturated		
Palmitoleic	16:1ω7	Fish and animal fats
Oleic	18:1ω9	All plant and animal fats
cis-Vaccenic	18:1ω7	Small amounts in animal fats
Eicosenoic	20:1ω9	Rapeseed and animal fats
Gadoleic	20:1ω11	Fish oils
Erucic	22:1ω9	Rapeseed, animal tissue
Cetoleic	22:1ω13	Fish oils
Nervonic	24:1ω9	Animal tissue (brain)
Hexacosenoic	26:1ω9	Minute amounts in animal tissues
Polyunsaturated		
Linoleic (LO)	18:2ω6	Plant oils: cottonseed, sesame, soybean, corn, safflower
α-Linolenic (LN)	18:3ω3	Plant oils: soybean, mustard, walnut, linseed
γ-Linolenic (GLA)	18:3ω6	Plant oils: evening primrose, borage, blackcurrant
Dihomo-γ linolenic (DGLA)	20:3ω6	Small amounts in animal tissues
Arachidonic (AA)	20:4ω6	Small amounts in animal tissues
Adrenic	22:4ω6	Small amounts in animal tissues
Eicosapentaenoic acid (EPA)	20:5ω3	Fish, fish oils
Docosapentaenoic (DPA)	22:5ω3	Fish, fish oils, animal tissues (brain)
Docosahexaenoic (DHA)	22:6ω3	Fish, fish oils, animal tissues (brain)

a combination of different fatty acids. It is important to appreciate that while one fatty acid, or class of fatty acids (e.g. saturated), might predominate in a particular food, most foods contain a wide range of fatty acids. Occasionally in naturally occurring glycerides, only one or two fatty acids are attached to a glycerol molecule. These are called monoacylglycerols (monoglycerides) and diacylglycerols (diglycerides). The major food sources of fatty acids and sources of triacylglycerols that contain them are shown in Table 4.2 and the detailed fatty acid composition of some fats and oils are given in Table 4.3.

Table 4.2 Fat and cholesterol content of some common foods

Food item	Common serving size	Total fat (g)	SFA (g)	MUFA (g)	PUFA (g)	Chol (mg)
		per 100 g edible portion				
Skimmed milk	1 cup (260 g)	0.4	0.3	0.1	0.0	4
Yoghurt	1 pot (150 g)	2.4	1.5	0.6	0.1	8
Cottage cheese	1/2 cup (120 g)	3.5	2.2	0.9	0.1	9
Whole milk	1 cup (260 g)	4.0	2.4	1.1	0.1	12
Ice cream	1 cup (143 g)	10.8	6.5	2.3	0.3	30
Cheddar cheese	1 × 2 cm cube (22 g)	35.2	22.3	8.4	0.8	107
Cream	1 tbsp (15 g)	40.0	24.9	10.1	1.3	104
Wholemeal bread	1 slice (22 g)	1.7	0.4	0.4	0.6	1
Toasted muesli	1 cup (110 g)	16.6	7.7	5.0	2.9	0
Egg	1 medium (32 g)	11.6	3.4	4.6	1.2	412
Baked potato	1 potato (90 g)	0.2	0.0	0.0	0.1	0
Potato crisps	1 packet (50 g)	33.4	14.3	13.8	3.8	1
Cauliflower	1 stem + flower (90 g)	0.2	0.0	0.0	0.1	0
Lentils	1/2 cup (100 g)	0.5	0.1	0.1	0.2	0
Peanuts	1/3 cup (50 g)	49.0	9.2	23.4	13.9	0
Cashew nuts	18 cashews (28 g)	51.0	8.3	25.4	15.1	0
Sole	1 fillet (51 g)	1.2	0.3	0.4	0.3	53
Mackerel	1 fillet (89 g)	2.9	0.8	0.8	0.9	53
Salmon (tinned)	1/2 cup (120 g)	8.2	2.0	3.1	2.1	90
Sausage	1 serving (79 g)	25.2	11.3	10.8	1.2	48
Beef blade steak (lean)	1 steak (216 g)	5.0	2.2	1.9	0.2	60
Beef mince	1/2 cup (130 g)	13.8	5.7	5.4	0.5	68
Chicken breast (lean, no skin)	1 breast (192 g)	5.5	1.7	2.5	0.6	66
Fried chicken	1 wing (37 g)	28.4	8.7	13.4	2.7	116
Pork loin steak (lean)	1 fillet (98 g)	2.3	0.9	0.9	0.2	68
Lamb midloin chop	1 chop (50 g)	5.7	2.5	2.0	0.2	66
Pizza	1 slice (57 g)	10.5	4.5	3.3	1.8	13

(Continued)

Table 4.2 Fat and cholesterol content of some common foods (*Continued*)

Food item	Common serving size	Total fat (g)	SFA (g)	MUFA (g)	PUFA (g)	Chol (mg)
		per 100 g edible portion				
Hamburger	1 burger (204 g)	15.6	5.7	5.4	2.4	22
Muesli bar	1 bar (32 g)	19.4	9.1	7.2	1.9	1
Biscuit	1 biscuit (12 g)	30.0	19.2	6.2	1.2	98
Salad dressing	1 tbsp (16 g)	48.3	7.0	11.1	28.1	0
Palm oil	1 tbsp (14 g)	98.7	44.7	41.1	8.2	0
Olive oil	1 tbsp (14 g)	99.6	16.6	65.3	11.8	0
Sunflower seed oil	1 tbsp (14 g)	99.7	11.7	21.1	61.9	0

Chol, cholesterol; MUFA, monounsaturated fatty acids; PUFA, polyunsaturated fatty acids; SFA, saturated fatty acids.

Table 4.3 Fatty acid composition of plant and animal fats

Food item	4:0	6:0	8:0	10:0	12:0	14:0	16:0	18:0	16:1	18:1	18:2ω6	18:3ω3	20:4ω6	20:5ω3	22:6ω3	20:1ω11	22:1ω13	22:5ω3
	Percentage of total acids																	
Plant fats																		
Olive	–	–	–	–	–	–	12	2	1	72	11	1	–	–	–	–	–	–
Palm	–	–	–	–	0	1	42	4	0	43	8	0	–	–	–	–	–	–
Canola	–	–	–	–	–	–	5	1	2	56	24	10	–	–	–	–	–	–
Safflower	–	–	–	–	–	–	8	3	0	13	76	0	–	–	–	–	–	–
Sunflower	–	–	–	–	–	0	6	6	0	33	53	0	–	–	–	–	–	–
Avocado	–	–	–	–	–	–	12	–	3	75	9	0	0	–	–	–	–	–
Soybean	–	–	–	–	0	0	10	4	0	25	52	7	–	–	–	–	–	–
Coconut	–	–	8	7	48	16	9	2	–	7	2	–	–	–	–	–	–	–
Animal fats																		
Butter	4	2	1	3	3	11	28	16	1	26	1	2	–	–	–	–	–	–
Beef	–	–	–	–	–	3	28	13	7	43	2	1	1	–	–	–	–	–
Chicken	–	–	–	–	–	1	27	7	7	41	14	1	1	–	–	–	–	–
Lamb	–	–	–	–	–	6	25	22	1	40	3	3	–	–	–	–	–	–
Pork	–	–	–	–	–	2	27	13	4	41	8	1	1	–	–	–	–	–
Salmon	–	–	–	–	–	5	19	4	6	23	1	1	1	8	11	8	5	3
Trout	–	–	–	–	–	2	37	13	5	17	1	–	–	3	11	2	2	2

4.1.2 Phospholipids

Phospholipids comprise a relatively small proportion of total dietary lipid. The four major phospholipids comprise a diglyceride in which the third position of the glycerol molecule is occupied by a phosphoric acid residue to which one of four different base groups is attached (choline, inositol, serine, or ethanolamine). Along with sphingomyelin, these four phospholipids make up more than 95% of the phospholipids found in the body and in foods. The structure of the most abundant phospholipid in nature, phosphatidylcholine (also known as lecithin), is shown in Fig. 4.3.

Phospholipids occur in virtually all animal and vegetable foods: liver, eggs, peanuts, soyabeans, and wheatgerm are very rich sources. The base group endows the phospholipid with a polar region soluble in water, while the fatty acids constitute a non-polar region, insoluble in water. This amphipathic nature—having both polar and non-polar characteristics—of the phospholipid enables it to act at the interface between aqueous and lipid media, so they make excellent emulsifying agents. The structural integrity of all cell membranes and lipoproteins is dependent, among other factors, on the amphipathic nature of the constituent phospholipids. Phospholipids are also an important source of essential fatty acids.

4.1.3 Sterols

Sterols are also built up from carbon, hydrogen, and oxygen, but in these lipid compounds (unlike triacylglycerols and phospholipids), the carbon, hydrogen, and oxygen atoms are arranged in a series of four rings with a range of side chains. Cholesterol is the principal sterol of animal tissues and is found only in animal foods, especially eggs, meat, dairy products, fish, and poultry. Cholesterol in food often has a fatty acid attached to it, thus forming a cholesterol ester (Fig. 4.4). Approximate quantities of cholesterol in some common foods are given in Table 4.2. The major sterols of plants (group name phytosterols) are β-sitosterol, campesterol, and stigmasterol. Cholesterol plays an important structural role in membranes and lipoproteins, and functions as a precursor of bile acids, steroid hormones, and vitamin D.

4.1.4 Other constituents of dietary fat

Dietary fats may also contain small quantities of other lipids including fatty alcohols, gangliosides, sulphatides, and cerebrosides, as well as vitamin A, vitamin E (tocopherols, tocotrienols), carotenoids (α- and β-carotene, lycopene, and xanthophylls), and vitamin D (see Chapters 14, 12, and 15, respectively).

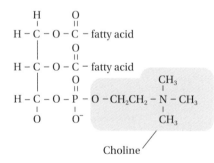

Fig. 4.3 Structure of phosphatidylcholine.

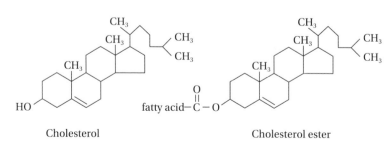

Cholesterol

Cholesterol ester

Fig. 4.4 Structure of cholesterol and cholesterol ester.

4.2 Dietary fats altered during food processing

The food industry incorporates fats and oils into margarines, biscuits, cakes, chocolates, pies, sauces, and other manufactured food products. In addition to using naturally occurring lipids, food manufacturers use fats and oils that have been altered by the process of hydrogenation, adding hydrogen atoms to the double bonds in mono- or polyunsaturated fatty acids in order to increase the degree of saturation of the fatty acids in the oil (i.e. reduce the number of double bonds) and consequently increase the melting point of the fat. Through this process, a polyunsaturated oil that is liquid can be converted into a fat that is solid at room temperature. Partial hydrogenation of oils is used by manufacturers to produce a fat consistency appropriate to the texture of the desired food and to prolong the stability and shelf-life of the food product. Until 10 years ago, margarines for home use normally contained partially-hydrogenated fats; in recent years, margarines are now manufactured without such fats using a process called inter-esterification and blending. Partial-hydrogenation also changes the configuration of some of the remaining double bonds from the natural *cis* configuration to a *trans* configuration. *cis*-Mono- and polyunsaturated fatty acids have the two hydrogen atoms attached to the carbons on the same side of the double bond and the molecule bends at the double bond. In *trans*-fatty acids, the hydrogens are placed on opposite sides of the double bond and the molecule stays straight at the double bond (Fig. 4.5). *trans*-Unsaturated fatty acids behave biologically like saturated rather than like *cis*-unsaturated fatty acids. The bulk of *trans*-fatty acids in hydrogenated fats are monounsaturated (elaidic acid, 18:1n-9 *trans*, is the *trans* equivalent of oleic acid).

Small quantities of *trans*-fatty acids are found naturally in fats from ruminant animals (e.g. cows and sheep) but most of the dietary intake of *trans*-fatty acids is derived from margarine and other manufactured foods containing hydrogenated fats. Unfortunately, in most countries information about the relative proportions of *cis*- and *trans*-fatty acids is not available for many foods, especially manufactured products, so it is not possible at present to quantify the total amount of *trans*-unsaturated fatty acids in the diet. *Trans*-fatty acids have in the past made up 5–10% of fatty acids in soft margarines but most now contain less than 1–2%. Hard margarines contain up to 40–50% of fatty acids in the *trans*-form and their use by food manufacturers continues to be common in processed foods such as cakes, pastry, pies, biscuits, and crackers (Box 4.1).

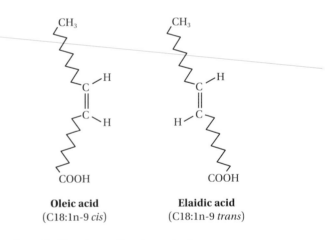

Oleic acid
(C18:1n-9 *cis*)

Elaidic acid
(C18:1n-9 *trans*)

Fig. 4.5 Structure of a *cis*- and a *trans*-monounsaturated fatty acid.

BOX 4.1 Trans-fatty acids

- Partial hydrogenation of oils is used by food manufacturers to produce a fat consistency appropriate to the texture of various food products and to prolong stability and shelf life. The process also changes the configuration of some double bonds from the natural *cis* configuration (i.e. the two hydrogen atoms attached to carbons on the same side of the double bond) to a *trans* configuration (i.e. the hydrogens are placed on opposite sides of the double bond).

BOX 4.1 *(Continued)*

- *trans*-unsaturated fatty acids (TFAs) are found naturally in very small amounts in fats from ruminal animals (e.g. cows and sheep). Most TFA is now *'hidden'* in processed foods such as cakes, biscuits, pies, pastries, and crackers. In the recent past, margarines for home use were also major sources but are now manufactured without such fats. Globally, few countries require food labelling of TFA.

- Clinical trials have shown that TFAs behave like saturated fat rather than like *cis*-unsaturated fatty acids in that they are associated with increases in serum total and low-density lipoprotein (LDL) cholesterol. In addition, they have the ability to reduce high-density lipoprotein (HDL) cholesterol.

- Epidemiological studies show convincingly that TFAs are associated with increased risk of coronary heart disease.

- In 2003 legislation introduced in Denmark made it illegal for any food to contain more than 2% of its fat content as industrially produced TFA. Doing so can result in a maximum penalty of 2 years' imprisonment.

- In 2006 labelling of TFA in food containing 0.5 g or more per serving became mandatory in the USA.

- In 2008 New York City *'banned'* the use of TFA in restaurant food, the TFA content must be less than 0.5 g per serving.

- These measures with potentially important health benefits have largely resulted from nutrition *'activists'* publicizing the results of experimental and epidemiological research.

4.3 Digestion, absorption, and transport

4.3.1 Digestion (Fig. 4.6)

Triacylglycerols must be hydrolysed to fatty acids and monoacylglycerols before they can be absorbed. In children and adults, the process starts in the stomach, where the churning action helps to create an emulsion. Fat entering the intestine is mixed with bile and further emulsified so that lipids are reduced to small bile acid-coated droplets that disperse in aqueous solutions and provide a sufficiently large surface area for the digestive enzymes to act. Bile acids facilitate the process of emulsification because they are amphipathic. Lipase enzymes secreted by the pancreas split by hydrolysis each triacylglycerol molecule, removing the two outer fatty acids, which can be absorbed with the remaining monoacylglyc-erol. Some monoacylglycerols (about 20%) are rear-ranged so that the lipase enzymes remove the third fatty acid. Phospholipids are hydrolysed by a phos-pholipase and cholesterol ester by cholesterol ester hydrolase. In the newborn, the pancreatic secretion of lipases is low, and fat digestion is augmented by lingual lipase secreted from the glands of the tongue and by a lipase present in human milk. The products of lipid digestion, along with other minor dietary lipids, such as fat-soluble vitamins, coalesce with bile acids into microscopic aggregates known as mixed micelles.

4.3.2 Absorption (Fig. 4.6)

Glycerol and fatty acids with a chain length of less than 12 carbon atoms can enter the portal vein sys-tem directly by diffusing across the enterocytes (cells lining the wall of the small intestine). On the other hand, monoglycerides, fatty acids, cholesterol, lysophospholipids, and other dietary lipids diffuse from the mixed micelles into the enterocytes of the small intestine, where they are resynthesized into triacylglycerols, phospholipids, and cholesterol esters in preparation for their incorporation into chylomicrons. In general, absorption is efficient, with greater than 95% of dietary lipid absorbed

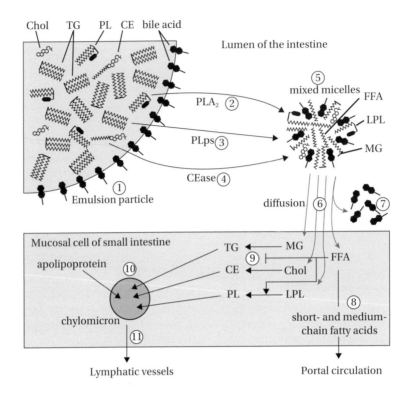

Fig. 4.6 Digestion and absorption of dietary lipids.
(1) Dietary lipid leaves the stomach and enters the upper region of the small intestine where bile acids, released from the gallbladder, surround and coat droplets of fat to form emulsion particles. The emulsion particles provide the surface area for the pancreatic enzymes to degrade the dietary lipids.
(2) Phospholipase A_2 (PLA_2) breaks down each phospholipid (PL) into a free fatty acid (FFA) and a lyso-phospholipid (LPL).
(3) Pancreatic lipase (PLps) converts triacylglycerol (TAG) into a monoglyceride (MG) and two free fatty acids.
(4) Cholesterol esterase (CEase) splits cholesterol ester (CE) into free cholesterol (Chol) and a free fatty acid.
(5) The products of lipid digestion coalesce with bile acids into mixed micelles.
(6) The mixed micelles move close to the mucosal cell surface, where the lipids diffuse down a concentration gradient into the mucosal cells.
(7) Bile acids are not absorbed here.
(8) Short- and medium-chain fatty acids move immediately into the portal circulation, where they are transported in the blood bound to albumin.
(9) To maintain the concentration gradient necessary for lipid diffusion, the breakdown products of lipid digestion are resynthesized into their parental lipids.
(10) The lipids are combined with apolipoproteins, synthesized in the mucosal cells, to form chylomicrons.
(11) Chylomicrons leave the mucosal cell via the lymphatic vessels.

(triacylglycerols, phospholipids, and fat-soluble vitamins). Cholesterol, other sterols, and β-carotene are only partially absorbed (less than 30%).

Diseases that impair the secretion of bile (e.g. obstruction of the bile duct), that reduce secretion of lipase enzymes from the pancreas (e.g. pancreatitis or cystic fibrosis), or that damage the cell lining of the small intestine (e.g. coeliac disease) can lead to severe malabsorption of fat. Under such circumstances, medium-chain triacylglycerols can be better tolerated and are often used as part of the dietary treatment.

4.3.3 Lipid transport (Fig. 4.7)

Since lipids are not soluble in water, it is necessary for them to be associated with specific proteins, the apolipoproteins, to make water-miscible complexes. Free fatty acids make up only about 2% of

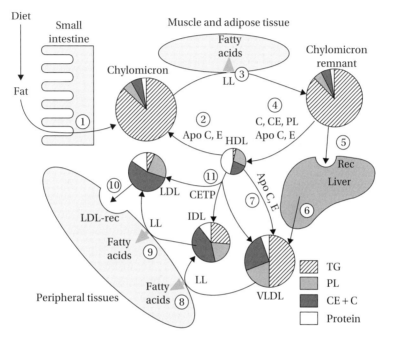

Fig. 4.7 Lipid transport and lipoprotein metabolism.
(1) Chylomicrons transport recently ingested fats into the blood.
(2) Upon entering the blood, chylomicrons pick up apoliproteins C and E (apo C, E) from high-density lipoprotein (HDL).
(3) Apolipoprotein C activates lipoprotein lipase (LL) on the walls of the capillaries causing triacylglycerol to be broken down to glycerol and three fatty acids. The fatty acids are taken up primarily by adipose and muscle tissue.
(4) During breakdown of triacylglycerol (TAG) some cholesterol (C), cholesterol ester (CE) and phospholipids (PL) along with apo C and E pinch off to form HDL.
(5) Following degradation of 70–80% of the chylomicron's TAG, the resulting chylomicron remnant binds to receptors (rec) on the liver cells and is removed from the circulation.
(6) Lipids synthesized in the liver and those delivered to the liver by chylomicron remnants are packaged into very-low-density lipoproteins (VLDL) and secreted into the blood.
(7) VLDL picks up apo C and E from HDL.
(8) LL, activated by apo C, breaks down VLDL TAG and the fatty acids are transferred to peripheral tissue (mainly muscle and adipose) resulting in the formation of intermediate-density lipoprotein (IDL).
(9) Nearly all of the TAG is removed from IDL, producing a cholesterol-rich LDL.
(10) Cholesterol is delivered to the cells when LDL binds to LDL-receptors (LDL-rec) and is taken up into the tissues.
(11) Cholesterol ester transfer protein redistributes cholesterol esters from HDL to VLDL, IDL, and LDL.

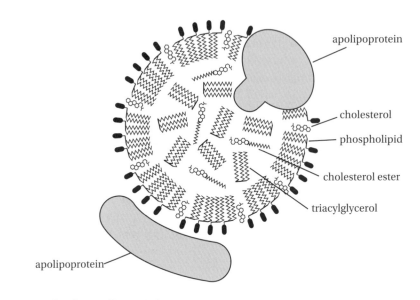

apolipoprotein

cholesterol

phospholipid

cholesterol ester

triacylglycerol

apolipoprotein

Fig. 4.8 Structure of a plasma lipoprotein.

total plasma lipid and are transported in the blood as complexes with albumin. The remainder of lipid in the plasma is carried as lipoprotein complexes (lipid + protein = lipoprotein). The structure of a lipoprotein is given in Fig. 4.8. They consist of a core of neutral lipid (triacylglycerol and cholesterol esters) surrounded by a single surface layer of polar lipid (phospholipid and cholesterol). Coiled chains of apolipoproteins extend over the surface. There are five classes of lipoprotein, which are identified according to their density (Table 4.4) and five major groups of apolipoprotein (apo A, apo B, apo C, apo D, and apo E), which play important roles in determining the functions of the lipoproteins. Each has a distinct physiological role (Table 4.5) and when present in inappropriate amounts (too high or too low) has different adverse health consequences.

Chylomicrons transport lipids of dietary origin, so they consist predominantly of triacylglycerols. Chylomicrons are abundant in the blood after eating food, particularly fatty food, but are scarce in fasting blood. The fatty acid composition of the lipids in chylomicrons is largely determined by the composition of the meal just eaten. Chylomicrons leave the enterocytes of the small intestine and enter the blood stream via lymph vessels. The enzyme lipoprotein lipase, located on the walls of capillary blood vessels, hydrolyses the triacylglycerols, allowing the free fatty acids to move into muscle or heart tissue, where they can be used for energy, or into adipose tissue where they can be stored. During a short life in the circulation (15–30 minutes) more than 90% of the triacylglycerol in the chylomicron is removed. The resulting chylomicron remnant is cleared from the circulation by the liver. The fat-soluble vitamins (A, D, E, and K) are delivered to the liver as part of the chylomicron remnant.

Very-low-density lipoproteins (VLDLs) are large triacylglycerol-rich particles made in the liver. They function as a vehicle for delivery of fatty acids to the heart, muscles, and adipose tissue, lipoprotein lipase again being needed for their liberation. Lipoprotein lipase in the heart has a much stronger affinity for triacylglycerol than that in the adipose tissue or muscle, so when triacylglycerol concentration is low, triacylglycerol is preferentially taken up by heart tissue. Following removal of much of the triacylglycerol from VLDL, the remaining remnant particles are intermediate-density lipoproteins (IDL), which are the precursors of low-density lipoprotein.

Low-density lipoprotein (LDL) is the end product of VLDL metabolism and its lipid consists

Table 4.4 Composition of human plasma lipoproteins

Class	Density	Composition (weight %)		Percentage of total lipid (weight %)					Major apoproteins
		Protein	Lipid	TAG	PL	CE	Chol	FFA	
Chylomicrons[a]	<0.95	2	98	88	8	3	1	–	AI, AIV, B-48, Cs, and E from HDL
Very-low-density lipoprotein (VLDL)[b] from HDL	0.95–1.006	10	90	56	20	15	8	1	B-100, Cs, and E
Intermediate-density lipoprotein (IDL)[c]	1.006–1.019	11	89	29	26	34	6	1	B-100, E
Low-density lipoprotein (LDL)[c]	1.019–1.063	21	79	13	28	48	10	1	B-100
Lipoprotein(a) [Lp(a)][b]	1.05–1.12	31	69	11	29	48	11	1	B-100, apo(a)
High-density lipoprotein HDL$_2$[a]	1.063–1.125	33	68	16	43	31	10	–	As, Cs, E
High-density lipoprotein HDL$_3$[b,c]	1.125–1.210	57	43	13	46	29	9	6	As, Cs, E
Albumin[b]	>1.281	99	1	–	–	–	–	100	Albumin

[a]Origin: intestine.
[b]Origin: liver.
[c]Origin: VLDL.

CE, cholesterol ester; chol, cholesterol; FFA, free fatty acids; PL, phospholipid; TAG, triacylglycerol (triglyceride).

Table 4.5 Functions of human plasma lipoproteins

Class	Function
Chylomicrons[a]	Transport dietary lipids from intestine to peripheral tissues and liver
Very-low-density lipoprotein (VLDL)[b]	Transports lipids from liver to peripheral tissues
Intermediate-density lipoprotein (IDL)[c]	Precursor of LDL
Low-density lipoprotein (LDL)[c]	Transports cholesterol to peripheral tissues and liver
Lipoprotein(a) (Lp(a))[b]	Uncertain. Associated with CHD risk
High-density lipoprotein HDL$_2$[a]	Removes cholesterol from tissues and transfers it to the liver or other lipoproteins
High-density lipoprotein HDL$_3$[b,c]	
Albumin[b]	Transports free fatty acids from adipose tissue to peripheral tissues

[a]Origin: intestine.
[b]Origin: liver.
[c]Origin: VLDL.

largely of cholesterol ester and cholesterol. Its surface has only one type of apolipoprotein, apo B100. LDL carries about 70% of all cholesterol in the plasma. LDL is taken up by the liver and other tissues by LDL receptors.

High-density lipoprotein (HDL) is synthesized and secreted both by the liver and intestine. A major function of HDL is to transfer apolipoproteins C and E to chylomicrons so that lipoprotein lipase can break down the triacylglycerols in the lipoproteins. HDL also plays a key role in the reverse transport of cholesterol, i.e. the transfer of cholesterol back from the tissues to the liver. HDL can be divided into two subfractions of different densities: HDL_2 and HDL_3.

Lipoprotein (a) (Lp(a)) is a complex of LDL with apolipoprotein (a).

4.3.4 Nutritional determinants of lipid and lipoprotein levels in blood

The fact that plasma lipid and lipoprotein levels are important predictors of coronary heart disease risk (discussed in Chapter 21) has led to a great deal of research into nutritional and other lifestyle factors that interact with genetic factors to determine their concentration in the blood (Table 4.6).

The chylomicron count and the fatty acid composition of chylomicron lipid are principally determined by the amount and type of fat eaten in the preceding meal. VLDL levels tend to be low in lean individuals and those who have regular physical activity. Obesity and an excessive intake of alcohol are associated with higher than average VLDL levels. An increased intake of carbohydrate

Table 4.6 Nutritional determinants of lipoprotein levels

Nutritional factor	VLDL	LDL	HDL	Notes
Obesity	↑	↑	↓	
Saturated fat				
Lauric (12:0)	–	↑	↑	
Myristic (14:0)	–	↑↑	↑	
Palmitic (16:0)	–	↑↑	↑	
Stearic (18:0)	–	–	–	
Monounsaturated fat				
Oleic (18:1 *cis*)	–	↓	↑	
Elaidic (18:1 *trans*)	–	↑↑	↓	
Polyunsaturated fat (ω-6)				HDL may ↓ if 18:2ω-6 is
Linoleic (18:2ω-6)	–	↓↓	(↑)	>10% of total energy
Polyunsaturated fat (ω-3)				↑ in LDL if initial LDL
α-Linolenic (18:3ω-3)	↓↓	(↑)	(↓)	is high
Eicosapentaenoic (20:5ω-3)	↓↓	(↑)	(↓)	↓ in HDL if fed in large
Docosahexaenoic (22:6ω-3)	↓↓	(↑)	(↓)	quantities

↑, ↓, increase or decrease;
↑↑, ↓↓, appreciable increase or decrease;
LDL, low-density lipoproteins; HDL, high-density lipoproteins; VLDL, very-low-density lipoproteins.

(especially sugars and starches) is generally associated with an increase in VLDL as a result of increased hepatic synthesis of triacylglycerols, though adaptation may occur if the high carbohydrate intake is sustained over a prolonged period. Populations with habitual high carbohydrate intakes (e.g. Asians or African people who consume their traditional diets and are healthy weight) do not have particularly high plasma VLDL concentrations. Consumption of eicosapentaenoic ($20:5\omega3$) and docosahexaenoic ($22:6\omega3$) acids as fish or fish oils lowers plasma VLDL levels. In routine clinical work, plasma triacylglycerol, rather than VLDL, is measured because the bulk of triacylglycerol levels in blood taken from fasting (10–12 hours) individuals tend to parallel levels of VLDL.

Levels of LDL and total plasma cholesterol are determined by an interaction of genetic factors and dietary characteristics. High intakes of saturated fatty acids, especially myristic and palmitic acids, and *trans*-fatty acids (e.g. elaidic acid) are associated with raised LDL-cholesterol, while high intakes of linoleic acid, the major polyunsaturated acid in foods, and to a lesser extent *cis*-monounsaturated fatty acids tend to reduce cholesterol levels. The precise mechanism has not been established, but high intakes of saturated fatty acids appear to decrease the removal of plasma LDL by LDL-receptors, whereas mono- and polyunsaturated fatty acids are associated with increased LDL receptor activity. Dietary cholesterol has a minor influence on plasma total and LDL-cholesterol, but this is enhanced when saturated fatty acids comprise a high proportion of dietary lipid (greater than 15% of energy) and cholesterol intake exceeds 300 mg/day. It is less clear whether dietary cholesterol plays a major role over the relatively low range of intakes now seen in many countries and when saturated fatty acid intake is reduced. Plant sterols (e.g. β-sitosterol) are very poorly absorbed and interfere with the absorption of cholesterol. This property of plant sterols has been utilized by incorporating them into margarines. Consumption of these margarines (25 g/day containing roughly 2 g plant sterols) can lower plasma total and LDL-cholesterol concentrations.

The ability of soluble forms of dietary fibre to reduce total and LDL-cholesterol is small compared with the effect of altering the nature of dietary fat. Dietary protein may also influence plasma lipids and lipoproteins: soybean protein particularly has some cholesterol-lowering properties. Vegetarians have lower levels of total and LDL-cholesterol in general than non-vegetarians, but it is not clear which characteristic of the vegetarian diet principally accounts for this effect.

Debate centres around whether saturated fatty acids should be replaced by wholegrain fibre-rich carbohydrate-containing foods or by fats and oils with a more favourable fatty acid profile (i.e. monounsaturated or polyunsaturated fatty acids with a *cis* configuration). However, provided energy balance is taken into account, it probably matters little whether appropriate carbohydrate-containing foods (see Chapter 3) or more acceptable fats and oils, or indeed a combination of both, provide replacement energy for saturated fats.

Dietary factors do not have much effect on HDL-cholesterol concentration. However, HDL-cholesterol can be slightly reduced by very high intakes of polyunsaturated fatty acids (e.g. when the dietary polyunsaturated fat to saturated fat ratio is greater than 1), or by increasing carbohydrate from more usual levels consumed (less than 45% of energy) in affluent societies to 60% or more of total energy, or by increasing *trans*-unsaturated fatty acids. The HDL-lowering effect of a high-carbohydrate diet may be reduced or prevented if the carbohydrate is high in soluble forms of non-starch polysaccharide. HDL levels tend to be raised by diets relatively high in dietary cholesterol and saturated fatty acids, although this 'positive' effect is offset by the larger increases in LDL-cholesterol caused by such diets. Increasing *cis* forms of monounsaturated fatty acids appears to be marginally better at maintaining HDL levels than polyunsaturated fatty acids when reducing saturated fat consumption. Most dietary studies have not included measurements of the subfractions of HDL. HDL-cholesterol is raised in people who take substantial amounts of alcohol (see Chapter 7).

4.4 Essentials of lipid metabolism

4.4.1 Biosynthesis of fatty acids

Saturated and monounsaturated fatty acids can be synthesized in the body from carbohydrate and protein. This process of lipogenesis occurs especially in a well-fed person whose diet contains a high proportion of carbohydrate in the presence of an adequate energy intake. Insulin stimulates the biosynthesis of fatty acids. Lipogenesis is reduced during energy restriction or when the diet is high in fat. Unsaturated fatty acids may be further elongated or desaturated by various enzyme systems (Fig. 4.9).

4.4.2 Essential fatty acids

Essential fatty acids are those that cannot be synthesized in the body and must be supplied in the diet to avoid deficiency symptoms. They include members of the ω-6 (linoleic acid) and ω-3 (α-linolenic acid) families of fatty acids. When the diet is deficient in linoleic acid, the most abundant unsaturated fatty acid in tissue, oleic acid, is desaturated and elongated to eicosatrienoic acid (20:3ω9), which is normally present in trace amounts. Increased plasma levels of this 20:3ω9 suggest a deficiency of essential fatty acids. Essential fatty acid deficiency is rare except in those with severe, untreated fat malabsorption or those suffering from famine. Symptoms include dry, cracked, scaly, and bleeding skin, excessive thirst due to high water loss from the skin, and impaired liver function resulting from the accumulation of lipid in the liver (i.e. fatty liver).

Linoleic acid and α-linolenic acid are not only required for the structural integrity of all cell membranes, but they are also elongated and desaturated, in limited amounts, into longer chain, more polyunsaturated fatty acids that are the precursors

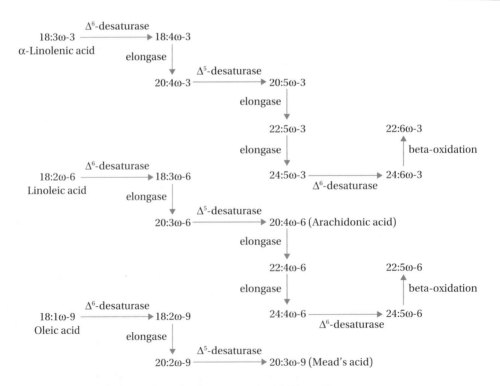

Fig. 4.9 Desaturation and elongation of polyunsaturated fatty acids.

to a group of hormone-like eicosanoid compounds, prostaglandins and leukotrienes (see Section 4.4.4). Linoleic acid (18:2ω-6) is converted to arachidonic acid (20:4ω-6), while α-linolenic acid (18:3ω-3) is converted to eicosapentaenoic (20:5ω-3) and docosahexaenoic (22:6ω-3) acids. A high ratio of linoleic to α-linolenic acid in the diet tends to reduce the amount of α-linolenic acid converted to eicosapentaenoic and docosahexaenoic acids.

There is some question as to whether the arachidonic, eicosapentaenoic, and docosahexaenoic acids incorporated into the body's tissues come predominantly from endogenous desaturation and elongation of dietary essential fatty acids or are obtained from the diet as preformed fatty acids. Whatever the answer, the body appears to have a capacity to desaturate and elongate essential fatty acids, because individuals following strict vegan diets (no animal foods) ingest plenty of linoleic and α-linolenic acids but only negligible amounts of arachidonic, eicosapentaenoic, and docosahexaenoic acids, yet have adequate levels of these latter fatty acids in their blood.

4.4.3 Membrane structure

Unsaturated fatty acids in membrane lipids play an important role in maintaining fluidity. The critically important metabolic functions of membranes such as nutrient transport, receptor function, and ion channels are affected by interactions between proteins and lipids. For example, the phosphoinositide cycle, which determines the responses of many cells to hormones, neurotransmitters, and cell growth factors and which controls processes of cell division, is influenced by the proportion of ω-6 to ω-3 fatty acids. Docosahexaenoic acid (22:6ω3) is uniquely abundant in brain tissue, it is the predominant polyunsaturated fatty acid in brain phospholipid, and it plays a critical role in the functions of the central nervous system.

4.4.4 Eicosanoids

Eicosanoids are biologically active, oxygenated metabolites of arachidonic acid, eicosapentaenoic

acid (EPA), or dihomo-γ-linolenic acid (20:3ω-6). They are produced in virtually all cells in the body, act locally, have short life spans, and act as modulators of numerous physiological processes including reproduction, blood pressure, haemostasis, and inflammation. Eicosanoids are further categorized into prostaglandins/thromboxanes and leukotrienes, which are produced via the cyclooxygenase and lipoxygenase pathways, respectively (Fig. 4.10). Considerable recent interest has centred around the cardiovascular effects of eicosanoids, in particular the role they play in thrombosis (i.e. vessel blockage). Thromboxane A_2 (TxA$_2$), synthesized in platelets from arachidonic acid, stimulates vasoconstriction and platelet aggregation (i.e. clumping), while prostacyclin I_2 (PGI$_2$), produced from arachidonic acid in the endothelial cells of the vessel wall, has the opposing effects of stimulating vasodilation and inhibiting platelet aggregation. The balance of these two counteracting eicosanoids affects overall thrombotic tendency.

Research, initially based on the observation that the Inuit (Eskimo) people of Greenland have very low rates of coronary heart disease, led to the demonstration that a high dietary intake of EPA (usually in fish oil) can profoundly influence the balance of thromboxanes and prostacyclins. Such diets lead to the substitution of EPA for arachidonic acid in platelet membranes. TxA$_2$ production decreases, not only because of lower levels of platelet arachidonic acid, but also because the increased levels of EPA in platelets inhibit the conversion of arachidonic acid to TxA$_2$. On the other hand, PGI$_2$ production in the endothelial cells is only slightly reduced and there is a sharp rise in the production of PGI$_3$ from EPA, which has equal vasodilatory and platelet-inhibiting properties. The overall changes in eicosanoid production contribute to reducing thrombotic risk.

Leukotrienes are important in several diseases involving inflammatory or hypersensitivity reactions including asthma, eczema, and rheumatoid arthritis. The effect of EPA consumption on leukotriene synthesis is to shift production from the more inflammatory 4-series leukotrienes, synthesized

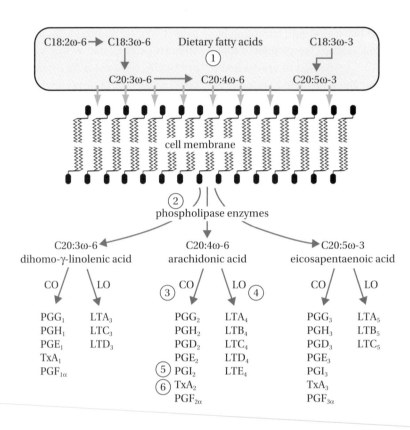

Fig. 4.10 Formation of eicosanoids.

(1) Dihomo-γ-linolenic acid (DGLA), arachidonic acid (AA), and eicosapentaenoic (EPA) acid, obtained ready-made in the diet or via desaturation and elongation of their respective parent ω-6 (linolenic acid) or ω-3 (linolenic acid) essential fatty acids, are incorporated into the phospholipids of cell membranes.

(2) When cells are stimulated by hormones or activating substances, phospholipase enzymes release DGLA, AA, and EPA into the interior of the cell.

(3) Once released from the cell membranes, DGLA, AA, and EPA can be converted via the cyclo-oxygenase pathway (CO) into prostaglandins (PG) and thromboxanes (Tx) of the 1, 2 and 3 series, respectively;

(4) or via the lipoxygenase pathway (LO) to leukotrienes (LT) of the 3, 4, and 5 series, respectively.

(5) In platelets, AA is converted primarily to the 2 series thromboxane (TxA_2), which stimulates platelet clumping and increases blood pressure.

(6) In the endothelial cells lining arterial vessels, AA is converted into the 2 series prostacylin (PGI_2), which counters the action of TxA_2 by inhibiting platelet clumping and decreasing blood pressure.

from arachidonic acid, to the less inflammatory 5-series leukotrienes synthesized from EPA. This metabolic effect helps to explain the improvements in some of the clinical symptoms experienced by rheumatoid arthritis sufferers who consume significant quantities of fish (i.e. EPA).

4.4.5 Effects of fatty acids on other metabolic processes

Fatty acids influence a range of other metabolic processes that have been less well studied in humans. Hydrolysis of some phospholipids results in the formation of biologically active compounds such as the platelet activating agent (PAF) from 1-alkyl, 2-acyl phosphatidylcholine. Different polyunsaturated fatty acids in the precursor phospholipid can modify PAF formation. ω-3 fatty acids influence the production of cytokines, including the interleukins and tumour necrosis factors, which are involved in regulation of the immune system. An exciting area of current research is the study of the effects of fatty acids on the expression of genes encoding enzymes that are involved in lipid metabolism, as well as the expression of genes involved in cell growth regulation.

4.4.6 Oxidation of fatty acids

Those fatty acids not incorporated into tissues or used for synthesis of eicosanoids are oxidized for energy. Oxidation of fatty acids occurs in the mitochondria of cells and involves a multiple-step process by which the fatty acid is gradually broken down to molecules of acetyl CoA, which are available to enter the tricarboxylic acid cycle and so to generate energy. The rate of oxidation of fatty acids is highest at times of low energy intake and particularly during starvation. As the acetyl CoA splits off, adenosine triphosphate (ATP) is generated, which is also a source of energy. Fatty acids of different chain lengths and degrees of saturation are oxidized via slightly different pathways, but the ultimate purpose of each is the production of acetyl CoA and the generation of energy. Ketone bodies are produced during times of particularly rapid fatty acid oxidation during the process of ketogenesis. An absolute insulin deficiency, such as is seen in severe uncontrolled insulin-dependent diabetes, results in a very high rate of production of ketones, and acidosis results because of accumulation of acetoacetic and β-hydroxybutyric acids. In healthy individuals with a functioning pancreas, the ingestion of glucose stimulates insulin secretion and thereby prevents or abolishes ketosis. This can be achieved by as little as 50–100 g of glucose daily. In the normal fasting individual, a modest increase in that level of ketone bodies stimulates insulin secretion. The insulin inhibits further ketogenesis and enhances peripheral ketone body use so that ketone body levels do not rise above 6–8 mol/L. (In severe diabetes, levels may be twice as high as this.) In prolonged starvation there is further ketone-body formation and a moderate degree of ketosis may result. However, ketoacidosis does not occur in the absence of insulin deficiency.

4.4.7 Lipid storage

Energy intake in excess of requirements is converted to fat for storage. Stored fat in adipose tissue provides the human body with a source of energy when energy supplies are not immediately available from ingested carbohydrate, fat, or glycogen stores. Triacylglycerols are the main storage form of lipids and most stored lipids are found in adipose tissue. The lipid is stored as single droplets in cells called adipocytes, which can expand as more fat needs to be stored. Most of the lipid in adipose tissue is derived from dietary lipid and the stored lipid reflects the composition of dietary fat. The triacylglycerol stores of adipose tissue are not static but are continually undergoing lipolysis and re-esterification.

4.4.8 Cholesterol synthesis and excretion

Cholesterol is present in tissues and in plasma lipoproteins as free cholesterol or combined with a fatty acid as cholesterol ester. About half the cholesterol in the body comes from endogenous synthesis and the remainder from the diet. It is synthesized in the body from acetyl CoA via a long metabolic pathway. Cholesterol synthesis in the liver is regulated near the beginning of the pathway by the dietary cholesterol delivered by chylomicron remnants. In the tissues, a cholesterol balance is maintained between factors causing a gain of cholesterol (synthesis, uptake into cells, hydrolysis of stored cholesterol esters) and factors causing loss of cholesterol (steroid hormone synthesis, cholesterol ester formation, bile acid synthesis, and reverse transport via HDL). The specific binding sites and receptors for LDL play a crucial role in cholesterol balance since they constitute the principal means by which LDL-cholesterol enters the cells. These receptors are defective in familial hypercholesterolaemia (see Section 20.4.1). Excess cholesterol is excreted from the liver in the bile either unchanged as cholesterol or converted to bile salts. A large proportion of the bile salts that are excreted from the liver into the gastrointestinal tract are absorbed back into the portal circulation and returned to the liver as part of the enterohepatic circulation, but some pass on to the colon and are excreted as faecal bile acids.

4.5 Health effects of dietary lipids

Most fatty acids can be made in the body, except for the essential fatty acids (EFAs) linoleic and α-linolenic acids, which must be obtained from the diet (see Section 4.4.2). The fact that specific deficiencies resulting from inadequate intakes of EFAs are very rare in adults, even in African and Asian countries where total dietary fat can provide as little as 10% of total energy, suggests that the minimum requirement is low. Amongst adults, EFA deficiency has only been reported when linoleic acid (18:2ω-6) intakes are less than 2–5 g/day or less than 1–2% of total energy. Most adult Western diets provide at least 10 g/day of EFA and healthy people have a substantial reserve in adipose tissues. Clinical manifestations of α-linolenic acid deficiency are rare in humans.

Amongst adults in Western countries, the major health issues concerning intake of fat centre around the role of excessive dietary saturated fat in coronary heart disease (Chapter 21) and whether total fat intake plays a role in obesity (Chapter 17) and certain cancers (Chapter 22). There is concern too regarding the optimal amounts and balance of ω-3 to ω-6 fatty acids with regard to coronary heart disease risk, as well as the effect this balance may have on inflammatory and immunological responses.

Human milk provides 6% of total energy as essential fatty acids (linoleic and α-linolenic acids); it also contains small amounts of longer chain, more polyunsaturated fatty acids such as arachidonic acid (AA; 20:4ω-6) and docosahexaenoic acids (DHA; 22:6ω-3). Commercial baby milk formulae contain comparable amounts of essential fatty acids and a number of brands—in some countries—contain AA and DHA. Infants fed exclusively with formula without AA and DHA have lower levels of these fatty acids in their plasma and red blood cells in comparison with breastfed infants. There is strong evidence that inadequate provision of AA and DHA to premature infants delays development of visual acuity (see Chapter 33).

Concern has been expressed that the desire to reduce total fat intake by some health-conscious parents in affluent societies might result in a diet high in complex carbohydrate and dietary fibre and containing insufficient energy for growth and development in childhood. These wide-ranging issues need to be taken into account when making nutritional and dietary recommendations.

4.6 Recommendations concerning fat intake

4.6.1 Minimum desirable intakes

In adults, it is necessary to ensure that dietary intake is adequate to meet energy needs and to meet the requirements for EFAs and fat-soluble vitamins. Adequate intakes are particular important during pregnancy and lactation. Thus, for most adults, dietary fat should provide at least 15% of total energy, and 20% for women of reproductive age. World Health Organization recommendations suggest that 2% of total daily energy is required from ω-6, and at least 0.5% energy from ω-3 polyunsaturated fatty acids. These levels are rather arbitrary and are based on the amounts required to cure EFA deficiency. Few countries recommend a specific ω-3 to ω-6 ratio, but a recommendation for eicosapentaenoic (EPA) and docosahexaenoic acids (DHA) is common. For example, WHO recommends 0.25–2 g per day of EPA plus DHA. Particular attention must be paid to promoting adequate maternal intakes of EFAs throughout pregnancy and lactation to meet the needs of the fetus and young infant in laying down lipids in their growing brains (which have a high content of DHA and AA).

For infants and young children, the amount and type of dietary fat are equally important. Breast milk fulfils all requirements (50–60% energy as fat, with appropriate balance of nutrients), and during weaning it is important to ensure that dietary fat intake does not fall too rapidly. At least until the age of 2 years, a child's diet should contain about 40% of energy from fat and provide similar levels of EFAs to breast milk. Infant formulae with AA and DHA in proportions similar to those found in breast milk are available in many countries.

It is necessary also to take into account associated substances, in particular several vitamins and antioxidants. These are considered in other chapters. In particular, vitamin E (Chapter 14) in edible oils is required to stabilize unsaturated fatty acids. Foods high in polyunsaturated fatty acids should contain at least 0.6 mg α-tocopherol equivalents per gram of polyunsaturated fatty acids. In countries where vitamin A deficiency is a public health problem, the use

of red palm oil should be encouraged wherever it is available.

4.6.2 Upper limits of fat and oil intakes

In most Western countries, dietary recommendations concerning fat intake have focused primarily around desirable upper limits of intake. The strongest reason for reducing intake of total fat from the typical Western intake of about 35% or more total energy is the widespread problem of obesity and the expectation that reducing fat intake to 30% or less of total energy will help to reduce the near epidemic proportions of the global health problem of overweight (Chapter 17).

Reducing total fat may also reduce the frequency of some cancers (Chapter 22) but the evidence here is more tenuous, and it may also be that the extent of fat reduction required to reduce cancer risk (to around 20% of total energy) is unlikely to be achievable in most Western countries in the foreseeable future. There is convincing evidence that replacing saturated fat with polyunsaturated fat will help to lower rates of coronary heart disease. The target is to reduce saturated fat intake in Western countries from current levels of 12% of energy or higher to 10% of energy or lower. This remains a particularly important dietary recommendation since the consumption of high-fat (mostly saturated) convenience foods is high in Western countries and is becoming increasingly common worldwide.

Further Reading

1. **Gurr, M.I., Harwood, J.L., and Frayn, K.** (2002) *Lipid biochemistry*, 5th edition. London, Blackwell Science.

2. **Mensink, R.P., Zock, P,L., Kester, A.D.M., and Katan, M,B.** (2003) Effects of dietary fatty acids and carbohydrates on the ratio of serum total to HDL cholesterol and on serum lipids and apolipoproteins: A meta-analysis of 60 controlled trials. *Am J Clin Nutr*, **77**, 1146–55.

Useful Websites

 To see topical and scientifically robust updates on nutrition associated with this textbook and web links to many of the journals in the Further Reading sections, please see the dedicated Online Resource Centre at **http://www.oxfordtextbooks.co.uk/orc/mann4e/**

5 Protein

Alan A. Jackson and Stewart Truswell

5.1 Normal growth and the maintenance of health

To maintain normal weight, function, and health in adults and growth in childhood requires a constant intake of oxygen, water, energy, and nutrients. In adults this intake is matched by an equivalent loss of elements as carbon dioxide, water, and solutes in urine, or solids in stool. In this way, a balance is achieved and body weight and composition are maintained relatively constant over long periods of time. In childhood there is positive balance associated with the net deposition of new tissue. If intake is less than that needed for normal function then there is loss of weight and function is compromised to a point where it eventually impairs health: in childhood, growth is curtailed or stops.

Proteins are fundamental structural and functional elements within every cell and undergo extensive metabolic interaction. This widespread metabolic interaction is intimately linked to the metabolism of energy and other nutrients. Following water, protein is the next most abundant chemical compound in the body. All cells and tissues contain proteins. For an adult man who weighs 70 kg, about 16% will be protein, i.e. about 11 kg. A large proportion of this will be muscle (43%), with substantial proportions being present in skin (15%) and blood (16%). Half of the total is present in only four proteins: collagen, haemoglobin, myosin, and actin, with collagen comprising about 25% of the overall total.

Proteins fulfil a range of functions and the amount of protein does not, in itself, provide any indication of the importance or relevance of the function. Indeed, some of the most important functionally active proteins might only comprise a small proportion of the total present, e.g. peptide hormones such as insulin, growth factors, or cytokines. The biochemical activity of proteins is an attribute of their individual structure, shape, and size. This in turn is determined by the sequence of amino acids within the polypeptide chains, the characteristics of the individual amino acids (size,

charge, hydrophobicity, or hydrophilicity) and the environment, which together determine the primary, secondary, and tertiary structure of the protein. The tertiary structure of the protein determines the nature of the biochemical reactions in which it will engage.

Proteins taken in the diet are broken down into amino acids in the processes of digestion and absorption. Absorbed amino acids contribute to the amino acid pool of the body, from which all proteins are synthesized. The proteins of the body exist in a 'dynamic state' as they are constantly turning over through the processes of protein synthesis and degradation (Fig. 5.1). On average, the rates of synthesis and degradation are similar in adults, so that the amount of protein in the body remains more or less constant over long periods of time, and nitrogen balance is achieved. During growth, protein synthesis exceeds protein degradation to enable net deposition of protein. The process of turnover is obvious for some proteins, e.g. enzymes, skin or mucosa, or digestive juices, but is also true for plasma proteins such as albumin or γ-globulins, and even structural proteins such as muscle and bone. There are many hundreds of proteins in the body, each of which is formed and degraded at a characteristic rate that may vary from minutes to days or even months. Each protein fulfils a specific function, which might be structural, protective, or enzymatic, or it might be involved in transport or an aspect of cellular communication (Box 5.1).

5.2 Protein status of the body

There is no single way in which the protein status of an individual can be determined. Different approaches provide information on different aspects. The amount of protein contained in the body cannot be measured directly. However, most of the nitrogen in the body is present as amino acids in protein, and most protein is present as lean tissue. Thus, the nitrogen content of the body can be determined by *in vivo* neutron activation analysis (an expensive research

procedure that requires special equipment and exposes the subject to radiation).

On the assumption that the protein content of tissues remains fairly constant, the determination of the lean body mass (which approximates the fat-free mass) also gives an index of the total protein content. Indirect measures of lean body mass include bioelectrical impedance, assessment of total body water, total body potassium, underwater

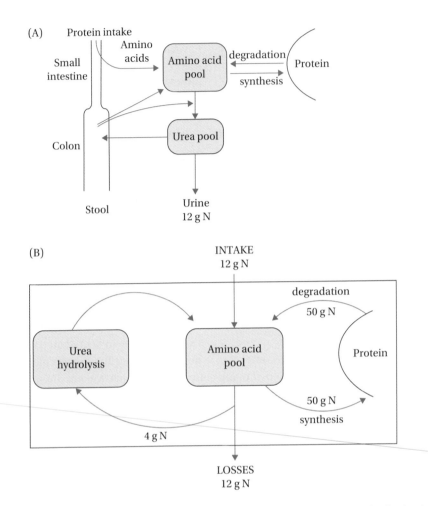

Fig. 5.1 (A) There is a dynamic interchange of protein, amino acids, and nitrogen in the body, which conceptually takes place through an amino acid pool. Amino acids are added to the pool from the degradation of body proteins and also from dietary protein, following digestion and absorption. There is the continuous breakdown of amino acids, with energy being made available when the carbon skeleton is oxidized to water and CO_2. The amino group goes to the formation of urea. Although urea is an end-product of mammalian metabolism, a significant proportion of the nitrogen is salvaged for further metabolic interaction following hydrolysis of urea by the flora resident in the colon. (B) The quantitative relations of these exchanges in normal adults expressed as grams of (amino) nitrogen (N) per day.

weighing, or fat-fold thickness (see Chapter 31). Organ and tissue size can be determined by imaging techniques. Muscle mass and changes in muscle content in clinical situations can be assessed from the urinary excretion of creatinine or the girth of limbs, such as the mid-upper arm circumference or thigh circumference. Determinations of the concentration of amino acids in plasma or the albumin concentration have been used as indirect indices of body protein status. However, each of these can be difficult to interpret (see Section 5.18.3).

Assessment of the function of the metabolically active tissues has been used as an index of protein status, for example muscle function tests, liver function tests, and tests of immune function. The content of the body is not static, and therefore measurements of the rates at which proteins are formed and degraded in the body and the rate at which

BOX 5.1 The pattern of amino acids that form proteins give them very different shapes and chemical and physical properties, thereby enabling them to carry out a wide range of functions within the body

Structural		Transport/communication	
Body:	skeleton and supporting tissues, skin, and epithelia	Plasma proteins:	albumin, transferrin, apolipoproteins
Tissue:	connective tissues and ground substance	Hormones:	insulin, glucagon, growth hormone
Cell:	cellular architecture	Cell membrane and receptors:	intracellular communications/ second messenger
Protective		**Enzymatic**	
Barrier:	non-specific defences/ turnover, keratins, skin, tears, mucin	Extracellular:	digestive, clotting; haemoglobin and O_2, CO_2 transport; acid base
Inflammation: Immune response:	acute phase response cellular and humoral	Metabolic pathways:	glycolysis, protein synthesis, citric acid cycle, urea cycle

nitrogen flows to the end products of metabolism provide one important approach to determining the mechanisms through which nitrogen equilibrium is maintained in health: positive balance is achieved during growth and negative balance is brought about during wasting conditions.

5.3 Proteins, amino acids, and other nitrogen-containing compounds

The structure and function of all proteins is related to their amino acid composition: the number and order of linkages, folding, intrachain linkages, and the interaction with other groups to induce chemical change, e.g. phosphorylation/dephosphorylation, oxidation and reduction of sulphydral groups. The amino acids are linked in chains through peptide bonds. The structure of individual amino acids and the patterns of their linkages give the unique properties to an individual protein. Proteins may have critical requirements for either a tight or loose association with micronutrients and this is particularly likely for enzymes in which catalytic activity might require the presence of cofactors or prosthetic groups in close association with the active centres.

For each protein, the amino acid composition is characteristic. For a protein to be synthesized requires that all the amino acids needed are available at the point of synthesis. If one amino acid is in short supply, this will limit the process of protein synthesis; such an amino acid is defined as the 'limiting amino acid'. There is no dietary requirement for protein *per se*, but protein is important for the individual amino acids it contains. There are 20 amino acids required for protein synthesis and these are all 'metabolically essential' (Box 5.2). Of the 20 amino acids found in protein, eight have to be provided preformed in the diet for adults and are identified as being 'indispensable' or 'essential' (isoleucine, leucine, lysine, methionine, phenylalanine, threonine, tryptophan, and valine).

BOX 5.2 There are 20 amino acids that are found as the constituents of proteins. All are 'essential' for metabolism, but not all have to be provided preformed in the diet, because they can be made in sufficient amounts from other metabolic precursors. If the situation arises where the formation in the body is not adequate to satisfy the metabolic needs, the amino acids become conditionally essential

Indispensable (essential) amino acids	Conditionally indispensable (essential) amino acids	Dispensable (non-essential) amino acids
Leucine (Leu)	Tyrosine (Tyr)	Glutamic acid (Glu)
Isoleucine (Ile)	Glycine (Gly)	Alanine (Ala)
Valine (Val)	Serine (Ser)	Aspartic acid (Asp)
Phenylalanine (Phe)	Cysteine (Cys)	
Threonine (Thr)	Arginine (Arg)	
Methionine (Met)	Glutamine (Gln)	
Tryptophan (Trp)	Asparagine (Asn)	
Lysine (Lys)	Proline (Pro)	
	Histidine (His)	

The other amino acids do not have to be provided preformed in the diet, provided that they can be formed in the body from appropriate precursors in adequate amounts and are identified as being 'dispensable' or 'non-essential'. The non-essential amino acids are not necessarily of lesser biological importance. They have to be synthesized in adequate amounts endogenously. Their provision in the diet appears to spare additional quantities of other (essential) amino acids or sources of nitrogen that would be required for their synthesis.

In early childhood, a number of amino acids, which are not essential in adults, cannot be formed in adequate amounts, because the demand is high,

BOX 5.3 Amino acids are the precursors for many other metabolic intermediates and products with structural and functional roles

Product/function	Examples
Nucleotides	Formation of DNA, RNA, ATP, NAD
Energy transduction	ATP, NAD, creatine
Neurotransmitters	Serotonin, adrenaline, noradrenaline, acetylcholine
Membrane structures	Head groups of phospholipids: choline, ethanolamine
Porphyrin	Haem compounds, cytochromes
Cellular replication	Polyamines
Fat digestion	Taurine, glycine-conjugated bile acids
Fat metabolism	Carnitine
Hormones	Thyroid, pituitary hormones

the pathways for their formation are not matured, or the rate of endogenous formation is not adequate (or some combination of these). These amino acids have been identified as being 'conditionally' essential, because of the limited ability of their endogenous formation relative to the magnitude of the demand (arginine, histidine, cysteine, glycine, tyrosine, glutamine, and proline). There may be disease situations during adult life when for one reason or another a particular amino acid, or group of amino acids, becomes conditionally essential.

Although most of the amino acids are found in proteins, many amino acids also have metabolic activities that are not directly related to the formation of proteins or they act as the precursors for other important metabolically active compounds (Box 5.3). Not all amino acids are found in proteins and there are a number of metabolically important amino acids that play no direct part in the formation of proteins (e.g. citrulline). There is a relatively small pool of free amino acids in all tissues. This is the pool from which amino acids for protein formation are derived and to which amino acids coming from protein degradation contribute; therefore, the amino acid pools have a very high rate of turnover.

There are many other nitrogen-containing compounds that are not proteins, polypeptides, or amino acids.

5.4 Dietary proteins, the amino acid pool, and the dynamic state of body proteins

Before proteins taken in the diet can be utilized, they have to be broken down to the constituent amino acids through digestion. The catalytic breaking of the peptide bond is achieved through enzymes, which act initially in the acid environment of the stomach, and the process is completed in the alkaline environment of the small intestine. There is a series of proteolytic enzymes that selectively attack specific bonds (Table 5.1). The products of digestion are presented for absorption as individual amino acids, dipeptides, or small oligopeptides. Absorption takes place in the small intestine as an energy-dependent process through specific transporters. There is evidence for the absorption of small amounts of intact protein—it is unlikely to be of great nutritional significance, but may be of potential importance in the development of allergies. The extent of absorption of whole proteins is not clear, nor whether this can take place through intact bowel or requires mucosal lesions.

The absorptive capacity of the bowel for amino acids has to be greatly in excess of the dietary intake, because there is a considerable net daily secretion of proteins into the bowel. The protein is contained in secretions associated with digestion and the enzymes contained therein, mucins, and sloughed cells. The amount varies, but estimates suggest a minimum of 70 g protein/day and possibly up to 200–300 g protein/day—i.e. the amounts are at least as great as the dietary intake. Therefore, dietary amino acids mix with and are diluted by endogenous amino acids. These dietary and endogenous amino acids are taken up into the circulation and distributed to cells around the body.

5.5 Protein turnover

When dietary amino acids are labelled with either stable or radioactive isotopes, their fate in the body can be determined. As a matter of course, there is retention of the labelled amino acids in the body, and the labelled amino acids can be recovered from the proteins of most tissues. This approach can be used as the basis for measuring the rate at which body proteins are synthesized and degraded. The

Table 5.1 Human protein digestion

Organ	Activation	Enzyme	Substrate	Product
Stomach	pH < 4	Pepsin	Whole protein	Very large polypeptides with C-terminal Tyr, Phe, Trp, also Leu, Glu, Gln
Pancreas	pH 7.5 Enterokinase secreted by small intestinal mucosa	Endopeptidases	Bonds with peptide chain	Peptide with basic amino acid at C terminus (Arg, Lys)
		Trypsin	Peptides	Peptide with neutral amino acid at C terminus
		Chymotrypsin	Peptides	Amino acids
		Exopeptidases	C-terminal bonds	Amino acids
		Carboxypeptidase	Successive amino acids at C terminus	
		Aminopeptidase	Successive amino acids at N terminus	

Note: Enzymes that digest proteins are secreted as inactive precursors (e.g. pepsinogen, trypsinogen, chymotrypsinogen) and are activated under appropriate conditions by the removal of a small peptide from the parent molecule.

relative rates of protein synthesis and degradation determine the overall nitrogen balance. For nitrogen balance (see 5.15), the rates of protein synthesis and protein degradation have to be equal. If synthesis exceeds degradation, then nitrogen balance is positive, and if degradation exceeds synthesis nitrogen balance is negative. Because overall balance is determined by the relative rates of synthesis and degradation, the achievement of balance itself provides no information on the absolute rates of either process. As shown in Fig. 5.2, negative nitrogen balance can result from a range of patterns of change in synthesis and degradation. As the factors that act on or control synthesis and degradation are different, interventions that are designed to modify balance or improve growth might act on one or the other process. On average, about 50% of protein synthesis takes place in the visceral tissues, with liver predominating (25%), and 50% takes place in the carcass, with muscle predominating (25%). Although the mass of liver is much less than the mass of muscle, the intensity of turnover in liver (fractional turnover, 100% per day) is much greater than that in muscle (fractional turnover, 18% per day).

5.6 Protein synthesis and degradation

The fact that the body constituents are in a dynamic state and that proteins are constantly being synthesized, and constantly being degraded, represents a major and fundamental aspect of the metabolic function of the body. Protein synthesis is an intracellular event, and the amount and pattern of

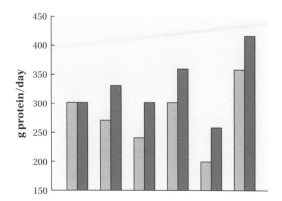

Fig. 5.2 Proteins in the body are constantly turning over (i.e. they are being synthezized and degraded). The net amount of protein is determined by the relative rates of synthesis and degradation, not the absolute rate. When the rate of protein synthesis (■) is equal to the rate of protein degradation (■), there is no change in the amount of protein (first column). Loss of protein and negative nitrogen balance will result when the relative rate of protein degradation exceeds the rate of protein synthesis. The five columns to the right show that this might be achieved either through a decrease in protein synthesis, an increase in protein degradation, or any combination of the two, at either high or low absolute rates of protein synthesis and degradation.

proteins being formed in a cell at any point in time are determined by the factors that control genomic expression, the translation of the message, and the control exerted on the activity of the synthetic machinery on ribosomes. Protein degradation is also an intracellular event and is thought to take place through three major pathways—the calcium-protease, ATP–ubiquitin, or lysozomal pathways.

In normal adults, about 4 g protein/kg body weight are synthesized each day: about 300 g protein/day in men and 250 g protein/day in women. In newborn infants, the rate is about 12 g protein/kg, falling to about 6 g/kg by 1 year of age. Basal metabolic rate is closely related to the size, shape and body composition of an individual, and the same is true for protein synthesis. In adults in a steady state, protein synthesis is matched by an equivalent rate of protein degradation, but in infancy and childhood, because of the net tissue and protein deposition associated with growth, protein synthesis exceeds protein degradation.

Dietary intake and the metabolic behaviour of the body show a diurnal rhythmicity. Food is normally ingested during the daytime. There is a diurnal pattern of nitrogen excretion in urine, which is more marked on higher protein intakes, with increased losses during the day and reduced losses during the night. On average over a 24-hour period, nitrogen equilibrium is maintained. However, as intake exceeds losses during the day and losses exceed intake during the night, there is a diurnal pattern of nitrogen balance, with balance being positive during the day and negative during the night. It is likely that nitrogen is retained in a number of forms during the day. There is evidence that protein deposition is most marked in the gastrointestinal tract, liver, and other visceral tissues, with lesser deposition in muscle. There are equivalent losses of these relatively labile pools of protein during the night. In situations of fasting or longer-term undernutrition, the early losses of protein appear to be from the liver and gastrointestinal tract, but after a short time the majority of the losses are borne by peripheral tissues such as muscle and skin.

Despite the diurnal swings in protein turnover, the effect of protein intake on the average whole-body protein synthesis is relatively modest, provided the intake exceeds the minimal dietary requirement. Below the minimal dietary requirement (about 0.66 g/kg/day), there is a relative fall in protein synthesis during the fed period.

5.7 Energy cost of protein turnover

Both protein synthesis and protein degradation consume energy, 4 kJ/g of protein of average composition. Protein degradation takes place through ATP-dependent pathways, which are both lysozomal and non-lysozomal. At the level of the whole body, the biochemical cost of peptide bond formation is estimated to be about 15–20% of the resting energy expenditure. There are additional energy costs to the body if protein turnover is to be sustained, as processes such as transport of amino acids into cells require energy. If the full energy costs of maintaining the system are included, then the physiological cost is probably in the region of 33% of resting energy expenditure.

There is a general interaction between the intake of dietary energy and nitrogen balance. Thus, although nitrogen balance and protein synthesis appear to be protected functions, modest increases in energy intake lead to positive nitrogen balance, and decreasing energy intake results in a transient negative nitrogen balance. In general, about 2 mg nitrogen is retained or lost for a change in energy intake of 4 kJ (1 kcal).

In childhood growth, net tissue deposition is a normal feature. During adulthood, the demands for net tissue formation occurs under three important circumstances: in women during pregnancy, during lactation, and during recovery from some wasting condition.

5.8 Growth

Growth consists of a complex of processes and changes in the body. There is an increase in stature and size and the proportions of the individual tissues change, resulting in changes in the composition of the body. These changes are related to the physiological maturation of function, which is an orderly series of changes in time. Maturation of function underlies development in general, and mental or intellectual development in particular. The orderly sequence of neurological maturation is directly linked into more complex behavioural changes, which under normal circumstances involve social interaction and the development of patterns of behaviour that are identified as social development.

At the level of cells and tissues, growth can be characterized as an increase in the number of cells (hypertrophy), an increase in the size of cells (hyperplasia), or a combination of the two processes (mixed hypertrophy and hyperplasia), which then leads to differentiation and specialization of function.

Net protein deposition is required for growth to take place and therefore protein synthesis must exceed protein degradation. There is an increase in protein synthesis, but there is also an increase in protein degradation, so that overall about 1.5–2.0 g protein are synthesized for every 1 g of net deposition. The apparent inefficiency of the system might be accounted for by:

1 a measure of flexibility to allow remodelling;

2 transcriptional and translational errors; and

3 wear and tear on the protein synthetic machinery.

5.9 Linear growth

Linear growth is a function of the growth and development of the long bones, and the deposition of a collagenous matrix (protein) within which the deposition of mineral crystals can take place. Ultimate adult height is determined by the genetic make-up of an individual, but at every stage of development there are factors that might operate to limit the extent to which this potential is achieved. Following an illness or deprivation, there may be recovery in height gain when the adverse influence is removed, but there may be a loss of some of the capacity for achieving the full genetic potential.

The hormones insulin, thyroid hormone, growth hormone, and insulin-like growth factors (IGFs) have all been shown to modulate linear growth within physiological ranges. Calcification is directly related to vitamin-D hormones, parathormone and osteocalcin.

An adequate intake of energy is an absolute requirement for growth, but is not in itself sufficient to achieve optimal growth in height—an adequate intake of protein and other nutrients is also required. Human and animal studies have identified a specific need for dietary protein, which is thought to have a direct effect on IGFs. Balance studies indicate the need for adequate calcium, phosphorus, zinc, and other micronutrients.

Adverse influences, such as infection, inflammation, and psychological and social factors may act either directly or indirectly, through nutritional considerations. Activity is an important trophic factor for the healthy development and calcification of bones.

Stunting, or linear growth retardation, is the major nutritional problem across the globe affecting socially and economically disadvantaged children within and between societies. There is clear evidence that stunted individuals have increased mortality from a variety of causes and an increased number of illnesses. Stunted individuals have a decrease in their physical work performance and impaired mental and intellectual function.

5.10 Protein turnover in muscle and its control

Muscle contains a large proportion of the protein in the body. Considerable interest has been shown in the growth of muscle, which is commercially important for the livestock industry. Muscle is one tissue most affected by wasting and, because it is relatively accessible, it has been the subject of more detailed study *in vivo* in humans than any other tissue. Hormones, the availability of energy and nutrients, and muscle activity (stretch) all make a contribution to the rate of muscle tissue deposition.

Protein turnover in muscle is responsive to the hormonal state. Insulin, growth hormone, and testosterone have overall anabolic effects, mainly by stimulating protein synthesis. Corticosteroids produce a decrease in synthesis and an increase in degradation. Thyroid hormones increase protein synthesis and degradation. However, at normal physiological levels they have a greater effect on synthesis than on degradation, thus exerting a net anabolic effect. At hyperthyroid levels, the increase in degradation exceeds the increase in synthesis and thus the hormone exerts an overall catabolic effect. β-Adrenergic anabolic agents such as clenbuterol promote muscle growth by decreasing protein degradation.

People on bed rest go into negative nitrogen balance and lose weight through wasting of muscle. Activity is required to maintain muscle mass and the pull of contracting muscles on bone serves to promote bone growth. Mechanical signals exert an effect on cellular function through direct effect on the intracellular cytoskeleton, through activated ion channels, and through second-messenger signal transduction processes. Prostaglandins (PGs) have a direct effect on muscle protein synthesis and degradation, with PGF_{2a} stimulating synthesis and PGE_2 stimulating degradation. The activity of phospholipase A2 makes arachidonic acid available for the synthesis of PGF_{2a} (blocked by indomethacin). The activity of phospholipase A2 is enhanced by stretch (activation of calcium) or insulin (cyclic AMP) and inhibited by glucocorticoids. Lipopolysaccharide exerts an influence on the release of arachidonic acid under the action of phospholipase A2, with the formation of PGE_2, which increases protein degradation through increased proteolysis within the lysozomes.

Stress, trauma, and surgery have all been shown to induce a negative nitrogen balance in rats and humans. In wasted individuals or people on low-protein diets, a catabolic response, with negative nitrogen balance, may not be evident. Those who do not show this response are more likely to die, giving the impression that the negative response is purposive and that under these circumstances the catabolic response is more important than conserving body protein.

5.11 Injury and trauma

Injury and trauma are characterized by an inflammatory or acute-phase response. This is a coordinated metabolic response by the body that appears to be designed to limit damage, remove foreign material, and repair damaged tissue. Under the influence of cytokines, there is a shift in the pattern of protein synthesis and degradation in the body. Substrate from endogenous sources is made available to support the activity of the immune system. In muscle, protein synthesis falls and protein degradation might increase, resulting in net loss of protein from muscle, with wasting. The amino acids made available by muscle wasting may provide substrate for protein synthesis in liver and the immune system. In the liver, there is a shift in the pattern of proteins synthesized, with a reduction in the formation of the usual secretory proteins, albumin, lipoproteins, transferrin, retinol-binding protein, and so on, and an increase in the formation of the acute-phase reactants, such as C-reactive protein, α-1-acid glycoprotein, and α-2-macroglobulin. In combination with a loss of appetite, the changes in protein turnover in liver and muscle result in a negative nitrogen balance. There is usually an increase in protein degradation overall, and the intensity of the increase is determined by the magnitude of the trauma. At the lower end of the scale, uncomplicated elective surgery is characterized by losses of less than 5 g/day. At the upper end of the scale, burn injury can lead to losses in excess of 70 g/day. The dietary intake appears to have an important influence on the extent to which protein synthesis can be maintained, and therefore the magnitude of the negative nitrogen balance and the severity of the consequent wasting.

5.12 Amino acids

The habitual dietary intake of about 80 g protein/day in adults is only one-quarter of the protein being formed in the body each day. The minimal dietary requirement for protein, about 35–40 g protein in adult men, is approximately one-tenth of the protein being formed in the body each day.

The pattern and amounts of amino acids required to support protein synthesis are determined by the amount and pattern of proteins being formed. It has been presumed that the overall pattern is dominated by proteins of mixed composition similar to that seen in muscle, but this is not necessarily true for all situations, especially in some pathological states. For example, the amino acid profile of collagen is very rich in glycine and proline, but poor in leucine and the branched-chain amino acids. During growth, where the demands for collagen formation are increased, the balance of amino acids needed is likely to be shifted towards a collagen pattern. During an inflammatory response, there is increased synthesis of the antioxidant glutathione and the zinc-binding protein metallothionein, both of which are particularly rich in cysteine. The demand for the most appropriate pattern of amino acids might vary with different situations. The nature of the demand may change from one time to another, being determined by the physiological state, such as pregnancy, lactation or growth, or the pathological state, such as infection, the response to trauma, or any other reason for an acute-phase response.

5.13 Amino acid turnover

The amino acid pool is the precursor pool from which all amino acids are drawn for protein synthesis and other pathways. It is helpful to identify the pool for each amino acid individually and to consider the general factors that are of importance (Fig. 5.3). For any amino acid, there are three inflows to the pool and three outflows. The flows from the pool to protein synthesis and other metabolic pathways represent the metabolic demand for the amino acid. Flow to amino acid oxidation is determined either by the need to use the amino acid as a source of energy, or as a degradative pathway for amino acids in excess of what can be used effectively at that point in time. This demand has to be satisfied from:

1 amino acids coming from protein degradation; or

2 *de novo* synthesis of amino acids; or

3 dietary amino acids.

It might be expected that in a steady state amino acids coming from protein degradation would represent a perfect fit for the proteins that are being synthesized, and hence there should be no general need for amino acids to be added to the system. However, this is not so. The amino acids released from protein degradation are different from those used in protein synthesis, because some amino acids are altered during the time they are part of a polypeptide chain. For example, amino acids might be methylated or carboxylated. These post-translational modifications relate to the structure and function of the mature protein. Lysine as part of a protein might be methylated to trimethyl lysine. When the protein is degraded, the released trimethyl lysine is of no value in future protein synthesis, but it can act as a metabolic precursor for the synthesis of carnitine. Carnitine plays a fundamental role in fatty acid metabolism. The endogenous formation of carnitine facilitates fatty acid oxidation and limits the need for a dietary source of carnitine, but an additional source of lysine is still needed for protein synthesis to be maintained. As lysine is an indispensable amino acid, and cannot be synthesized endogenously in quantities sufficient to satisfy the metabolic need, lysine has to be obtained preformed in the diet.

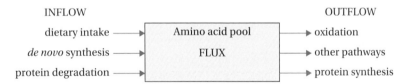

Fig. 5.3 The dynamic turnover of any amino acid in the body can be characterized by a model in which there is a single pool of an amino acid. Inflows to the pool are from three potential sources: protein degradation, the diet, and *de novo* synthesis. There are three outflows from the pool: to protein synthesis, to other metabolic pathways, and to oxidation with the breakdown of the amino acid.

5.14 Amino acid formation and oxidation

The *de novo* synthesis of an amino acid requires that its carbon skeleton can be made available from endogenous sources, and this skeleton then has an amino group effectively added in the right position. The sulphur moiety has to be added for the sulphur amino acids. In mammalian metabolism, some amino acids are readily formed from other metabolic intermediates, for example transaminating amino acids, alanine and glutamic and aspartic acids, derived from intermediates of the citric acid cycle, pyruvate, α-ketoglutarate, and oxaloacetate. These amino acids are important in the movement of amino groups around the body and also in gluconeogenesis (e.g. the glucose–alanine cycle between the liver and the periphery) or renal gluconeogenesis from glutamine during fasting. Some dispensable amino acids derive directly from an indispensable amino acid (e.g. tyrosine from phenylalanine) and the endogenous formation of the amino acid is determined by the availability of the indispensable amino acid. Methionine and cysteine are amino acids that contain a sulphydryl group, with considerable chemical activity. Although methionine can be formed in the body from homocysteine, this is part of a cycle (methionine cycle) that generates methyl groups for metabolism and in which there is no net gain of methionine (Fig. 5.4). Homocysteine has an alternative metabolic fate, towards the formation of cysteine. In this pathway, the sulphhydryl group derived from methionine is made available to a molecule of serine with the formation of cysteine; the carbon skeleton derived from methionine is subsequently oxidized. Cysteine is the precursor for taurine, which, with glycine, is required for the formation of bile salts from bile acids. Thus, cysteine can be formed in the body provided there is sufficient methionine and serine available. However, the pathway for cysteine formation has not fully matured in the newborn, making cysteine a conditionally essential amino acid at this time.

For some amino acids, the pathway for their formation appears complex and tortuous, involving a complex pathway that is shared between a number of tissues. The renal formation of arginine is an example (Fig. 5.5). Arginine is the precursor of nitric oxide, which has important metabolic functions as a neurotransmitter, in maintaining peripheral vascular tone and is one of several oxidative radicals formed during the oxidative burst of leukocytes. Arginine is also the direct precursor of urea, the main form in which nitrogen is excreted from the body. Arginine is formed in two main sites, the kidney and the liver. Arginine formed in the kidney is available for the rest of the body, whereas that formed in the liver is cleaved to urea and ornithine in the urea cycle. In both locations the arginine is

made from citrulline, but whereas in liver the citrulline is generated locally in the mitochondria, in kidney it is imported. The imported citrulline has been formed in the gastrointestinal tract, one of the end products of the oxidation of glutamine. The glutamine itself has been generated in muscle from the branched-chain amino acids. During digestion and

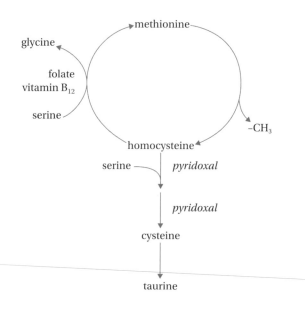

Fig. 5.4 The methionine cycle. Methionine has to be provided in the diet, and, like other amino acids, is required for protein synthesis. In addition, it has a number of other important functions. Apart from acting as a signal for protein synthesis, it is the precursor for cysteine and other reactions in which methyl groups are made available to the metabolism. In donating its methyl group, methionine forms homocysteine, which can be reformed to methionine using a single carbon group, derived either from serine or betaine (a breakdown produce of choline). Homocysteine is a branch point in metabolism as it also has another important fate, the formation of cysteine and taurine. In these pathways, the sulphydryl group is transferred to the carbon skeleton of serine. Thus, serine is used for the further metabolism of homocysteine, down either pathway. Increased amounts of homocysteine in the circulation are associated with increased risk of cardiovascular disease.

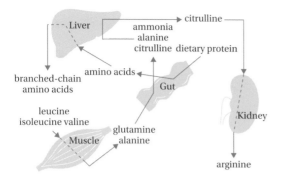

Fig. 5.5 There is a complex system of inter-organ cooperation for many aspects of amino acid metabolism and the partitioning of different functions between organs is of critical importance for effective metabolic control. Arginine is formed in significant amounts in both liver and kidney, but that formed in the liver goes to urea formation in general, whereas that formed in the kidney is exported and available for the needs of the rest of the body in, for example, the generation of nitric oxide. Arginine is formed from citrulline in the kidney, with the citrulline being derived from the gastrointestinal tract, where its formation is linked to the utilization of glutamine. Glutamine itself is formed in large amounts in muscle, in part from the breakdown of the branched-chain amino acids, leucine, isoleucine, and valine. The branched-chain amino acids coming from dietary protein are, as a group, handled in a special way; following absorption they tend to pass through the liver without being metabolized and are preferentially taken up by the muscles.

absorption of the amino acids taken in protein in a meal, most are first taken up by the liver, but more of the branched-chain amino acids pass directly through the liver and are taken up preferentially by muscle, where they give rise to glutamine. This complex pattern of metabolic interchange enables control to be exerted and, in particular, creates a mechanism through which two important sets of metabolic interaction of arginine are separated and therefore can be controlled independently.

Other amino acids, such as glycine, are required as the building blocks for more complex compounds

in relatively large amounts (haemoglobin and other porphyrins, creatine, bile salts, and glutathione), but the pathways that enable the formation of large quantities of the amino acid are not clear.

It has generally been considered that the carbon skeleton of the indispensable amino acids cannot be formed at all in the body. However, recent evidence shows that colonic bacteria synthesize these amino acids for their own use, with some being available to the host in amounts that may be physiologically useful.

In a number of inborn errors of metabolism, the enzymes involved in the oxidation of amino acids do not function normally, and there is considerable accumulation of an amino acid or its breakdown products. The extent to which the body can tolerate an excess of any single amino acid might vary, but almost always sustained, high, increased levels of amino acids in the body exert toxic effects. Therefore, the body goes to some lengths to maintain very low levels. The catabolic pathways for individual amino acids are active, although the activity may decrease on very low protein intakes. For the indispensable amino acids in particular, the amounts of individual amino acids usually found in diets are in excess of the usual requirements. This may be the reason why the body has not selected to maintain the pathways for their formation. The dietary requirement for the indispensable amino acids determines the minimal physiological requirement for protein and has been used for defining protein quality, protein requirements, and the recommendations for protein for populations. For the dispensable amino acids, the body is able to tolerate larger amounts of the amino acid, but also control can be exerted at two levels—the rate of formation and the rate of oxidation—and therefore toxicity may be less likely. On a daily basis, for a person in balance, an equivalent amount of protein or amino acids is oxidized as it is taken in the diet. Therefore, for a person consuming 80 g protein each day, the equivalent of 80 g of amino acids will be oxidized to provide energy, with the amino group going to the formation of urea. Thus, the proportion of total energy derived from protein each day is similar to the relative contribution of protein to the energy in the diet.

5.15 Nitrogen balance

About 16% of protein is amino nitrogen, and therefore by measuring this nitrogen (e.g. by the Kjeldahl method) and multiplying it by 6.25, the approximate protein content of a food or tissue can be obtained. Nitrogen balance identifies the overall relationship between the nitrogen removed from the environment for the body and the nitrogen returned to the environment. The intake is almost completely dietary, mainly as protein, but also in part as other nitrogen-containing compounds, such as nucleic acids and creatine in meat. Nitrogen can be lost from the body through a number of routes, but 85–90% is lost in urine and 5–10% in stool, with skin and hair or other losses making up the remainder. Nitrogen is lost as soluble molecules in urine as urea (85%), ammonia (5%), creatinine (5%), uric acids (2–5%), and traces of individual amino acids or proteins. There may be large losses of nitrogen through unusual routes in pathological situations (e.g. through the skin in burns, as haemorrhage or via fistulae).

$$B = I - (U + F + other)\ g\ nitrogen/day$$

where B = nitrogen balance, I = nitrogen intake, U = urinary nitrogen and F = faecal nitrogen.

The achievement of nitrogen balance in response to a change in either intake or losses is brought about largely by a change in the rate at which urea is excreted in the urine. A reduction in the dietary intake of protein is matched by an equivalent reduction in the urinary excretion in urea, which returns nitrogen equilibrium within 3–5 days. Faecal losses of nitrogen on habitual intakes are usually 1–2 g nitrogen/day, or about one-tenth of the intake. However, faecal nitrogen may increase considerably on diets that are rich in non-starch polysaccharides or fibre. There is then a reduction in the excretion of urea in urine equivalent to the increase in faecal nitrogen. Increased cutaneous losses, through excessive sweating, exudation, or burns, are associated with a proportionate decrease in urinary urea.

In a system that is constantly turning over, the retention of body protein is a necessary condition for maintaining the integrity of the tissues and tissue protein. Any limitation in the availability of energy or a specific nutrient will lead to a net loss of tissue and negative nitrogen balance through increased losses of nitrogen. Thus, the major control over the protein content of the body is established by modifications in the rate at which nitrogen is lost from the body. Balance is re-established by a change in the rate of nitrogen excretion, which for most part means a change in the rate at which urea is excreted. Therefore, it is important to consider in some detail factors that might exert control or influence over the formation and excretion of urea.

5.16 Urea metabolism and the salvage of urea nitrogen

Urea is formed in the liver in a cyclical process on a molecule of ornithine (Fig. 5.6). Within the mitochondrion, carbamyl phosphate (from ammonia and carbon dioxide) condenses with ornithine to form citrulline. The citrulline passes to the cytosol, where a further amino group is donated from aspartic acid, with the eventual formation of arginine (which has three amino groups). This is hydrolysed with the formation of urea and the regeneration of ornithine. Urea is lost to the body by excretion through the kidney. In the kidney, urea fulfils an important physiological role in helping to generate and maintain the concentrating mechanism in the countercurrent system of the loops of Henle. The rate of loss of urea through the kidney is influenced by the activity of the hormone vasopressin on the collecting ducts. Urea is reabsorbed from urine in the collecting duct, so nitrogen is potentially

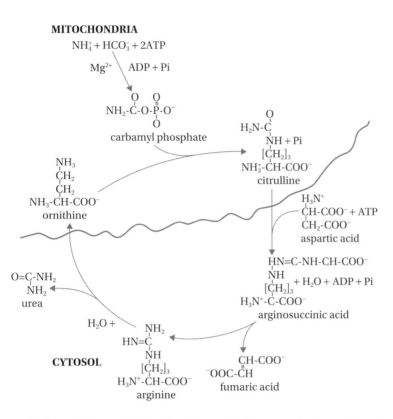

MITOCHONDRIA

$NH_4^+ + HCO_3^- + 2ATP$

Mg^{2+} ADP + Pi

carbamyl phosphate

ornithine

citrulline

aspartic acid

arginosuccinic acid

urea

CYTOSOL

arginine

fumaric acid

Fig. 5.6 The urea cycle. Urea is formed in the liver in a cyclical process between the mitochondria and the cytosol. A molecule of ornithine and the synthesis of a molecule of carbamyl phosphate from ammonia and CO_2 is the starting point with the ultimate formation of arginine, which is hydrolysed to reform ornithine and a molecule of urea. The cycle utilizes three molecules of ATP for each revolution.

retained in the system. Under all normal circumstances, more urea is formed in the liver than is excreted in the kidney. About one-third of the urea formed passes to the colon, where it is hydrolysed by the resident microflora. About one-third of the nitrogen from urea released in this way is returned directly to urea formation, but the other two-thirds are incorporated into the nitrogen pool of the body, presumably as amino acids. In other words, urea-nitrogen has been salvaged. There are specific urea transporters in the collecting duct that are upregulated on low-protein diets. Similar transporters exist in the colonocyte leading to coordinated regulation of increased retention of urea in the kidney with increased movement of urea into the colon.

In situations where the body is trying to economize on nitrogen, the proportion of urea-nitrogen lost in the urine is decreased, and the proportion salvaged through the colon is increased. This happens when the demand for nitrogen for protein synthesis increases, as in growth, or when the supply of nitrogen is reduced, as on a low-protein diet. In situations of very rapid growth, in early infancy or during catch-up from wasting conditions, the salvage of urea-nitrogen may reach very high levels, compared with the dietary intake. In normal adults, increased salvage is seen as the intake falls from habitual levels of intake (around 75–80 g protein/day) to a protein intake around the minimum requirement (35–40 g/day). On the lower protein intake, balance is maintained by a reduction in the rate of urea excretion and an increase in urea-nitrogen salvage. Below this level of protein intake, nitrogen balance is not maintained, urea excretion increases, and salvage falls. Thus, a central part of adapting to low-protein diets is an enhancement of the salvage of urea-nitrogen.

In this way, nitrogen may be retained within the system in a functionally useful form.

The optimal intake of protein is likely to be that which provides appropriate amounts of the different amino acids to satisfy the needs of the system. There is no evidence that the ingestion of large amounts of protein in itself confers any benefit. Indeed, the system may be stressed by the need to catabolize the excess amino acids that cannot be directed to synthetic pathways and have to be excreted as end products. High-protein intakes increase renal blood flow and glomerular filtration rate. In individuals with compromised renal function, this may increase the risk of further damage.

5.16.1 Low-protein therapeutic diets

The two clinical situations in which control of protein intake and metabolism are of considerable potential importance are renal failure and hepatic failure. In hepatic failure, there is a limitation in the liver's ability to detoxify ammonia through the formation of urea. In renal failure, the ability to excrete the urea is impaired. In each situation, reduction of the intake or modification of the metabolism of protein or amino acids is an important part of treatment.

5.17 The nature of protein in the diet

The majority of foods are made of cellular material and therefore in the natural state contain protein. Processing of foods may alter the amounts and relative proportions of some amino acids, for example the Maillard reaction and browning reduces the available lysine (its ε-amino group forms a bond with sugars that cannot be digested). The pattern of amino acids in animal cells is similar to the pattern in human cells and therefore the match for animal protein foods is good; plant materials may have very different patterns of amino acids. This difference has in the past led to the concept of first-class and second-class proteins, for animal and plant foods, respectively. However, diets are hardly ever made up of single foods. In most diets, different foods tend to complement each other in their amino acid pattern, so any potential imbalance is likely to be more apparent than real for most situations. Thus, the mixture of amino acids provided in most diets matches the dietary requirements for normal humans fairly well.

5.18 How much protein do we need?

5.18.1 From obligatory losses

One approach is to measure the losses of nitrogen on a protein-free diet adequate in energy. Urinary nitrogen (mostly urea) decreases rapidly for the first 5 days and then settles at a new low level. For adults, the 1973 committee of the Food and Agriculture Organization (FAO) and World Health Organization (WHO) estimated:

- urine loss: 37 mg/kg;
- faecal loss: 12 mg/kg;
- skin loss: 3 mg/kg;
- miscellaneous loss: 2 mg/kg.

This gives a total of 54 mg × 6.25, which is 0.34 g protein/kg/day.

This is an average requirement, so the recommended daily intake (RDI) (+2 standard deviations) should be 0.44 g protein/kg or 29 g protein for a 65 kg adult.

However, this assumes an impossible 100% efficiency of metabolizing dietary protein and empirically it is not possible to achieve equilibrium nitrogen balance on 29 g protein/day. When protein intake is reduced, the many enzymes of amino acid catabolism rapidly decline in activity. Metabolic conditions for absorbed amino acids are far from normal in protein starvation. However, on an ordinary diet they are actively oxidizing and transaminating the amino acids. Thus, although the factorial method using obligatory losses is useful for some other essential nutrients with simple metabolism, it cannot provide us with realistic requirement numbers for protein.

5.18.2 From nitrogen balance

International and national recommendations for protein intake are based on this method. If protein intake is insufficient, the nitrogen balance is negative (below zero or equilibrium balance). However, above an adequate protein intake the balance becomes negative for a few days, if protein intake is changed from high-adequate to moderate-adequate. This has to be allowed for by testing at intakes near the expected requirement and allowing about 5 days for adjustment at each intake level. Nitrogen balance experiments need much attention to detail. Nitrogen intakes tend to be overestimated (people do not swallow every last crumb) and nitrogen losses tend to be underestimated (some urine may be spilt; skin losses are very difficult to measure). The energy intake must neither be too much nor too little because any deviation moves the balance more positive or more negative, respectively.

Rand *et al.* (2003) selected well-designed balance experiments in healthy adults in several different countries. The protein intake was at two or more levels and near the expected requirement; each intake was for 10–14 days and only the last 5 days were used for calculating the balance. Energy intake was based on the subjects' usual diets. The subjects needed to have a quiet and unvarying life during the experiments and they lived in a special metabolic unit.

The amount of protein for nitrogen equilibrium in 235 subjects in 10 studies was estimated by meta-analysis to be 105 mg nitrogen/kg/day (×6.25 = 0.65 g protein/kg/day). However, this is an estimated

average requirement (EAR). For the RDI, 2 standard deviations were added (and here the numbers were available, not estimated) giving 132 mg nitrogen/kg or (×6.25) 0.83 g protein/kg. For someone who weighs, say, 65 kg this is 54 g protein per day. The protein should be of good quality, that is not too low in any of the indispensable amino acids.

5.18.3 Amino acid requirements

The indispensable (or essential) amino acids are not all present in the same amounts in body tissues; individual tissues differ in amino acid pattern and in turnover rates (which also affect requirements). Our foods also have different amino acid patterns, and those near to the pattern of human requirements of indispensable amino acids have the best nutritive or biological value.

The first estimates of amino acid requirements by W.C. Rose (in men) (1957), R.M. Leverton and others (in women), and S.E. Snyderman (in infants) in the 1950s used nitrogen balances. The adult subjects were usually college graduate students in the USA. They had to eat a diet of pure corn starch, sugar and syrup, butter, and oil, made into wafers or pudding, plus vitamin tablets and mineral salts. Instead of dietary protein they were given a mixture of pure L-amino acids. They were also allowed a little apple or grape juice (very low in protein), and lettuce and carrot. Average adult requirements from nitrogen balances are in Table 5.2.

In subsequent years researchers have reasoned that these requirements (from Rose, 1957) are too low. They add up to only 5.5 g, yet essential amino acids make up one-third to half the total amino acids in dietary proteins and 11–17 g protein would be quite inadequate. There were technical problems with the experiments. Rose's subjects received more dietary energy than expected. In the women's experiments, balance did not always reach equilibrium and nitrogen losses in skin were not taken into account.

Young *et al.* (1999) estimated essential amino acid requirements by an ingenious approach—biochemical evidence of increased oxidation of an

Table 5.2 Early and recent estimates of essential amino acid requirements of healthy human adults (mg/kg/day)

	N balance method (1)	^{13}C amino acid oxidation method (2)
Isoleucine	10	19
Leucine	14	42
Lysine	12	38
S-amino acids	13	19
Phenylalanine	14	33
Threonine	7	20
Tryptophan	3.5	5
Valine	10	24
Total	83.5	200

Source: (1) Joint FAO/WHO (1973) *Energy and Protein Requirements*. Report of a Joint FAO/WHO Ad Hoc Expert Committee. *WHO Tech Rep Ser*, **522**. Geneva, World Health Organization. (2) Food and Nutrition Board, Institute of Medicine (2002) *Dietary reference intakes for energy, carbohydrate, fiber, fat, fatty acids, cholesterol, protein and amino acids (macronutrients)*. Washington, DC, National Academy Press.

requirement (the indicator amino acid oxidation method; Table 5.2).

When one essential amino acid is inadequate, protein synthesis using all the amino acids is impaired, so there is both increased oxidation of all amino acids and increased urea production, increased urinary nitrogen, and negative nitrogen balance. In these stable isotope experiments, the diet also consists of protein-free starch, sugar, fat, and oil in cookies with multivitamins and minerals. The L-amino acids are given in a mixture, providing the expected requirement of all essential amino acids and also non-essential amino acids. Only the intake of the test essential amino acid is varied. Typically each experiment lasts 7 days; each subject is tested at three levels of the test amino acid. On day 7, the ^{13}C-labelled indicator amino acid (e.g. leucine) is given by constant intravenous infusion over 24 hours and $^{13}CO_2$ is collected and measured to indicate oxidation of the indicator amino acid. These experiments are very expensive and require gas chromatography mass spectrometry.

The Institute of Medicine (2002) has accepted the amino acids in the right-hand column of Table 5.2 in its dietary reference intake report for macronutrients. To grade the amino acid pattern of dietary proteins, either this pattern can be used or the amino acid pattern of whole hen's egg (which has the highest biological value of all the dietary proteins). These two amino acid patterns are similar when compared at the same total of essential amino acids.

indictor amino acid, labelled with the stable isotope ^{13}C, when intake of the test amino acid is below

5.19 How much protein do we eat?

The amount of protein eaten each day is determined by the total food intake and the protein content of the food. In general the proportion of energy derived from protein is between 11% and 15% of the total energy of the diet, which is generous for all normal purposes.

Fig. 5.7 shows the estimated amount of food available to different populations around the world on average. There is a two-fold difference overall between the technologically developed countries and the underdeveloped countries. The protein available from non-meat sources is very similar for all countries, around 50 g protein/head/day, varying by less than ±10% for the extremes. In contrast, the protein available from meat sources varied 10-fold between the extremes. Virtually all of the variation in protein availability between different countries was determined by the availability of meat protein. Within a population there are differences among individuals in the amount of protein taken.

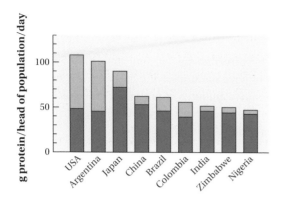

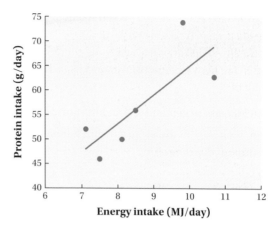

Fig. 5.7 The amount of protein available to the population can be assessed (g protein/head of population/day) and divided into meat protein (■) and non-meat protein (■). For countries of widely different characteristics, the availability of non-meat protein falls within a narrow range (within ±10%), whereas the availability of meat protein varies widely, over a 10-fold range (meat includes fish).

To a large extent this will be determined by the total food intake. Fig. 5.8 shows the relationship between protein intake and energy intake amongst a group of young women vegetarians. The proportion of energy derived from protein was similar for each woman. Those who were most active had the greatest intake of energy and the highest protein intake. Those who were relatively sedentary had a protein intake that approached the maintenance level.

In young children, energy expenditure per unit body weight is high, and therefore energy intake per unit body weight is high. In consequence, as a proportion of total energy, the dietary protein requirement for normal growth is relatively low. For example, for an infant weighing 10 kg at 1 year of age

Fig. 5.8 Under most normal circumstances, the total food intake of a person is determined by their energy expenditure, which sets their energy requirement. The energy requirement consists of a reasonably fixed component, basal metabolic rate (BMR), and a variable component, which is determined primarily by the level of physical activity. The protein content of most diets provides between 10% and 15% of dietary energy and therefore the total protein intake is closely related to the total energy intake and hence the level of physical activity. MJ, megajoules.

and growing at a normal rate, for an energy intake of 95 kcal/kg/day and a protein requirement of 1.5 g/kg/day, the proportion of total energy coming from protein would be 6.3%. The highest relative requirement for protein is in sedentary individuals. For example, for a 70-year-old woman who weighs 80 kg, who is lying relatively immobile in bed, the proportion of total energy coming from protein would have to be 20%, which is not readily achievable on a normal diet.

5.20 Dietary protein deficiency and protein-deficient states

For the diets consumed by most populations, the intake of protein is adequate, provided that the overall intake of food is not limited (e.g. by inactivity or unavailability). However, for some diets in which the density of protein to energy is low, and/or where the quality of amino acids is low, there may be situations related to relative inactivity when the ability to satisfy the protein intake is marginal.

Protein-deficient states, where the content of protein in the body is reduced, are most likely to be the result of:

- an increase in demand (e.g. in infection or stress);

- an increase in losses (e.g. with haemorrhage, burns, or diarrhoea); or

- a failure of the conservation systems (e.g. with impairment of urea salvage in the colon).

In correcting the deficient state, it is as important to remove the underlying cause as it is to provide adequate amounts of protein or amino acids in the diet. For the effects of protein-energy malnutrition in children, see Chapter 19.

5.21 Imbalance

In the midst of famine, severely undernourished people have a poorer appetite, take longer to mobilize oedema fluid, and are more likely to die when the protein content of their diet is similar to that consumed in western Europe or North America than when they are given a diet that is unusually low in protein (Collins *et al.*, 1998). In seriously shocked and traumatized individuals, intravenous protein in the form of albumin is associated with higher mortality (Cochrane Injuries Group Albumin Reviewers, 1998). Pregnant women given protein-dense diets give birth to smaller babies, and preterm infants provided with high-protein diets may have poor brain development. Proteins are consumed in the diet as a source of amino acids and nitrogen—essential for life—but when the pattern of consumption is only a poor fit for the needs of the body, the imbalance can lead to serious ill health.

5.22 Inborn errors of amino acid metabolism

There are about 100 uncommon or rare aminoacidopathies due to a genetic mutation that affects the function of an enzyme or transporter involved in the metabolism of one (or more) amino acid. The outstanding example is phenylketonuria.

5.22.1 Phenylketonuria (PKU)

The aromatic amino acid, phenylalanine, is essential for protein synthesis and also over half of it is converted by phenylalanine hydroxylase (PAH) to tyrosine, another important amino acid. When PAH is not functioning, because of a mutation of its gene on chromosome 12, phenylalanine can only go down minor pathways to phenylpyruvic acid, which passes into the urine as phenylketonuria.

PKU was discovered by Følling in 1934. In an institution for mentally retarded people the urine of a few cases gave a green colour with ferric chloride, due to phenylketone. PKU leads to irreversible, severe mental retardation unless the elevated blood phenylalanine is brought down in the first few weeks of the infant's life, and kept down throughout childhood and beyond. In developed countries all newborns are screened routinely, with a heelprick for elevated plasma phenylalanine above 250 μmol/L.

Management has to start with a low-phenylalanine milk, 'Lofenalac', and go on to low-protein natural foods plus special medical foods that are low in phenylalanine and contain extra tyrosine. The diet has to be titrated against plasma phenylalanine levels, weekly in early infancy. On the other hand, if the phenylalanine level is too low, deficiency of this essential amino acid impairs growth from protein malnutrition. Dietetic treatment of PKU is specialized and demanding for parents and child.

PKU is a Mendelian recessive, occurring in about 1 in 10 000 infants.

5.22.2 Other amino acid disorders

Cystinuria is one of the earliest recognized inborn errors of metabolism. There is a defect in transport across membranes of cystine and dibasic amino acids (lysine, arginine). The only clinical effect is urinary tract stone formation because the increased urinary cystine has low solubility. This is an uncommon cause of urinary tract stones. On microscopy of the urine, flat hexagonal crystals of cystine are diagnostic.

Homocystinuria is usually due to a defect in the enzyme that converts homocysteine, a metabolite of methionine, to cystathionine (and hence to cysteine). People with homocystinuria may have skeletal deformities, arachnodactyly, and dislocated lenses. They may also have premature vascular disease (see Chapter 21).

Hartnup disease has a pellagroid skin rash and intermittent neurological symptoms. The inherited defect is in renal transport of the neutral amino acids, so there is aminoaciduria. The most critical is loss of tryptophan. Symptoms are much improved with high dose nicotinamide and a high-protein diet. Hartnup was the name of the first family described.

Further Reading

1. **Borgonha, S., Regan, M., Oh, S.-H., Condon, M., and Young, V.R.** (2002) Threonine requirement of healthy adults, derived with a 24-hour indicator amino acid balance technique. *Am J Clin Nutr*, **75**, 698–704.

2. **Brosnan, J.T.** (2001) Amino acids, then and now—a reflection on Sir Hans Krebs' contribution to nitrogen metabolism. *IUBMB Life*, **52**, 265–70.

3. **Cochrane Injuries Group Albumin Reviewers** (1998) Human albumin administration in critically ill patients: Systematic review of randomized controlled trials. *BMJ*, **317**, 235–40.

4. **Collins, S., Myatt, M., and Golden, B.** (1998) Dietary treatment of severe malnutrition in adults. *Am J Clin Nutr*, **68**, 193–9.

5. **Joint FAO/WHO** (1973) *Energy and Protein Requirements*. Report of a Joint FAO/WHO Ad Hoc Expert Committee. *WHO Tech Rep Ser*, **522**. Geneva, World Health Organization.

6. **Food and Nutrition Board, Institute of Medicine** (2002) *Dietary reference intakes for energy, carbohydrate, fiber, fat, fatty acids, cholesterol, protein and amino acids (macronutrients)*. Washington, DC, National Academy Press.

7. **Millward, D.J., and Jackson, A.A.** (2004) Protein/energy ratios of current diets in developed and developing countries compared with a safe protein/energy ratio: Implications for recommended protein and amino acid intakes. *Public Health Nutr*, **7**, 387–405.

8. **Rand, W.M., Pellett, P.L., and Young, V.R.** (2003) Meta-analysis of nitrogen balance studies for estimating protein requirements in healthy adults. *Am J Clin Nutr*, **77**, 109–27.

9. **Rose, W.C.** (1957) The amino acid requirements of adult man. *Nutr Abst Rev*, **27**, 631–47.

10. **Stewart, G., and Smith, C.P.** (2005) Urea nitrogen salvage mechanisms and their relevance to ruminants, non-ruminants and man. *Nutr Res Rev*, **18**, 49–62.

11. **Waterlow, J.C.** (1999) The mysteries of nitrogen balance. *Nutr Res Rev*, **12**, 25–54.

12. **Young, V.R., and Ajami, A.** (1999) The Rudolph Schoenheimer Centenary Lecture. Isotopes in nutrition research. *Proc Nutrition Soc*, **58**, 15–32.

Useful Websites

To see topical and scientifically robust updates on nutrition associated with this textbook web links to many of the journals in the Further Reading sections, please see the dedicated Online Resource Centre at **http://www.oxfordtextbooks.co.uk/orc/mann4e/**

6

Energy

Andrew M. Prentice

Energy is the primary currency of nutrition. Mammals require energy to stay warm and to drive all the processes of life itself. All of this energy is derived from the chemical combustion of food, a process requiring oxygen and producing carbon dioxide and water. It is the need to maintain an adequate supply of energy that is the major stimulus of food intake, and this appetite drive has an important influence on the intake of all other nutrients.

In humans, dietary energy is derived from four major food types: carbohydrate, fat, protein, and alcohol. These are termed macronutrients and each can be composed of numerous subtypes that have a slightly different energy content. Generation of energy from the various macronutrients requires different chemical processes, and

for each of them there are optional pathways that can be used in different metabolic circumstances. For instance, glucose can initially be utilized by muscle without oxygen (anaerobically) when a short burst of movement is required, or with oxygen (aerobically) for longer periods of activity. Ultimately all energy is derived through the process of oxidative phosphorylation that occurs in mitochondria. The biochemical pathways involved in these processes are summarized elsewhere (e.g. Cox, 2005). This chapter outlines the energy value of foods and how they may be calculated, and summarizes human energy needs and how these can be measured. It concludes by briefly summarizing the mechanisms by which energy balance is regulated.

6.1 The energy value of food

6.1.1 Chemical energy

The chemical energy of food is simply the total amount of energy that would be liberated by the food if it were combusted in oxygen (i.e. its heat of

combustion). This can be measured directly in a bomb calorimeter whereby the heat liberated by burning a small sample of the food is accurately recorded. This total chemical energy of food is also referred to as its *gross energy* (GE).

6.1.2 Metabolizable energy

A portion of the GE of food is unavailable for human metabolism for a variety of reasons. First, not all of it can be digested and absorbed by the body (e.g. some components of dietary fibre, or the central parts of hard grains and nuts) and the energy will be lost in faeces. The proportion of GE that is actually absorbed across the digestive tract is termed *digestible energy* (DE). Second, even this DE is not fully available to the body because a number of the oxidative pathways are incapable of proceeding to completion. These are mostly confined to protein metabolism. For instance, amino acids are only oxidized as far as urea or ammonia. These compounds still contain energy, which is lost in the urine, and for which it is necessary to make a final adjustment in order to calculate the actual energy available for metabolism, known as *metabolizable energy* (ME).

6.1.3 Methods for assessing metabolizable energy intake

When very precise values are required in experimental studies of energy metabolism, it is possible to make direct measurements of ME, though this is extremely tiresome for the subjects and investigators alike. The method requires the accurate collection of duplicate portions of all foods consumed in proportion to the amount of each component of the diet that was eaten. Each food can then be analysed separately by bomb calorimetry, or the whole diet can be homogenized together and a small aliquot of the homogenate measured. The same process must be performed for all the faeces and urine collected

Table 6.1 Example of measuring the metabolizable energy of a diet

Subjects	
• Young women	
Methods	
• Provision of a diet of known composition over 7 days in a metabolic suite	
• Bomb calorimetry of duplicate portions of the diet and of all faeces and urine	
Measured values	
• Duplicate portions of diet (a)	9900 kJ/day
• Faeces (b)	710 kJ/day
• Urine (c)	420 kJ/day
Derived values	
• Gross energy of food (a)	9900 kJ/day
• Digestible energy (a – b)	9190 kJ/day
• Digestibility coefficient [100(a – b)/a]	92.8%
Metabolizable energy (a – b – c)	8770 kJ/day
4.184 kJ = 1 kcal	

Table 6.2 Example of calculating the metabolizable energy of a diet

Subjects		
• Young women		
Methods		
• Weighed food records over 7 days		
• Food composition tables		
• Use of Atwater factors		
– carbohydrate	17 kJ/g	
– fat	37 kJ/g	
– protein	17 kJ/g	
– alcohol	29 kJ/g	
Derived values		
• Carbohydrate	245 g/day	4165 kJ/day
• Fat	90 g/day	3330 kJ/day
• Protein	75 g/day	1275 kJ/day
• Alcohol	0 g/day	0 kJ/day
Metabolizable energy		8770 kJ/day

throughout the period that the diet is eaten. Table 6.1 gives an example of the calculations used.

The ME of diets can also be calculated if the composition of the diet is accurately known. The composition can be obtained by chemical analysis of foods, or most frequently by reference to tables of food composition, which themselves have been derived from chemical analysis of a wide range of commonly consumed foods. Many countries have their own food tables reflecting their national diet. Once the macronutrient composition of a food or diet is known, the energy content is computed using standard conversion factors (Table 6.2). These were first derived by W.O. Atwater (and hence are frequently referred to as Atwater factors) in a series of experiments with human volunteers in which the conversion factors from GE to DE to ME were determined. It should be stressed that ME values of diets derived from food tables are somewhat imprecise since there may be variations in the actual composition of listed foods and because the Atwater factors are approximate values derived from people consuming a 'standard' Western diet. It should be noted that the conversion factor for carbohydrates refers to the amount of carbohydrate in a food when expressed as available monosaccharides, since dietary fibre and nonstarch polysaccharides have a lower digestibility.

6.2 Measurement of energy expenditure

The ability to measure human energy expenditure has been important in many aspects of nutritional science, ranging from very precise studies into how energy balance is regulated, to large-scale estimations of the energy needs of populations. There are numerous techniques available, each of which has advantages and disadvantages. It is important carefully to match the technique used to the situation at hand. Table 6.3 summarizes the major methods and lists their key features.

Table 6.3 Methods for measuring human energy expenditure

Method	Measurement principle	Advantages	Disadvantages	Applications
Direct calorimetry				
Whole-body chamber	Subject confined within a small-to-moderately sized chamber. Measures heat loss.	Historically had faster response time than indirect calorimetry (now no longer true). Good environment for strictly controlled studies.	Extreme technical complexity. Very high construction and running costs. Studies confined to small subject numbers. Artificial environment.	Initially used to validate the principle of indirect calorimetry. Some distinct applications in studying heat dynamics of exercise. Now largely obsolescent.
Body suit	Subject wears an insulated metabolic suit. Measures heat loss.	As above.	As above.	As above.

Table 6.3 (*Continued*)

Method	Measurement principle	Advantages	Disadvantages	Applications
Indirect calorimetry				
Whole-body chamber	Subject confined within a small-to-moderately sized chamber. Measures oxygen consumption (and frequently also measures CO_2 production). Calculates EE from energy equivalence of oxygen consumed. Calculates macronutrient oxidation from RQ after adjustment for urinary nitrogen losses.	Very precise and repeatable. Provides minute-by-minute data. Measurements over 1–14 days. Good environment for strictly controlled studies. Measures macronutrient oxidation rates in addition to total EE. Represents gold standard.	Technically challenging. High production and running costs. Studies confined to relatively small subject numbers. Artificial environment.	Fundamental studies of the mechanisms regulating human energy balance. Includes effects of exercise, diet, physiological states such as pregnancy, and pharmacological effects of compounds intended to affect energy expenditure.
Bedside methods	Supine subject has Perspex hood placed over their head or entire bed covered with a plastic tent. Measures oxygen consumption (and frequently also measures CO_2 production). Calculations as for whole-body indirect calorimetry.	Accurate and reliable data. Commercially available versions with integrated gas meters, computers and display systems. User-friendly. Measurements possible over several hours. Good for measuring BMR. Can measure macronutrient oxidation rates in addition to total EE.	Relatively expensive. Requires periodic calibration.	Short-term studies of energy expenditure such as BMR or diet-induced thermogenesis. Can be used with hospital patients.
Ventilated hood methods	As for bedside methods, but subjects can be standing (e.g. on cycle ergometer).	As above.	As above.	As above, and for exercise studies.

(*Continued*)

Table 6.3 Methods for measuring human energy expenditure (*Continued*)

Method	Measurement principle	Advantages	Disadvantages	Applications
Douglas bag method	Subject wears mouthpiece with one-way valve and nose clip. Collects expired air directly into an impermeable 'Douglas' bag then measures volume and gas concentrations of bag contents. Calculations as for whole-body indirect calorimetry.	Simple and robust. Provides reliable results. Inexpensive.	Prompt analysis required after gas collection to avoid gas leakages and diffusion. Only suitable for short periods of study. Inconvenient and uncomfortable for subjects. Interferes with normal activity.	Short-term studies of EE such as BMR or diet-induced thermogenesis. Can be used for ambulatory studies of work and exercise. Can be used with hospital patients.
Ambulatory methods	Subject wears mouthpiece with one-way valve and nose clip, or ventilated mask, and carries gas analysis 'respirometer' strapped to their back. Measures oxygen consumption. Calculations as for whole-body indirect calorimetry but usually without CO_2 measurement and hence RQ.	Smaller and more compact than Douglas bag method. Relatively simple and robust. Yields reliable results.	Discomfort to subject after prolonged wearing of apparatus. Some versions require separate analysis of gas concentrations. Some versions are expensive.	Useful for studies of light to moderate physical activity in near-to-natural conditions.
Stable isotope methods				
Doubly labelled water	Assesses CO_2 turnover from differential rate of disappearance of ^2H and ^{18}O. Calculates EE from CO_2 production and an assumption about RQ.	Gold standard method for assessing habitual EE in free-living subjects. Measurements over 10–20 days.	^{18}O isotope is very expensive. High capital investment for mass spectrometer. Technically and mathematically challenging. Requires certain assumptions that can lead to errors if not correctly applied.	Studies of free-living EE in all subjects. Especially valuable for use in children as minimal subject cooperation is required.

Table 6.3 (*Continued*)

Method	Measurement principle	Advantages	Disadvantages	Applications
Labelled bicarbonate	Assesses CO_2 turnover from rate of disappearance constantly infused ^{13}C bicarbonate. Calculates EE from CO_2 production and an assumption about RQ.	Requires no cumbersome apparatus except for a mini-pump to infuse the bicarbonate. Can assess expenditure over a shorter time frame than doubly labelled water.	High capital investment for mass spectrometer. Technically and mathematically challenging. Requires certain assumptions that can lead to errors if not correctly applied.	Especially applicable in clinical studies where a shorter time frame is required.
Heart-rate monitoring	Electrodes collect minute-by-minute heart-rate data and store on computer chip. EE can be calculated from individual calibration curves generated for each subject, or unconverted data can be used in a semi-quantitative manner.	Inexpensive and easy to use for both subject and investigator. Provides minute-by-minute data over periods of 7 days or longer.	Calibration of each subject is a cumbersome and time-consuming process. Can become tiresome to subjects if worn for long periods.	Generally used for large-scale epidemiological studies where comparative values are more important than absolute expenditure values (for instance, in studies of activity levels and health).
Movement sensors	Sensors collect minute-by-minute movements of the body and store on computer chip. EE can be calculated from individual calibration curves generated for each subject, or unconverted data can be used in a semi-quantitative manner.	As above.	As above.	As above.

(*Continued*)

Table 6.3 Methods for measuring human energy expenditure (*Continued*)

Method	Measurement principle	Advantages	Disadvantages	Applications
Time-and-motion studies and factorial method	Daily activities are recorded by subjects themselves or by an observer. EE calculated by reference to standard tables for the energy cost of activities.	Very inexpensive if subjects record their own activities. Provides good data on types of activities.	High subject burden if self-recording. May cause alteration in activity patterns to simplify recording.	Many applications. For instance, has frequently been used (with fieldworkers doing the recording) to study work and activity patterns among farmers etc. in developing countries.

EE = energy expenditure, RQ = respiratory quotient, BMR = basal metabolic rate.
Full details of all techniques can be found in Murgatroyd *et al.* (1993).

6.2.1 Direct calorimetry

Principle Direct calorimetry, as the name implies, directly measures the *heat loss* from a subject. The first such study was conducted during a Parisian winter over two centuries ago by the father of energy metabolism, Antoine Lavoisier, when he measured the amount of water melted by a guinea pig kept in a small chamber surrounded by ice. By knowing the specific heat of melting ice, he was able to compute the heat liberated by all the metabolic processes within the animal.

Equipment Modern human direct calorimeters employ the same principle but use complex thermocouple sensors and heat exchangers to measure the subject's radiative heat loss (heat lost through radiation as from any hot object), conductive heat loss (heat carried away by air passing over the skin and warming as it does so), and evaporative heat loss (heat lost as the specific heat of evaporation of perspiration). This can be achieved in a chamber ranging in size from just large enough to cover a man on a cycle ergometer to a moderately sized room. Attempts were also made to use an insulated body suit, but this proved too cumbersome. Direct calorimeters are extremely difficult and expensive to construct. Their main function has been to

demonstrate that indirect calorimetry (which measures *heat production*; see below) gives precisely the same answers. There is a slight lag period between heat production and heat loss due to the temporary storage of heat in the body (for instance, when exercising a subject will become hot and some of the heat produced will take some minutes to exit the body as it cools down again). However, as long as time lag is accounted for, the two methods give precisely the same result. Because of the technical complexity of direct calorimeters, no more than a handful are still in commission worldwide.

6.2.2 Indirect calorimetry

Principle Indirect calorimetry measures *heat production* by assessing oxygen consumption and (optionally) carbon dioxide production. Variations between different versions of the technique essentially come down to the method by which the exhaled respiratory gases are collected from the subject (Table 6.3). In one form or another, indirect calorimetry is now the usual method for measuring human energy expenditure. It is much easier to perform than direct calorimetry and is less expensive. It can also be used to estimate the relative contribution of each of the macronutrients to the total energy expenditure—a major advantage over direct calorimetry.

Table 6.4 Constants used in indirect calorimetry

	Fat	Carbohydrate[a]	Protein	Alcohol
Oxygen consumption (L/g)	2.101	0.746	0.952	1.461
Carbon dioxide production (L/g)	1.492	0.746	0.795	0.974
Respiratory quotient	0.710	1.000	0.835	0.667
Energy equivalence of oxygen (kJ/L)	19.61	21.12	19.48	20.33
Energy density (kJ/g)	39.40	15.76	18.55	29.68

[a]As monosaccharide equivalents.

Table 6.4 lists the basic constants used to calculate energy expenditure by indirect calorimetry. The most important of these are the energy equivalence of each litre of oxygen consumed, which ranges between 19.48 kJ/L for protein and 21.12 kJ/L for carbohydrate—a difference of 8%. However, the body rarely combusts single macronutrients and for most practical purposes it can be assumed that it is combusting a mixture of fuels, similar to the diet that a person is consuming, and therefore a generalized value of 20.3 kJ/L oxygen is frequently used. In most circumstances, this assumption will lead to an error of less than 3%. To achieve a greater accuracy, as would be required for detailed physiological studies of human energy regulation, it is necessary also to measure carbon dioxide production to calculate the *respiratory quotient* (RQ = carbon dioxide produced/oxygen consumed) and the urinary nitrogen output in order to estimate protein oxidation. If alcohol has been consumed, it is further necessary to estimate its contribution to energy expenditure by making separate measurements of the rate of decline of blood alcohol levels. Once all these variables are known, it is possible to use the precise values for the energy equivalence of oxygen.

Indirect calorimetry can be used to assess the mixture of fuels oxidized as follows. First, since protein and alcohol oxidation can be assessed as described above, it is possible to calculate their contributions to a subject's total oxygen consumption and carbon dioxide production using the values in Table 6.4. The remaining gas exchange is due to carbohydrate and fat oxidation and can be expressed as the nonprotein, nonalcohol RQ (frequently termed the nonprotein RQ (NPRQ) since most measurements are made in the absence of alcohol consumption). The following equation shows that the RQ for carbohydrate (glucose) oxidation is precisely 1.0 since 1 mole of carbon dioxide is liberated for each mole of oxygen consumed:

$$C_6H_{12}O_6 + 6O_2 = 6CO_2 + 6H_2O + heat$$

A similar calculation can be performed for fatty acid oxidation (e.g. palmitic acid, $C_{16}H_{34}O_2$) and reveals that the average for different fats yields an RQ of 0.701 (Table 6.4). Thus, if the NPRQ is calculated to be 1.00, then only carbohydrate is being combusted, and if it is 0.701 then only fat is being combusted. Values between these indicate that a mixture of fat and carbohydrate is being combusted, the proportions of which can be calculated from nomograms or simultaneous equations. These are the basic principles. In practice there are many complexities to the calculations and many special circumstances when adjustments must be made in order to obtain correct estimates. Readers interested in applying the techniques are referred to more advanced texts, such as that by Livesey and Elia (1988).

Equipment Table 6.3 lists the various types of equipment that can be used for indirect calorimetry, together with their major advantages and disadvantages.

The classic (now rarely used) method uses the Douglas bag (Fig. 6.1). This is a large bag (usually with a 100-litre volume) that is impermeable to gases. The subject wears a nose clip and breathes through a mouthpiece connected to a one-way valve that allows them to inhale fresh air and exhale into the bag. At the end of the experiment—which has to be short (up to 15 minutes) because of limited capacity in the bag—the volume of expired air is measured with a gas meter. The oxygen and carbon dioxide contents are analysed. Oxygen consumption is calculated from the difference between oxygen in the ambient (inspired) and expired air, multiplied by the ventilation rate.

For short-term measurements during exercise, the Kofrani–Michaelis respirometer used to be used (Fig. 6.1) because it measures expired air volume as it is produced, and therefore only a small sample of the expired air needs to be retained for subsequent gas analysis. New generations of these machines with similar working principles include the Oxylog and Cosmed K2. These portable respirometers were designed for short-term measurements at rest and during exercise in 'field' situations but can also be used in laboratory settings.

Ventilated hood systems (Fig. 6.1) avoid the discomfort of a face mask. With this equipment, air flows over the subject's head (which is within a transparent Perspex or plastic hood) while they lie or sit quietly. The system is suited for situations in which the subject's gas exchange is measured in a laboratory or hospital setting for periods of between 30 minutes and several hours. There are a number of commercially available ventilated hood systems specially designed for use in a hospital setting.

Whole-body calorimeters (also called respiration chambers) represent the most sophisticated option and are chiefly used for detailed physiological experiments. Whole-body calorimeters are furnished airtight rooms (frequently about 10–15 m^3) in which subjects can live for periods of 1–14 days. Respiratory gas exchange is measured continuously using small samples of air drawn from the inlet and outlet vents of the chamber. Subjects can carry out all the activities of a relatively sedentary life, as well as controlled exercise on a cycle ergometer or tread-mill. Food and drink are passed in through one air-lock and waste products out through another. Whole-body calorimeters are extremely accurate and precise.

6.2.3 Isotopic tracer methods

Doubly labelled water method

Principle The disadvantage of the methods described above is that none of them can capture information on the total habitual energy expenditure of someone living their normal life. In the mid-1980s it became possible to do this using the doubly labelled water ($^2H_2{}^{18}O$) method (Speakman and Nagy, 1997).

The principle of the method is illustrated in Fig. 6.2. The subject drinks an accurately weighed amount of water labelled with the harmless, nonradioactive isotopes of deuterium (^2H) and oxygen-18 (^{18}O) and then provides a series of saliva or urine samples for the next 10–20 days (the optimal duration depends on their activity level). These are analysed by mass spectrometry to assess the disappearance of the isotopes from the body (Fig. 6.3). The ^2H labels the body's water pool, and its disappearance from the body (k_2) provides a measure of water turnover (rH_2O). The ^{18}O labels both the water and the bicarbonate pools, which are in rapid equilibrium with each other. The disappearance of ^{18}O (k_{18}) provides a measure of the combined turnover of water and bicarbonate ($rH_2O + rCO_2$). Therefore, bicarbonate turnover can be calculated by difference ($k_{18} - k_2$) and is equivalent to the subject's carbon dioxide production rate. The value $k_{18} - k_2$ is represented by the difference in slope between the two isotope disappearance curves shown in Fig. 6.3. Carbon dioxide production can be converted to energy expenditure using classical indirect calorimetric calculations.

In practice, there are many theoretical and mathematical complications in the technique, but these can be overcome by using appropriate procedures, and the method has been cross-validated against energy expenditure measured within a whole-body

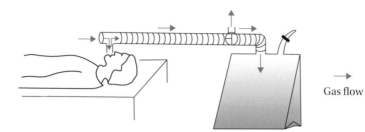

The Douglas bag

Gas flow

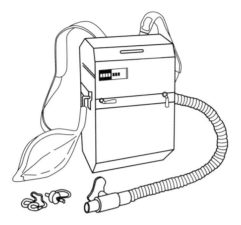

The Kofrani–Michaelis respirometer

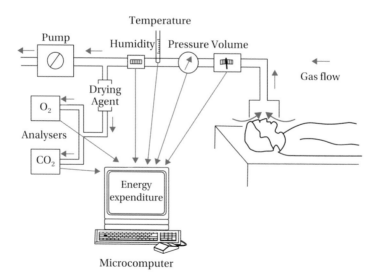

A ventilated-hood indirect calorimeter

Fig. 6.1 Most commonly used devices for indirect calorimetry.

Source: Garrow, J.S., and James, W.P.T. (eds) (1993) *Human nutrition and dietetics*, 9th edition. Edinburgh, Churchill Livingstone.

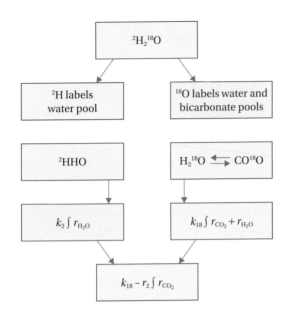

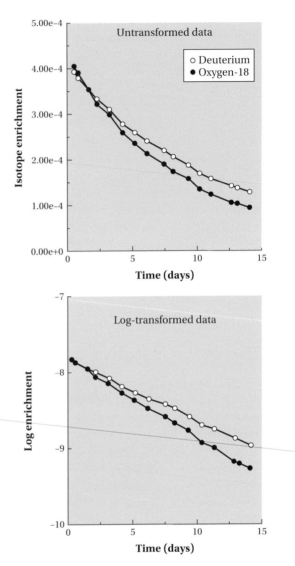

Fig. 6.2 Principle of the doubly labelled water. Production rates are represented by r and rate constants (calculated from the slope of the isotope disappearance curves shown in Fig. 5.3) are represented by k.

Source: Murgatroyd, P.R., Shetty, P.S., and Prentice, A.M. (1993) Techniques for the measurement of human energy expenditure: a practical guide. *Int J Obesity*, 17, 549–68.

chamber. It is now recognized as the gold standard method for assessing total energy expenditure (TEE) in freeliving people. By combining it with an assessment of basal metabolic rate (BMR), it becomes possible to estimate the energy costs of activity and thermogenesis (A&T = TEE − BMR) and as thermogenesis represents a small and rather constant proportion of A&T, in practice it provides a good measure of a person's activity level.

Equipment Doubly labelled water measurements require a mass spectrometer to analyse the levels of ^2H and ^{18}O. Because ^{18}O is so costly, it is necessary to use very small amounts that only raise the subject's levels a little above the natural background level. Hence, the mass spectrometer has to be extremely precise and the measurements are technically challenging. There are only a few specialist centres

Fig. 6.3 Examples of isotope disappearance curves from the doubly labelled water method.

Source: Murgatroyd, P.R., Shetty, P.S., and Prentice, A.M. (1993) Techniques for the measurement of human energy expenditure: a practical guide. *Int J Obesity*, 17, 549–68.

worldwide with the capacity to do the measurements and computations.

Labelled bicarbonate method

Principle The principle of the labelled bicarbonate method is similar to the doubly labelled water method insofar as it assesses carbon dioxide production from the rate of turnover of the body's bicarbonate pool. In the labelled bicarbonate method, this is achieved through a constant subcutaneous infusion of ^{13}C-labelled bicarbonate using a minipump strapped to the subject. As with doubly labelled water, samples of urine or saliva can be used to assess ^{13}C levels, which reach a steady state at a level proportional to the rate at which the subject's carbon dioxide production washes out the infused label. The method is suitable for relatively short-term assessments of up to about 24 hours and is ideally suited for use in hospitalized patients. In practice, however, this method has been rarely used.

Equipment The method requires a mass spectrometer capable of assessing ^{13}C enrichment.

6.2.4 Heart rate methods

Principle There is a linear relationship between energy expenditure and heart rate for all levels of expenditure above resting levels. The slope and intercept of this relationship vary among individuals according to age, sex, and fitness levels, so must be determined in each person by a calibration experiment using a treadmill or cycle ergometer in which heart rate can be measured at different work rates. Once this is known, it is possible to convert records of a person's heart rate into an estimate of TEE. The method has been validated within whole-body calorimeters and shown to have little bias, and hence is excellent for assessing group values. However, its precision is limited to about ±1 MJ per day. It should be noted that heart rate traces can provide very reliable assessments of activity patterns and of interindividual differences without actually having to convert the output into energy expenditure. This is true also of the actometers described below.

Equipment There are various commercially available ambulatory heart rate monitors that can be worn by a subject for long periods and that collect minute-by-minute data on a computer chip.

These data can be uploaded straight into software that computes energy expenditure.

6.2.5 Movement sensors (actometers)

Principle The principle of actometers is very similar to that for heart rate but a measure of movement in three dimensions (so called 'tri-axial') is substituted for heart rate. Modern actometers are an advance over simple instruments such as pedometers because they can capture movement in all directions and can assess the intensity of movement. As with heart rate, it is necessary to calibrate each individual against an alternative indirect calorimetric procedure in order to calculate energy expenditure.

Equipment There are a number of commercially available ambulatory actometers that operate in a similar way to heart rate monitors by accumulating minute-by-minute data over periods of up to a week.

6.2.6 Time-and-motion studies

Principle Frequently it is desirable just to obtain a relatively rough-and-ready estimate of peoples' energy expenditure, for instance to estimate a population's average energy requirements. Time-and-motion studies (often called activity diaries) can be used for this purpose. If subjects are literate, they can be asked to record their own activity patterns over short intervals (e.g. 5 or 15 minutes) throughout the day. It is necessary to have illiterate subjects followed and observed by trained field workers. Each activity is then ascribed an energy cost from standard tables. It will be appreciated that there are many approximations involved in such a process and it also carries a high burden for the subjects that can lead to inaccurate record keeping. In its most approximate form, this sort of calculation is used by the World Health Organization (WHO) and Food and Agriculture Organization (FAO) in their system for calculating the estimated average energy requirements of a population (FAO/WHO/UNU, 2004; James and Schofield, 1990).

Equipment The method only requires record sheets, a watch, and tables of the energy cost of different activities.

6.3 Human energy needs

The body's energy needs can be divided into three main components: basal metabolism, diet-induced thermogenesis, and physical activity. Children, or adults recovering from illness and weight loss, require additional energy for the growth of new tissue, and pregnant and lactating women require additional energy to sustain the growth of their offspring.

6.3.1 Basal metabolism

Definition Basal metabolism represents the energy required to sustain the basic processes of life, which include breathing, circulation, tissue repair and renewal, and ionic pumping. In humans, basal metabolism generally produces enough heat to maintain thermoregulation without any need to specifically generate additional heat. In most people (except the very active), basal metabolism is the largest component of daily energy expenditure, representing up to 70% of all energy used.

Measurement BMR is a specific term that describes energy expenditure measured under the following highly standardized conditions: subjects should be lying completely still and should be emotionally relaxed immediately after waking in the morning; they must have fasted for the previous 12–14 hours and must not have performed heavy physical activity on the previous day; they must be healthy and free from fever; and the measurement must be made at thermoneutral temperature. The great advantage of applying such standardized conditions is that it permits comparisons among individuals and among different studies. Measurements made under similar conditions, but not quite

meeting all of the above stipulations, are frequently referred to as resting metabolic rate. BMR is most frequently measured using a ventilated hood system but can also be assessed easily as part of a whole-body calorimetry protocol. The results as kJ/minute are frequently multiplied up over 24 hours and expressed as MJ/day. Because BMR is relatively predictable on the basis of a subject's age, sex, weight, and height, a number of predictive equations are available from which a reasonable approximation on a person's BMR can be obtained without having to measure it (Table 6.5) (FAO/WHO/UNU, 2004; James and Schofield, 1990).

Factors affecting basal metabolism An individual's BMR is largely determined by their body size and body composition, and differences in these variables can explain the fact that women have a lower BMR than men and that BMR declines with age. The major determinant of BMR is the amount of lean tissue (often referred to as lean body mass (LBM) or fat-free mass, since this is much more metabolically active than adipose tissue. BMR is therefore frequently expressed per kg LBM. Muscle is the major contributor to lean tissue, and in its resting basal state it has a moderately high energy expenditure. Visceral organs, especially the heart and liver, have an even higher metabolic rate, and hence the total basal metabolism is determined also by the composition of the lean tissue in terms of the proportion of muscle to visceral organ mass. On average, women have a lower BMR than men because they are smaller and, even if matched for weight, they have a lower proportion of lean tissue than men. Older people have a lower BMR because ageing is associated with a gradual substitution of lean tissue by fat. BMR is high in children largely

Table 6.5 Equations for estimating BMR from body weight

Age (years)	No.	BMR (MJ/day)	SEE	BMR (kcal/day)	SEE
Males					
<3	162	0.249 kg – 0.127	0.292	59.512 kg – 30.4	70
3–10	338	0.095 kg + 2.110	0.280	22.706 kg + 504.3	67
10–18	734	0.074 kg + 2.754	0.441	17.686 kg + 658.2	105
18–30	2879	0.063 kg + 2.896	0.641	15.057 kg + 692.2	153
30–60	646	0.048 kg + 3.653	0.700	11.472 kg + 873.1	167
≈60	50	0.049 kg + 2.459	0.686	11.711 kg + 587.7	164
Females					
<3	137	0.244 kg – 0.130	0.246	58.317 kg – 31.1	59
3–10	413	0.085 kg + 2.033	0.292	20.315 kg + 485.9	70
10–18	575	0.056 kg + 2.898	0.466	13.384 kg + 692.6	111
18–30	829	0.062 kg + 2.036	0.497	14.818 kg + 486.6	119
30–60	372	0.034 kg + 3.538	0.465	8.126 kg + 845.6	111
≈60	38	0.038 kg + 2.755	0.451	9.082 kg + 658.5	108

Weight is expressed in kg.

SEE, standard error of the estimate.

Source: FAO/WHO/UNU (2004) *Human energy requirements. FAO Technical Report Series 1*. Rome, Food and Agricultural Organization.

because they have a higher proportion of visceral organ mass to total mass.

BMR declines when people are in negative energy balance. There are two components to this decline. The first is a decrease (of up to 20%) in the metabolic rate per kg LBM; this is an adaptive mechanism to spare energy in starvation and is mediated by alterations in thyroid status. The second is due to the fact that LBM itself declines with longer-term energy deficiency. There has been considerable controversy for over a century as to whether BMR is increased when people overconsume energy, and whether this constitutes a homeostatic mechanism ('adaptive thermogenesis') for stabilizing body weight. The current consensus, based on detailed whole-body calorimeter studies and doubly labelled water measurements is that such a mechanism does not exist, and that any increases in BMR can be accounted for by the increase in lean tissue mass that occurs with overfeeding.

BMR also changes as women pass through the various phases of reproduction and it even alters by a few per cent during the menstrual cycle. In pregnancy, BMR increases in proportion to the amount of new tissue accrued by the mother in the form of the fetus, placenta, and uterus. In thin women and in those short of food in pregnancy, BMR is suppressed in the early stages of gestation; this appears to be an adaptation to help women reproduce in marginal conditions.

Certain stimulants (e.g. caffeine) and pharmacological agents (e.g. ephedrine) also affect BMR. Drug companies have been trying to develop compounds that will increase metabolic rate as possible anti-obesity agents (e.g. through stimulating the β3-adrenoreceptors) but so far they have either had minimal effects in humans or have had unacceptable side effects on heart rate or blood pressure.

Certain clinical conditions also affect BMR, especially fevers. Alterations in thyroid function can have a pronounced effect on BMR: hypothyroidism decreases BMR and hyperthyroidism increases it. Before specific hormone assays were available, measurements of BMR were widely used in the diagnosis of thyroid disorders.

6.3.2 Diet-induced thermogenesis

Definition Diet-induced thermogenesis (DIT), often also called the thermic effect of food, represents the additional energy required to absorb, digest, transport, interconvert, and store the constituents of a meal. This is wasted energy that must be lost because no physiological process can be 100% efficient. It amounts to under 10% of total intake.

Experimental approach DIT is usually measured using a ventilated hood. With subjects resting, fasting energy expenditure is first measured for a short period in order to establish their baseline. Then they are fed a standard test meal and remain under the hood for a further 3–4 hours. Energy expenditure increases as the body processes the meal and then declines back to the initial baseline. DIT is assessed as the incremental area under the curve for energy expenditure.

Factors affecting diet-induced thermogenesis DIT is affected by the size and composition of the meal consumed. Protein tends to cause a higher DIT than fat and carbohydrate, though in practice these differences are trivial within the normal range of the mixed diets consumed by humans.

6.3.3 Physical activity

Definition Energy expenditure caused by movements or performing physical work is generally classified under the overall heading of physical activity. This includes both conscious movements and subconscious ones (fidgeting).

Experimental approach The energy expended on standardized activities, such as walking at a fixed pace on a treadmill or cycling on a cycle ergometer, can be measured by Douglas bag, or a portable respirometer or in a whole-body chamber. Everyday activities are usually measured using a portable respirometer and in the past these have been used for numerous studies of occupational physical activity, such as farming, factory work, and coal mining. Tables have been compiled that summarize these values, together with values for the energy costs of the everyday activities of life, and these can be used to make an approximation of a person's total energy expenditure (Durnin and Passmore, 1967; FAO/WHO/UNU, 2004). The energy cost of activities is usually expressed as kJ/minute, or as a multiple of BMR (termed the physical activity level (PAL)). The advantage of the latter is that it makes an automatic internal adjustment for differences between subjects of different weights, sexes, and ages, since these variables are already factored into the BMR.

Factors affecting the energy costs of physical activity Clearly the total cost of physical activity is largely dependent on the amount of activity a person chooses to undertake. Within this, the specific cost of the individual activities will be influenced by the person's size, the speed of the activity, the times taken resting, the skill with which the activity is performed, and the efficiency of the muscles. Perhaps surprisingly, the efficiency with which muscles can convert food energy (glucose and fatty acids) into useful work is very constant among individuals and averages only about 25%.

The energy cost of weight-bearing activities such as walking up stairs or uphill is directly proportional to a person's body weight, but in non-weight-bearing activities such as cycling a person's body weight has less influence on the overall energy cost.

Differences in physical activity represent the major source of variability in the energy needs of different people. At the lowest end of the range are the bed-bound sick and the very elderly. These will have a PAL of about $1.35 \times$ BMR. At the other end of the range are elite endurance athletes such as Tour de France cyclists who can sustain PAL values of almost $3 \times$ BMR. People in the developing world who are engaged in hard physical labour, for instance at the peak of the farming season, sustain activity levels equivalent to about $2 \times$ BMR. In modern society where sedentary occupations are combined with very inactive leisure time pursuits such as TV viewing, the average PAL is around $1.55 \times$ BMR. Children tend to have spontaneously high levels of energy expenditure (often up at about $1.8 \times$ BMR) that decline as they go through puberty, especially in girls.

6.3.4 Growth

Maintaining an adequate energy intake is essential at times of growth, and energy deficiency leads to stunting, wasting, and ultimately to severe malnutrition (see Chapter 19). In fact, in humans the marginal energy costs of growth (i.e. over and above the other daily energy needs) are surprisingly small because human growth is extraordinarily slow—an evolutionary adaptation that allows plenty of time for the growth, organization, and training of our large brain. Growth is fastest in the fetus, the very young neonate, and during the adolescent growth spurt, but even at these periods the energy required for normal growth rarely exceeds 5% of the daily energy need.

Faster tissue deposition rates than these can occur in people recovering from a severe illness, from severe childhood malnutrition, or from starvation. These very rapid rates are often accompanied by an inappropriate composition of new tissue with a higher proportion of fat tissue than is desirable. Generally these deviations in body composition are corrected naturally after several months of weight stability. Growing children may also show episodic growth, particularly those in developing countries who are frequently affected by infections. During the recovery phase after an illness, children can have very high energy needs. These are often not met by poor-energy and protein-deficient diets in developing countries, leading to a gradual falling away from optimal growth rates and nutritional status.

6.3.5 Pregnancy and lactation

The marginal extra energy costs of pregnancy and lactation are also quite low in humans due to the slow growth of the offspring. In pregnancy, a mother requires only around 10% extra energy, and in lactation only about 25% (see Chapter 32 for more detail). There is good evidence that when women are short of energy they display a range of energy-sparing mechanisms, both metabolic and behavioural, that can help ensure the success of reproduction.

6.4 Mechanisms for regulating energy balance

Energy balance is a dynamic state that constantly alters between positive deviations during meals and negative deviations during the intervals between meals. The challenge for the body is to ensure that these small deviations cancel out over time (except during periods of intentional growth when a slight positive energy balance is required). This regulation is achieved largely in the hypothalamus, which receives a wide range of neural and endocrine signals from the rest of the body; it integrates these through a complex network of interacting neural pathways. The

hypothalamus then sends efferent neural signals to regulate appetite and energy expenditure. The short-term signals indicating energy sufficiency include blood glucose, amino acid, and fatty acid levels, together with stomach- and gut-derived hormones, and vagal signals from the liver. The long-term signals consist of hormones secreted by adipose tissue in proportion to the amount of fat that is stored there. Primary among these is leptin. Plasma concentrations of leptin are directly proportional to fat stores, but are also strongly influenced by the direction of change in the fat stores. Leptin acts as the body's fuel gauge, allowing the brain to assess its energy reserves and their rate of change and hence it plays a vital role in regulating appetite and energy expenditure, tissue growth, reproduction, and various other physiological processes.

It used to be thought that differences in energy expenditure were major determinants of a person's energy balance. For instance, over several decades there was a popular theory that obese people must have extraordinarily efficient metabolisms and low energy requirements. In the reverse direction, it was thought that many weight-losing clinical conditions such as AIDS and Alzheimer's disease were caused by a hypermetabolism that raised energy needs. Studies using the doubly labelled water method have now shown that there is little truth in these theories and that most deviations in energy balance can be traced to differences in food intake. Most differences in energy expenditure can be adequately explained by differences in age and reproductive state, body size, body composition, and physical activity levels. There is, however, some flexibility in the efficiency of energy expenditure, particularly in times of weight loss or starvation, when metabolic rate can decline by about 20%.

This realization that most of the regulation of energy balance is achieved on the intake side of the energy balance equation has had a profound impact on research in the field, and there has been astonishing progress over the past decade in understanding the neurohormonal regulation of appetite. There is still much to be learnt about how these longer-term regulatory mechanisms modulate the influence of short-term internal appetite cues (such as low glucose levels or surges in the appetite-stimulating hormone, ghrelin) and external appetite cues (such as the sight and smell of food or advertising). Nonetheless, these advances hold great promise for the development of therapeutic compounds to assist in the treatment of conditions such as obesity and anorexia nervosa.

Further Reading

1. **Blaxter, K.** (1989) *Energy metabolism in animals and man.* Cambridge, Cambridge University Press.
2. **Cox, S.** (2005) Energy: Metabolism. In: Caballero, B., Allen, L.H., and Prentice, A.M. (eds) *Encyclopedia of human nutrition*, 2nd edition. London, Elsevier. pp. 106–14.
3. **Durnin, J.V.G.A. and Passmore, R.** (1967) *Energy, work and leisure.* London, Heinemann.
4. **FAO/WHO/UNU** (2004) *Human energy requirements. FAO Technical Report Series 1.* Rome, Food and Agricultural Organization.
5. **Garrow, J.S. and James, W.P.T.** (eds) (1993) *Human nutrition and dietetics*, 9th edition. Edinburgh, Churchill Livingstone.
6. **James, W.P.T. and Schofield, E.C.** (1990) *Human energy requirements: A manual for planners and nutritionists.* Oxford, Oxford University Press.
7. **Livesey, G., and Elia, M.** (1988) Estimation of energy expenditure, net carbohydrate utilization, and fat oxidation and synthesis by indirect calorimetry: Evaluation of errors with special reference to the detailed composition of fuels. *Am J Clin Nutr*, **47**, 608–28.
8. **Murgatroyd, P.R., Shetty, P.S., and Prentice, A.M.** (1993) Techniques for the measurement of human energy expenditure: A practical guide. *Int J Obesity*, **17**, 549–68.
9. **Speakman, J.R. and Nagy, K.** (1997) *Doubly-labelled water: Theory and practice.* Amsterdam, Kluwer Academic.

Useful Websites

To see topical and scientifically robust updates on nutrition associated with this textbook and web links to many of the journals in the Further Reading sections, please see the dedicated Online Resource Centre at **http://www.oxfordtextbooks.co.uk/orc/mann4e/**

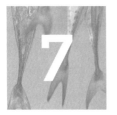

7 Alcohol

Stewart Truswell

Alcohol is the only substance that is both a drug affecting brain function and a nutrient (sometimes providing 5–10% of people's calorie intake). It is dispensed with food, not in a pharmacy. Alcohol is associated with happy times—weddings and celebrations; it is also a cause of misery. The dose determines the effect!

Alcohol is normally consumed not pure ('neat') but in aqueous solution in alcoholic beverages that were first developed thousands of years ago. Beer was first drunk by the Sumerians and Babylonians, around 4000 years ago and has been brewed ever since. Wine is mentioned occasionally in the Old Testament (in Genesis 9, Noah planted a vineyard and got drunk), and was important in the life of classical Greece and Rome. It featured in Jesus' first miracle at the marriage feast in Cana and at his last supper, and passed into the central part of the Christian mass. Alcoholic beverages were also developed in prehistoric times in East Asia, e.g. sake fermented from rice, and in Africa beers from fermented millet or maize. Alcoholic beverages were thus independently discovered in different parts of the world by prehistoric sedentary agriculturalists who were growing barley, rice, or grapes. But the indigenous peoples of Oceania (Polynesians and Australian Aborigines) and of America (American Indians) did not know alcohol until the arrival of the Europeans and had not established ways of using and controlling it.

From the basic fermented beverages alcohol can be concentrated by the process of distillation (which was brought to Europe by the Arabs). Brandy and whisky first appeared in the fifteenth century.

7.1 Production of alcoholic beverages

Alcohol is produced by alcoholic fermentation of glucose. The specific enzymes are provided by certain yeasts, *Saccharomyces*. The biochemical pathway first follows the usual 10 steps of anaerobic glycolysis to pyruvate, as in animal metabolism (see Chapter 3). Yeast contains the enzyme, pyruvate decarboxylase, not present in animals. This converts pyruvate to acetaldehyde, then alcohol dehydrogenase converts acetaldehyde to ethanol. The overall reaction is:

$$C_6H_{12}O_6 + cofactors + ATP \rightarrow 2\ C_2H_5OH + 2CO_2$$

Grapes are unusual among fruits in containing a lot of sugar, nearly all glucose (around 16%), so providing an excellent substrate for alcoholic fermentation. Starch is a polymer of glucose. Before it can ferment to alcohol it has to be hydrolysed to its constituent glucose units. Beers are made by malting the starch in barley. To do this the barley is spread out, moist and warm, and allowed to germinate for several days. Enzymes are generated in the sprouting grain that break down the stored starch into glucose. The barley is then heated and dried. This kills the embryo, which stops using sugar. For *sake* the starch is in rice. It is first treated with a mould, *Aspergillus oryzae*, that grows on the rice and secretes an amylase to yield glucose.

Beer contains around 5% alcohol (unless alcohol-reduced), wines contain around 10% alcohol (unless fortified) and spirits are about 30% alcohol. Alcoholic beverages also contain variable amounts of unfermented sugars and dextrins (in beers), small amounts of alcohols other than ethyl (e.g. propyl alcohol), moderate amounts of potassium, almost no sodium, small amounts of riboflavin and niacin but no thiamin, and sometimes vitamin C. They also contain a complex array of flavour compounds, colours (natural anthocyanins in red wines), phenolic compounds, a preservative (e.g. sodium metabisulphite), and sometimes additives. A standard drink (e.g. ½ pint beer, see Table 7.1) provides 10 g of ethanol.

Table 7.1 Volume of various alcoholic beverages providing approximately 10 g ethanol

Type of drink	Usual % ethanol[a] v/v (by volume)	Vol. that provides approx. 10 g ethanol
Low alcohol beer	2–3%	568 ml = 1 (UK) pint = 20 oz
Average beer	4–5%	285 ml = 1/2 (UK) pint = 10 oz
Average wine[b]	10%	120 ml = 4 oz
Fortified wine (e.g. sherry, port)	20%	60 ml = 2 oz
Spirits (e.g. whisky, gin, vodka, brandy)	40%	30 ml = 1 oz

[a]*Note:* These are approximations. The exact percentage of alcohol should be on the label of the bottle. The specific gravity of ethanol is 0.790. To convert to g/100 ml multiply by 0.79 (or 0.8).
[b]Wine bottles usually contain 750 ml = 6¼ standard drinks.

7.2 Metabolism of alcohol

Ethanol is readily absorbed unchanged from the jejunum; it is one of the few substances that is also absorbed from the stomach. It is distributed throughout the total body water (moving easily through cell membranes), so that after having one drink its 10 g of alcohol is diluted in about 40 litres of water in an adult, giving a peak concentration of 0.025 g/dL in the blood and in the rest of body water. For comparison, the permitted limit of blood alcohol for driving in many countries is double this—0.05 g/dL (11 mmol/L)—and the driving limit varies from 0.02 g/dL in Sweden to 0.08 g/dL in the British Isles (Fig. 7.1). Alcohol is nearly all metabolized in the liver, but a small amount is already metabolized as it passes through the stomach wall (first pass metabolism). A small amount of alcohol passes unchanged into the urine and an even smaller (but diagnostically useful) amount is excreted in the breath.

There are three possible pathways for alcohol metabolism in man. The major pathway in most people starts with alcohol dehydrogenase (ADH), a zinc-containing enzyme in the cytoplasm of the liver (Box 7.1). The ADH step is the rate-limiting step in alcohol metabolism. ADH occurs in slightly different forms and some individuals have more active ADH than others. It may seem surprising that humans naturally possess this enzyme for dealing with beer and wine, to which our hunter-gatherer ancestors were not exposed. However, some alcohols are produced naturally inside the body by fermentation in the large intestine (e.g. small amounts of methyl alcohol from pectin), and they occur in over-ripe fruits. The next step is conversion of acetaldehyde to acetate by aldehyde dehydrogenases (ALDHs), which are present in the cytoplasm and mitochondria (Box 7.2). In most people, there is no

BOX 7.1

$$CH_3CH_2OH + NAD \rightarrow CH_3CHO + NADH + H^+$$

Ethanol   ADH   Acetaldehyde

BOX 7.2

$$CH_3CH_2OH + NAD + H_2O \rightarrow CH_3COOH + NADH + H^+$$

Acetaldehyde   ALDH   Acetic acid

build up of acetaldehyde, but nearly 50% of Chinese, Korean, and Japanese people have an inactive variant of one of the ALDHs, so after moderate intake of alcohol their blood acetaldehyde increases. This causes facial flushing and headache; sickness in homozygotes.

In long-term heavy drinkers the microsomal ethanol oxidizing system (MEOS) with cytochrome P450 becomes a second important route for alcohol metabolism. The microsomes proliferate (are induced) in heavy drinkers. As with ADH, ethanol is converted to acetaldehyde. A third minor pathway for conversion of ethanol to acetaldehyde is via catalase in peroxisomes.

On average, people can metabolize about 5 g of ethanol per hour (i.e. half a standard drink). The rate varies about two-fold between individuals. Alcohol absorption can be slowed by having a meal, or even milk, in the stomach but there is no agent that increases the rate of alcohol metabolism. Smaller people are likely to have smaller livers and so metabolize less alcohol per hour. Women on average have smaller livers than men, a lower percentage of total body water (in which to distribute the alcohol) and also have less first pass gastric alcohol dehydrogenase, so that they are less tolerant of alcohol than men. East Asian people may suffer from headaches and flushing at quite low intakes of alcohol because of acetaldehyde accumulation. This may limit their intake.

A drug used to control alcohol addiction, disulfiram (Antabuse) antagonizes ALDH. People taking it experience unpleasant symptoms (headache, nausea, flushing) as a result of acetaldehyde accumulation when they have a drink.

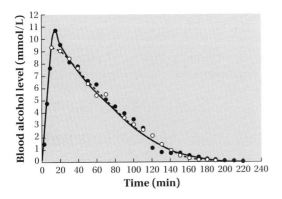

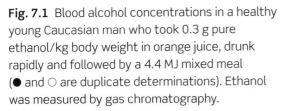

Fig. 7.1 Blood alcohol concentrations in a healthy young Caucasian man who took 0.3 g pure ethanol/kg body weight in orange juice, drunk rapidly and followed by a 4.4 MJ mixed meal (● and ○ are duplicate determinations). Ethanol was measured by gas chromatography.

7.3 Effect of alcohol on the brain

Pharmacologists classify ethanol as a central nervous system depressant, in the same group as volatile anaesthetic agents. With increasing levels of blood alcohol people pass through successive stages of alcohol intoxication (Table 7.2). At the biochemical level alcohol affects a number of neurochemical processes simultaneously. γ-Aminobutyric (GABA) systems (inhibitory) are more active. Activity of the stimulatory glutamate N-methyl-D-aspartate receptor system is reduced. Dopamine is released and contributes to the reward effects of alcohol. The serotonergic system is stimulated. Reversal of all these effects occur in the alcohol withdrawn syndrome.

Ingestion of alcohol has effects in other systems of the body. There is peripheral vasodilation and increased heart rate. The imbiber may feel warm but be losing more heat than usual. Alcohol inhibits hypothalamic osmoreceptors, hence there is reduced pituitary antidiuretic hormone secretion so there is diuresis (an increased urine output) which can lead to dehydration, especially after drinking spirits.

Table 7.2 Successive stages of acute alcohol intoxication

Blood alcohol concentration (g/dL)	Stage	Effects
Up to 0.05	Feeling of wellbeing	Relaxed, talks a lot
0.05–0.08	Risky state	Judgement and finer movements affected
0.08–0.15	Dangerous state	Slow speech, balance affected, eyesight blurred, wants to fall asleep, likely to vomit, needs help to walk
0.2–0.4	Drunken stupor	Dead drunk, no bladder control, heavy breathing, unconscious (e.g. deep anaesthesia)
0.45–0.6	Death	Shock and death

7.4 Energy value of ethanol

The gross chemical energy of ethanol can be measured outside the body in a bomb calorimeter, and the value is between the energy value of carbohydrates and that of fat, about 30 kJ or 7.1 kcal/g.

However, in a metabolic ward, with food intakes strictly controlled, Lieber (1992) replaced 50% of subjects' energy (calorie) intake by isocaloric amounts of ethanol (they had been accustomed to high alcohol intakes). Instead of gaining weight, they lost weight. Free-living heavy drinkers are not usually overweight. It appears that above a certain intake ethanol provides less than 7 kcal/g. Alcohol increases the basal metabolic rate (thermogenesis) and it is thought that metabolism of alcohol by liver microsomes yields less energy than the ADH route.

In heavy drinkers, 10–30% (or more) of energy intake comes from alcohol, but alcoholic beverages contain no protein and very few micronutrients, so this nutrient-poor source of calories displaces other foods that normally provide essential nutrients. Appetite may be suppressed in heavy drinkers, either by alcoholic gastritis or by associated smoking. Alcohol dependency is an important cause of conditioned (or secondary) nutritional deficiency—the drinker may have access to enough foods and their nutrients but is not eating them.

Nutrients that are typically depleted in alcoholics include thiamin, folate, niacin, and several inorganic nutrients (see Section 7.6).

Nutrition surveys that do not take alcohol intake into account cannot represent their subjects' full nutrient intake.

7.5 Direct consequences of alcohol intake

7.5.1 Acute intoxication

Acute intoxication can lead to road and other accidents, or domestic and other violence. Intoxicated people can suffer and inflict a range of injuries. Occasionally people consume such a large dose of alcohol that they die with lethal blood levels. The breathalyser was developed to reduce road traffic accidents. In many countries, a driver stopped at random by a police check who has a breathalyser reading corresponding to a blood level of 0.05 g/dL (0.02 to 0.08 in different countries) has his driver's licence suspended. This measure has reduced traffic accidents and contributed to the decline of alcohol consumption in a number of developed countries.

7.5.2 Hangovers

The excess intake of alcohol the night before may not yet have all been cleared from the blood. Dehydration may be present from diuresis and, with some drinks (e.g. brandy), toxic effects of small amounts of methanol and higher alcohols contribute to the symptoms.

7.5.3 Chronic alcoholism

Some people become dependent or addicted to alcohol and cannot face the world unless they have some alcohol in their blood throughout the day. Thus they maintain an intake of alcohol per day larger than their liver's capacity to metabolize it.

7.5.4 Alcohol withdrawal syndrome

Alcohol addicts who have maintained some alcohol in their blood continuously for weeks or even longer suffer withdrawal symptoms if an accident or illness abruptly removes them from their alcohol supply. There are tremors of the hands, anxiety, insomnia, and tachycardia. *Epileptic convulsions* can occur and, in severe cases there is agitation, mental confusion, and hallucinations. This is *delirium tremens*, a severe illness.

7.5.5 Binge drinkers

One-night binge drinkers expect to get drunk (see Box 7.3). Men imbibe 80 g of alcohol (4 pints of beer) or more and women somewhat less.

BOX 7.3 Different patterns of alcohol consumption

- The inexperienced drinker (e.g. an adolescent) who misjudges the dose and has an accident.
- The person who doesn't drink during the week but drinks to excess and gets drunk on payday or Saturday night (one-night binge).
- The person who enjoys a controlled one or two drinks with dinner most days.
- The person who has too many drinks each day (most after work) but more or less maintains their (increasingly inefficient) usual life.
- The person who drinks very heavily for weeks.

The other pattern of alcohol excess is that a person drinks heavily for weeks. Consequently, as alcohol displaces much of the usual food intake there can be an acute deficiency of micronutrients with the smallest reserve in the body, usually thiamin (see Wernicke–Korsakoff syndrome, Chapter 13).

7.6 Medical consequences of excess consumption

7.6.1 Liver disease

Alcohol causes liver damage in three stages. The least severe is fatty liver. Metabolism of large amounts of ethanol in the liver produce an increased ratio of NADH/NAD; this depresses the citric acid cycle and oxidation of fatty acids, and favours triglyceride synthesis in the liver cells. It used to be thought that the fatty liver was due to an associated nutritional deficiency, but fatty liver has been observed (using needle biopsy of the liver) in volunteers who took a moderately large intake of alcohol but with all nutrients provided under strictly controlled conditions in hospital. The symptoms of fatty liver are not striking. On abdominal examination a doctor can feel that the liver is somewhat enlarged, and this shows with ultrasound; biochemical changes can be seen in a blood sample (see Section 7.9).

Alcoholic hepatitis (inflammation of the liver) is more serious. This type is not caused by a virus but by prolonged excess alcohol intake. There is loss of appetite, fevers, tender liver, jaundice, and elevation in the plasma of enzymes produced in the liver (e.g. aminotransferases (transaminases), γ-glutamyl transpeptidase, and alkaline phosphatase). If the patient continues drinking, this can progress to cirrhosis.

Alcoholic cirrhosis may be associated with chronic alcoholism. When the liver has to metabolize large amounts of alcohol over a long time, membranes inside the cells become disordered; mitochondria show ballooning. In its fully developed form, irregular strands of fibrous tissue criss-cross the liver, replacing damaged liver parenchymal cells. These effects may be due to acetaldehyde or to free radical generation by neutrophil polymorph white cells in the liver. Cirrhosis seems to occur in people who have managed to consume large amounts of alcohol over many years but carried on a reasonably regular life and were able to eat and afford the alcohol. The amount of alcohol needed to cause cirrhosis is difficult to establish exactly because many people understate their alcohol consumption, especially heavy drinkers. It is greater than 40 g of ethanol per day in women and 50 g in men over years, usually much more.

Not all cases of chronic hepatitis and cirrhosis are caused by alcohol excess. Some are caused by hepatitis viruses (B or C) and there are other less common causes (see Sections 10.7 and 11.2.8). Prolonged excessive alcohol intake is, however, the most common cause of liver cirrhosis and rates of mortality due to cirrhosis are an important indicator of population levels of harm from alcohol. In western Europe, France had the highest mortality from cirrhosis in 1960 but by 2000 Austria and then Scotland had the highest rates.

7.6.2 Metabolic effects

Moderate regular drinkers who are apparently well may have increased plasma triglycerides (an overflow from the overproduction of fat in the liver). Plasma urate is raised because of reduced renal excretion probably due to increased blood lactate, which follows alcohol ingestion.

7.6.3 Fetal alcohol syndrome

Women who drink alcohol heavily during early pregnancy can give birth to a baby with an unusual facial appearance (small eyes, absent philtrum, thin upper lip), prenatal and postnatal growth impairment, central nervous system dysfunction, and often other physical abnormalities. Mothers of children with the fetal alcohol syndrome were heavy drinkers during their pregnancy and most were socially deprived. More moderate drinkers may have babies that are small for dates but otherwise normal. Some authorities insist that pregnant women should avoid all alcohol, but in a careful prospective study in Dundee, Scotland, Florey's group (Sulaiman *et al.*, 1988) found that, after adjustment for the effect of smoking, social class, and mother's size, there was no detectable effect on pregnancy of alcohol consumption below 100 g/week (i.e. one standard drink a day).

7.6.4 Wernicke–Korsakoff syndrome

In heavy drinkers who consume large amounts of alcohol and virtually stop eating for 3 or more weeks, brain function can be affected by acute thiamin deficiency. Ethanol uses up thiamin for its metabolism, yet alcoholic beverages provide no thiamin; there is no rich food source of thiamin and body stores are very small (see Chapter 13). In Wernicke's encephalopathy, the patient is quietly confused—not an easy state to recognize in an alcoholic. The diagnostic feature, if the sufferer is brought to medical attention, is that the eyes cannot move properly (ophthalmoplegia). When Wernicke's encephalopathy is treated with thiamin, the ophthalmoplegia and confusion clear but the patient may be left with a loss of recent memory, the inability to recall what has happened recently (Korsakoff's syndrome). It has been suggested that when an alcoholic has a partner who provides food, containing some thiamin, Wernicke–Korsakoff syndrome (WKS) is less likely. The incidence has been high in Australia. Korsakoff's psychosis can be permanent. It is one cause of alcohol-related brain damage. As a preventive measure bread is fortified with thiamin since 1991, as it had been for a long time (for other reasons) in the USA, UK, and most other developed countries. WKS has become uncommon in Australia. Wernicke's encephalopathy uncommonly occurs in people who have not taken alcohol, e.g. with persistent vomiting of pregnancy, hyperemesis gravidarum.

7.6.5 Other nutritional deficiencies in alcoholics

In societies with adequate food supply, vitamin deficiencies are rare but do occur in heavy drinkers. Chronic thiamin or other B-vitamin deficiency may be responsible for a peripheral neuropathy in the legs, with reduced function of the motor and sensory nerves and diminished ankle jerks. Folate metabolism is commonly impaired in alcoholics, and megaloblastic anaemia may be seen. Vitamin A metabolism is abnormal where there is alcoholic liver disease: the liver does not store retinol normally or synthesize retinol-binding protein adequately. There can, consequently, be reduced plasma retinol and night blindness. Among inorganic nutrients, plasma magnesium and zinc can be subnormal in alcoholics.

7.6.6 Predisposition to some types of cancer

The risk of cancer of the mouth and pharynx is increased, especially when high alcohol intakes are combined with smoking. Other cancers associated with high alcohol consumption are those of the oesophagus or liver (primary cancer of the liver is a complication of cirrhosis), the rectum (in some beer drinkers), and possibly breast cancer.

7.6.7 Gastrointestinal complications

Chronic gastritis and gastric or duodenal ulcers may be associated with excessive alcohol consumption. Acute pancreatitis is a severe complication.

7.6.8 Impaired immunity

Heavy alcohol consumption impairs immunity and increases susceptibility to pneumonia and tuberculosis.

7.6.9 Hypertension

The prevalence of raised arterial blood pressure increases with usual alcohol intakes above three or four drinks per day. Prompt falls of moderately elevated blood pressures have been well documented in heavy drinkers admitted to hospital for detoxication. Increased prevalence of hypertension explains the greater risk of stroke from cerebral haemorrhage in heavy alcohol drinkers. Heavy intakes of alcohol simulate secretion of corticotrophin-releasing hormone. Increased cortisol and sympathetic activity may explain the increased blood pressure. Limiting alcohol consumption is a standard part of lifestyle modification recommended for people with hypertension.

7.7 Alcohol and coronary heart disease

Opposed to the deleterious effect of alcohol on blood pressure is its apparent effect in reducing the risk of coronary heart disease (CHD); one of the major causes of death in affluent communities. Over 20 large prospective studies in several countries have all found that-light-to moderate alcohol consumption appear to protect against CHD (Table 7.3). At postmortem examination, pathologists have long known to expect little or no atheroma in the arteries of people dying of alcoholic complications. However, the discovery that light-to-moderate drinking is negatively associated with CHD emerged only in the 1990s (Doll, 1997). It was surprising to find a major health benefit of drinking alcohol. A study in Rotterdam also found that consumption of 1 or 2 drinks per day was inversely associated with coronary artery calcification (Vliegenthart *et al.*, 2004).

The longest established mechanism for this protective effect (known since 1969) is that alcohol consumption increases plasma high-density lipoprotein (HDL) cholesterol, a well-established protective factor for CHD (see Chapter 21). This increase of HDL in moderate drinkers is not sufficient to explain fully their lower risk of CHD.

There is also evidence that alcohol drinking reduces the tendency to thrombosis. It is not possible to test this directly, but alcohol reduces aggregation of platelets *in vitro*, in response to collagen and ADP.

Wines, especially red wines contain flavonoid antioxidants, principally catechins and anthocyanins. These are better absorbed from alcoholic drinks than from vegetables and fruits. Sir Richard Doll (1997) suggested the extra benefit (in some countries) of wine over beer and spirits can be accounted

Table 7.3 Relative risks of total mortality and mortality from coronary heart disease (CHD) in 276, 802 men in the USA (aged 40–59 years at entry) in a 12-year follow-up

	Drinks per day							
	0	<1	1	2	3	4	5	6+
Total death rate	1.00	0.88	0.84	0.93	1.02	1.08	1.22	1.38
CHD death rate	1.00	0.86	0.79	0.80	0.83	0.74	0.85	0.92

Source: Boffetta, P., and Garfinkel, L. (1990) Alcohol drinking and mortality among men enrolled in an American Cancer Society Prospective Study. *Epidemiology*, **1**, 342–8.

for by differences in the pattern of drinking. No epidemiological study has conclusively shown a benefit of red over white wine (Klatsky *et al.*, 1997).

This health benefit of alcohol consumption on CHD only applies to older people in developed countries. Even in this group, the benefit is almost balanced by deaths related to alcohol from other diseases. In the younger majority in developed countries and at all ages in developing countries, CHD hardly ever occurs: the effects of alcohol are almost all adverse (Fig. 7.2).

The cardioprotective effect of regular light-to-moderate drinking does not apply to episodic heavy drinking. A meta-analysis confirms that binge drinking confers no cardioprotective effects (Lieber, 1992). In Russian cities excessive vodka drinking has been the cause of more than half of all deaths in people 15–54 years of age, some of which are certified as ischaemic heart disease. Russia's death rate from CHD has risen to be the highest in the world, while mortalities have been declining in Western countries.

7.7.1 Type 2 diabetes

In prospective cohort studies, it appears that small intakes of alcohol may also reduce the risk of developing type 2 diabetes (Koppes *et al.*, 2005). In a meta-analysis of 15 studies in 369 000 individuals followed over 10 years those who stated their daily alcohol consumption as 20–30 g had a relative risk of diabetes around 0.70. Higher intakes were not protective. The mechanism could be by increased insulin sensitivity.

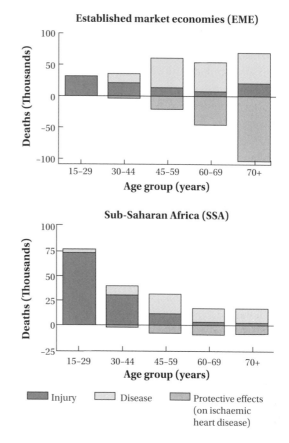

Fig. 7.2 Male deaths attributable to and averted by alcohol in established market economies (developed countries) compared with sub-Saharan Africa.

Source: Murray, C.J.L., and Lopez, A.D. (eds) (1996) *The global burden of disease*. For WHO and World Bank. Cambridge MA, Harvard University Press.

7.8 Global burden of diseases related to alcohol

In the different WHO regions of the world, alcohol-attributable deaths (percentage of all deaths) in men (in 2004) were 11% in Europe, 9% in Americas, and 8.4% in the West Pacific. They were 3.9% in South-east Asia, 3.7% in Africa, and only 1.0% in the eastern Mediterranean region. Mortalities in women were around 17% of men's rates.

Disabilities attributable to alcohol, expressed as disability-adjusted life years (DALYs) as a proportion of all DALYs by sex and region, in men (in 2004) were 17.3% in Europe, 14.2% in the Americas, 11.8% in west Pacific countries, 4.7% in South-east Asia, 3.4% in Africa, and 0.9% in eastern Mediterranean countries. DALYs from alcohol in women were around 18% of rates in men, i.e. 4.4% down to 0.1% in the different regions.

Thus one component of our diet, of our overall food and drink, the alcohol, though providing conviviality and social lubrication yet is a serious cause of premature death and disease, except in Moslem countries. In poor developing countries, alcohol consumption has been increasing. For example, Thailand's alcohol consumption has increased 33 times in the past 40 years and 8.1% of disability-adjusted life years lost in that country are now attributable to alcohol (Gilmore, 2009).

It is estimated that in 200 three-digit disease codes in the International Classification of Diseases, alcohol is a component cause. And there are also 30 three- or four-digit codes that are alcohol-specific.

Health authorities in several countries are particularly concerned about increasing numbers of young people who go out binge drinking to excess on Friday or Saturday nights (Pincock, 2003). This includes teenage girls, some of whom mistakenly believe they can tolerate the same excess intakes as their male companions (Frezza *et al.*, 1990).

7.9 Recognizing the problem drinker

There are different types of alcohol abuse. An 'alcoholic' is a group term for any person whose drinking is leading to harm. This harm may be alcohol dependence or physical disease or social harm.

People drinking more than others or more than they feel they should are very likely to underestimate their alcohol intake when asked. The spouse or other family member may give a very different answer. Health professionals are trained to suspect when someone is drinking too much and researchers use tactfully drafted questionnaires. Alcohol can be smelt on the breath and measured quantitatively in the breath, blood, or urine within hours of drinking. If a person has not been recently drinking there are changes in the blood which are suggestive of long-term excessive alcohol intake:

1 increased plasma γ-glutamyl transferase (GGT) activity;

2 increased plasma carbohydrate-deficient transferrin;

3 increased red cell volume (mean corpuscular volume);

4 increased plasma (fasting) triglycerides (i.e. very low-density lipoproteins);

5 increased plasma aminotransferases (transaminases);

6 increased plasma urate.

These vary in sensitivity and specificity. 1, 2, 4, and 5 occur in the liver. Increased urate is a result of increased plasma lactate. Increased red cell volume is sometimes due to folate depletion; its cause in most cases is not yet clear.

7.10 Is alcoholism a disease or the top end of a normal distribution?

Alcoholism is a costly problem in most communities because of associated diseases, accidents, loss of earning, medical expenses, and social misery.

There are two philosophical approaches. One is the medical model which sees alcoholism as a disease in individuals who should be treated by the health professions. The other is the society model: the more alcohol sold and consumed, the larger will be the number of alcoholics. There are sections of society (e.g. some occupations, deprived minorities) who are at increased risk and there are social practices that contribute to alcohol abuse.

Clearly, primary care physicians cannot communicate with or control the majority of heavy drinkers, until they present with complications. At this stage, brief medical advice can be effective.

Ledermann (1956) put forward the hypothesis that in a homogeneous population the distribution of alcohol consumption is a logarithmic normal curve and that the number of people who drink a certain amount can be calculated if the average consumption is known (Fig. 7.3). This theory predicts that major complications of alcoholism in a country will be related to average national consumption. Governments rely on this principle in maintaining substantial taxes on alcohol, restricted outlets and hours, lower age limits, and other measures to reduce its free availability.

Governments have a responsibility to work to limit excessive alcohol consumption. Here, public health can be in conflict with the great lobbying power of the alcohol industry-brewers, hotels, bars, restaurants, and wine growers.

Six well-established policies can be effective if governments are strong enough to implement them:

• taxation, making alcohol more expensive and this should be based on alcohol content (no discounts);

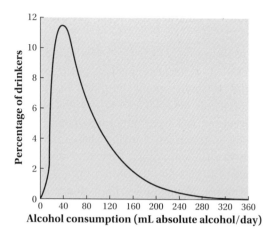

Fig. 7.3 Hypothetical curve proposed by Ledermann (1956). In a homogeneous population, alcohol consumption is distributed in a logarithmic normal curve.

Source: Smith, R. (1982) In *Alcohol problems: ABC of alcohol. Alcohol and alcoholism*, p. 29. London, BMJ.

• drinking-driving legislation—and enforcement;

• banning advertising;

• limiting availability, number of outlets, opening and closing times, minimum purchase age preventing illicit alcohol production;

• providing help for hazardous drinkers.

Education campaigns on their own are not effective.

7.11 Genetic liability to alcohol dependence?

Occurrence of alcoholism in families could be learnt rather than genetic. From comparing monozygotic with dizygotic twins the heritability of amount and frequency of alcohol drinking appears to be about 0.36 (i.e. one-third of the way along the scale from purely environmental to purely genetic). But studies on twins cannot completely exclude environmental effects. Adoption studies have shown that the sons of alcoholic fathers are four times more likely to become alcoholics than the sons of fathers who were not alcoholics. The search is on to find one or more variations of brain metabolism which makes people more likely to become alcohol-dependent. There have been several claims (e.g. abnormality of brain handling of dopamine or serotonin) but none as been convincingly confirmed.

7.12 Acceptable intakes of alcohol

The usual way in which alcohol is mentioned in national sets of dietary guidelines (see Chapter 37) is 'drink alcohol in moderation, if at all' or 'if you drink alcoholic beverages, do so in moderation'.

Because women have lower rates of metabolizing alcohol, advice on safe drinking levels has to be different for men and women. Recommendations are expressed in standard drinks that (in many countries) contain 10 g of pure alcohol. Note that standard drinks are normally served in the pub, but at home people tend to be more generous. In men, two or three standard drinks per day (20–30 g alcohol) (i.e. 140–210 g alcohol/week), are usually biologically safe, but no more than two drinks before driving and a minority of men should not take this much, or even any alcohol (e.g. people with liver disease, taking other sedative drugs, with a history of alcohol dependence). In women, the biologically safe intake is one or two drinks (10–20 g alcohol) per day (i.e. 70–140 g alcohol/week). In pregnancy, intake should be one drink or less, likewise if a woman thinks she might be pregnant. Children should not take alcohol, but in some cultures they are offered a small drink of wine with the family's main meal and some believe this can be a good training in moderation in consumption of alcohol. The quantities of various alcoholic beverages providing 10 g ethanol are shown in Table 7.1.

Further Reading

1. **Anderson, P., Chisholm, D., and Fuhr, D.C.** (2009) Effectiveness and cost-effectiveness of policies and programmes to reduce the harm caused by alcohol. *Lancet*, **373**, 2234–46.
2. **Boffetta, P., and Garfinkel, L.** (1990) Alcohol drinking and mortality among men enrolled in an American Cancer Society Prospective Study. *Epidemiology*, **1**, 342–8.
3. **Doll, R.** (1997) One for the heart. *BMJ*, **315**, 1664–8.
4. **Frezza, M., di Padova, C., Pozzato, G., Teroin, M., Baraona, E., and Lieber, C.S.** (1990) High blood alcohol levels in women. The role of decreased gastric alcohol dehydrogenase activity and first-pass metabolism. *N Engl J Med*, **322**, 95–9.
5. **Gilmore, I.** (2009) Action needed to tackle a global drink problem. *Lancet*, **373**, 2174–4.
6. **Hall, W. and Zador, D.** (1997) The alcohol withdrawal syndrome. *Lancet*, **349**, 1897–900.
7. **Klatsky, A.L., Armstrongm, M.A., and Friedman, G.D.** (1997) Red wine, white wine, liquor, beer, and risk for coronary artery disease hospitalization. *Am J Cardiol*, **80**, 416–20.
8. **Koppes, L.L.J., Dekker, J.M., Hendricks, H.F.J., Bouter, L.M., and Heine, R.J.** (2005) Moderate alcohol consumption lowers the risk of type 2 diabetes. *Diabetes Care*, **28**, 719–25.
9. **Ledermann, S.** (1956) *Alcool, alcoolisme, alcoolisation.* Paris, Presse Universitaires de France.
10. **Leon, D.A., and McCambridge, J.** (2006) Liver cirrhosis rates in Britain from 1950 to 2002. *Lancet*, **367**, 52–6.
11. **Lieber, L.S.** (ed.) (1992) *Medical and nutritional complications of alcoholism. Mechanisms and management.* New York and London, Plenum.
12. **Murray, C.J.L. and Lopez, A.D.** (eds) (1996) *The global burden of disease.* For WHO and World Bank. Cambridge MA, Harvard University Press.
13. **Pincock, S.** (2003) Binge drinking on rise in UK and elsewhere. *Lancet*, **365**, 1126–7.
14. **Rehm, J., Mathers, C., Popova, S., Thavorncharoensap, M., Teerawattananon, Y., and Patra, J.** (2009) Global burden of disease and injury and economic cost attributable to alcohol use and alcohol-use disorders. *Lancet*, **373**, 2223–33.
15. **Schukit, M.A.** (2009) Alcohol-use disorders. *Lancet*, **373**, 492–501.
16. **Smith, R.** (1982) In *Alcohol problems: ABC of alcohol. Alcohol and alcoholism*, p. 29. London, BMJ.

17. **Sulaiman, N.D., Florey, C. du V., Taylor, D.J., and Ogston, S.A.** (1988) Alcohol consumption in Dundee primigravidas and its effects on outcome of pregnancy. *BMJ*, **296**, 1500–3.
18. **Vliegenthart, R., Hok-Hay, S.O., van den Elzen, A.P.M., *et al*.** (2004) Alcohol consumption and coronary calcification in a general population. *Arch Int Med*, **164**, 2355–60.
19. **Zaridze, D., Brennan, P., Boreham, J., *et al*.** (2009) Alcohol and cause-specific mortality in Russia: A retrospective case-control study of 48,557 adult deaths. *Lancet*, **373**, 2201–14.

Useful Websites

To see topical and scientifically robust updates on nutrition associated with this textbook and web links to many of the journals in the Further Reading sections, please see the dedicated Online Resource Centre at **http://www.oxfordtextbooks.co.uk/orc/mann4e/**

Part 2

Organic and inorganic essential nutrients

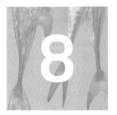

8 Water, electrolytes, and acid–base balance

Zoltán H. Endre

8.1 Body water

8.1.1 Importance of water

In 1913, Lawrence Henderson explained how peculiar properties resulting from a hydrogen-bonded structure make water an essential constituent of all known forms of life. It is, remarkably, liquid in the range of 'ordinary' temperatures at which biochemical reactions can occur in solution or at active sites of enzymes in contact with water. Its high specific heat moderates temperature gradients; its high latent heat allows efficient cooling by evaporation and protects against damage by frost. A dielectric constant that is large enough to reduce by 80 times the forces between charges immersed in it makes water a superb solvent for ionic compounds. It is also a good solvent for most organic compounds (apart from fats and hydrocarbons) and, even when the active sites of enzymes are in clefts that exclude water molecules, most reactants must arrive and most products move away in aqueous solution.

8.1.2 Amount and distribution in the body

The extent to which freely diffusible substances (e.g. ethanol, urea, isotopic forms of water) are diluted after being ingested or injected shows that adult persons contain about 35–45 L of water, which makes up approximately 60% of the body weight. Two-thirds of this body water is located inside cells as the intracellular fluid (ICF), though fat cells contain none. One-third of body water is extracellular. The extracellular fluid (ECF) is distributed in various body compartments, such as blood vessels (the intravascular volume), body cavities, and between cells in organs and tissues (the interstitial space). The ECF is further divided into intravascular (plasma) and interstitial fluid plus the small (usually) volume of fluid in epithelial-lined cavities (transcellular fluid) such as joint fluid, cerebrospinal fluid, pleural and peritoneal cavities, ocular fluid, and bladder urine. These relationships are illustrated in Fig. 8.1.

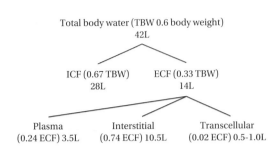

Total body water (TBW 0.6 body weight)
42L

ICF (0.67 TBW)   ECF (0.33 TBW)
28L   14L

Plasma   Interstitial   Transcellular
(0.24 ECF) 3.5L   (0.74 ECF) 10.5L   (0.02 ECF) 0.5-1.0L

Fig. 8.1 Distribution of total body water. Typical volumes for a 70 kg man are illustrated. ECF, extracellular fluid; ICF, intracellular fluid; TBW, total body water.

The volumes quoted are approximate. No two people are identical; different methods yield results that are similar but not the same. The interstitial fluid bathes the cells—in the overcrowded and somewhat salty pond we carry with us for them. In 1878, Claude Bernard called the ECF the 'milieu interieur' (the 'internal environment') of the cells; it nourishes them, supplies their needs, and takes away their waste products. The circulating blood keeps the ECF 'stirred' so that it can transport heat and substances in solution from one cell to other cells and between cells inside the body and the external environment.

8.1.3 Body fluids

Water crosses cell membranes easily and rapidly through aquaporin (AQP) 1 channels to balance the concentrations of osmotically active substances inside and outside cells. The concentration of materials (osmoles) dissolved in the ICF and ECF compartments differ because there are differences in permeability, transporters, and pumps for the individual solutes. If differences in concentration are maintained, then these solutes are regarded as 'effectives osmoles', since they regulate the volume of the compartment.

The ECF contains mainly sodium ions (Na^+), small but important concentrations of potassium (K^+), calcium (Ca^{2+}), and magnesium (Mg^{2+}) ions, and the anions, chloride (Cl^-), and bicarbonate (HCO_3^-). For electroneutrality, positively charged ions (cations) must always be balanced by an equal number of negatively charged ions (anions). The ICF contains mainly potassium ions (mostly balanced by organic phosphate and the negatively charged groups on proteins), small amounts of sodium, magnesium, bicarbonate, chloride, and calcium (see Table 8.1). Despite large differences in ECF and ICF sodium and potassium concentrations,

Table 8.1 Muscle cell fluid and blood plasma to illustrate intracellular fluid and extracellular fluid

Muscle cell fluid (mmol/L water)				Plasma (mmol/L water)			
K^+	150	Cl^-	5	K^+	4	Cl^-	104
Na^+	10	HCO_3^-	10	Na^+	140	HCO_3^-	28
Mg^{2+}	10			Mg^{2+}	1.0		
Ca^{2+}	10^{-4}	Org P^-	130	Ca^{2+}	2.4	$H_2PO_4^-$	1
pH	7.1	Prot[17-]	2	pH	7.4	Prot[17-a]	1
Osmolality*	287 mosmol/kg cell water			287 mosmol/kg plasma water			

Note: Because only about 95% of plasma is water, laboratory results per litre of plasma are lower than these. Average cell fluid is only about 80% water. Total calcium concentrations are shown. See text for discussion of ion concentrations.

*The concentration of osmoles is usually expressed per kg of water (approximately 1 L), and termed osmolality, although osmolarity (particles per L) is often used interchangeably with osmolality.

[a] Protein 17- refers to the 17 negative charges associated with albumin at normal ph.

the cell membranes are somewhat permeable to sodium and potassium. Cells must therefore use a large part of the energy from their metabolism to pump out sodium that diffuses in and to recover potassium that leaks out. Because water distribution depends on the number of particles restricted to ICF or ECF, sodium and potassium ions, respectively, account for the *effective* osmolality and volumes of these compartments. Even at rest, cells are very busy! They use about 40 kg adenosine triphosphate each day to supply the energy for maintenance and up to 0.5 kg per minute during maximal exertion!

The 'free' or ionized concentrations of ions is the fraction available to interact with other ions and is often much lower than the total concentration. This is particularly important for calcium, which is extensively involved in intracellular signalling reactions that control processes as divergent as muscle contraction and initiation of apoptosis, a form of programmed cell death. In plasma, the ionized Ca^{2+} concentration is reduced to about half the total concentration by protein binding. The intracellular or (ionized) Ca^{2+} concentration is even more restricted to about 100 nmol/L (i.e. 10^{-7} mol/L or 10^{-4} mmol/L) by binding within subcellular organelles such as endoplasmic reticulum or sarcolemma and to calcium-binding proteins such as calmodulin.

The kidneys adjust the excretion of water to keep osmolality constant and reabsorb (or excrete) sodium and water to control blood pressure and they maintain acid–base balance by excretion of titrateable acids and ammonium. The kidneys thus regulate both the concentration of sodium and the volume of the ECF. The kidneys excrete surplus potassium, indirectly facilitating cellular regulation of intracellular volume as the cells regulate the amount of potassium they contain.

8.1.4 Water balance

The fact that most people maintain much the same weight implies that total body water is kept constant, with gains balanced by losses. Weighing is therefore the best way to measure day-to-day changes in the amount of water in the body.

Regulation of water balance Changes in ECF sodium concentration result primarily from changes in total body water and water concentration. Water movement between the ICF and ECF occurs with changes in total body water in order to maintain osmolar balance. Thus, the ICF volume will increase as the ECF sodium concentration decreases and vice versa. Loss of water makes body fluids more concentrated. All the cells lose water and shrink as the osmotic pressure of the ECF rises. Special cells in the hypothalamus at the base of the brain respond to shrinking in two ways: (a) by sending messages that excite the sensation of thirst, and (b) by releasing into the blood antidiuretic hormone (ADH, also called vasopressin), that allows the renal tubules to reabsorb water from dilute urine and return it to the blood. The volume of urine immediately decreases as ADH stimulates the insertion of AQP2 water channels into the luminal cell membrane of the distal part of the nephron, the collecting duct. If gains of water exceed losses, the cells swell, the thirst message is switched off, ADH release stops, the AQP2 channels are recycled, and the collecting duct cells become impermeable to water. This immediately results in a flow of dilute urine ('water diuresis') that quickly gets rid of excess water. This is what happens after drinking a glass of water, for example. Intense exercise, (e.g. marathon running), anaesthetic gases, and some drugs, (e.g. methylenedioxymethamphetamine, ecstasy) all stimulate release of ADH. There are also nervous paths from receptors in the heart and large central blood vessels that stimulate thirst and release of ADH when the volume of blood shrinks, or stop the release of ADH when blood volume is restored. As highlighted, the kidney normally responds rapidly to changes in ADH concentration. However, the renal response can be suppressed by some drugs such as lithium carbonate.

Water balance: magnitude of gains and losses of water

Intake

1 'Solid' food: 1.0 L/day (from water present in food as it is eaten).

2 Metabolic water (water produced by oxidation of hydrogen in food): ~400 mL/day.

3 Beverages: 1.0 L/day or more (voluntary intake may be much more, especially since bottled water has become a fashion statement).

Total: 2.4 L/day

Output (Note: most of these are unavoidable losses from the body.)

1 *'Insensible' water loss.* This is evaporative loss (~800 mL/day) following (a) transepidermal diffusion (water diffusing through skin, about 400 mL/day in the adult) and (b) evaporation from the moist surface of the lung in contact with air (respiratory loss, variable in amount and dependent on activity and the dryness of the ambient air, about 500 mL/day at sea level in a temperate climate and much more from the lungs with increased ventilation during exercise, especially at high altitudes). More than 2.0 L/day may be lost in altitudes above 6000 m. The first successful ascent of Mount Everest depended partly on allowing for the magnitude of this loss. Note that this is loss of pure water with no associated solute (sodium) loss.

2 *Sweat*: 100 mL/day, but litres may be secreted by sweat glands to get rid of heat.

3 *Faeces*: normally 100 mL/day; with choleric diarrhoeas, this may reach 10 or 12 L/day.

4 *Urine*: The 'obligatory' urine volume is the least water required to carry the day's soluble waste (osmotic load) in the most concentrated urine the kidneys can make. With normal kidneys able to concentrate the urine four times as concentrated as plasma ($4 \times {\sim}300 = 1200$ mosmol/L), this is about 600 mL. It increases to 2.4 L if kidneys cannot make urine more concentrated than plasma. Urine volume may be more than 10 L in patients with diabetes insipidus who fail to produce ADH or whose kidneys do not respond to it.

Wild animals are at greater risk from predators when they stand still to drink or urinate and often seem to drink only enough to replace unavoidable losses. People usually drink more and rely on water diuresis to match output to their voluntary intake.

Both excesses and deficiencies of body water can occur, and both may threaten life. The normal compensations for these changes are summarized in Table 8.2.

Table 8.2 Compensation for changes in water balance

WATER LOSS leads to:	WATER INGESTION leads to:
Increased:	Decreased:
Antidiuretic hormone	Antidiuretic hormone
Angiotensin II	Angiotensin II
Aldosterone	Aldosterone
Urine osmolality	Urine osmolality
Decreased:	Increased:
Urine volume (oliguria)	Urine volume (diuresis)
Urine sodium	Urine sodium

8.1.5 Deficiency of body water

Dehydration describes a state of negative fluid balance that may be caused by numerous disease entities. Diarrhoeal illnesses are the most common causes, especially in children. Worldwide, dehydration secondary to diarrhoeal illness is the leading cause of infant and child mortality. The effects of water loss depend on the electrolyte composition of the fluid lost, since this will affect the osmolality (also called tonicity) of the ECF. Loss of pure water will raise the tonicity of the ECF (so-called hypertonic dehydration). Loss of water accompanied by loss of salt (NaCl) in the usual ECF (plasma) concentration will leave ECF tonicity unchanged (isotonic or isosmotic loss/dehydration) and is the most common type. Loss of fluid containing higher than ECF electrolyte composition will reduce the tonicity of the ECF (hypotonic dehydration). Since the terms hyper- and hypo-tonic are sometimes confused in relation to 'dehydration', they are probably best avoided, and the focus should be on describing exactly what is lost.

Loss of 'pure' water may be caused by reduced intake, increased losses, or both. Even when intake is zero, unavoidable insensible losses continue and may be increased from the skin and lungs by activity and fever or from the gastrointestinal tract by diarrhoea or vomiting (or by nasogastric suction after surgery). If 'pure' or very hypotonic water is lost from the ECF, the osmolality of all body fluids increases, stimulating the hypothalamus to secrete ADH, which allows formation of a concentrated urine. In addition, kidney reabsorption of sodium increases (the urine sodium concentration decreases) so that both water and sodium are retained in the body. Sodium concentration in sweat and intestinal and other secretions is also reduced as more aldosterone is secreted from the adrenal cortex in response to the lower volumes of plasma and ECF. This response has survival value—the high osmotic pressure maintains thirst and the output of ADH, minimizing urinary loss. Because of the increased ECF osmolality, water moves from cells (the ICF) into the ECF; the cells shrink, exaggerating the apparent volume depletion. This shift helps to sustain the volumes of ECF and circulating blood, and this takes precedence over the regulation of osmolality.

A note on 'dehydration' The distinctions in types of dehydration are obviously important in treatment, which involves repairing the deficit with appropriate fluid management. The term 'dehydration' is best avoided in dealing with altered sodium states (see Section 8.2) and possibly best avoided altogether. While ECF volume depletion is often termed dehydration, to many dehydration refers to a lack of water alone, in which case plasma sodium may increase as already described. In both of these conditions treatment involves supplying water with or without additional electrolytes. In contrast, a low plasma sodium is always associated with water retention by the kidney due to an absolute or relative excess of ADH, and management often involves fluid restriction!

Symptoms The cardinal manifestation of severe water deficiency is thirst; dry cracking skin, confusion, seizures, and coma may follow. See Box 8.1 for information on effects of water loss in an open barren environment.

> **BOX 8.1** Survival without water
>
> Amount of body water lost:
>
> - 1–5% body weight: thirst; vague discomfort; economy of movement; no appetite; flushed skin; impatience; increased pulse rate; nausea.
> - 6–10% body weight: dizziness; headache; laboured breathing; tingling in limbs; absence of saliva; blue body (cyanosis); indistinct speech; inability to walk.
> - 11–12% body weight: delirium; twitching; swollen tongue; inability to swallow; deafness; dim vision; shrivelled skin; numb skin.
>
> 'A man can exist for days without food, but only for 2–5 days without water.'
>
> Source: Hildreth B (1979). How to survive in the bush, on the coast, in the mountains of New Zealand. Government Printer, Wellington.

Fresh water may be as unavailable at sea as it is in deserts. The dry mouth, swollen tongue and delirium with hallucinations are admirably described by Samuel Taylor Coleridge in The Rime of the Ancient Mariner (1798).

And every tongue through utter drought,
    Was withered at the root;
We could not speak, no more than if
    We had been choked with soot.
With throats unslaked, with black lips baked,
    We could not laugh nor wail;
Through utter drought all dumb we stood!
    I bit my arm, I suck'd the blood,
And cried, 'A sail! a sail!'

During World War II, R.A. McCance (Professor of Experimental Medicine at Cambridge in England) was chairman of a subcommittee of the British Admiralty concerned with safeguarding the lives of hundreds of men cast adrift in lifeboats or rafts after their ships were sunk by enemy action. The reports showed that those who drank sea water had a mortality of 39% compared with 3.3% for those who did not. He studied volunteers in life rafts in temperate, arctic, and tropical seas, and came to the conclusion that sea water could not be used to supplement limited supplies of fresh water. Sea water has a higher salt concentration, typically a 'salinity' of 3.5% (35 g/L) giving a sodium concentration of 469 mmol/L, than human kidneys can achieve (about 270 to 300 mmol/L). As kidneys therefore need to excrete more water to eliminate the salt than the water gained by drinking seawater, drinking seawater will generally make dehydration worse. Any temporary improvement in circulation and feeling when water is withdrawn from cells is overshadowed by shortened survival. It is of no ultimate advantage to feel better on Monday and die on Tuesday if it happens that your party is not going to be rescued until Wednesday.

Treatment The remedy for primary water deficiency is water—as the predominant symptom of thirst indicates. It is important to realize that this is not confined to oceans and deserts; it can occur in hospital wards if thirst fails or cannot be satisfied. Unconscious patients do not experience thirst; others may be too confused or too weak to drink water set beside them. Thirst, water diuresis, and the response to ADH tend to become attenuated with advancing years, highlighting that many older people are increasingly at risk of dehydration.

8.1.6 Excess of body water

An excessive amount of water in the body is rarer than deficiency, because water diuresis protects against excess, and normal kidneys can usually excrete water as fast as the gut can absorb it (except after massive water or fluid ingestion). However, water diuresis can fail:

1 *in anuria* (zero urine) or *oliguria* (reduced urine output) with impaired renal function, as the kidneys cannot respond to absence of ADH;

2 *with inappropriate release of ADH*: e.g. with head or chest tumours, trauma, or infection. ADH release is also stimulated by pain, some anaesthetics, some drugs (including ecstasy), and ADH-like substances are secreted by some cancers, especially small-cell carcinoma of the lung.

If patients under these conditions are given much more than the 1 L per day, which they need to replace unavoidable losses, ECF osmolality and sodium concentration fall and water goes into cells, which swell. Weakness and cramps develop. Swelling of brain cells (cerebral oedema) leads to disturbances of consciousness and behaviour, and may progress to convulsions and death, so-called 'water intoxication'. Note that an excess of pure water does not cause generalized oedema (see Sodium excess).

Low osmolality and low plasma sodium concentration (hyponatraemia) can occur without an excess of total body water (e.g. if the water, but not the salt, lost in profuse sweating is replaced). Muscle cramps are then a major feature—previously known as miners' cramps and stokers' cramps, as they were common in English coal mines and ships. J.B.S. Haldane showed in 1928 that extra salt prevents or cures these cramps; as with miners in hot mines, some military rations in hot climates are supplemented with high-salt foods to replace the salt lost in sweat.

8.2 Sodium and extracellular fluid

8.2.1 Significance and functions of sodium

Salt has long been a valuable commodity and part of the fabric of human life and culture. We pay salaries, from *salarium*, the allowance for a Roman soldier to buy salt. We question whether a man is worth his salt. We often crave salt and some animals in arid regions trek vast distances to salt licks to get the sodium they need in order to excrete potassium from their high-potassium vegetable diet.

Common salt is sodium chloride (NaCl). Each gram contains 17.1 mmol of sodium, which is the principal cation in most extracellular fluids and is responsible for 95% of ECF osmolality. The ECF sodium concentration, at ~140 mmol/L in man and most animals, helps to determine the membrane potentials of most cells and the action potentials underlying the transmission of nerve impulses and the contraction of muscles. Since ECF sodium concentration is tightly regulated, it may be argued that the sodium concentration maintains the ECF (at 1 L for every 150 mmol, or 9 g of NaCl) that our cells live in. Consistent with this, disorders where plasma (ECF) sodium concentration is high or low (the dysnatraemias) are also disorders of water balance, not just sodium regulation.

8.2.2 Amount and distribution of sodium in the body

Adults contain about 5600 mmol of sodium (325 g NaCl). About half of that (2800 mmol) is dissolved in the extracellular fluids, with 300 in cells and 2500 in bone mineral. Half of the sodium in the bones is exchangeable with isotopically labelled Na, the rest is deeper and less accessible. Thus in classical analyses of dissolved bodies, more sodium was found than with modern measurements, which are based on isotopic dilution during life.

8.2.3 Sodium balance

Intake Diet: 70–250 mmol/day, but varies with habit, taste, and custom.

1 Natural foods contain 0.1–3.0 mmol sodium per 100 g: fruits 0.1 mmol/g; vegetables 0.3 mmol/g; meat, fish, and eggs about 3.0 mmol/100 g. 2. Processed foods contain far more: bread around 20 mmol/100 g; cheese 30 mmol/100 g; salted butter 40 mmol/100 g; raw lean bacon as much as 80 mmol/100 g.

People add widely varying amounts of salt to their cooking or at the table. Discretionary salt intake is usually much lower than that obtained from manufactured and processed or take-away food products.

Output

1 *Faeces*: normally 5–10 mmol/day.

2 *Sweat*: 20–80 mmol/day. Extremely variable (see section 8.2.4 below).

3 *Urine*: variable. Normally similar to but a little less than dietary intake.

The kidneys are capable of excreting between 1 and 500 mmol/day. They normally keep the amount in the body constant by excreting the excess of intake over the sum of other losses. Homer Smith's one-time remark that the composition of the body depends 'not on what the mouth takes in but on what the kidneys keep' aptly sums up their control of sodium balance.

The rate of excretion of sodium depends on the balance between glomerular filtration rate (GFR × sodium concentration) and tubular reabsorption (usually greater than 99%). When blood and ECF volumes fall, GFR is reduced by constriction of glomerular vessels (autoregulation) and reabsorption is increased by several factors. One major factor is aldosterone, secreted from the adrenal cortex. When blood pressure or volume is reduced and sympathetic nerves are activated, renin is released from the kidney; this enzyme forms angiotensin I from angiotensinogen in the plasma. Angiotensin-converting enzyme in blood and some tissues converts this to angiotensin II, which stimulates adrenal cortex production of aldosterone. In turn, aldosterone stimulates sodium and water reabsorption and simultaneous potassium loss in the distal nephron. Angiotensin II itself also stimulates sodium reabsorption. When blood volume increases, these sodium-conserving mechanisms are inhibited, GFR increases, and tubular sodium reabsorption is reduced; sodium reabsorption is also inhibited by atrial natriuretic peptide during volume expansion.

8.2.4 Sodium depletion

Deficiency of sodium does not simply result from deficient intake, for the kidneys can make the urine almost sodium-free. Abnormal losses causing depletion may arise from:

1 *Sweat*: up to as much as 15 L/day. Sweat is hypo-tonic, but with a sodium concentration of 50 mmol/L. 15 L of sweat contains the same amount of salt as 5 L of normal ECF; so even after osmolality is corrected by replacing water, the volume of the ECF will be reduced by 5 L unless the sodium is replaced.

2 *Intestinal fluid*: 10 L/day of intestinal secretions are normally reabsorbed. However, with diarrhoea, absorption is depressed and intestinal fluid secretion often increased. Losses may reach 18 L/day in cholera, and the fluid lost is almost isotonic, equivalent to its own volume of ECF.

3 *Urine*: The kidneys normally act to guard the body's stores of sodium. Diuretics and osmotic diuresis (e.g. with the load of glucose and ketone acids in diabetes) commonly remove large amounts of sodium in the urine. In adrenal insufficiency, e.g. in Addison's disease, the adrenal cortex fails to produce aldosterone, and the kidneys fail to conserve sodium (but retain potassium).

Most commonly osmolality is maintained and 1 L of water is lost with every 150 mmol of sodium, so that this volume depletion is largely confined to the ECF. As ECF volume depletion increases, blood pressure decreases and there may be a threat to life from circulatory failure, better known as 'shock'.

Symptoms Early symptoms of ECF volume depletion include dry mouth and tongue, loose skin that lacks turgor and sunken eyes, and, eventually, a rapid weak ('thready') pulse and low blood pressure complete the picture described as 'shock'. Packed cell volume, the concentrations of haemoglobin and plasma albumin, and blood viscosity all increase as the volume of plasma decreases. When oxygen transport to tissues is badly impaired, cells swell, taking up sodium and water; this further reduces the volume of ECF and may set up a vicious cycle, further reducing blood pressure and oxygen delivery.

Treatment Salt as well as water are required to treat this desperate state. Water given alone or by infusing glucose solutions will disappear into the cells with the risk of cerebral oedema (water intoxication). Isotonic saline ('normal', 0.9 g/L, 150 mmol/L NaCl) supplies sodium, chloride, and water in the proportions needed.

8.2.5 Experimental human salt deficiency

McCance subjected himself, and some other healthy people, to forced sweating for 2 hours each day while they ate a low-salt diet and drank only distilled water. They lost about 1 kg/day for 3 or 4 days, while plasma sodium concentrations remained normal. After that, the loss of sodium continued, but not the loss of weight; plasma sodium concentration fell and water moved into the cells. Their faces shrank, they lost their appetite and sense of taste, and they became very weak, weary, and muddleheaded and experienced a general sense of exhaustion, reduced initiative, delayed excretion of water loads, and almost continuous muscle cramps. Many of McCance's symptoms resembled those of severe Addison's disease, although the adrenal glands were presumably overactive! They endured these miseries for a week or two, and then enjoyed a rapid cure by eating salty fried herrings and licking the salt out of the pan! McCance's fascinating description in the third of his Goulstonian lectures (McCance, 1936) is a nutritional classic.

8.2.6 Sodium excess

An increased intake of salt does not usually increase the amount in the body, because the kidneys normally excrete the extra sodium and keep the volume of ECF constant. However, the kidneys can be misdirected or malfunction, and retain too much sodium. Examples (with some contributory factors) include:

1 Patients with cirrhosis and cardiac failure share the pathophysiology of decreased 'effective' arterial blood volume (EABV), resulting from

hypoalbuminaemia and splanchnic vasodilatation in cirrhosis and from decreased cardiac output in cardiac failure. This decrease in EABV results in stimulation of the renin–angiotensin–aldosterone system, and secondary sodium and water retention.

2 Patients with a reduced plasma albumin, e.g. from reduced retention within the plasma combined with loss in the urine in the nephrotic syndrome, or resulting from reduced synthesis in late cirrhosis, or from severe malnutrition also develop a reduced EABV, with stimulation of the renin–angiotensin–aldosterone system. The reduction in albumin decreases plasma oncotic pressure resulting in enhanced movement of plasma out of the intra- into the extravascular (interstitial) compartment of the ECF. However, the plasma volume is not always low, indicating that there are other incompletely understood factors involved.

The concept of EABV is important in understanding why the kidney retains sodium and water. EABV is an abstract term that refers to the adequacy of the arterial blood volume to 'fill' the capacity of the arterial vasculature. EABV is normal when the ratio of cardiac output to peripheral resistance maintains venous return and cardiac output at normal levels. EABV can be reduced, therefore, by factors which reduce actual blood volume (haemorrhage, dehydration), increase arterial vascular capacitance (cirrhosis, sepsis), or reduce cardiac output (cardiac failure). EABV can be reduced in the setting of low, normal, or high actual blood volume. Whenever EABV falls, the kidney is triggered to retain sodium and water. The mechanisms involved are: (a) reduced renal blood flow; (b) increased proximal tubular sodium and water reabsorption (angiotensin II); (c) increased distal tubular sodium and water reabsorption (aldosterone); and (d) increased ADH activity. When EABV is reduced, renal blood flow is reduced and volume receptors in large arteries are activated, leading to increased renal sympathetic tone and further decreased renal blood flow. Decreased renal blood flow stimulates the renin–angiotensin–aldosterone system, as already described.

Retained sodium increases osmolality in the ECF, provoking thirst and release of ADH, which immediately reduces renal 'free' water clearance (in antidiuresis). With normal osmoregulation, 1 L of water is retained with each 150 mmol of sodium (9 g NaCl). If just water is retained, it distributes throughout the total body water compartment and oedema will not usually form. However, if sodium is retained as well, it is confined to the extracellular spaces. The increased osmolality due to sodium retains water in the ECF. If the extra salt and water is not retained in the vasculature (e.g. if capillary pressure is raised or colloid oncotic pressure is low from lack of albumin), then it escapes into the interstitial spaces. Hence, blood volume is not expanded and the signals to retain sodium are not turned off. The excess sodium and water accumulates as generalized oedema, an excessive accumulation of fluid, usually beneath the skin, but sometimes in other compartments (see Fig. 8.1). Generalized oedema can occur with low, normal, or high serum sodium concentration. Thus, serum sodium concentration does not alone reflect total body sodium. An increased total body sodium can occur with a low, normal, or high serum sodium concentration.

Excessive ECF fluid can impair normal organ function. Oedema of the skin, particularly in the lower limbs can be painful, interferes with normal circulation, impairs wound healing, and increases the likelihood of infection. Ascites can impair breathing, decrease venous blood return to the heart, and promote intraperitoneal infection. Pulmonary oedema interferes with respiratory gas exchange and is a major cause of morbidity and mortality. Furthermore, oedema is a sign of an underlying disease process that needs to be treated.

Treatment Apart from treating the underlying disease process, treatment involves decreasing salt and water intake and/or promoting salt and water excretion, usually with diuretics (although these can make EABV worse). Extremely low-salt diets are unpalatable; however, some attempt to restrict salt should be made: processed foods are amongst the worst offenders and should be avoided. Diuretics inhibit reabsorption of sodium by the renal tubules. See Table 8.3 for a summary of disturbances in the water content of the body.

Table 8.3 Summary of disturbances in the amount of water in the body

Disturbance	Cause	Osmotic pressure (plasma [Na])	Volume change	Manifestation
Excess water	Water only	Reduced	ICF↑ ECF ↑	Cerebral oedema
	Excess Na	Normal	ECF ↑	Generalized oedema
Dehydration	Water loss	Increased	ICF↓ ECF ↓	Thirst
	Na loss	Normal	ECF ↓	Circulatory failure

ECF, extracellular fluid; ICF, intracellular fluid.

8.3 Potassium

8.3.1 Significance and functions of potassium

Potassium is the predominant cation in the cells of both animals and plants. Its salts, mainly organic, are responsible for most of the osmolality of animal cells and they determine their volume. Intracellular enzymes have evolved to require an environment rich in potassium. Cell membranes are much more permeable to potassium than sodium. Hence, the ratio of the intracellular concentration to the extracellular concentration of potassium largely determines the resting potentials of cells and the transient action potentials, which transmit messages and activate nerve cells and muscle fibres.

An increase in the low extracellular concentration of potassium lowers the concentration ratio of intracellular potassium to extracellular potassium; this depolarizes membranes and blocks transmission, whereas a decrease in extracellular potassium concentration increases the ratio, hyperpolarizes membranes, and raises the threshold for excitation. Consequently, the tight control of the low concentration of potassium in the ECF is critically important—large increases or decreases (twofold to threefold) can paralyse muscles and stop the heart.

8.3.2 Amount and distribution in the body

An average adult human's body contains about 3800 mmol of potassium; most of this (about 3200 mmol) is in the cells. Indeed, a total body count of the natural isotope, potassium-40, can yield an estimate of cell mass. About 300 mmol is contained in the skeleton and only 80 mmol is in solution in the extracellular fluids. Hence, if the cells increased their content by only 1.25% (40 mmol) at the expense of the ECF, the external concentration would be halved, with potentially serious consequences for neuromuscular and cardiac function.

8.3.3 Potassium balance

Intake Diet: around 100 mmol/day.

1 Meat is animal muscle and vegetables contain plant cells, hence all foods contain potassium. There are no large differences between natural and processed foods, as there are for sodium.

2 Wholemeal flour, meats, and fish: 7–9 mmol/100 g.

3 Common vegetables: 5–9 mmol/100 g.

4 Milk, eggs, and cheese: 4–6 mmol/100 g.

5 Fruit: 5–8 mmol/100 g (citrus fruits, bananas, and dry fruits have high potassium concentrations, e.g. oranges have 5 mmol/100 g, so orange juice is a useful source of potassium).

The lowest values are for salted butter at 0.5 mmol/100 g and apples at 0.3 mmol/100 g. Hence, ordinary mixed and vegetarian diets contain adequate amounts of potassium. It is difficult to devise a diet that is deficient, but it is easy to find one that is excessive for patients with kidney failure who have trouble excreting potassium and may die from the consequences of uncontrolled hyperkalaemia.

Output

1 *Faeces*: about 10 mmol/day.

2 *Urine*: 90 mmol/day.

This can be varied widely to match alterations in intake. The kidneys hold the balance by adjusting the amount in the urine. They can excrete potassium rapidly if extracellular potassium concentration rises and can conserve it when scarce, though not as avidly or as briskly as sodium. The renal priority is to keep the critically important concentration of potassium in the ECF within its normal range of 3.5–5 mmol/L.

8.3.4 Regulation of extracellular concentration

The most important factors are:

1 *Active uptake by cells*: This is maintained by ongoing metabolism and is promoted by insulin and by ECF acidosis. Potassium must be supplied to prevent a lethal fall in extracellular potassium concentration when patients with diabetic ketoacidosis treated with insulin and glucose begin to rebuild the severely depleted stores of glycogen and potassium in their muscles.

2 *Excretion by the kidneys*: The bulk of the potassium in the glomerular filtrate is reabsorbed from proximal tubules; what appears in the urine is mostly lost by distal tubular cells as they preferentially reasborb sodium in response to stimulation by aldosterone. The rate of renal excretion is increased by:

i increased extracellular potassium concentration;

ii aldosterone;

iii faster flow through distal tubules: the transcellular diffusion gradient sets the concentration of potassium in the tubular fluid (the transtubular potassium gradient), so that excretion is proportional to the flow;

iv increased sodium delivery or concentration in the distal tubular fluid; potassium diffuses into the tubular lumen partly in exchange for reabsorbed sodium. This can be promoted by more proximally acting diuretics that fundamentally work by inhibiting sodium reabsorption by various mechanisms.

8.3.5 Potassium depletion

Deficiency of potassium requires a failure of renal conservation, abnormal losses, or both.

1 Net absorption from the gastrointestinal tract is reduced or even negative (i.e. potassium is lost) if there is significant vomiting, aspiration of stomach contents, or diarrhoea, when lost fluid often contains more potassium than normal intestinal secretions. Colonic potassium loss will be further stimulated by aldosterone. Thus, abuse of purgatives can cause potassium depletion.

2 The kidneys usually excrete some potassium and this excretion is increased by adrenal steroids (e.g. aldosterone), diuretics, or acidosis. In diabetic ketoacidosis, there is movement of intracellular potassium to the ECF; increased renal excretion is driven by the high extracellular concentration, and the osmotic diuresis provoked by large amounts of ketones and glucose.

3 Most disturbances of acid–base balance increase the rate of excretion of potassium. Cells accumulate hydrogen ions in preference to potassium

(they effectively buffer the hydrogen ions). Thus ECF acidosis will bring potassium out of cells, raising extracellular concentrations, so potassium removed from renal cells is excreted and lost. Alkalosis promotes uptake of potassium from plasma into cells including renal tubular cells, from which potassium can be lost into the urine. Thus, alkalosis as well as acidosis can deplete the body of potassium.

Symptoms The symptoms of potassium deficiency are often mild, vague, and non-specific, and include fatigue and ill-defined malaise with weakness especially of skeletal and intestinal muscles; the post-operative form of this is called an ileus. Cardiac arrhythmias are also common and characteristic changes may be visible in an electrocardiogram (ECG). Hypokalaemia can interfere with the kidney's maximum concentrating ability, which may promote further loss.

Treatment Oral potassium replacement is the norm except when serum concentration is dangerously reduced or when patients are receiving intravenous fluids. Intravenous potassium supplementation must be carried out cautiously because of the risk that a sudden high extracellular potassium concentration can produce cardiac asystole. Oral replacement with food (e.g. bananas) is safe in less urgent cases.

8.3.6 Excess of body potassium

Potassium is not stored in the body; there is no overstocking of cells corresponding to oedema. Localized excesses in the form of high concentrations of potassium in ECF are dangerous, but these are rare in the absence of renal failure (acute or chronic kidney injury). The kidneys may fail to protect against excessive concentrations:

1 *In shock*, cells deprived of oxygen cannot retain potassium, and kidneys without adequate blood flow cannot excrete it.

2 *In crush injuries*, crushed muscles release potassium and also myoglobin, which can injure the kidneys, leading to acute failure.

3 *In anuria* (from any cause), excretion is impossible, and an increasing concentration of potassium in the plasma as cells break down may be a more pressing indication of the need for dialysis than a rising concentration of blood urea.

4 *In Addison's disease*, when adrenal mineralocorticoid secretion is deficient, extracellular potassium concentration may be moderately increased without an increase in total body potassium because the kidneys fail to conserve sodium but retain potassium.

Note that high (like low) ECF potassium can produce changes in an ECG, producing large peaked T waves, broadening of the QRS complex, and flattening of the P wave. These changes are a sign that treatment of the hyperkalaemia is urgently required. This can be performed by some combination of driving potassium into cells with insulin and glucose administration or with alkali (as bicarbonate) and removal of potassium from the body using chelating agents (such as oral resonium), loop diuretics, or dialysis. The ECG changes can be temporarily stabilized by intravenous calcium gluconate.

8.4 Acid–base balance

8.4.1 Regulation

The maintenance of acid–base balance implies keeping the body fluids mildly alkaline (i.e. plasma and other ECF at pH 7.35–7.45; cells about pH 7.1). This alkalinity is essential for cells in exciteable tissues (nerves, muscles, and heart). It is usually achieved by:

1 controlling excretion of carbon dioxide by the lungs (about 13 000 mmol/day); this removes the weak organic acid, carbonic acid, H_2CO_3; and

2 excretion of smaller amounts of non-volatile acid (hydrogen ions) or regeneration of alkali (bicarbonate) by the kidneys.

The kidneys control the numerator and lungs the denominator of the Henderson–Hasselbalch equation:

$$pH = 6.1 + \log \frac{[HCO_3^-]\quad \leftarrow kidneys}{0.03 P_{CO_2}\quad \leftarrow lungs \text{ and respiratory system}}$$

Normally, bicarbonate (HCO_3) concentration is kept around 24 mmol/L and the partial pressure of carbon dioxide near 40 mmHg; hence, pH must be:

$$6.1 + \log (24/(0.03 \times 40)) = 6.1 + \log (24/1.2)$$
$$= 6.1 + \log 20 = 6.1 + 1.3 = 7.4.$$

In response to chronic acidosis, the kidneys can upregulate glutaminase, which promotes ammonia secretion (from glutamine) and this facilitates additional hydrogen ion excretion as ammonium.

Respiratory and renal diseases are the common causes of altered acid–base balance. Considering only dietary factors, it has been known for more than 100 years that meat diets leave excess acid and vegetarian diets excess alkali in the body to be dealt with. Claude Bernard, in 1865, noticed that rabbits that happened to be starved produced acid urine instead of the usual alkaline urine characteristic of herbivorous animals. He deduced that starvation made them temporarily carnivorous, living on their own flesh, and found that he could make their urine alkaline or acid at will by giving them grass or meat to eat. He did the same with a horse. Metabolic acidosis is usually associated with impaired renal acid excretion, respiratory acidosis with a reduced respiratory rate causing CO_2 retention. Metabolic alkalosis is uncommon, while respiratory alkalosis from hyperventilation is quite common.

8.4.2 Dietary considerations

Meat diets yield sulphuric acid from S-amino acids, and phosphoric acid from nucleoproteins and phospholipids. Mixed diets leave about 70 mmol/day of hydrogen ions to be excreted (the so-called titrateable acids). Food faddists may label sour fruits as 'acid foods' but the organic acids they contain are either not absorbed or are mostly oxidized to water and carbon dioxide. Most of this is breathed out, although a little remains in the body as bicarbonate; hence, these acids, taken in as potassium salts, leave an excess of potassium bicarbonate, which tends to make the blood more alkaline! Table 8.4 gives examples of food acids and their metabolic rates, and it can be seen that these dietary acids pose no threat to the body's mild alkalinity.

Organic acids that can pose threats are:

1 acetoacetic and other keto acids, particularly produced in diabetic ketoacidosis; smaller, less important amounts during fasting;

2 lactic acid produced in severe muscular exercise or from tissues inadequately supplied with oxygen (e.g. in shock when blood pressure is very low).

Table 8.4 Acids in fruits and their metabolic fate

Food source	Acid	Fate
Citrus, pineapples, tomatoes, summer fruits	Citric	Oxidized to CO_2 and HO_2
Apples, plums, tomatoes	Malic	Oxidized to CO_2 and HO_2
Cranberries, blueberries	Benzoic	Excreted as hippuric acid
Grapes	Tartaric	Not absorbed
Strawberries, rhubarb, spinach	Oxalic	Not absorbed; forms calcium oxalate in the gut

Source: Modified from Passmore, R. and Eastwood, M.A. (1988) *Davidson and Passmore's human nutrition and dietetics*, 8th edition. Edinburgh, Churchill Livingstone.

8.4.3 Renal bicarbonate regeneration

Filtered bicarbonate is reabsorbed by the secretion of hydrogen ions in the proximal and distal tubules. This reaction forms carbonic acid, which is converted to CO_2 and water. The CO_2 diffuses back into renal cells; and forms intracellular bicarbonate which is secreted into the plasma, restoring buffer balance. Additional bicarbonate can be generated by promoting ammonia secretion, which leads to excretion of further hydrogen ions. Since electro-neutrality must be maintained, a molecule of bicarbonate is generated for every extra hydrogen ion excreted. The kidney thus makes bicarbonate by

secreting acid, with 1 mmol of bicarbonate added to the plasma for each 1 mmol of hydrogen ions secreted into the urine. Similarly, additional secreted hydrogen ions convert filtered buffers, especially phosphate, into their acid forms in acid urine. Hydrogen ions are also excreted as ammonium. Thus 1 mmol of additional bicarbonate is added to the plasma for every 1 mmol of hydrogen ion excreted as acid buffer or ammonium. In alkalosis, the concentration of bicarbonate in the plasma may be so high that there is more in the glomerular filtrate than the total rate of hydrogen ion secretion can cope with; the excess bicarbonate then escapes in alkaline urine and lowers the concentration in the plasma.

Further Reading

1. **Bray, J.J., Cragg, P.A., Macknight, A.D.C., and Mills, R.G.** (1999) *Lecture notes on human physiology*, 4th edition. Oxford, Blackwell Scientific Publications.
2. **Halperin, M.L., Kamel, K.S., and Goldstein M.B.** (2010) *Fluid, Electrolyte, and Acid-Base Physiology. A problem-based approach*. 4th edition. Philadelphia, Saunders Elsevier.
3. **Hildreth, B.** (1979) *How to survive in the bush, on the coast, in the mountains of New Zealand.* Wellington, Government Printer.
4. **McCance, R.A.** (1936) Medical problems in mineral metabolism. *Lancet*, **227**, 823–30.
5. **Passmore, R., and Eastwood, M.A.** (1988) *Davidson and Passmore's human nutrition and dietetics*, 8th edition. Edinburgh, Churchill Livingstone.
6. **Wrong, O.** (1993) Water and monovalent electrolytes. In: Garrow, J.S., and James, W.P.T. (eds) *Human nutrition and dietetics*, 9th edition. Edinburgh, Churchill Livingstone, pp. 146–61.

Useful Websites

To see topical and scientifically robust updates on nutrition associated with this textbook and web links to many of the journals in the Further Reading sections, please see the dedicated Online Resource Centre at **http://www.oxfordtextbooks.co.uk/orc/mann4e/**

This chapter has been modified and updated from that written by Professor James Robinson (deceased), which appeared in the first three editions of *Essentials of Human Nutrition*.

9 Major minerals: calcium and magnesium

Susan A. Lanham-New, Ohood Hakim, Ailsa Goulding, and Andrea Grant

9.1 Calcium
Susan A. Lanham-New, Ohood Hakim, and Ailsa Goulding

Calcium (Ca) is a unique mineral that is an essential constituent of all forms of life. The skeleton contains approximately 99% of the body's total calcium and we need adequate dietary calcium intake (as well as vitamin D) to facilitate normal growth and maintain healthy bones and teeth (Box 9.1). Calcium is a divalent cation, with an atomic weight of 40 (equivalents: 40 mg Ca = 1 mmol Ca). Calcium is the fifth most abundant element in our bodies. It is the main mineral in bone, being stored as hydroxyapatite, $Ca_{10}(OH)_2(PO4)_6$. One of the key roles of our skeletal system is to protect the vital organs. Furthermore, the skeleton provides a store of minerals from which calcium and phosphorus may be continually withdrawn or deposited according to physiological needs. The content of total body calcium differs widely among individuals at all ages because some people grow better skeletons than others. This is due to a combination of genetic/familial factors; as well as nutritional and other influences (Fig. 9.1).

In stark contrast, both intracellular and extracellular calcium concentrations are tightly controlled within narrow limits by the calciotrophic hormones.

BOX 9.1 Nutrition and bone

Essential for growth and maintenance of strong bones and teeth, healthy nerve and muscle function, blood clotting, and hormone release. Calcium intake is needed daily to offset the obligatory losses seen in urine and faeces. When dietary supply is insufficient, bone calcium stores are resorbed via parathyroid hormone (PTH). Food sources include dairy products, soy products, leafy green vegetables, bread, tap water in hard water areas, nuts and seeds, and dried fruits. Vitamin D improves alimentary calcium absorption. High calcium intakes and ensuring replete vitamin D status are both useful in slowing osteoporotic bone loss and reducing the risk of falling. Calcium balance is maintained by the calciotrophic hormones (PTH, calcitonin, and calcitriol (1,25-dihydroxyvitamin D).

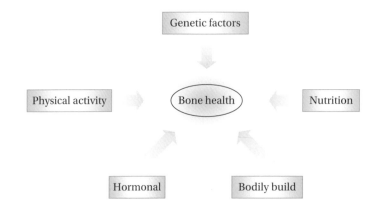

Fig. 9.1 Endogenous versus exogenous factors influencing bone health. Bone health is determined by a combination of endogenous and exogenous factors.

This is critical to human survival because interactions of calcium ions with proteins alter molecular activity. Ordered movement of ionic calcium plays an essential role in regulation of muscle contraction, nerve conductivity, ion transport, enzyme activation, blood clotting, and secretion of hormones and neurotransmitters. Life without calcium is not possible and small fluctuations in plasma calcium concentrations may have serious consequences. Hypocalcaemia and hypercalcaemia are common medical emergencies. Low blood calcium (hypocalcaemia) may cause seizures and tetany (musculoskeletal spasms and twitching, particularly in the fingers and face) and tingling and numbness due to increased neuromuscular activity. High blood calcium (hypercalcaemia) results in thirst, mild mental confusion and irritability, loss of appetite, and general fatigue and weakness. Polyuria and constipation are common. when concentration of calcium is high, calcium salts may precipitate in soft tissues and kidney stones may subsequently form.

9.1.1 Bone metabolism

There are two types of bone: dense cortical bone (80% of the skeleton), often referred to as compact bone, and spongy trabecular bone (20% of the skeleton), often referred to as cancellous bone. The skeleton undergoes constant renovation, rather like a building site! (Fig. 9.2) Old worn bits are being chiselled out or resorbed by multinucleate cells called osteoclasts, while new teams of cells called osteoblasts busily rebuild excavation holes with strong new bone. These activities take place within a bone-remodelling unit. Bone cell activity affects biochemical markers: blood levels of alkaline phosphatase, N-terminal propeptide of human procollagen type I, and osteocalcin reflect formation; urinary hydroxyproline, deoxypyridinoline and pyridinoline, C-terminal peptide (CTx), and N-terminal peptide (NTx) indicate resorption. Osteoblasts buried deep in bone mineral are called osteocytes; they seem to sense weight bearing and may help to regulate bone-remodelling responses to exercise. The different bone cells communicate actively. A complex, exquisitely sensitive 'internet' of chemical messages appears to control their differentiation and activity, but our understanding of this bone language remains limited. When osteoblasts and osteoclasts are matched, or coupled, bone mass is in a steady state. The amount of bone destroyed by osteoclasts is replaced by an equal amount of new bone. When bone remodelling becomes uncoupled, and resorption exceeds formation, bone is lost. Bone mass can be measured accurately *in vivo* using dual-energy X-ray absorptiometry (DEXA scanning, which provides an area density, units g/cm^2) or computerized tomography (CT scanning, which provides a volumetric density, units: g/cm^3). Quantitative ultrasound is a

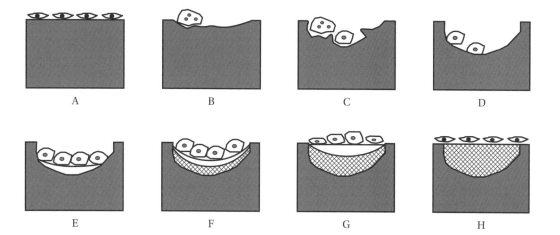

Fig. 9.2 Bone remodelling sequence. Early in the remodelling sequence osteoclasts are attracted to a quiescent bone surface (A) and excavate an erosion cavity (B, C). Mononuclear cells smooth off the erosion cavity (D), a subsequent site for the attraction of osteoblasts, and synthesize an osteoid matrix (E). Continuous new bone matrix synthesis (F) is followed by calcification (G) of the newly formed bone. When complete, lining cells once more overlie the trabecular surface (H).

useful tool for assessing risk of osteoporotic fracture, cheaper than DEXA and CT, and involves no ionizing radiation. However, unlike DEXA, it cannot be used to diagnose osteoporosis as defined by the World Health Organization (WHO, 1994).

9.1.2 Metabolic bone disorders

Children with vitamin D deficiency develop rickets, and adults, osteomalacia (see Section 15.1). Children do not calcify bone normally and their bones contain osteoid (unmineralized bone). Because this bone is weak, children with rickets often show bowed limbs.

Rickets is still seen in developing countries and amongst immigrant populations in more affluent Western societies, where osteoporosis is the most frequently seen bone disease. Osteoporosis is defined by the WHO as a 'progressive systemic skeletal disease characterized by low bone mass and micro-architectural deterioration of bone tissue, with a consequent increase in bone fragility and susceptibility to fracture'. Osteoporosis is caused by substantial loss of bone. Despite too little bone, what

remains is normally calcified. Osteoporotic bones are thin and break easily, especially in the wrist, spine, and hip. The thinner the bone density, the higher the risk of fractures.

9.1.3 Calcium stores

Bone stores It is often observed in the clinic that when plump people are being weighed they say 'I've got big bones'. However, bones are strong, rather than weighty. Bones of an average adult constitute 14% of body weight, and bone mineral 4%. Men accumulate more skeletal calcium (1200 g) than women (1000 g). Approximately one-fifth of this (21%) is in the skull, half (51%) in the arms and legs, and the remainder (28%) in the trunk (ribs 9%; pelvis 8%; spine 11%).

Peak bone mass The 'heaviest' bone mass that an individual achieves is called their peak bone mass (PBM). This is generally reached by 18–20 years of age, although some researchers conclude that the age could be as high as late twenties. The age at which PBM is attained varies between individuals as there are fast and slow bone losers in older age. To achieve average PBM values, men require a positive daily calcium gain of 160 mg and women 130 mg for every single day of the first 20 years of their lives! Ethnic and familial studies and studies of monozygotic and dizygotic twins show that there are strong genetic influences on PBM attainment. These may account for up to 80% of the variability in adult bone density. The variance in PBM is wide, with values ranging between 20% higher and 20% lower than average. The variance does not change in the third and fourth decades of life, indicating that young adults with low density do not catch up bone density over time. Thus, if a good PBM is not attained by the late twenties, it is unlikely to ever be achieved.

Calcium in extraskeletal stores and body fluids

These stores are small (15 g), comprising teeth (7 g), soft tissues (7 g), and plasma and intracellular fluids (1 g). Cytoplasm concentrations are one thousand times lower than those in plasma. Breast milk contains a high level of calcium (350 mg/L or 8.8 mmol/L) and a lactating mother transfers around 260 mg daily to her baby. Plasma calcium concentration is 2.2–2.6 mmol/L (8.8–10.4 mg/dL). Half of this is bound to protein (37% to albumin and 10% to globulin), 47% is free or ionized, and 6% is complexed to anions (phosphate, citrate, bicarbonate). Ionized calcium is biologically active. Levels are regulated by the PTH–vitamin D axis and calcitonin.

Control of plasma calcium

When ionized plasma calcium concentrations fall, PTH is secreted to increase calcium input from the kidney, bone, and gut (Fig. 9.3). In the kidney, PTH augments the tubular reabsorption of calcium, decreases tubular reabsorption of phosphate and bicarbonate, and stimulates conversion of $25(OH)D_3$ to $1,25(OH)_2D_3$ (calcitriol). In bone, PTH promotes release of calcium and phosphate into blood. The effects of PTH on kidney and bone are direct and rapid and are assisted by $1,25(OH)_2D_3$. The ability of PTH to raise alimentary calcium and phosphate absorption is mediated solely by calcitriol. When normal plasma calcium concentrations are restored, PTH secretion decreases, the flow of calcium from bone subse-quently diminishes, urinary calcium rises, and $1,25(OH)_2D_3$ synthesis is closed down. This system is extremely robust and PTH and calcitriol influence each other's synthesis. The specific role of vitamin D is discussed in Section 15.1.

Calcitonin, a hormone secreted by the thyroid gland, helps to fine-tune plasma calcium regulation. It lowers calcium by inhibiting bone resorption and is secreted when ionized blood calcium levels rise above normal, probably helping to curb blood calcium fluctuations after meals. Calcitonin plays a smaller role in plasma calcium homeostasis than either PTH or calcitriol. Interestingly, patients who have had surgery on the thyroid gland maintain levels extremely well. In contrast, patients lacking either PTH or active vitamin D metabolites develop hypocalcaemia. Magnesium deficiency also causes hypocalcaemia because magnesium is a cofactor for PTH secretion. Restoring magnesium corrects the problem in alcoholics and patients with steator-rhoea. Total plasma calcium rarely falls below 1.25 mmol/L (5 mg/dL) because calcium ions from bone mineral constantly exchange with extracellular fluid. This is why bone is referred to as a giant 'ion exchanger' facility in the body.

Obligatory losses of calcium

Significant amounts of calcium 'leak' from the body. These unavoidable obligatory losses occur through the skin (generally less than 20 mg/day via epithelial cells and sweat), in the faeces (unabsorbed digestive juice calcium may contain 80–120 mg/day), and in urine. Obligatory urinary calcium loss varies between 40 and 200 mg/day, depending on how effectively calcium is reabsorbed from the glomerular filtrate. Renal tubules reabsorb more than 98% of the 10 000 mg calcium filtered daily by the glomeruli. Dietary salt (NaCl), protein, and caffeine are all know to aggravate obligatory urinary calcium loss.

9.1.4 Calcium balance and absorption

If more calcium is retained in the body than excreted, a person is said to be in positive calcium balance.

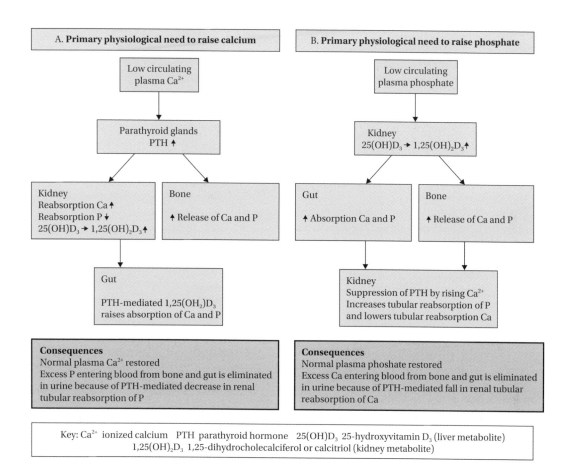

Fig. 9.3 Coordinated actions of parathyroid hormone and calcitriol in target organs regulate levels of calcium and phosphate in plasma. Ca^{2+}, ionized calcium; PTH parathyroid hormone; $25(OH)D_3$, 25-hydroxyvitamin D_3 (liver metabolite); $1,25(OH)_2D_3$, 1,25-dihydrocholecalciferol or calcitriol (kidney metabolite).

Negative calcium balance occurs if more calcium is excreted than ingested in the diet. Zero calcium balance implies that amount of calcium absorbed daily from food exactly matches amounts lost in the faeces and urine and from the skin (Fig. 9.4).

Alimentary calcium absorption
Alimentary calcium absorption is not as efficient as renal tubular calcium reabsorption. Absorption is normally less than 70% (and usually less than 30%) of calcium entering the gut. Net calcium absorption (the difference between calcium ingested by mouth and calcium excreted in the faeces) can be determined by traditional metabolic balance techniques. To ensure avoidance of negative calcium

balance, net absorption must fully offset calcium losses from urine and skin. However, measurement of net calcium absorption considerably underestimates total calcium absorbed from the intestine into blood because some faecal calcium (endogenous faecal) is derived from calcium resecreted into the intestine in the digestive juices, rather than from unabsorbed food calcium. True alimentary calcium absorption (amount actually absorbed from the gut) is measured with radioisotopes or stable isotopes, ^{42}Ca and ^{44}Ca.

Factors affecting the bioavailability of calcium in the intestine
Variations in the efficiency of absorption are predominantly determined

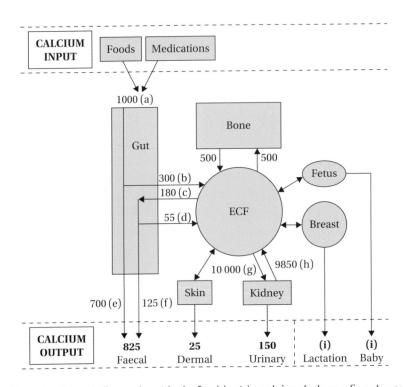

Fig. 9.4 Illustration of calcium influxes (mg/day) of subject in calcium balance (input = output). ECF, extracellular fluid; (a), total calcium ingested by mouth; (b), dietary calcium absorbed; (c), calcium in digestive secretions; (d), reabsorbed endogenous calcium; (e), unabsorbed dietary calcium; (f), endogenous faecal calcium excretion; (g), calcium load filtered at glomerulus; (h), calcium reabsorbed from glomerular filtrate (>98%); (i), losses only incurred in pregnancy (full-term baby has 25–30 g calcium) or lactation (160–300 mg/day in breast milk).

by two factors: (1) vitamin D metabolites; and (2) rate of transit of gut contents through the intestine. Calcitriol improves calcium absorption (see Chapter 15). However, some is absorbed even in vitamin D-deficient states, as some calcium is absorbed by passive concentration-dependent diffusion. The duodenum absorbs calcium most avidly, but larger quantities of calcium are absorbed by the ileum and jejunum, mainly due to food components spending longer in these areas. Some calcium is also absorbed from the colon, and surgical resection can impair absorption. Carbohydrates, such as lactose, improve calcium absorption by augmenting its passive diffusion across villous membranes. Diets rich in oxalate, fibre, and phytic acid are reputed to depress alimentary absorption by complexing calcium in the gut. However, it

appears that their overall effects seem small, possibly because bacterial breakdown of uronic acid and phytates in the colon frees calcium for absorption. Poor bioavailability of calcium from spinach is attributed to the high oxalate content. Dietary phosphorus increases the endogenous secretion of calcium into the gut. There is also evidence that calcium absorption diminishes in both sexes in the seventh decade of life because of lower renal synthesis of calcitriol and intestinal resistance to calcitriol, which contribute to the genesis of senile osteoporosis (see Section 9.1.6).

Factors influencing urinary calcium loss
Urinary calcium excretion rises when the filtered load of calcium increases or tubular reabsorption decreases. Acidifying agents, dietary sodium, protein,

and caffeine raise excretion. Phosphorus, alkaline agents (bicarbonate, citrate), and thiazide diuretics lower excretion. Variations in salt intake explain much of the day-to-day fluctuation in urinary calcium. A useful pointer is that one teaspoonful of salt (100 mmol NaCl) raises urinary calcium by 40 mg calcium/day, and this occurs even on a low calcium intake. Purified sulphur-containing amino acids (methionine and cysteine) cause significant calciuria but phosphate in whole proteins mitigates their calciuric effect when consumed in foods. There is evidence that even vegetarians with an alkaline urine excrete less urinary calcium than meat-eaters, who have an acid urine.

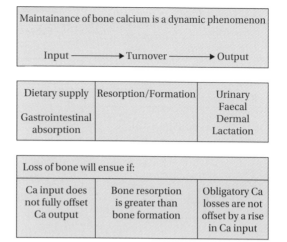

Maintainance of bone calcium is a dynamic phenomenon		
Input ⟶	Turnover ⟶	Output

Dietary supply Gastrointestinal absorption	Resorption/Formation	Urinary Faecal Dermal Lactation

Loss of bone will ensue if:		
Ca input does not fully offset Ca output	Bone resorption is greater than bone formation	Obligatory Ca losses are not offset by a rise in Ca input

Fig. 9.5 Illustration of the ways in which bone loss can be caused. Maintainance of bone calcium is a dynamic phenomenon.

9.1.5 Dietary calcium

The calcium stores in our bodies are built and maintained by extracting and retaining calcium from food. Our dietary needs vary according to gender, ethnicity, age, and magnitude of obligatory calcium loss. Table 9.1 provides details of the new (30th November 2010) recommendations for calcium (and vitamin D) by the US Food and Nutrition Board of the Institute of Medicine (IOM). It is essential, at all stages, to consume and absorb enough dietary calcium to satisfy physiological calcium needs. This is because some bone will be mobilized to maintain blood calcium levels whenever losses of calcium exceed that of alimentary calcium absorption (Fig. 9.5)

Threshold concepts Few individuals consume too much calcium from natural foods; however, many eat too little. This may subsequently affect their skeletons detrimentally, especially in childhood, when skeletal needs are high, and in later life when alimentary absorption of calcium deteriorates. There is a threshold intake for calcium below which skeletal calcium accumulation is a function of intake, and above which skeletal accumulation does not further increase, irrespective of further increases in intake. In other words, 'enough' calcium is good, but 'extra' calcium will not increase bone formation.

Recommended nutrient intake Considerable controversy exists worldwide regarding the optimal daily dietary intake of calcium for individuals to: (1) achieve optimal PBM attainment; (2) maintain adult bone mass; and (3) prevent bone loss in later life. There may be ethnic and genetic differences in calcium requirements. Those experts who argue for lower intakes point out that large sections of the population manage to grow and maintain bone on calcium intakes well below current US recommended dietary allowance (RDA). As shown in Table 9.1, new recommendations for calcium and vitamin D published on 30 November 2010 by the US IOM maintain the levels set by the 1997 Food and Nutrition Board of the IOM. For the 1–3 year age group, calcium recommendations have been increased from 500 mg/day to 700 mg/day, and for the 4–8 year age group, from 800 mg/day to 1000 mg/day. It is noteworthy that many people find difficulty in consuming more than 1000 mg calcium daily from natural foods. A possible (and better way) to boost the calcium economy would be to lower dietary salt intake, since this will reduce obligatory loss of calcium and improve calcium balance. Vitamin D supplementation is essential for housebound elderly individuals.

Table 9.1 US dietary recommendations for calcium and vitamin D

Life stage group	Age	Calcium (mg/day)		Vitamin D (mg/day)	
		RDA/AI	UIL	RDA/AI	UIL[a]
Infants	(0–6 m)	200*	1000	400*	1000
	(6–12 m)	260*	1500	400*	1500
Children	(1–3 y)	700	2500	600	2500
	(4–8 y)	1000	2500	600	3000
Males	(9–13 y)	1300	3000	600	4000
	(14–18 y)	1300	3000	600	4000
	(19–30 y)	1000	2500	600	4000
	(31–50 y)	1000	2500	600	4000
	(51–70 y)	1000	2000	600	4000
	(>70 y)	1200	2000	800	4000
Females	(9–13 y)	1300	3000	600	4000
	(14–18 y)	1300	3000	600	4000
	(19–30 y)	1000	2500	600	4000
	(31–50 y)	1000	2500	600	4000
	(51-70 y)	1200	2000	600	4000
	(>70 y)	1200	2000	800	4000
Pregnancy	(14–18 y)	1300	3000	600	4000
	(19–30 y)	1000	2500	600	4000
	(31–50 y)	1000	2500	600	4000
Lactation	(14–18 y)	1300	3000	600	4000
	(19–30 y)	1000	2500	600	4000
	(31–50 y)	1000	2500	600	4000

RDA, recommended dietary allowance; AI, adequate intake; UIL, tolerable upper intake level; ND, not determined.

[a]UIL for magnesium represents intake from pharmacological agents only and does not include intake from food or water.

Institute of Medicine (IOM) (30th November 2010) *Dietary reference intakes for calcium and vitamin D*. Washington, DC, National Academy Press.

Food sources of calcium

Foods vary greatly in their calcium content. Milk has an especially high calcium content (Table 9.2). Other excellent sources of calcium include cheeses and yoghurt. In many Western countries, dairy products supply up to two-thirds of the total daily intake of calcium. Soymilk substitutes are also excellent suppliers of calcium. Good sources of calcium include nuts, canned fish with bones, leafy vegetables and dried fruit. In some countries, foods are fortified with mineral calcium salts.

Table 9.2 Calcium content of some common foods

Calcium sources	Serving size		mg Ca/ serving
Excellent sources			
Milk, whole	1 cup	250 mL	276
Milk, reduced fat 2%	1 cup	250 mL	293
Yoghurt, plain-whole milk	1 cup	8 oz	275
Soymilk	1 cup	250 mL	255
Cheddar cheese		1 oz	204
Swiss cheese		1 oz	221
Good sources			
Ice cream, French vanilla	1/2 cup	66 g	113
Almonds/walnuts	24 nuts	1 oz	75
Canned sardines with bones		3 oz	325
Canned salmon with bones		3 oz	181
Baked beans	1 cup		124
Broccoli/peas	1/2 cup		31–47
Cabbage/spinach—cooked	1/2 cup		36–122
Dried figs	2 figs		62

Source: USDA National Nutrient Database for Standard Reference, release 22, 2009.

Dietary advice to increase calcium intake (while following nutritional guidelines for lowering fat intake) includes:

- Have a serving of either yoghurt or milk daily for breakfast.
- Always have low-fat milk available in the fridge but use the full-fat varieties for children.
- Choose low-fat dairy products when shopping.
- Add cheese chunks or a sprinkling of nuts/seeds to salads/vegetables.
- Eat pieces of cheese, nuts/seeds, or green vegetables as snacks.
- Add grated cheese or milk when serving soups and pasta.
- Use canned fish with bones in sandwich spreads.
- Try tofu chunks with salads and casseroles.
- Add a little skimmed milk powder to recipes when baking.
- Serve vegetables in white sauces made with milk.
- Use yoghurt in place of cream with desserts.

When individuals choose the calcium-rich foods they like, satisfactory intake of calcium may be sustained throughout all the life stages.

Calcium supplementation and food fortification Individuals who find it difficult to eat enough calcium may benefit from mineral supplements. At risk are those with very low calorie intakes, milk allergies, or symptomatic lactose malabsorption. They may need to consume foods fortified with calcium (soybean and citrus drinks, breakfast cereals) or take supplements, which are as well absorbed as food calcium.

Calcium intoxication Ingestion of large amounts of alkaline calcium salts (the new US IOM reference nutrient intakes for calcium and vitamin D recommend an upper limit for Ca of between 2000 and 3000 mg/day from age 1 year to >70 years) can override the ability of the kidney to excrete unwanted calcium, causing hypercalcaemia and metastatic calcification of the cornea, kidneys, and blood vessels. People consuming huge quantities of calcium carbonate in antacids are prone to this intoxication (milk-alkali syndrome). Patients taking vitamin D, or its metabolites, may suffer similar symptoms. Very large amounts of vitamin D are known to be toxic (see Section 15.1.10). The new US IOM upper intake level for vitamin D from age 9 years to >70 years is now set at 4000 IU.

9.1.6 Factors affecting bone growth and attrition

Normal growth Both boys and girls display similar linear gains in calcium up to the age of about 10 years (Fig. 9.6). Their total body calcium then averages 400 g, indicating a daily increment of 110 mg over this period. Skeletal growth is accelerated at puberty. Spinal density matures earlier in girls, who go through puberty earlier than boys (UK average is 12.2 years for girls and 14.1 years for boys). Total body calcium doubles in girls between the ages of 10 and 15 years (an average gain of 200 mg daily). Boys have two extra years of prepubertal bone gain before their pubertal growth spurt, when they deposit over 400 mg calcium daily in bone. Children do not have higher calcium absorption than adults. Obligatory losses are also high and there are concerns that many children consume too little calcium to meet their skeletal needs. Indeed, in the UK, the National Diet and Nutrition Surveys show that intakes below the lower reference nutrient intake for calcium (400 mg/day) for boys and girls aged 11–18 years are greater than 10–15%. In teenagers, bone mass can be increased by supplementation. However, the gain may be temporary and catch-up may occur in children who consume less calcium. It may just take children longer to attain their skeletal potential on moderate calcium intakes than on very high intakes.

Exogenous factors such as calcium intake, physical activity, and sex steroid status influence bone accrual. Cigarette smoking and excess alcohol affect bone mass adversely. High levels of weight-bearing physical activity, adequate dietary calcium, and sex steroids favour bone accrual. Regular moderate exercise should be recommended for youngsters. Children with good lean body mass have the best bone mass (Fig. 9.7). In teenagers with anorexia nervosa and athletic amenorrhoea, low oestrogen status causes poor PBM. Girls who recover from these conditions continue to show thin spinal bone years after plasma oestrogen levels have returned to normal.

Fit but fragile phenomena More than a century ago, a German scientist, Julius Woolf, stated the theory now called 'Woolf's Law: 'bone accommodates the forces applied to it by altering its amount and distribution of mass.' More recently, this concept has been refined to a general theory of bone mass regulation, known as the mechanostat model. It is well known that in the absence of weight-bearing exercise bone loss will occur at both axial and appendicular skeletal sites. Whilst bone mass has been shown to be higher in athletes involved in various sports, there is increasing concern for the bone health of women engaged in high-intensity physical training, for whom amenorrhoea is a common characteristic. Some such sports also demand extremely low body weights and there is high reported incidence of anorexia nervosa amongst participants. The combination of amenorrhoea and anorexia is of detriment to bone mass and there is now good evidence to show that they 'underachieve' their PBM potential and thus are at considerably increased risk of osteoporosis. This picture of undernutrition, amenorrhoea, and osteoporosis is defined as the 'female athletic triad' and in 1997, the American College of Sports Medicine published a position stand to 'encourage the prevention, recognition and management of this syndrome' (Otis et al., 1997) (Fig. 9.8). The exact mechanisms involved in PBM reduction are unclear, but some data suggest suppression of osteoblasts rather than increased osteoclastic activity. Of further interest is

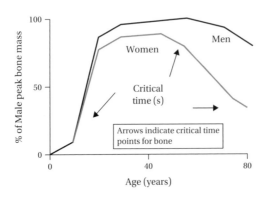

Fig. 9.6 Changes in skeletal mass throughout the life cycle.

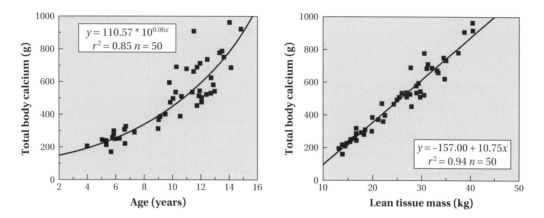

Fig. 9.7 Total body calcium changes in 50 growing girls aged 3–15 years, in relation to age ($r = 0.92$) and lean tissue mass ($r = 0.97$).

Source: A. Goulding.

the finding that in gymnasts, despite a high prevalence of oligo- and amenorrhoea, bone mass shows a higher than predicted value. In a 3-year longitudinal study undertaken at the University of Surrey, UK in gymnasts and controls, despite evidence of late age of menarche and/or amenorrhoea in the gymnast group, bone density was as much as 25% higher in these girls compared with age-matched and pubertal age-matched controls (Fig. 9.9), probably because extreme weight-bearing in gymnastics compensates.

Bone attrition

Bone mineral density declines after middle life. Falling levels of sex steroids cause trabecular loss, while calcium deprivation speeds

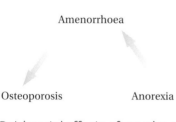

Fig. 9.8 Detrimental effects of exercise on the skeleton—the Female Athletic Triad.

Source: Otis CL, Drinkwater B, Johnson M, Loucks A, and Wilmore J. (1997) American College of Sports Medicine position stand. The female athletic triad. *Med Sci Sport Exerc*, **29**, i–ix.

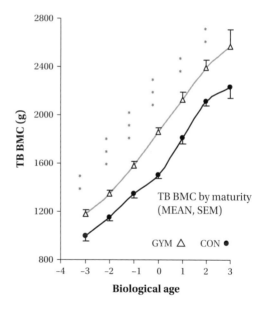

Fig. 9.9 Positive effect of impact loading exercise on PBM attainment. Values are mean ± standard error of the mean adjusted for height and weight. **, $P < 0.01$; ***, $P < 0.001$.

Source: Nurmi-Lawton, Baxter-Jones, A.D., Mirwald, R.L., et al. (2004) Evidence of sustained skeletal benefits from impact-loading exercise in young females: a 3-year longitudinal study. *J Bones Miner Res*, **19**, 314–22.

cortical loss. Effects of oestrogen deprivation are particularly pronounced at the menopause, with the rate of bone loss averaging 1–2% of bone over a 5–10 year period, although we know that there are fast and slow bone losers (Fig. 9.7). Bone losses are considerable: from youth to old age, women lose half their trabecular bone and a third of their cortical bone, while men lose a third of their trabecular bone and a fifth of their cortical bone. Low bone mass in the elderly may be due to poor PBM, to subsequent excessive loss of bone, or to both factors. Bone density will fall below the fracture threshold at a younger age in people with low PBM than in those with high PBM. Variations in the genetic inheritance of factors affecting mineral metabolism and bone cells probably affect PBM, rate of bone loss, and, hence, their susceptibility to bone fracture. Individuals inheriting different polymorphisms of the vitamin D receptor gene may differ in their dietary requirements for calcium and vitamin D and in their bone density. In future, public health strategies may target dietary advice at women with a genetic predisposition to low PBM attainment or increased peri/postmenopausal bone loss. For example, calcium intake has been found to be a determinant of bone mineral density in perimenopausal/early postmenopausal women with the 'bb' vitamin D receptor genotype but not those with the 'BB' genotype, a finding that is exclusive to those women not taking exogenous oestrogen. Modest alcohol intake (1–2 units per day) has been shown to be associated with reduced bone loss in perimenopausal women carrying the 'p' allele of the oestrogen receptor genoptype. Nutrient–gene interactions in the field of bone health is an area of considerable interest and research.

Bone fractures and osteoporosis

Weak bones break more easily than strong ones. Thus, low bone density increases fracture risk, even in youth. In childhood, up to a third of all fractures affect the distal forearm. Fractures at this site are particularly common in early puberty, when bone is remodelling fast and calcium requirements are especially high. Children who break their wrists have lower bone density than those without fractures. Increasing calcium intake and physical activity during growth help to strengthen their skeletons and avoid fractures (see Box 9.2).

BOX 9.2

Case 1. A boy who habitually avoided milk products because he disliked the taste was seen at 6.5 years and 2 years later. At 7.8 years he broke his forearm falling less than standing height on carpet, playing with his sister. Although his total body calcium at 8.5 years was 582 g and his DXA bone mineral density (BMD) values were slightly above average (111% of expected values), he had experienced rapid, inappropriate weight gain, possibly because he ate almond croissants daily for breakfast and exercised little. In 2 years he had gained 14.1 kg (11.2 g fat per day) and his body mass index (BMI) had risen from the 75th to >95th percentile for age. At 8.5 years he had the average weight of a 12-year-old (41.2 kg) but ultradistal radius BMD suitable only for a 10-year-old. He thus fell heavily on insufficient bone. Obesity, milk avoidance, and inactivity can increase fracture risk in growing children.

Osteoporosis is a serious and expensive public health problem, particularly in women. It causes significant pain and morbidity among elderly people (see Section 9.1.2). The incidence of osteoporotic fractures is expected to increase in future because people are living longer. In 1990, there were 1.16 million estimated hip fractures worldwide. By the year 2025, it is projected that there will be 1.66 million hip fractures in men and 2.78 million in women due to osteoporosis.

At present, the best way to avoid osteoporotic fractures in later life is to grow a good skeleton, to achieve optimal genetic skeletal mass, and then to retain this as long as possible. Every effort should therefore be made to ensure life-long consumption, absorption, and retention of sufficient calcium to do this (see Box 9.3).

Case 2. A 73-year-old woman (ht 152 cm, wt 48 kg, BMI 20.8 kg/m2) referred for investigation had been diagnosed lactose intolerant at age 7 years. She then avoided dairy products all her life without consuming other calcium-rich foods, but was active and a keen gardener. DXA scans taken 65 years after diagnosis of lactose intolerance confirmed severe osteoporosis and a low total body calcium content of only 488 g (half the young adult value of 960 g). Her BMD T scores were: −5.63 (wrist); −3.10 (hip); −5.71 (spine); −3.89 (total body). She was promptly placed on bone-conserving medication to reduce fracture risk. This case shows that sustained dietary calcium deprivation is detrimental to bone health. T score compares BMD with normal young adult.

9.1.7 Other possible health effects (positive and negative) of calcium

Relatively high intakes of calcium appear to be protective against hypertension, especially when consumed in low-fat dairy products in a diet high in fruit and vegetables and low in salt. The series of DASH (Dietary Approaches to Stop Hypertension) trials showed that consumption of low-fat dairy products resulted in further reductions in blood pressure when added to a diet with the other blood pressure-lowering attributes. Furthermore, such a diet is associated with decreased urinary calcium excretion and reduced bone resorption.

The consumption or absorption of other substances may be influenced by calcium intakes. Milk products contain considerable fat. However, fat-reduced dairy products are available for the cholesterol conscious and those worried about obesity. There are concerns that high dietary calcium may lower iron absorption, but few data confirm that this effect is found in the general population. High levels of calcium also aggravate the inhibitory effect of phytic acid on zinc absorption. Calcium binds gut oxalate so supplements do not induce kidney stones. Calcium may lower absorption of tetracyclines.

Population subgroups listed below, who have special nutritional needs and who may be vulnerable to calcium deprivation, should be targeted to improve calcium economy and hence safeguard bone health. Such groups include:

- people with habitually low dietary calcium intakes;
- people with food allergies or lactose malabsorption;
- adolescents building maximal bone;
- girls with anorexia nervosa or athletic amenorrhoea;
- the calorie-conscious (slimmers often avoid dairy foods);
- people with very low dietary energy intakes;
- pregnant women (last trimester) and lactating women;
- people with high intakes of common salt;
- people with heavy alcohol consumption and smokers;
- patients with malabsorption syndromes;
- patients taking corticosteroid medication;
- patients with renal disease;
- elderly people;
- people confined indoors who get no vitamin D from sunlight.

There has been recent interest in the possibility that calcium supplements may increase risk of myocardial infarction and other cardiovascular events. A meta-analysis published in 2010 showed that use of Ca supplements (without vitamin D) was associated with an increased risk of myocardial infarction and the authors suggest a reassessment of calcium supplementation in the management of osteoporosis (Bolland *et al.*, 2008; 2010). These conclusions have been criticized on the grounds that data from randomized controlled trials were misrepresented (Sabbagh and Vatanparast, 2009) and the Women's Health Initiative (WHI) study, criticized widely for poor study design and compliance, was overemphasized.

Definitive conclusions require more research. Further meta-analysis work is currently underway to see if the effects are present in supplementation studies of Ca and vitamin D combined. It is key to point out that the link between increased calcium intake from supplements and risk of myocardial infarction applies to calcium supplements and not calcium from the diet.

Further Reading

1. **Bolland, M.J., Barber, P.A., Doughty, R.N.**, *et al.* (2008) Vascular events in healthy older women receiving calcium supplementation: Randomized controlled trial. *BMJ*, **336**, 262–66.
2. **Bolland M.J., Avenell A., Baron J.A.**, *et al.* (2010) Effect of calcium supplements on risk of myocardial infarction and cardiovascular events: Meta-analysis. *BMJ*, **341**, c3691.
3. **Darling, A.L., Millward, D.J., Torgerson, D.J., Hewitt, C.E., and Lanham-New, S.A.** (2009). Dietary protein and bone health: A systematic review and meta-analysis. *Am J Clin Nutr*, **90**, 1674–92, editorial **90**, 1142–3.
4. **Goulding, A.** (2001) Bone mineral density and body composition in boys with distal forearm fractures: A dual energy X-ray absorptiometry study. *J Pediatr*, **139**, 509–15.
5. **Holick, M. and Dawson-Hughes, B.** (2004) *Nutrition and bone health*. USA, Humana Press.
6. **Lanham-New, S.A.** (2008) Importance of vitamin D and calcium in the maintenance of bone health and prevention of osteoporosis. *Proc Nutr Soc*, **67**, 163–76.
7. **Lanham-New, S.A.** (2008) The balance of bone health: Tipping the scales in favour of the potassium case. *J Nutr*, **138**:172S–7S.
8. **Lanham-New, S.A. and Gannon, R.H.T.** (2007) Fruit and vegetable link to bone health. In: Lanham-New, S.A., O'Neill, T., Sutcliffe, A., and Morris, R. (eds) *Prevention and treatment of osteoporosis*. Oxford, Clinical Publishing. pp 35–49.
9. **Lanham-New, S.A., Thompson, R.L., More, J., Brooke-Wavell, K., Hunking, P., and Medici, E.** (2007) Importance of vitamin D, calcium and exercise to bone health with specific reference to children and adolescents. *Nutrition Bulletin*, **32**, 364–77.
10. **Lanham-New, S.A., Al-Ghamdi, M., and Jalal, J.** (2011) Nutrition and bone health. In: Allen, L. (ed) 10th *edition of the encyclopedia of human nutrition*. New York, Elsiever.
11. **Loveridge, N. and Lanham-New, S.A.** (2009) Healthy ageing: Bone health. In: Stanner, S., Thompson, R., and Buttriss J.L. (eds) *BNF taskforce on healthy ageing—the role of nutrition and lifestyle*. Oxford, British Nutrition Foundation, Wiley-Blackwell, pp. 352–75.
12. **Matkovic, V.** (2005) Calcium supplementation and bone mineral density in females from childhood to young adulthood: A randomized controlled trial. *Am J Clin Nutr*, **81**, 175–88.
13. **New, S.A. and Bonjour, J.-P.** (2003) *Nutritional aspects of bone health*, 1st edition. Cambridge, UK, Royal Society of Chemistry.
14. **Nurmi-Lawton, Baxter-Jones, A.D., Mirwald, R.L.**, *et al.* (2004) Evidence of sustained skeletal benefits from impact-loading exercise in young females: A 3-year longitudinal study. *J Bones Miner Res*, **19**, 314–22.
15. **Otis, C.L., Drinkwater, B., Johnson, M., Loucks, A., and Wilmore, J.** (1997) American College of Sports Medicine position stand. The Female Athlete Triad. *Med Sci Sport Exerc*, **29**, i–ix.
16. **Sabbagh, Z. and Vatanparast, H.** (2009) Is calcium supplementation a risk factor for cardiovascular disease in older women? *Nutr Rev*, **67**, 105–8.
17. **USDA National Nutrient Database for Standard Reference** (2009) Release 22.
18. **WHO** (1994) *Study group on assessment of fracture risk and its application to screening and postmenopausal osteoporosis*. Report of a WHO Study Group. Technical Report, Series 84. Geneva, Switzerland, World Health Organization.

9.2 Magnesium
Susan A. Lanham-New, Ohood Hakim, and Andrea Grant

Since the early 1930s when McCollum first observed magnesium deficiency in rats and dogs, magnesium has been an intriguing mineral to research. It has both physiological and biochemical functions and important interrelationships, especially those with the cations calcium, potassium, and sodium. Magnesium is also involved with second messengers, PTH secretion, vitamin D metabolism, and bone functions.

9.2.1 Distribution and functions

Approximately, 60–65% of the body content, i.e. 1 mol (25 g), of magnesium in an adult person is found in the skeleton. Like calcium, it is an integral part of the inorganic structure of bones and teeth. However, unlike calcium, magnesium is the major divalent cation in the cells, accounting for most of the remaining magnesium, with 27% in the muscles and 7% in other cells. Intracellular magnesium is involved in energy metabolism, acting mainly as a metal activator or cofactor for enzymes requiring adenosine triphosphate, in the replication of DNA and the synthesis of RNA and protein. Hence it appears to be essential for all phosphate-transferring systems. Several magnesium-activated enzymes are inhibited by calcium, while in others, magnesium can be replaced by manganese. The remaining 1% of the body content of magnesium is in the extracellular fluids. Plasma concentrations of magnesium are about 1 mmol/L of which, as with calcium, about one-third is protein bound. Magnesium and calcium have somewhat similar effects on the excitability of muscle and nerve cells, but calcium has a further important function in signalling, which requires its concentration in the cells to be kept extremely low.

9.2.2 Metabolism

Magnesium is predominantly absorbed from the small intestine, both by a facilitated process and by simple diffusion. Absorption can vary widely and on average about 40–60% of dietary intake is absorbed. Excretion is mainly through the kidneys and increases with dietary intake. The kidney is extremely efficient in conserving magnesium; when the intake decreases, the urine can become almost magnesium-free. The intestinal and renal conservation and excretory mechanisms in normal individuals permit homeostasis over a wide range of intakes.

9.2.3 Dietary sources of magnesium

Similar to potassium, magnesium is present in both animal and plant cells and is also the mineral in chlorophyll. Green vegetables, cereals, legumes, and animal products are all good sources. In contrast to calcium, dairy products tend to be low in magnesium, with cow's milk containing 120 mg Mg/L (5 mmol/L) compared with 1200 mg Ca/L (30 mmol/L). The calcium, phosphate, and protein in meat and other animal products reduce the bioavailability of magnesium from these sources. Average magnesium intake is about 320 mg (13 mmol) per day for males and 230 mg (10 mmol) per day for females.

9.2.4 Magnesium deficiency

Since magnesium is the second most abundant cation in cells after potassium, dietary deficiency is unlikely to occur in people eating a normal varied diet. In his classical studies in the 1960s, Shils found it difficult to produce experimental magnesium deficiency (Shils, 1969). This research demonstrated the interrelationships between magnesium and the other principal cations, calcium, potassium, and sodium. The plasma concentration of magnesium decreased progressively, as did serum potassium and calcium, whereas the serum sodium remained normal even though sodium was being retained (Table 9.3). Functional effects, including

Table 9.3 Magnesium depletion and accompanying changes

	Blood chemistry	Metabolic balances
Magnesium	Plasma Mg ↓	Mg negative
Potassium	Serum K ↓	K negative
Calcium	Serum Ca ↓	Ca positive
Sodium	Serum Na no change	Na positive

personality changes, abnormal neuromuscular function, and gastrointestinal symptoms, were restored to normal only by repletion of magnesium. Hypomagnesaemia can precipitate hypocalcaemia because magnesium is required for the secretion of PTH.

Several clinical conditions are associated with magnesium deficiency (Table 9.4) and most frequently result from losses of magnesium from the kidney or gastrointestinal tract. Magnesium depletion induces neuromuscular excitability and may increase the risk of cardiac arrhythmias and cardiac arrest.

9.2.5 Magnesium excess

Excessive dietary intakes of magnesium appear unharmful to humans with normal renal function. Hypermagnesaemia is uncommon and is almost impossible to achieve from food sources alone. Magnesium supplementation is useful clinically to treat pregnancy-induced hypertension (pre-eclampsia and eclampsia). Many people also take oral magnesium supplements (such as Epsom salts) to prevent constipation, because they appear to have a cathartic effect.

9.2.6 Magnesium status

Serum magnesium concentration is the most frequently used index of magnesium status. Plasma is not used because anticoagulants may be contaminated with magnesium.

9.2.7 Recommended nutrient intakes

US Food and Nutrition Board of the IOM recommended intakes of magnesium within the different age groups shown in Table 9.5. The recommendations

Table 9.4 Clinical conditions associated with occurrence of magnesium deficiency

- Habitual or sustained low dietary supply/intake (<250 mg/day)
- Poor alimentary absorption—malabsorption syndromes (such as Crohn's disease), short bowel syndrome, laxative abuse
- Excessive body losses—via sweat or urine (genetic disorders, diabetes, alcohol abuse, diuretics)
- Increased requirement—pregnancy or lactation
- Hospitalized patients—65% of intensive care patients are hypomagnesaemic
- Endocrine disorders, such as parathyroid disorders and hyperaldosteronism

Table 9.5 US dietary recommendations for magnesium

Life stage group		Magnesium (mg/day)	
		RDA/AI	UIL[a]
Infants	(0–6 m)	30*	ND
	(6–12 m)	75*	ND
Children	(1–3 y)	80	65
	(4–8 y)	130	110

Life stage group		Magnesium (mg/day)	
Males	(9–13 y)	240	350
	(14–18 y)	410	350
	(19–30 y)	400	350
	(31–50 y)	420	350
	(51–70 y)	420	350
	(>70 y)	420	350
Females	(9–13 y)	240	350
	(14–18 y)	360	350
	(19–30 y)	310	350
	(31–50 y)	320	350
	(51-70 y)	320	350
	(>70 y)	320	350
Pregnancy	(14–18 y)	400	350
	(19–30 y)	350	350
	(31–50 y)	360	350
Lactation	(14–18 y)	360	350
	(19–30 y)	310	350
	(31–50 y)	320	350

Table 9.5 US dietary recommendations for magnesium (*Continued*)

RDA, recommended dietary allowance; AI, adequate intake; ND, not determined; UIL, tolerable upper intake level.

[a]UIL for magnesium represents intake from pharmacological agents only, and does not include intake from food or water.

Source: Food and Nutrition Board, Institute of Medicine (1997) *Dietary reference intakes for calcium, phosphorus, magnesium, vitamin D and fluoride*. Washington, DC, National Academy Press.

for the United Kingdom's are 300 mg/day for men and 270 mg/day for women.

9.2.8 Magnesium effects on bone

Magnesium deficiency has been shown to cause cessation of bone growth, decreased osteoblastic and osteoclastic activity, osteopenia, and increased bone fragility. There is also evidence from population-based, cross-sectional studies of a positive association between magnesium and bone mass/markers of bone metabolism, including the Aberdeen Prospective Osteoporosis Screening Study (APOSS) cohort and the Framingham population cohort. Recently, Carpenter *et al.* (2006) in a well-designed randomized controlled trial (RCT), showed that magnesium supplementation (300 mg elemental Mg per day in two divided doses) versus placebo given orally for 12 months significantly increased hip bone mineral content (BMC) in peri-adolescent girls (aged 8–14 years) who habitually consume a low magnesium intake (<220mg/day). Few other good Mg supplementation studies exist and it is an area for urgent further research given the growing recognition that population groups have sub-optimal intakes of magnesium.

Acknowledgement

The section on magnesium was originally written by the late Professor Marion Robinson and then subsequently by Andrea Grant. Much of the material by Dr Grant remains unaltered, with only updates provided.

Chapter 9 Major minerals: calcium and magnesium

Further Reading

1. **Carpenter, T.O., Delucia M.C., Zhang J.H., et al.** (2006) Randomized controlled study of effects of dietary magnesium oxide supplementation on bone mineral content in healthy girls. *J Clin Endrocin Metab*, **91**, 4866–72.

2. **Committee of Medical Aspects of Food Policy (COMA)** (1991) Magnesium. In: *Dietary reference values for food and energy and nutrients for the UK*. Report 41. London, HMSO, pp. 146–9.

3. **Fleet, J.E. and Cashman, K.D.** (2001) Magnesium. In: Bowman, B.A. and Russell, R.M. (eds) *Present knowledge in nutrition*, 8th edition. Washington, DC, ILSI, pp. 292–301.

4. **Food and Nutrition Board, Institute of Medicine** (1997) *Dietary reference intakes for calcium, phosphorus, magnesium, vitamin D and fluoride.* Washington, DC, National Academy Press.

5. **Holick, M. and Dawson-Hughes, B.** (2004) *Nutrition and bone health.* USA, Humana Press.

6. **Knochel, J.P.** (1998) Disorders of magnesium metabolism. In: *Harrison's principles of internal medicine*, 14th edition. New York, McGraw Hill, pp. 2263–6.

7. **New, S.A. and Bonjour, J.-P.** (2003) *Nutritional aspects of bone health.* 1st edition. Cambridge, UK, Royal Society of Chemistry.

8. **Shils, M.E.** (1969) Experimental production of magnesium deficiency in man. *Ann NY Acad Sci*, **162**, 847–55.

Useful Websites

To see topical and scientifically robust updates on nutrition associated with this textbook and web links to many of the journals in the Further Reading sections, please see the dedicated Online Resource Centre at **http://www.oxfordtextbooks.co.uk/orc/mann4e/**

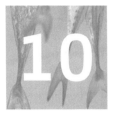

Iron

A. Patrick MacPhail

Iron deficiency is the most frequently encountered nutritional deficiency in man. WHO has ranked it very high among the preventable risks of disability in the world. Paradoxically, iron overload is also a major clinical problem in some populations. Both iron deficiency and iron overload have serious consequences and are major causes of human morbidity.

Iron owes its importance in biology to its remarkable reactivity (see Box 10.1). Of paramount importance is the reversible one-electron oxidation–reduction reaction that allows iron to shuttle between ferrous (Fe^{2+}) and ferric (Fe^{3+}) forms. This reaction is exploited by most iron-dependent enzyme systems involving electron transport, oxygen carriage, and iron transport across cell membranes. It is also responsible for the toxicity seen in acute and chronic iron overload. These contradictory properties are managed by highly specialized and conserved proteins involved in the storage and transport of iron and in regulating the concentration of intracellular iron.

In recent years there has been an explosion of knowledge about the proteins of iron metabolism and the genes that produce them, filling many gaps in our understanding and, at the same time, creating new questions that have still to be answered.

10.1 Basic iron metabolism

The total body iron content is about 50 mg/kg (3–4 g per person). It is convenient to think of body iron as distributed between four interconnected compartments. Over 60% is in the red cell compartment, mainly in haemoglobin, while about 25% is in the storage compartment, mainly in the liver. The remainder is distributed between myoglobin in muscles (8%) and in enzymes (5%). A small amount (about 3 mg) is in transit in the circulation bound to the plasma transport protein, transferrin.

- Iron is highly reactive and specialized proteins have evolved to protect organisms from damage when iron is in transit (transferrin) and when stored (ferritin).

- Ferrous iron (Fe^{2+}) crosses cell membranes but ferric iron (Fe^{3+}) is stored and transported. Iron transporters are associated with ferric reductases (Dcytb and DMT1) and ferroxidases (hephaestin and ferroportin) to achieve this.

- Iron itself controls the expression of many proteins essential for its distribution and storage (hepcidin, ferritin, DMT1, transferrin receptor, ferroportin).

10.1.1 Iron absorption

The mechanism by which iron is absorbed from the gut is not clearly understood, but recent work has uncovered the existence of a number of genes coding for proteins involved in the control of iron absorption and transport of iron across membranes. Four phases of iron absorption are recognized. In the *luminal phase*, food iron is solubilized, largely by acid secreted by the stomach, and is presented to the proximal duodenum, where most iron absorption takes place. Factors that maintain the solubility of iron in the face of rising pH, such as valency (ferrous iron is better absorbed), mucin secreted by the cells lining the gut (mucosa), and chelators (ascorbic acid), appear to be important in this phase. In addition, other foods present in the meal may promote or inhibit iron absorption (see Section 10.3). The second phase, *mucosal uptake*, depends on iron binding to the brush border of the apical cells of the duodenal mucosa and the transport of iron into the cell (Fig. 10.1). Two forms of dietary iron, haem and non-haem iron, need to be accommodated. The mechanism by which haem iron, derived mainly from myoglobin and haemoglobin in food, is transported into the cell is not clear (1 in Fig. 10.1). Non-haem iron, derived from a wide

variety of foods, has to be in the ferrous form (Fe^{2+}) before it can be transported across the cell membrane by the *divalent metal transporter* (DTM1) (3 in Fig. 10.1). The reduction from ferric to ferrous iron is probably achieved by a membrane-bound ferrireductase called *duodenal cytochrome b* (Dcytb) (2 in Fig. 10.1). Protons, required by DMT1, are supplied by gastric acid flowing into the proximal duodenum, where DMT1 is most highly expressed. This explains why proton pump inhibitors reduce non-haem iron absorption. In the third *intracellular phase*, iron, whether derived from haem or non-haem sources, is either stored in the storage protein, *ferritin*, or is transported directly to the opposite (inner) side of the mucosal cell and released. In the *release phase*, iron is oxidized to the ferric form by a membrane-bound ferroxidase, *hephaestin* (5 in Fig. 10.1), and released by a specialized iron transporter, *ferroportin 1* (4 in Fig. 10.1) into the portal circulation, where it is bound to the transport protein, *transferrin*. Both iron uptake and particularly iron release by the mucosal cell are inversely related to the amount of iron stored in the body and directly related to the rate of erythropoiesis. The mechanism by which this is achieved is discussed in Sections 10.1.3–4.

10.1.2 Internal iron exchange

Once released from the mucosal cell, iron enters the portal circulation and is bound to the transport protein, *transferrin* (Fig. 10.1) which keeps iron non-reactive in the circulation. While transferrin is able to distribute iron to most tissues, 80% of the iron in circulation is transported directly to the bone marrow, where it is incorporated in haemoglobin. The mechanism of transferrin uptake by the young red cells, and all active cells, involves a specific *transferrin receptor* (TfR1) (7 in Fig. 10.1) expressed on the surface of the cell. The iron–transferrin–TfR1 complex is taken into the cell by receptor-mediated endocytosis. A fall in the pH within the endosome causes the iron to be released from transferrin. This Fe^{3+} is reduced to Fe^{2+} by another ferrireductase,

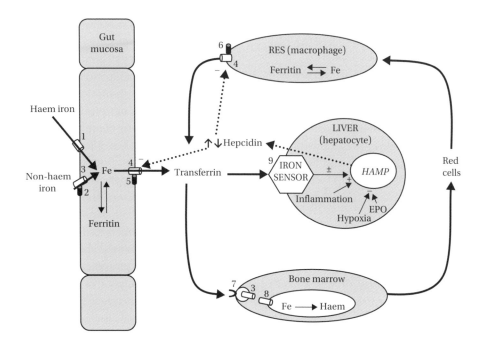

Fig. 10.1 The iron circuit and the central role of the liver. Iron, absorbed from the lumen of the small intestine (left), passes through the mucosal cell and enters the circulation, where it is bound to transferrin and redistributed to tissues. Most goes to the bone marrow for the production of haemoglobin in red cells which circulate and after 120 days are engulfed by macrophages of the reticuloendothelial system (RES). Iron in the RES is either stored in ferritin or redistributed back to transferrin. Most of the iron in circulation comes from the recycling of haemoglobin iron via the RES. Control of iron release by ferroportin from both absorption and recycling is mediated by hepcidin, which binds to ferroportin, inhibiting iron release. Several factors modulate the transcription of the *HAMP* gene to increase (high iron, inflammation) or decrease (low iron, anaemia, hypoxia, erythropoiesis [EPO]) hepcidin expression. 1, Haem-iron transporter; 2, duodenal cytochrome b (Dcytb), a ferrireductase, converts Fe^{3+} to Fe^{2+} to facilitate transfer by (3) divalent metal transporter (DMT1), which transports non-haem iron (Fe^{2+}) into cells; (4) ferroportin 1, iron transporter on the basolateral surface of the mucosal cell and the macrophage (reticuloendothelial system, RES), transports Fe^{2+} out of cells and is regulated by hepcidin; (5) hephaestin and (6) caeruloplasmin are ferroxidases, converting Fe^{2+} to Fe^{3+} for binding to transferrin; (7) transferrin receptor 1 (TfR1) binds with iron-loaded transferrin and transfers both into cells; (8) mitoferrin transports iron into the mitochondrion, the site of haem synthesis; (9) 'Iron sensor' represents the complex interaction of at least ten proteins (including transferrin, HFE, transferrin receptors 1 and 2, and haemojuvalin (HJV)) in and on the surface of the hepatocyte, which senses iron status and modulates the expression of hepcidin and hence the function of ferroportin.

STEAP3, and then transported through the vesicle membrane into the cell by DMT1 (3 in Fig. 10.1). The transferrin–TfR1 complex, now devoid of iron, is cycled back to the cell surface, where the apotransferrin (transferrin without iron) is released back into the circulation and is available to transport more iron. In order to be incorporated into protoporphyrin IX by ferrochelatase the iron in the erythroid cell must enter the mitochondrion. A specific transporter, *mitoferrin* (8 in Fig. 10.1), plays a crucial role in achieving this.

At the end of its lifespan, the red cell is engulfed by macrophages of the reticuloendothelial system (RES), located mainly in the liver, spleen, and bone marrow. The iron is separated from haem and stored in ferritin or as *haemosiderin* (a denatured form of ferritin). Ferrous iron is released back into the circulation via *ferroportin* (4 in Fig. 10.1), converted to ferric iron by *caeruloplasmin* (6 in Fig. 10.1), and again picked up by transferrin.

It should be noted that most of the iron entering the circulation comes from recycled red cells via the RES and not from iron absorption (ratio about 20:1). There is normally only one way into the iron circuit and there is no way out except through blood loss or, in pregnancy, to the fetus. In reality, a small amount of iron is lost, mainly through loss of blood and surface cells of the gut, urinary tract, and skin. In men, this amounts to about 1 mg/day and the loss is relatively easily balanced by iron absorption. In women, additional losses through menstruation (0.5 mg/day), and the cost of pregnancy (2 mg/day) and lactation (0.5 mg/day), make it more difficult to balance the loss through iron absorption (see Section 10.1.5).

10.1.3 Control of iron recycling: circulating iron and hepcidin

Elegant experiments using radio-iron in the 1950s by Bothwell and Finch showed that the body responds to changes in iron requirements by increasing or decreasing iron absorption and iron release from the RES. The recent discovery of the iron transporter ferroportin and its regulator *hepcidin* has greatly enhanced our understanding of how this may be achieved (Fig. 10.1). Hepcidin, a small, 25-amino-acid peptide, is secreted by hepatocytes under the influence of several known mechanisms, and its expression is modulated by changes in the transcription of the *HAMP* gene.

First, changes in iron status appear to be sensed, probably through the saturation of transferrin, by two distinct pathways (the 'iron sensor', 9 in Fig. 10.1). Their relationship to each other is not fully understood but their central role is illustrated by the severe disturbances of iron homeostasis that result from mutations in any of the genes coding for these proteins. The pathway that has been best characterized involves HJV, the stability of which is influenced by transferrin saturation. HJV is a co-receptor for a group of growth factors known as bone morphogenic proteins (BMPs). Binding of BMP sets off a cascade of events which results in phosphorylation of intracellular signalling molecules (SMAD) which bind to the *HAMP* promoter to increase hepcidin expression. Disturbances in this pathway lead to severe iron overload early in life.

The other pathway involves the HFE protein, and mutations in the gene (*HFE*) that codes for this protein are responsible for the majority of cases of hereditary haemochromatosis (HH) (see Section 10.6). HFE, transferrin receptor 1 (TfR1), and its homologue TfR2 are known to be closely associated on the cell surface and, through binding of circulating transferrin to TfR2, appear to be able to sense iron status and modulate *HAMP* transcription accordingly by an as-yet unknown mechanism. The result of both systems is a change in the rate of transcription of *HAMP*, the gene responsible for encoding hepcidin. Hepcidin, released into the circulation, in turn binds to ferroportin, causing the iron transporter to be internalized and degraded, thus inhibiting iron release. This feedback mechanism causes increased iron release when iron is scarce or in high demand, and switches off iron release when it is plentiful.

It has long been known that inflammation has a profound effect on iron metabolism. Again, Bothwell and Finch showed that inflammation induced by injection of turpentine resulted in hypoferraemia (low plasma iron), impaired iron absorption, and impaired iron transport to the fetus. It is now understood that these effects are mediated through increased secretion of hepcidin and thus impaired iron release by ferroportin. As part of the immune response, cytokines, particularly IL-6, increase transcription of *HAMP*, bypassing the iron sensor mediated effect. Injection of IL-6 results in a rapid rise in hepcidin and a profound fall in plasma iron. If this is sustained, the resulting iron starvation inhibits erythropoiesis (red cell production) and leads to anaemia. While other factors such as shortened red cell survival and direct inhibition of the bone marrow contribute to the *anaemia of chronic disorders*, hepcidin-induced hypoferraemia is the central cause. The advantage to the body of the hypoferraemia induced by inflammation appears to be the limitation of iron supply to an invading organism.

Other mechanisms have been shown to inhibit *HAMP* transcription, and therefore hepcidin expression, leading to uninhibited iron release by ferroportin (Fig. 10.1). These operate in situations where erythropoiesis would benefit from an increase in iron supply. Factors operating in this manner include hypoxia operating directly through hypoxia inducible transcription factor (HIF) and erythropoiesis through erythropoietin (EPO).

10.1.4 Control of iron recycling: intracellular iron

While hepcidin controls the entry of iron into the circulation, and hence its distribution, the level of intracellular iron within the cytosol of the cell controls the expression of some important proteins involved in the movement of iron in and out of cells. Control is largely at the level of the translation of messenger RNA (mRNA) to protein, although iron-related changes in transcription also occur. Control of translation is mediated by iron-responsive proteins (IRP1 and IRP2), which bind to specific stem loop structures, called iron-responsive elements (IRE) of the mRNA. In the iron-deficient state, the IRP binds to an IRE in the 5′ untranslated region of some mRNAs (e.g. ferritin and ferroportin), inhibiting translation and to IREs in the 3′ untranslated region of other mRNAs (e.g. transferrin receptor and DMT1), stabilizing the mRNA. In the presence of iron, the binding is lost, ferritin and ferroportin

mRNA are translated while the mRNA of transferrin receptor, and DMT1 becomes unstable and cannot be translated. The way in which the two IRPs sense iron levels differs. IRP1 contains an iron sulphur cluster (Fe–S) which, when iron is plentiful, changes the shape of the protein, facilitating binding to the IRE while IRP2, which lacks a Fe–S cluster, is rapidly degraded. When iron is scarce, IRP1 opens and is no longer able to bind to the IRE while IRP2 becomes stable. The result of these complex reciprocal arrangements is that when the level of iron is low, more transferrin receptor and more DMT1 are translated, facilitating the movement of iron into the cell, while when the level of iron in the cell rises, the need for iron storage is met by increased translation of ferritin mRNA, and iron export is facilitated by increased ferroportin translation.

10.1.5 Iron balance

Iron requirements must be balanced by iron supply if iron deficiency or iron overload are to be avoided. Several factors combine to influence iron balance (Fig. 10.2). Obligatory iron losses, the requirements

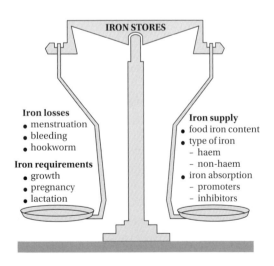

Fig. 10.2 Iron balance. Iron losses and requirements for growth (left) are balanced by iron supplied in the diet (right). Surplus iron is stored and can be drawn upon to supplement increased losses or requirements.

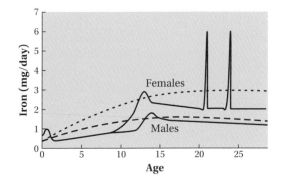

Fig. 10.3 Iron requirements for males and females vary during life. A Western diet rich in meat and iron promoters (- - -) is able to meet iron requirements of the majority of females at all ages except in infancy, at the peak of pubertal growth spurt, and onset of menstruation and during pregnancies. In contrast, a cereal-based diet without meat or iron promoters and with excess inhibitors of iron absorption (– – –) is not able to meet the requirements of most childbearing women and some men.

of growth and pregnancy, as well as pathological losses due to excessive menstrual and other bleeding must be balanced against iron supply. Iron supply is influenced by the amount and type of iron in food and the combination of various inhibitors and promoters of iron bioavailability. These requirements are buffered by iron which can be mobilized from stores. The body's iron requirements and the ability of the diet to meet the demand vary during life (Fig. 10.3). In infancy, during the pre-adolescent growth spurt, and in women during reproductive life, particularly during pregnancy, the iron requirements may exceed the iron supply, making iron deficiency more common during these periods. Individuals consuming a diet of low iron bioavailability are even more at risk.

10.2 Iron in food

Iron supply is greatly influenced by the composition of the diet. Two broad categories of iron are present in food: *haem iron* derived mainly from haemoglobin and myoglobin in meat, and *non-haem iron* in the form of iron salts, iron in other proteins, and iron derived from processing or storage methods. Haem iron enters the mucosal cells by a different mechanism and is better absorbed than non-haem iron. It is also less influenced by the body's iron status and, because the iron is protected by the haem molecule, it is not affected by other constituents in the diet.

Non-haem iron compounds are found in a wide variety of foods of both plant and animal origin. The iron is present in metalloproteins (e.g. ferritin, haemosiderin, and lactoferrin), soluble iron, iron

bound to phytates in plants, and contaminant iron such as ferric oxides and hydroxides introduced in the preparation and storage of food and by contamination from soil. The bioavailability of these forms of non-haem iron, unlike haem iron, is influenced by other constituents of the diet. Forms of iron that are similarly affected are said to enter a 'common pool'. The importance of this concept is that fortificant iron added to food will be subjected to the same inhibitory and promotive influences as the intrinsic food iron and will therefore have similar bioavailability. This concept, however, does not hold true for all forms of added iron. For example, most ferric salts, whether contaminant or added as fortificants, do not enter the common pool and have very low bioavailability.

10.3 Promoters and inhibitors of iron absorption

The relative concentrations of promoters and inhibitors of iron absorption in foods are responsible for the wide range of bioavailability that has been demonstrated (Table 10.1). The most important *promoters* of non-haem iron absorption are ascorbic acid (vitamin C) and meat. Other organic acids (e.g. citric acid) and some spices have also been shown to enhance iron absorption. The major *inhibitors* of iron absorption are phytates and polyphenols, common constituents of cereals and many vegetables.

Ascorbic acid is thought to enhance iron absorption by converting ferric to ferrous iron and by chelating iron in the lumen of the gut. This keeps iron in a more soluble and absorbable form and prevents binding to inhibitory ligands. It follows that the bioavailability of non-haem iron from foods with significant ascorbic acid content is high. Moreover, the addition of ascorbic acid to meals with potent inhibitors increases non-haem iron absorption.

The factor in meat responsible for enhancing non-haem iron absorption has not been identified. The enhancing effect is not shared by proteins derived from plants or other animal proteins such as milk, cheese, and eggs. For example, substitution of beef for egg albumin as a source of protein in a test meal resulted in a fivefold increase in iron absorption. Present evidence suggests that peptides rich in the amino acid cysteine may play a role in the enhancement of non-haem iron absorption.

Polyphenols commonly found in many vegetables and in some grains are potent inhibitors of non-haem iron absorption. There is a strong inverse relationship between the concentration of polyphenols in foods and the absorption of iron from them. Many of the foods with low iron bioavailability listed in Table 10.1 are rich in polyphenols. Among the best-known polyphenols is tannin, found in tea and other beverages, which has a profound inhibitory

Table 10.1 Relative bioavailability of non-haem iron in foods

Food	Bioavailability		
	Low	Intermediate	High
Cereals	Most cereals Whole wheat flour	Corn flour White flour	
Fruits	Apple Banana Peach Strawberry	Cantaloupe Mango	Guava Citrus Pawpaw Tomato
Vegetables	Aubergine Legumes	Carrot Potato	Beetroot Broccoli Pumpkin
Beverages	Tea Coffee	Red wine	White wine
Nuts	All		
Animal proteins	Cheese Egg Cow's milk		All meat Poultry Breast milk

effect on iron absorption. Polyphenols also form strongly coloured compounds with iron, which is a major problem in food fortification. This phenomenon can be illustrated by dropping a few crystals of ferrous sulphate into a cup of tea.

Phytates, found mainly in the husks of grains, are also major inhibitors of iron absorption. In this regard, iron absorption from unpolished rice is significantly worse than from polished rice, while increasing the bran content of a meal produces a dose-related depression in iron bioavailability. Both meat and ascorbic acid are able to overcome this inhibitory effect.

10.4 Recommended dietary intake

The concept of a recommended dietary intake of iron is difficult to reconcile with the wide range of bioavailability (Table 10.1 and Box 10.2). The total iron content of a diet is a meaningless, although commonly employed measure of its nutritional adequacy, and may provide a false sense of nutritional security. For example, foods with high iron content due to large quantities of contaminant iron, or inappropriate fortificant iron, may be nutritionally worthless because of the low bioavailability of the iron. On the other hand, haem iron, making up only 10–15% of the total ingested iron, may account for a third of the iron actually absorbed. Similarly, the iron absorbed from a meal containing non-haem iron may be doubled if the meal is taken with a glass of orange juice (30 mg ascorbic acid) or reduced to a third if taken with tea. However, it is possible to divide diets into ones of low, intermediate, and high

Table 10.2 FAO/WHO recommended daily iron intake for individuals consuming diets of low, intermediate, and high iron bioavailability. Requirements are given for absorbed iron.

Group	Age (years)	Requirements of absorbed iron (µg/kg/day)	Recommended intake (mg/day)		
			Low (5%)	Intermediate (10%)	High (15%)
Children	0.25–1	120	21	11	7
	1–2	56	12	6	4
	2–6	44	14	7	5
	6–12	40	23	12	8
Boys	12–16	34	36	18	12
Girls	12–16	40	40	20	13
Adult men		18	23	11	8
Adult women					
Menstruating		43	48	24	16
Post-menopausal		18	19	9	6
Lactating		24	26	13	9

Source: FAO/WHO (1988) *Requirements of vitamin A, iron, folate and vitamin B-12*. Report of a Joint FAO/WHO Consultation. FAO Food and Nutrition Series, no 23. Rome: Food and Agriculture Organization.

Although human milk contains less iron than cow's milk, the iron in human milk is much more bioavailable (estimated absorption up to 50%). The US Institute of Medicine considers that the iron provided by exclusive breastfeeding is adequate to meet the needs of infants up to the age of 6 months.

iron bioavailability. These correspond to iron absorption of about 5%, 10%, and 15% in subjects with depleted iron stores.

A diet of low bioavailability (<5%) with a high inhibitor content, negligible amounts of enhancers, and little haem iron is based largely on unrefined cereals and legumes. Such diets are typical of many developing countries and supply about 0.7 mg of available iron daily, which is insufficient to meet the needs of most women, growing children, and some men. A diet of intermediate bioavailability (about 10%) includes limited amounts of foods that promote iron absorption and supplies enough absorbed iron (about 1.5 mg) to meet the needs of 50% of women. A diet of high iron bioavailability (>15%) contains generous amounts of food rich in promoters and haem iron. The inhibitor content is low as cereals are often highly refined. Such diets, typical of many developed countries, supply sufficient iron (>2.1 mg/day) for most adults but still cannot match the daily amounts of absorbed iron required in the second half of pregnancy (5 mg/day).

The Food and Agriculture Organization/World Health Organization (FAO/WHO) recommendations (Table 10.2) based on estimates that apply to the 95th percentile of the population, are an attempt to take variations in bioavailability and requirements into account.

10.5 Iron deficiency

In the past, iron deficiency was thought to be due largely to blood loss rather than insufficient iron supply. Credence for this view was given by the obvious effects of pathological blood loss and the high prevalence of iron deficiency in the developing world, where hookworm infestation is endemic. However, it is now apparent that the poor bioavailability of iron in largely unrefined cereal-based diets is a major cause of iron deficiency in most developing countries. The impact of such diets is obviously enhanced when pathological blood loss or increased physiological iron demand is also present. These factors explain the geographical and gender variation in the prevalence of iron-deficiency anaemia (IDA), which is most common in Asia, where up to 60% of women and over 30% of men are anaemic, while in Europe and North America less than 5% of females and 2% of males are anaemic. The preponderance of females can be explained by increased physiological loss of iron in menstruation and pregnancy and to their lower food, and therefore iron, intake.

The development of iron deficiency is characterized by sequential changes in the amount of storage iron in the various iron compartments of the body. The measurement of iron in these compartments is discussed in Section 10.7. In the first stage, iron stores become depleted, but there is enough iron to meet the needs of red cell production. When iron stores are exhausted, the amount of iron in the circulation starts to fall, and red cell production becomes compromised (iron-deficient erythropoiesis). In the final stage, iron stores are exhausted, the amount of iron in the circulation is very low, red cell production is drastically reduced and anaemia develops. The point at which the function of iron-containing enzymes becomes impaired is uncertain, but probably depends on the rate of renewal of the enzymes and the growth of the tissues involved.

While blood loss and the diet are of fundamental importance in causing iron deficiency, other factors need to be considered. Gastrointestinal diseases, not necessarily causing bleeding, may hinder iron absorption and are important causes of IDA refractory to oral iron therapy. Atrophic gastritis and gastrectomy reduce acid output vital for iron solubilization and functioning of DMT1 (see Section 10.1.1). Coeliac disease, associated with antibodies directed against small intestinal epithelium, is a cause of iron malabsorption. Recent work has shown that eradication of *Helicobacter pylori* infection improves response to oral iron. As the genetics of more proteins of iron metabolism are unravelled, inherited causes of iron deficiency in humans are beginning to emerge. Hereditary iron-refractory IDA is due to mutations in the gene coding for matripase-2 (*TMPRSS6*), part of the HJV pathway (see Section 10.1.3), which result in increased hepcidin and inhibition of iron recycling. Mutations in DMT1 causing severe congenital iron deficiency because of impaired membrane iron transfer, previously described in mice and rats, has now been found in humans (3 in Fig. 10.1).

Iron deficiency has been associated with a number of pathological consequences of which anaemia is the most obvious. Severe anaemia is associated with weakness, impaired effort tolerance, and, eventually, heart failure. There is no doubt that even mild IDA limits work performance and studies in Indonesia and Sri Lanka have linked it to reduced productivity. In children, IDA, particularly in infancy, is associated with impaired psychomotor development, the effects of which may be irreversible. Although well-designed trials are lacking, iron supplementation in infancy appears to improve cognitive function. In pregnancy, IDA is associated with prematurity, low birth weight, and increased perinatal mortality, as well as an increased risk of iron deficiency in the infant after 4 months of age. Changes in the gastrointestinal tract (atrophy of the mucosa of the mouth, oesophagus, and stomach) and the skin and nails (spoon-shaped nails) are well described but infrequent. Other less well-recognized abnormalities include inability to adapt to cold and impaired immunity.

10.6 Iron overload

Excessive amounts of iron may accumulate in the body and result in organ damage. The *acute* ingestion of a large amount of bioavailable iron, usually in the form of ferrous sulphate tablets, will exceed both the ability of the mucosa to control iron absorption and the capacity of transferrin to bind iron in the circulation. The acute iron toxicity that results is thought to be due to the generation of free radicals by free iron, both in the gut and in the circulation. Most of the victims are children, who develop severe abdominal pain, vomiting, metabolic acidosis, and cardiovascular collapse. Severe poisoning, requiring urgent chelation therapy, may follow ingestion of more than 30 mg of iron/kg.

Chronic iron overload develops insidiously and the recent discovery of novel genes coding for proteins involved in iron sensing and transport (see Section 10.1) have greatly increased our understanding of iron overload. *Haemochromatosis* is the name given to inherited forms of iron overload in which abnormalities of hepcidin and ferroportin function play a central role (Table 10.3). Type 1 is the most common form, and is found almost exclusively in people of north-western European origin, reaching a homozygous prevalence of 1.2–1.4% in Ireland and Denmark. Types 1–3 share common features but differ in severity and age of onset. In these types, iron floods the circulation because of uninhibited release of iron by ferroportin due to the absence of hepcidin (see Section 10.1). Transferrin becomes saturated with iron and free, toxic, non-transferrin-bound iron is rapidly taken up by the liver, heart, pancreas, and other organs where excessive iron accumulates over years. The damage to these organs is due to free radicals induced by iron and can result in liver cirrhosis, liver cancer, heart failure, arthritis, and endocrine disease (diabetes and impotence). Removal of haemoglobin by repeated bleeding is an effective treatment because iron stores have to be mobilized to replace the lost haemoglobin. Interestingly, recent epidemiological studies have shown that the majority of people homozygous for

Table 10.3 Classification of haemochromatosis

Type	Protein (see Fig. 10.1)	Gene (common mutation)	Clinical picture
1 Classic (adult)	HFE (9)	*HFE* (C282Y in > 80%)	Hepcidin deficiency. Recessive inheritance. Severe iron overload with organ damage (liver, heart, pituitary). Type 1 has variable expression. Parenchymal iron distribution (hepatocytes, cardiac muscle, endocrine tissues) with little or no iron in reticuloendothelial tissues (spleen, bone marrow). High transferrin saturation (>50%), high serum ferritin (can be thousands ng/L).
2 Juvenile	A Haemojuvelin (9) B Hepcidin	*HFE2* *HAMP*	
3 Non-HFE (adult)	Transferrin receptor 2 (9)	*TFR2*	
4 Dominant	Ferroportin (4)	*SLC40A1*	Dominant inheritance. Variable effects from severe to trivial. Reticuloendothelial iron distribution (spleen, Kupfer cells, bone marrow), parenchymal loading late and in severe cases. High serum ferritin, transferrin saturation normal, later high.

the common mutation of type 1 haemochromatosis (C282Y) do not go on to develop the full-blown clinical features, probably because more than one iron-sensing pathway is available (see Section 10.1.3).

Two other clinically important forms of iron overload, sometimes called secondary, should be mentioned. *African dietary iron overload* is caused by the ingestion, over many years, of large amounts of highly bioavailable iron in low-alcohol beer brewed in iron containers. Recent evidence suggests that there is also a genetic predisposition, possibly related to the ferroportin gene since the distribution of iron is the same as that seen in haemochromatosis type 4. In severe cases, the toxic effects of iron are similar to those seen in the other forms of haemochromatosis. *Secondary iron overload* occurs in the so-called 'iron-loading anaemias' of which thalassaemia major is the most common. Excessive amounts of iron are absorbed over a relatively short period because of the inhibition of hepcidin expression caused by the increased turnover of red cells (EPO in Fig. 10.1). This effect can be reduced by regular blood transfusion, while the iron burden can be reduced by iron chelation therapy. The iron overload occurs rapidly and most victims die from iron-induced heart failure if not treated. A similar syndrome is seen in patients with bone marrow failure, kept alive by repeated blood transfusions.

10.7 Assessment of iron status

The iron status of an individual, or a population, can be gauged by measuring the amount of iron in each of the body iron compartments. The progression from normal through to IDA can be measured by sequential changes in the biochemical markers that reflect the iron status of each compartment. No single biochemical index can assess all the stages of iron depletion.

- During *iron depletion*, storage iron in the liver and in the reticuloendothelial cells of the spleen and bone marrow is progressively reduced and can be detected by a parallel fall in serum ferritin concentration. The function of circulating ferritin, which carries almost no iron, is not known, but there is a near-linear relationship between iron stores and serum ferritin. The serum ferritin concentration falls below 12 µg/L (12 ng/mL) when the iron stores are exhausted. Iron depletion is the only cause of a serum ferritin below this level. Other measurements of iron status are normal at this stage.

- In *iron-deficient erythropoiesis*, iron stores are exhausted (serum ferritin <12 µg/L) and iron supply to the marrow is insufficient to meet the needs of haemoglobin production. This stage is detected by a low serum iron concentration and transferrin saturation below 16%, although the haemoglobin concentration is still within the normal range. The *serum iron* (normal range 9–27 µmol/L) is also low when the entrance of iron into the circulation is inhibited by hepcidin, as in inflammation. The transferrin saturation (normal range 20–45%) is a more physiological measure of iron in circulation, since this is the means by which the secretion of hepcidin is controlled (see Section 10.1.3).

- In *iron-deficiency anaemia*, the supply of iron to the marrow is so reduced that the concentration of haemoglobin falls below normal. The cut-off value below which anaemia is diagnosed varies according to age and gender (below 110 g/L in children younger than 6 years and in pregnant women; below 120 g/L in women and adolescents under 15 years; and below 130 g/L in adult men). There are obviously many other causes of anaemia besides iron deficiency (e.g. vitamin B_{12} and folate deficiency, chronic infection, and intrinsic diseases of the bone marrow). The diagnosis of anaemia due to iron deficiency therefore requires that other measurements of iron status are also in the iron-deficient range (serum ferritin <12 µg/L and transferrin saturation <16%). In addition, in established IDA, the red cells become small (microcytosis) and pale (hypochromia). These changes can be detected by examination of a blood film or by a fall in the mean cell volume (MCV) below 85 fL and in the mean cell haemoglobin concentration (MCHC) below 27 pg.

- The diagnosis of *iron overload* is also measured by a combination of measurements of iron status. A raised serum ferritin concentration (>400 µg/L) and transferrin saturation greater than 60% are highly suggestive of types 1–3 haemochromatosis (Table 10.3). As a rough guide, 100 µg/L of serum ferritin is equivalent to a gram of storage iron and the normal range is usually given as 50–400 µg/L in men or 300 µg/L in women. In haemochromatosis, serum ferritin levels greater than 1000 µg/L (iron stores ten times normal) are associated with organ damage. Unfortunately, circulating ferritin is an acute phase reactant and increases when inflammation is present, making serum ferritin an unreliable estimate of iron stores in this situation. Some of this increase is a reflection of iron trapped in stores through the action of increased levels of hepcidin on ferroportin (see Section 10.1.3). In addition, tissue destruction is associated with high levels of serum ferritin because of the release of tissue ferritin into the circulation. Iron stores can also be measured by chemical estimation of iron in biopsies of liver or bone marrow or, more recently, by electromagnetic resonance. Very high levels of serum iron are seen in situations where hepcidin is low or absent (haemochromatosis and in acute iron poisoning), in which case the capacity for transferrin to hold iron becomes impaired (at 60 to over 100%) and free non-transferrin-bound iron becomes detectable in the plasma (see Section 10.6).

- The changes in the measurements of iron status that often accompany inflammation (see Section 10.1.3) are often confused with iron deficiency. In fact these changes represent a shift of iron from the red cell compartment to stores caused by inhibition of iron release by hepcidin, while the total amount of iron in the body is actually unchanged. The serum iron is low (*hypoferraemia of inflammation*) while the transferrin saturation may be low or normal. In prolonged inflammation, the haemoglobin falls and the red cells may develop changes suggestive of IDA. Because iron is trapped in stores, the serum ferritin is high and is out of keeping with the low serum iron. This high serum ferritin is not indicative of iron overload. Similar changes have been described in obesity (*hypoferraemia of obesity*) but whether this is due to inflammation alone is not clear. The diagnosis of iron deficiency in the presence of inflammation is often difficult. A hint that iron deficiency may also be present is provided by a serum ferritin in the low normal range since the total iron is diminished. The only sure way to resolve this is to assess iron stores and erythropoiesis in the bone marrow.

- Other tests which may be used to infer iron status rely on the levels of proteins of iron metabolism that are controlled by iron itself. A neglected, and simple test that can be done on a drop of blood, is the concentration of *free erythrocyte protoporphyrin* (FEP), which gives information similar to the transferrin saturation. The production of haem is dependent on the supply of iron to the marrow. When iron supply is restricted, free protoporphyrin, a precursor of haem, accumulates in red cells. A transferrin saturation lower than 16% is associated with an FEP greater than 1.24 μmol/L red cells. The FEP is, however, also elevated in lead poisoning and in inflammation.

Tissue iron depletion can also be measured by the concentration of soluble *transferrin receptor* in plasma or serum. The expression of transferrin receptors on the surface of all cells is determined by the level of intracellular iron (see Section 10.1.4). In cellular iron depletion, the concentration of soluble transferrin receptor in the plasma rises but, unlike the serum ferritin concentration, the level is less affected by inflammation. The ratio of serum transferrin receptor to log serum ferritin may be useful in distinguishing iron deficiency from inflammation as the cause of anaemia. The recent development of methods to measure the concentration of hepcidin in urine and plasma, which are high in inflammation and low in iron deficiency (10.1.3), may prove helpful in this regard.

10.8 Treatment and prevention of iron deficiency

Iron-deficiency anaemia in individuals is best treated by the oral administration of ferrous iron salts. The cheapest and most effective is ferrous sulphate, which is usually given in a dose of one tablet (65 mg of iron) two or three times a day. The increase in haemoglobin concentration that can be expected with optimal doses of ferrous sulphate is about 2 g/L/day. Gastrointestinal side effects of oral iron therapy are common, which has led to a plethora of different oral iron compounds being available. Most differ in their formulation in an attempt to limit side effects, the most popular being slow-release preparations. None has been shown to be convincingly better than ferrous sulphate and all will correct iron deficiency in time. The addition of ascorbic acid, while enhancing food iron availability, does little to improve therapeutic efficacy and probably increases the side effects. In persons intolerant of, or refractory to oral iron therapy (see Section 10.5), it is possible to give iron by intravenous injection.

The treatment and prevention of iron deficiency in high-risk groups and the population at large presents many problems. *Supplementation* refers to the administration of iron compounds in the form of tablets or syrups usually targeted to high-risk groups such as children and pregnant women. Again, the major problem encountered is the high prevalence of side effects and its impact on compliance. Giving smaller or less frequent (weekly) doses prolongs the time to response considerably, while supply and distribution limit efficacy. Food *fortification* offers a more cost-effective approach through the fortification of staples such as cereals or condiments (salt, fish sauce, or soy sauce). Target groups (such as infants and children) can be reached by iron fortification of infant formulas and cereals. While there is abundant evidence that iron fortification of food can be effective, the process is fraught with practical difficulties. Apart from the logistic problems in the manufacture of iron-fortified food and its distribution, so important in the developing world, the major dilemma is that bioavailable iron compounds are highly reactive and cause unacceptable changes in the taste and colour of the food vehicle. Insoluble salts, such as ferric orthophosphate and elemental iron powders, while producing less changes in food, are poorly absorbed. Strategies that have been employed to overcome these barriers include encapsulating ferrous salts, reducing the phytate content of cereals, and adding a promoter to cereals fortified with a ferric salt. This last has been used successfully in the fortification of infant formulas and cereals with iron and ascorbic acid but is only effective when oxidation of the ascorbic acid can be prevented by keeping the product dry, avoiding heat and exposure to air until shortly before use.

The iron chelate, sodium ferric EDTA (NaFeEDTA) escapes the effects of inhibitors, particularly phytates, and, in this setting, the iron is two to three times better absorbed than from ferrous sulphate. Judicious choice of the food vehicle can avoid unwanted colour changes. Field trials have shown NaFeEDTA to be an effective fortificant. In one study, the prevalence of iron deficiency in women was reduced from 22% to 5% over a 2-year period. The Joint FAO/WHO Expert Committee on Food Additives (JECFA) considers NaFeEDTA safe for use in supervised fortification programmes, and extensive programmes are currently underway in Vietnam (fish sauce) and China (soy sauce and wheat flour). Similar claims have been made regarding the amino acid chelate ferrous bisglycinate, which has the advantage of being considered a natural compound and as 'Generally Recognized as Safe' (GRAS) by the FDA but is more costly. Despite these limitations, fortification of food with iron is commonplace in the industrialized world. Paradoxically, these fortification programmes have often been carried out in a haphazard way, with little attention being paid to the bioavailability of the fortificant or the efficacy of the programme.

Elemental iron, widely used as a fortificant in Western countries, has a very low bioavailability. In the developing world, iron fortification programmes face additional problems. Foods are seldom centrally processed, making fortification a difficult logistical problem. Furthermore, the diets are largely cereal-based and lack natural promoters of iron absorption, which means that the added iron will be poorly absorbed. This topic has been extensively reviewed by SUSTAIN (Hurrell *et al.*, 2004; SUSTAIN, 2004).

Further Reading

1. **Adams, P.C. and Barton, J.C.** (2007) Haemochromatosis. *Lancet*, **370**, 1855–60.
2. **Anderson, G.J., Frazer, D.M., and McLaren, G.D.** (2009). Iron absorption and metabolism. *Curr Opin Gastroenterol*, **25**,129–35.
3. **Andrews, N. C.,** (2008). Forging a field: The golden age of iron biology. *Blood*, **112**, 219–30.
4. **Ganz, T.** (2011). Hepcidin and iron regulation, 10 years later on. *Blood*, **117**, 4425–33.
5. **Goodnough, L.T.** (ed.) (2009). Iron deficiency and metabolism. *Seminars in hematology*, **46**, 325–94.
6. **Hershko, C.** (2005) Iron diseases. *Best Pract Res Clin Haematol*, **18**, 157–380.
7. **Hurrell, R.F., Lynch, S., Bothwell, T.H., et al.** (2004) Enhancing the absorption of fortification iron. *Int J Vitam Nutr Res*, **74**, 387–401 (the whole of volume 74, number 6 is devoted to technologies to enhance iron fortification).
8. **FAO/WHO** (1988) *Requirements of vitamin A, iron, folate and vitamin B-12*. Report of a Joint FAO/WHO Consultation. FAO Food and Nutrition Series, no 23. Rome: Food and Agriculture Organization.
9. **SUSTAIN** (2004) Innovative ingredient technologies to enhance iron absorption. Proceedings of a SUSTAIN workshop. *Int J Vitam Nutr Res*, **74**, 385–475.
10. **Zimmermann, M.B., and Hurrell, R.F.** (2007) Nutritional iron deficiency. *Lancet*, **370**, 511–20.

Useful Websites

To see topical and scientifically robust updates on nutrition associated with this textbook and web links to many of the journals in the Further Reading sections, please see the dedicated Online Resource Centre at http://www.oxfordtextbooks.co.uk/orc/mann4e/

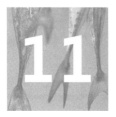

Trace elements

Samir Samman, Sheila Skeaff, Christine Thomson, and Stewart Truswell

11.1 Zinc
Samir Samman

11.1.1 Historical perspective

Experimental zinc deficiency was demonstrated in laboratory animals but the likelihood of deficiency in humans was considered remote because of the ubiquitous nature of zinc in the food supply and the relative difficulty in creating zinc-deficient animal models. Zinc deficiency was first recognized in humans in 1958.

11.1.2 Distribution and function

Zinc is one of the IIB series of metals with a molecular weight of 65.4 (Fig. 11.1). It is the most common catalytic metal ion in the cytoplasm of cells. Adult humans contain between 1.2 and 2.3 g of zinc, which is distributed in all tissues. The highest concentrations of zinc are observed in the choroid of the eye and the prostate gland but most of the body zinc is in bones and muscles. In liver cells, zinc is associated with all subcellular fractions. The plasma concentration of zinc is approximately 15 µmol/L, of which a third is bound to α2 macroglobulin and the rest to albumin. However, only 10–20% of the zinc in blood is found in the plasma: the rest is in red blood cells, associated mainly with carbonic anhydrase. The red cell membrane contains some zinc. Semen has 100-fold the zinc concentration of plasma.

A number of genes are regulated by zinc through the presence of short DNA sequence motifs known as metal-responsive elements. Some genes are positively affected; others negatively; and some are affected only by extremes of zinc status (deficiency or excess). Some of the genes identified include those involved in the regulation of redox signalling, fatty acid synthesis and degradation, platelet activation, and the regulation of homocysteine concentrations.

Zinc 'fingers' have been identified in the human genome. These are small proteins that have a zinc ion coordinated with a combination of cysteine and

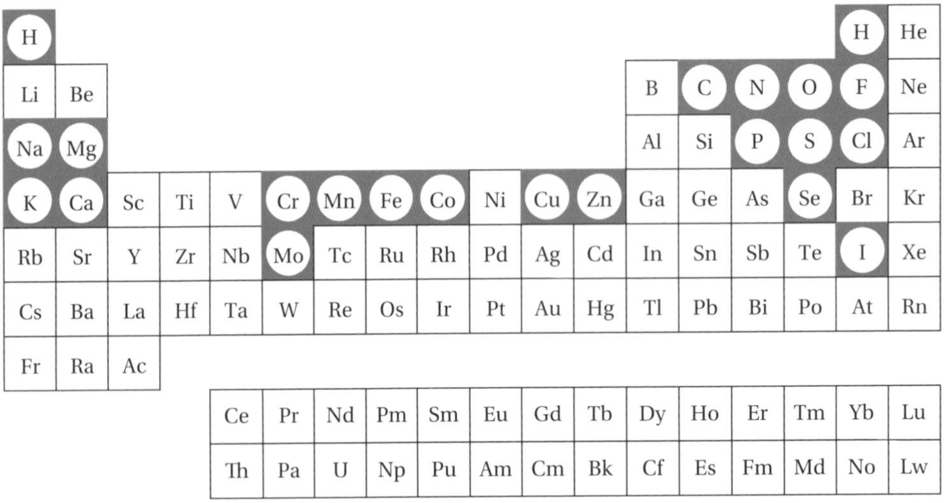

Fig. 11.1 Periodic table of the elements. Those essential for man are encircled in black. In addition, boron, silicon, nickel, arsenic, and vanadium are still under consideration as ultratrace elements.

histidine residues. The proteins, which may contain up to 30 fingers, interact with DNA, RNA, and other cellular proteins. Thus they have a widespread role in cellular metabolism.

Zinc also plays a role in stabilizing macromolecules and cellular membranes and it can function as a site-specific antioxidant. It can bind to or be in close proximity to thiol groups of proteins and reduce their reactivity. Zinc is a constituent of a large number of mammalian enzymes (more than 150), where it functions at the active site or as a structural component or both. Carbonic anhydrase was the first discovered zinc metalloenzyme; other enzymes include carboxypeptidase, alkaline phosphatase, transferases, ligases, lyases, isomerases, DNA/RNA polymerase, reverse transcriptase, and superoxide dismutase. Therefore zinc is involved in a number of major metabolic processes, including protein and nucleic acid synthesis. Zinc is essential for the synthesis and action of insulin. It also helps to stabilize the proinsulin and insulin hexamers by forming complexes with them.

11.1.3 Absorption and excretion

Zinc is absorbed mainly from the duodenum but some is absorbed lower down the small intestine. The mode of absorption involves both saturable and passive mechanisms. A number of zinc transporters has been identified: ZiPs (at least 15 different ones) promote zinc influx into cells, whilst ZnTs (ZnT1–9) promote efflux across membranes. The distribution of different ZnTs and ZiPs is tissue-specific. The exact site of zinc absorption depends on the form of zinc and the presence or absence of other nutrients that may form complexes with zinc or impact on intestinal transit time. Once absorbed, zinc is transported to the liver bound to albumin.

The major route of zinc excretion is by the intestine, followed by the kidneys and the skin. Faecal zinc originates from unabsorbed dietary sources as well as zinc which is excreted into the intestine along with the digestive juices (endogenous excretion). Smaller amounts of zinc are excreted in the urine or shed in skin cells. In addition, sexual activity in males contributes to zinc losses. In well-controlled metabolic ward studies, it has been shown that each ejaculate can contain up to 0.5 mg of zinc, probably derived from secretions of the prostate gland. Although conservation of zinc occurs during experimental zinc deficiency, the amount of zinc in ejaculates remains relatively high, thus representing a significant loss of zinc, particularly in people with low intakes. Hence the role of zinc in men is analogous to iron in women in that it is lost as part of normal sexual function.

11.1.4 Deficiency

Zinc deficiency was first observed in adolescents in Iran and Egypt (see Box 11.1). The first case was a 21-year-old male subject who resembled a 10-year-old boy. His main food was unleavened bread from unrefined wheat flour and he ate a considerable amount of clay. Other cases had hookworm infections and ate mostly unleavened wheat bread and beans. Unleavened bread prepared from unrefined wheat flour has a high phytate content which interferes with zinc absorption. Further investigations identified zinc as the limiting nutrient which was responsible for numerous symptoms including growth retardation, hypogonadism, and delayed sexual maturation. Other manifestations of zinc deficiency that have been reported subsequently include diverse forms of skin lesions, impaired wound healing, loss of taste (hypogeusia), behavioural disturbances, night blindness, and immune deficiency. These symptoms do not always occur together and seem to depend on the setting. For instance, in patients on total parenteral nutrition (if it lacks zinc), there is mental confusion, depression, eczema, and alopecia. In young children, zinc deficiency is expressed as a reduction in appetite, poor taste acuity, and poor growth.

Zinc deficiency is estimated by WHO to be one of the ten biggest factors that contribute to burden of disease in developing countries. In children, zinc deficiency contributes up to 15% of diarrhoea deaths, 10% of malaria deaths, and 7% of pneumonia deaths. Meta-analyses have shown that zinc supplementation of infants and young children reduces rates of diarrhoea and respiratory infections. Despite these important findings in developing countries, there is no strong evidence that zinc lozenges are effective in treating symptoms of the common cold in developed countries.

Night blindness, a significant symptom of vitamin A deficiency, can be due to deficiency of zinc, which is a coenzyme for the conversion of retinol to retinaldehyde by retinol dehydrogenase. Zinc deficiency has been observed in association with protein energy malnutrition in infants with marasmus or during their recovery. Zinc supplements supplied to malnourished children during recovery promote weight gain and synthesis of lean tissue and reduce common comorbidities. Anorexia nervosa in some ways resembles marasmus; however, the role of zinc in anorexia nervosa is unclear. It is likely that zinc deficiency develops in some anorexic patients through a generally inadequate diet which sustains the disorder and prevents adequate weight gain. However, zinc does not appear to play a causal role.

In pregnancy, plasma zinc has been reported to be low and, although this can be attributed partly to physiological changes unrelated to zinc depletion, the intakes of pregnant women are often below the recommendations. Adaptations in pregnancy such as increased absorption and reduced endogenous losses may help meet the requirement. Apart from possible reduction in induction of labour, caesarean section, and pre-term delivery and in some cases increases in birth weight and head circumference, zinc supplementation does not appear to have a significant or consistent effect on pregnancy outcome. Such inconsistencies may be related to small sample sizes, differing zinc status of pregnant women and inadequate study design.

Biochemical abnormalities of zinc deficiency include a reduction in plasma zinc concentrations, protein synthesis, activity of metalloproteins, resistance to infection, collagen synthesis, and platelet aggregation. In view of the large number of zinc finger proteins and the interaction between zinc and DNA, it has been hypothesized that zinc primarily restricts gene expression, rather than the enzyme activities.

Conditions which predispose to deficiency are related to:

(i) decreased intake, possibly associated with an eating disorder;

(ii) decreased absorption and/or bioavailability due to a high intake of an inhibitor (e.g. phytate), as noted in the first reported case of human zinc deficiency;

(iii) decreased utilization secondary to other conditions such as alcoholism;

(iv) increased losses in conditions such as diarrhoea and excessive vomiting, which may also be associated with an eating disorder;

(v) increased requirement associated with growth, pregnancy and lactation. The latter is recognized by a small increase in the recommended dietary intake for some countries.

11.1.5 Bioavailability and food sources

Zinc is available widely in the food supply but its bio-availability from different foods is highly variable. Zinc in animal products, crustacea, and molluscs is more readily absorbed than from plant foods. Rich sources of zinc include: oysters, red meat, lamb's liver, and cheese. Cereal grains, legumes, and nuts are rich in phytate, which reduces zinc absorption. The zinc content of refined cereals is lower than unrefined cereals but because the bran, which contains most of the phytate has been removed, the bio-availability is greater. Although a number of factors are known to influence the bioavailability of zinc, a reliable algorithm to calculate available zinc remains to be worked out. The molar ratio of phytate:zinc has been proposed as a predictor of zinc bioavailability and ratios greater than 15 have been associated with suboptimal zinc status. The phytate × calcium:zinc in the diet has been suggested as a marker of zinc bioavailability; however, there is limited data on the phytate content of foods. WHO has put forward three categories of bioavailability (Table 11.1).

The extent of adaptation to foods with low bioavailability of zinc is not fully understood and is confounded by the interaction with other nutrients. Current methods used for studying zinc bioavailability in humans include metabolic balance studies and radioisotope and stable isotope techniques. The radioisotope techniques are limited by ethical considerations such as long radioactive halflives and the amount of radiation exposure to subjects. Use of stable isotopes circumvents this issue but this technique requires costly instrumentation and demanding analytical procedures.

11.1.6 Nutrient reference values

The recommended dietary intake for zinc is 11–14 mg/day for men in different committee

Table 11.1 Dietary determinants of zinc bioavailability

Estimated absorption	Type of diet
Low (<15%)	Diets high in unrefined cereal grain
	Phytate:Zn molar ratio >15
	Calcium >1 g/day
Moderate (15–35%)	Mixed diet containing animal or fish protein
	Phytate:Zn molar ratio <10
High (35–55%)	Refined diets, low in cereal fibre
	Phytate:Zn molar ratio <5
	Dietary protein primarily from animal foods

Source: Updated from WHO (1996) *Trace elements in human nutrition and health*. Geneva, World Health Organization.

reports, 8 mg for women, with 3 and 4 mg extra for pregnancy and lactation, respectively. The upper intake level (UIL) is 40 mg/day.

11.1.7 Biochemical tests for status

The plasma zinc concentration represents less than 1% of the body pool of zinc and hence its measurement provides a limited amount of information about zinc status of individuals. Zinc from the plasma is taken up by the liver in response to cytokines released during stress and infection. In addition, plasma zinc concentrations fall in pregnancy, with injuries and in diseases such as liver cirrhosis and pernicious anaemia. Plasma zinc also undergoes diurnal variation, with a U-shaped curve over a 24-hour period. Peak concentrations are found in the mornings and trough concentrations in the mid-evening. Despite its limitations, the concentration of zinc in plasma is the most commonly used diagnostic indicator and the balance of evidence shows that the concentration falls in deficiency and rises in sufficiency (or with supplementation). A smaller number of studies suggest that urinary zinc and hair zinc concentrations also are reliable biomarkers of zinc status.

11.1.8 Toxicity

The ingestion of very high doses (>1 g zinc), results in a metallic taste in the mouth, nausea, fever, lethargy, and gastric distress. This acute response occurs with deliberate supplementation, occupational exposure, or food poisoning. Rapid infusion of intravenous feeding solutions containing zinc can cause similar symptoms. Very large doses have resulted in death.

Zinc supplements (50–150 mg zinc) decrease plasma high-density lipoprotein cholesterol (HDL-C) concentrations, thus increasing the risk of cardiovascular disease in normolipidaemic individuals. The major effect, however, is due to the adverse interaction between zinc and copper absorption. Zinc induces the synthesis of metallothionein, a sulphur-rich protein that binds copper with high affinity. In chronic toxicity, copper status is compromised, resulting in a decrease in copper-related functions, including the reduction in copper metalloenzyme activity and anaemia. The decrease in copper absorption is advantageous under some circumstances. It is required in the treatment of patients with (Kinnear) Wilson's disease and zinc supplementation is part of the management strategy. The UIL for adults is 40 mg zinc/day.

Further Reading

1. **Fischer Walker, C.L., Ezzati, M., and Black, R.E.** (2009) Global and regional child mortality and burden of disease attributable to zinc deficiency. *Eur J Clin Nutr*, **63**, 591–7.
2. **Gibson, R.S.** (2005). *Principles of nutritional assessment.* 2nd ed. Oxford, Oxford University Press.
3. **International Zinc Nutrition Consultative Group** (2009) *Systematic reviews of zinc interventions strategies.* Technical Document 2. Brown K.H., Hess S.Y. (guest eds). *Food Nutr Bull*, **30**, S5–184.
4. **Lowe, N.M., Fekete, K., and Decsi, T.** (2009) Methods of assessment of zinc status in humans: A systematic review. *Am J Clin Nutr*, **89**, 2040S–51S.
5. **World Health Organization** (1996) *Trace elements in human nutrition and health.* Geneva, World Health Organization.
6. **World Health Organization** (2004) *Vitamin and mineral requirements in human nutrition.* Geneva, WHO.

11.2 Copper
Samir Samman

11.2.1 Historical perspective

The essential role of copper was realized in 1926 and soon after it was shown that it is required for the synthesis of haemoglobin in rats. In 1962 copper deficiency was reported in humans.

11.2.2 Distribution and function

Copper is one of the IB series of metals with a molecular weight of 63.5. It is one of the most effective cations for binding to organic molecules. It is commonly used in biological reactions that involve electron transfer.

Adult humans contain about 100 mg Cu, which is distributed in concentrations of about 1.5 µg/g in the skin, skeletal muscle, bone marrow, liver, and brain. Studies in animals suggest that the copper content may decrease with age. The plasma concentration is 15 µmol/L (similar to zinc); up to 90% of this is associated with caeruloplasmin. Other Cu proteins include many of the oxidases, metallothionein, α-fetoglobulin, superoxide dismutase, and transcuprein.

Copper has diverse functions including erythropoiesis, connective tissue synthesis (via lysyl oxidase), oxidative phosphorylation, thermogenesis, and superoxide dismutation. As well as transporting copper, caeruloplasmin is one of the acute phase proteins and via its ferroxidase activity, catalyses the oxidation of ferrous iron. This latter reaction is essential for the mobilization of iron as a complex with transferrin. It is believed to be the mechanism by which copper is able to regulate the homeostasis of iron.

11.2.3 Absorption and excretion

Dietary copper is reduced to Cu^{1+} and transported across the apical membrane of the enterocyte by a specific transporter known as copper transporter 1 (Ctr1). Copper is incorporated into cellular protein (including enzymes), but the majority is released from the basolateral membrane of the intestinal cell to portal blood. Copper is transported to the liver by albumin and transcuprein. In the liver, copper is incorporated into caeruloplasmin and subsequently circulates to other tissues.

The efficiency of copper absorption depends on the individual's copper status. The efficiency of absorption increases in cases of deficiency or when dietary copper intake is low. Copper is excreted mainly via the gastrointestinal tract. Less is excreted in the urine and from the skin.

11.2.4 Bioavailability and food sources

Copper has a wide distribution in the food supply but in particular it is found in foods of animal sources, legumes, nuts, and the water supply (copper pipes). Copper absorption is enhanced by organic nutrients such as amino acids and in particular, histidine. Conversely, absorption is inhibited by excesses of other divalent cations such as zinc and iron. Studies in animals suggest that vitamin C may have an adverse effect on copper absorption, but the results of trials in humans are not conclusive. Phytic acid and dietary fibre do not appear to inhibit copper absorption.

11.2.5 Deficiency

Copper deficiency is relatively rare. It has been observed in protein energy malnutrition, in patients on long-term copper-free total parenteral nutrition, and in premature infants fed cow's milk or unfortified formula. Symptoms include anaemia, neutropenia, skeletal demineralization, decreased skin tone, connective tissue aneurysms, hypothermia, neurological symptoms, and depigmented hair.

Defects in copper metabolism have been identified. Menkes' disease, an X-linked progressive brain disease, was established as related to copper following the recognition by Australian researchers that patients with the disease have kinks in their hair which was similar to the kinks in the wool of sheep grazing on copper-deficient soils. The characteristics of the hair together with low concentrations of plasma copper and caeruloplasmin are features of the disease. Intestinal absorption of copper is defective.

Patients who lack plasma caeruloplasmin have been identified. Recent findings in patients with acaeruloplasminiaemia have confirmed the essential role of this copper protein in iron metabolism. Symptoms associated with acaeruloplasminiaemia include decreased copper and iron in plasma, increased iron concentrations in tissues, and impaired copper absorption.

11.2.6 Nutrient reference values

No estimated average requirement or dietary reference intake has been estimated for copper. An adequate intake for adults is approximately 1.2 (for women), 1.7 (for men) mg/day, with another 0.3 mg recommended for lactation. The UIL should not exceed 10 mg/day.

11.2.7 Assessment of copper status

Serum copper is the most useful biomarker of copper status. The assessment of marginal deficiency remains a challenge. However, it appears that the activity of some copper-dependant enzymes (e.g. serum diamine oxidase) respond to increases in dietary or supplemental copper and have the potential to reflect copper status. Frank copper deficiency can be determined by the measurement of plasma copper concentrations and plasma caeruloplasmin. The haematocrit decreases and there is microcytic hypochromic anaemia.

11.2.8 Toxicity

The amounts of copper in the diet (including water) are not likely to be toxic because of the ability to maintain homeostasis by decreasing absorption and increasing excretion. Acute toxicity has been reported as a result of accidental ingestion of large doses of copper or in industrial accidents. The symptoms of small doses include vomiting and nausea, while larger doses induce hepatic necrosis and haemolytic anaemia. Chronic toxicity is relatively rare.

Wilson's disease, Indian childhood cirrhosis, and idiopathic copper toxicosis are disorders that predispose individuals to copper overload. Wilson's disease is a rare inborn error of metabolism with a reported incidence of 1:30 000. It is an autosomal recessive disease that gives rise to hepatolenticular degeneration (juvenile cirrhosis, coarse tremor, browning around the cornea). Less well quantified are the incidences of Indian childhood cirrhosis, reported initially in India but also in other parts of the world in non-Indian children, and idiopathic copper toxicity. There is little evidence to support the efficacy of copper restriction for the management of Wilson's disease and other copper storage diseases. The primary intervention has to be pharmacological (chelation) therapy to increase urinary copper excretion.

Further Reading

1. **Harvey, L.J., Ashton, K., Hooper, L., Casgrain, A., and Fairweather-Tait, S.J.** (2009) Methods of assessment of copper status in humans: A systematic review. *Am J Clin Nutr*, **89**, 2009S–24S.
2. **Prohaska, J.R.** (2008) Role of copper transporters in copper homeostasis. *Am J Clin Nutr*, **88**, 826S–9S.
3. **World Health Organization**. (2004) *Vitamin and mineral requirements in human nutrition*. Geneva, WHO.

11.3 Iodine
Sheila Skeaff and Christine D. Thomson

Iodine was one of the first trace elements to be identified as essential. As early as 2700 BC, the Chinese were treating goitre by feeding seaweed, marine animal preparations, and burnt sponge (all rich in iodine). In the first half of the nineteenth century, the incidence of goitre was linked with low iodine content of food and drinking water, and by the late nineteenth century the geographic distribution of endemic goitre and cretinism was recognized to extend around the world. In the 1920s, iodine was shown to be an integral component of the thyroid hormone thyroxine, which is required for normal growth and metabolism, and later, in 1952, of triiodothyronine.

11.3.1 Chemical structure and functions of iodine

Iodine functions as an integral part of the thyroid hormones, the prohormone thyroxine (T_4), and the active form 3,5,3′-triiodothyronine (T_3), which is the key regulator of important cell processes. The thyroid hormones are required for normal growth and development of individual tissues such as the brain and central nervous system and maturation of the whole body, as well as for energy production and oxygen consumption in cells, thereby maintaining the body's metabolic rate.

If thyroid hormone secretion is inadequate (i.e. hypothyroidism), the basal metabolic rate is reduced and the general level of activity of the individual is decreased. Normal growth and development will also be impaired.

The regulation of thyroid hormone synthesis, release, and action is a complex process involving the thyroid, the pituitary, the brain, and peripheral tissues. The hypothalamus regulates the plasma concentrations of the thyroid hormones by controlling the release from the pituitary of thyroid-stimulating hormone (TSH, thyrotropin) through a negative feedback mechanism related to the level of T_4 in the blood. If blood T_4 falls, the secretion of TSH is increased, which enhances the activity of the thyroid and consequently the output of T_4 into the circulation. This fine control of T_4 secretion is important, as either an excess or a deficit in the hormone is detrimental to normal function. If the level of circulating T_4 hormone is not maintained because of severe iodine deficiency, TSH remains elevated, and both these measures are used for diagnosis of hypothyroidism due to iodine deficiency.

11.3.2 Body content

Iodine occurs in the tissues in both inorganic (iodide) and organically bound forms. The adult human body contains about 15–50 mg iodine, with 70–80% of this found in the thyroid gland, which has a remarkable concentrating power for iodine, and the remainder is mainly in the circulating blood.

11.3.3 Metabolism

The metabolism of iodine is closely linked to thyroid function, since the only known function for iodine is in the synthesis of thyroid hormones. Iodine is an anionic trace element that is rapidly absorbed in the form of iodide and taken up immediately by the thyroid gland. The thyroid gland is a globular, butterfly-shaped gland located at the base of the neck. It is composed of spherical follicles lined with thyroid cells filled with colloid. A sodium-iodide symporter protein located on the basal membrane of the thyroid cell actively transports iodide into the thyroid cell. Iodide then migrates to the apical membrane of the thyrocyte and crosses into the follicular lumen. Two enzymes, thyroperoxidase and hydrogen peroxidase, oxidize iodide, which is attached to tyrosyl residues of thyroglobulin (Tg) to form mono-iodotyrosine (MIT) and di-iodotyrosine (DIT). MIT and DIT are coupled to make T_3 or T_4 within the thyroglobulin (Tg) molecule. Tg enters the thyrocyte by endocytosis of the colloid and is proteolysed, releasing T_3 and T_4, which subsequently enter the circulation. Within the blood, more than 99% of the thyroid hormones are bound to plasma proteins. At receptors on the surfaces of target cells in organs around the body, T_4 is converted to T_3 by various iodothyronine 5′-deiodinase enzymes. The half-life of T_4 is approximately 7 days but only 24 hours for T_3. The majority (~80%) of T_3 is formed extrathyroidally from deiodination of T_4. The thyroid gland needs to trap around 60 µg iodide per day to maintain an adequate supply of T_4. Excess inorganic iodine is readily excreted in the urine.

11.3.4 Deficiency

Iodine deficiency is recognized as a major international public health problem because of the large number of populations living in iodine-deficient environments, characterized primarily by iodine-deficient soils. WHO estimates that 2 billion people have inadequate iodine nutrition; 285 million of these are school children. At least 20 million may suffer from mental defect that is preventable by correction of iodine deficiency. Basil Hetzel coined the term iodine-deficiency disorders (IDD), which refers to the wide spectrum of adverse effects that iodine deficiency can have on growth and development (Table 11.2). Goitre, a swelling of the thyroid gland (as shown in Fig. 11.2), is the most obvious

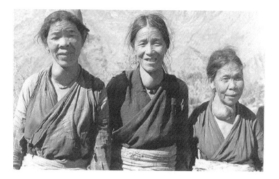

Fig. 11.2 Three women of the Himalayas with stage 11 goitres (courtesy of Professor Creswell Eastman and *Thyroid Manager*).

Table 11.2 Spectrum of the iodine-deficiency disorders (IDD)

Fetus	Abortions
	Stillbirths
	Congenital anomalies
	Increased perinatal mortality
	Increased infant mortality
	Neurological cretinism: mental deficiency, deaf mutism, spastic diplegia, squint
	Myxoedematous cretinism: mental deficiency, dwarfism, hypothyroidism
	Psychomotor defects
Neonate	Neonatal hypothyroidism
Child and adolescent	Retarded mental and physical development
Adult	Goitre and its complications
	Iodine-induced hyperthyroidism
All ages	Goitre
	Hypothyroidism
	Impaired mental function
	Increased susceptibility to nuclear radiation

Source: WHO/NHD (2001) *Assessment of iodine deficiency disorders and monitoring their elimination: A guide for programme managers*. 2nd edn. Geneva, World Health Organization.

and familiar feature of iodine deficiency, and is the body's adaptive response to inadequate dietary iodine. A number of changes take place in the thyroid gland, including hyperplasia of the thyroid cells, resulting in an increase in the size of the gland, and a more efficient use of available iodine to produce thyroid hormones.

Cretinism The most damaging consequences of iodine deficiency are on fetal and infant development. Thyroid hormones (therefore iodine) are essential for normal development of the brain, and insufficient levels may result in permanent mental retardation of the fetus or newborn child. Iodine deficiency is the world's greatest single cause of preventable brain damage and mental retardation. The most severe effect of fetal iodine deficiency is endemic cretinism, which occurs when a pregnant women is severely iodine deficient particularly in the first trimester. In general, cretins are mentally defective, with other physical abnormalities. Clinical manifestations differ with geographical location and two types of cretinism have been observed. In *myxoedematous cretinism*, features of hypothyroidism are present (dry skin, hoarse voice) with stunted growth and mental deficiency (Fig. 11.3). In the *nervous or neurological type of cretinism*, mental retardation is present, as well as hearing and speech defects and characteristic disorders of stance and gait, while hypothyroidism is absent. In myxoedematous cretinism, thyroid hormone treatment can lead to some

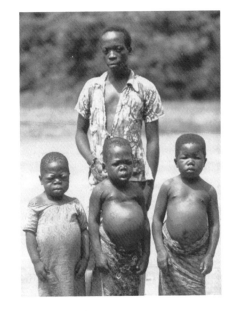

Fig. 11.3 Myxoedematous endemic cretinism in the Democratic Republic of Congo. Four inhabitants aged 15–20 years: a normal man and three females with severe longstanding hypothyroidism with dwarfism, retarded sexual development, puffy features, dry skin, and severe mental retardation (courtesy of Professor Creswell Eastman and *Thyroid Manager*).

improvement (iodine cannot help—the thyroid gland is atrophic). Mixed forms of cretinism are seen in some areas.

Mild to moderate iodine deficiency There are also detrimental effects of less obvious iodine deficiency on mental performance of school children, which may have considerable social consequences that are detrimental to national development. A meta-analysis of 18 studies estimated that the mean IQ scores of children living in moderately to severely iodine-deficient areas were 13.5 points lower than children living in iodine sufficient areas. Another meta-analysis of 37 studies in China confirmed this finding, finding a mean difference of 10 IQ points. Both meta-analyses primarily used data from cross-sectional studies. Only two well-conducted randomized controlled trials have been undertaken in this area. Albanian schoolchildren with moderate iodine deficiency given a bolus dose

of iodized poppyseed oil showed an improvement in four out of seven cognitive tests after 24 weeks. A similar study in New Zealand schoolchildren with mild iodine deficiency who took a daily iodine supplement for 28 weeks showed an improvement in two out of four cognitive tests compared to placebo children. The cerebral effect was not mirrored by total thyroid hormone levels.

The major cause of IDD is inadequate dietary intake of iodine from foods grown in soils from which iodine has been leached by glaciation, high rainfall, or flooding. Goitre is usually seen where the intake is less than 50 μg/day and cretinism where the mother's intake is 30 μg/day or less. However, thyroid function may also be impaired after exposure to antithyroid compounds in foods and drugs—called goitrogens (e.g. thiocyanate)—which prevent the uptake of iodine into the thyroid gland. Selenium has the potential to play a part in the outcome of iodine deficiency in two ways. First, the selenium-containing iodothyronine 5′-deiodinases regulate the synthesis and degradation of T_3. Second, selenoperoxidases protect the thyroid gland from hydrogen peroxide produced during the synthesis of thyroid hormones. In countries where iodine deficiency is not endemic, hypothyroidism is typically due to autoimmune disease.

11.3.5 Measures to prevent iodine deficiency

Iodization of salt has been the primary method for combating iodine deficiency since the 1920s, when it was first successfully used in Switzerland. Since then, introduction of iodized salt in a number of other countries has resulted in the elimination of goitre in these regions. Universal salt iodization (USI) for use by food industry as well as retail salt for use in the home, the iodization of all salt for human and animal consumption, is the recommended strategy for prevention of IDD. However, the success of iodization depends on whether all salt is iodized. Despite the WHO recommendation, few countries have implemented USI; the exception is China, who has successfully used USI since 1993 with a consequent reduction in goitre rate in children from 20%

to 6%. Indeed, USI has been so successful that in 2010 the Chinese government called for a lowering of the amount of iodine in salt from 20–60 mg/kg to 20–30 mg/kg in response to a study showing many Chinese now have excessive iodine intakes.

In regions with severe iodine deficiency, the use of iodized vegetable oil that contains 200–400 mg of iodine, given either as an injection or orally, has been successfully used to improve iodine status for at least 1 year. In 2007 WHO and UNICEF recommended that pregnant and lactating women and children < 2 years, who do not have access to iodized salt and live in areas of moderate to severe iodine deficiency, should be given oral doses of iodized oil annually. In countries where iodine intakes are higher, but still not adequate, daily iodine supplements are recommended, containing 150–250 μg.

11.3.6 Towards elimination of iodine deficiency: global action

Iodine deficiency is recognized as a major international public health problem because of the large populations at risk in iodine-deficient environments. The International Council for the Control of Iodine Deficiency disorders (ICCIDD) (http://www.iccidd.org/) formed in 1986 and is working closely with other international organizations to develop national programmes to prevent and control IDD. A Global Action Plan to eliminate IDD as a major public health problem by the year 2000 was adopted in 1990 by the United Nations system. Elimination of IDD by 2000 was also the goal of the World Summit for Children in 1990, and this goal was reaffirmed in 1992 by delegates from 160 countries at the International Conference on Nutrition in Rome. Reports indicate that there has been substantial progress towards the elimination of iodine deficiency in the past two decades through the development of the WHO Global Database on Iodine Deficiency and the USI policy. However, in order to reach the goal of global elimination of IDD, continued efforts are needed to monitor at-risk populations and to strengthen and maintain salt iodization

programmes. Australia and New Zealand are a case in point, where a lack in surveillance systems and changes in food patterns has resulted in the re-emergence of mild iodine deficiency from the early 1990s, necessitating the mandatory fortification of commercial breads with iodized salt in 2009.

11.3.7 Assessment of iodine status

The assessment of nutritional status of iodine is important in relation to a population or group living in an area or region that is suspected to be iodine deficient. To date, the most important information comes from measurement of the urinary iodide and the prevalence of goitre and cretinism. ICCIDD board member and iodine expert Dr Michael Zimmermann has recently suggested three additional strategies to target vulnerable groups at risk of IDD: measuring newborn thyroid-stimulating hormone; measuring urinary iodine in infants; and using dried blood spot thyroglobulin in children.

Urinary iodine excretion Approximately 90% of iodine intake is excreted in the urine and therefore 24-hour excretion of iodine reflects dietary intake and may be used for estimating the intake. However, 24-hour urine samples are difficult to collect in the field, and non-fasting casual or spot urine specimens are usually collected. The ease of obtaining a casual urine sample from subjects is offset by the large variability of such samples at the level of the individual. Thus, the median urinary iodine concentration of a group is used as a biomarker for the assessment of iodine nutrition; urinary iodine cannot be used to assess iodine status in an individual. An optimal median urinary iodine concentration between 100 and 200 μg/L corresponds to an intake of approximately 150–200 μg/day. Table 11.3 gives median urinary iodine concentrations associated with levels of iodine nutrition. Urinary iodine, however, is a sensitive indicator of recent iodine intake but not of thyroid function. Furthermore, where goitrogens are preventing the uptake of iodine into the thyroid gland and synthesis of thyroid hormones, urinary

Table 11.3 Epidemiological criteria for assessing iodine nutrition based on median urinary iodine concentrations in a group

Median urinary iodine (μg/L)	Iodine intake	Iodine nutrition
<20	Insufficient	Severe iodine deficiency
20–49	Insufficient	Moderate iodine deficiency
50–99	Insufficient	Mild iodine deficiency
100–199	Adequate	Optimal for children and adults, including breastfeeding women
>150	Adequate for pregnant women	Optimal for pregnant women
200–299	More than adequate	Risk of iodine-induced hyperthyroidism within 5–10 years following introduction of iodized salt in susceptible groups
>300	Excessive	Risk of adverse health consequences (iodine-induced hyperthyroidism, autoimmune thyroid diseases)

Source: WHO/UNICEF/ICCIDD (2007) *Assessment of iodine deficiency disorders and monitoring their elimination: A guide for programme managers*. 3rd edn. Geneva, WHO.

iodine may be normal and therefore not a suitable marker for iodine status.

Assessment of thyroid size and goitre rate

The prevalence of goitre reflects a population's history of iodine nutrition, but it does not properly reflect its present iodine status, because thyroid size decreases only slowly after iodine repletion. Goitre assessment is made by inspection, palpation, or more recently by ultrasonography. The recommended target group for monitoring goitre rate is school children. Normative values proposed by the WHO and the ICCIDD for thyroid volume by ultrasonography are based on data obtained from a large international sample of iodine-replete school-age children. The percentage of children with thyroid glands greater than the 97th percentile of normative values characterizes mild (5–19%), moderate (20–29%), and severe (≥30%) deficiency.

Thyroid hormones

The level of thyroid hormones provides an indirect measure of iodine nutritional status. When iodine in the diet is limited, TSH increases while T_4 concentration decreases; however, these changes are relatively transient because the iodine gland can respond to low iodine intakes. Typically alterations in TSH and T_4 concentration outside the reference range are only observed in moderate iodine deficiency, while T_3 concentrations only decline in severe deficiency. Thus, the assessment of TSH, T_4, or T_3 are not particularly useful or sensitive for determining iodine status in adults, especially in areas of moderate to mild iodine deficiency. WHO has advocated the use of neonatal TSH to assess iodine status for many years; however, technical issues have hindered its widespread use. Serum thyroglobulin is a more sensitive indicator of mild iodine deficiency and iodine repletion than TSH or T_4, as levels are elevated in subjects with mild iodine deficiency.

For population studies, both TSH and thyroglobulin are recommended surveillance measures and can be determined in blood spots on filter paper or serum samples. The percentage of neonates with TSH values greater than 5 μIU/mL whole blood defines the level of deficiency: mild (3–19%), moderate (20–39%), and severe (≥40%). Similarly, thyroglobulin values of 10–19, 20–39, or ≥40 ng/mL serum in groups of school-age children represent mild, moderate, and severe deficiency, respectively.

11.3.8 Dietary intakes of iodine

Iodine intakes vary considerably depending on geographical location, dietary habits, and salt iodization. Adequate dietary intakes of iodine are around 100–150 µg/day, with intakes of 220–270 µg/day recommended in pregnancy and lactation.

Foods of marine origin, such as sea fish, shellfish, seameal, and seaweeds, are rich in iodine and reflect the greater iodine concentration of sea water compared with fresh water. The iodine content of plants and animals depends on the environment in which they grow, but generally, vegetables, fruit, and cereals grown on soils with low iodine content are poor sources of iodine.

Because the mammary gland concentrates iodine, dairy products are usually a good source, but only if the cows get enough iodine. Iodine contamination of dairy products from iodophors and bread from iodates (used as bread improvers) have made major contributions to the daily intake. The use of iodophors as sanitizers in the dairy industry, now declining, has resulted in variable but considerable amounts of residual iodine in milk, cheese, and other milk products in the past. Other adventitious sources of iodine include kelp tablets and drugs and beverages or foods containing the iodine-containing colouring erythrosine.

Iodized salt is another source of iodine and has been the most extensive means of improving iodine nutrition. The amount added varies widely in different regions. In Canada and the USA, salt is iodized to a concentration of 77 ppm iodine as potassium iodide, so that the daily recommended intake might be obtained from 2 g salt. Most other countries add 10–40 ppm iodide to salt. However, in some countries both iodized salt and non-iodized salt is available. In developed countries, much of the salt intake now comes from processed foods; which often do not contain iodized salt.

11.3.9 Interactions

The utilization of absorbed iodine is influenced by goitrogens, which interfere with the biosynthesis of the hormones. Goitrogens are found in vegetables of the genus brassica: cabbage, turnip, swede, brussel sprouts, and broccoli, in some staple foods such as cassava, maize, millet, and lima beans that are used in developing countries; and in some parts of the world goitrogens can be found in the water. Goitrogens can become a problem where people whose iodine intakes are only marginal eat these staple foods, particularly if they are not well cooked. Most goitrogens are inactivated by heat, but not when milk is pasteurized.

11.3.10 Requirement and recommended dietary intakes

Goitre occurs when iodine intakes are less than about 50 µg/day, and cretinism when maternal intake is 30 µg/day or less. Minimum requirement to prevent goitre, based on the urinary excretion associated with a high incidence of goitre in a population, is approximately 1 µg/kg body weight/day. However, recommended dietary intakes are based on physiological requirements, which are in turn based on a number of indicators, including thyroidal radioiodine accumulation and turnover, iodine balance studies, urinary iodide excretion, thyroid hormone measures, and thyroid volume. From these data, a physiological requirement of around 100 µg/day is indicated, and a rather large safety margin is generally advised to ensure an adequate intake. In most countries, the recommended intake is in the range 150–200 µg/day. This is adequate to maintain normal thyroid function that is essential for growth and development. Because of the increased requirements for thyroid hormones during pregnancy and the importance of adequate iodine for the fetus and neonate, recommended intakes for pregnant and lactating women are considerably higher at 200–230 µg/day for pregnancy and 200–290 µg/day for lactation.

11.3.11 Toxicity

Intakes between 50 and 1100 µg/day are considered safe. The effects of high iodine intake on thyroid function are variable and depend on the health of the thyroid gland. Dietary intakes of up 1100 µg/day have few long-term effects when the thyroid is healthy. Daily intakes of 2000 µg iodine should be regarded as excessive or potentially harmful. Such intakes are unlikely to be obtained from diets of natural foods except where they are exceptionally high in marine fish or seaweed, such as in Japan or where foods are contaminated with iodine from iodophors.

Other large sources of iodine include iodine-containing drugs, radiographic contast media, and the use of kelp supplements that can contain very high but variable amounts of iodine.

Excess intakes of iodide can cause enlargement of the thyroid gland, just as deficiency can, as well as hypothyroidism and elevated TSH and increased incidence of autoimmune thyroid disease. People who have underlying autoimmune disease such as Grave's disease or Hashimoto's thyroiditis, or who have lived in areas of previous severe iodine deficiency but still have nodular goitres, may be more sensitive to an increase in iodine. Iodine-induced thyrotoxicosis (Jod–Basedow syndrome), characterized by a high pulse rate, weight loss, perspiration, and tremor, has been observed following iodization programmes. However, cases of thyrotoxicosis disappear alongside the disappearance of goitre as the iodine status of the population improves.

Further reading

1. **Chen, Z.-P., and Hetzel, B.S.** (2010) Cretinism revisited. *Best Pract Res Clin Endocrinol Metab,* **24,** 39–50.
2. **Hetzel, B.S.** (1989) *The story of iodine deficiency: An international challenge in nutrition.* Oxford, Oxford University Press.
3. **Preedy, V.R., Burrow, G.N., and Watson, R.R.** (eds) (2009) *The comprehensive handbook of iodine.* London, UK, Academic Press.
4. **WHO/NHD** (2001) *Assessment of iodine deficiency disorders and monitoring their elimination: A guide for programme managers.* 2nd edn. Geneva, World Health Organization.
5. **WHO** (2004) *Iodine status worldwide: WHO global database on iodine deficiency.* Geneva, WHO.
6. **WHO/UNICEF/ICCIDD** (2007) *Assessment of iodine deficiency disorders and monitoring their elimination: A guide for programme managers,* 3rd edn. Geneva, WHO.
7. **Zimmermann, M.B.** (2009) Iodine deficiency. *Endocrine Rev,* **30,** 376–408.
8. **The IDD newsletter** is very interesting, with illustrated stories about iodine deficiency and work to reduce it, in different countries round the world. It is published by ICCIDD and appears four times a year. To contact, email icciddnewsletter@ilw.agri.ethz.ch.

11.4 Selenium
Christine D. Thomson

Selenium first attracted interest in the 1930s as a toxic trace element that caused loss of hair and blind staggers in livestock that consumed high-selenium plants

in South Dakota. In 1957, selenium was shown to be essential for mammalian life when traces of this mineral prevented liver necrosis in vitamin E-deficient rats, and later to prevent a variety of economically important diseases in domestic animals, such as white muscle disease in cattle and sheep, hepatosis dietetica in swine, and exudative diathesis in poultry. The demonstration in 1973 of a biochemical function for selenium as an integral component of the seleno-enzyme glutathione peroxidase (GPx) was followed by identification of several other selenoproteins, all of which were found to contain selenocysteine. The importance of selenium in human nutrition was highlighted in reports in 1979 of selenium deficiency in a patient in New Zealand on total parenteral nutrition and of the selenium-responsive condition Keshan disease in China. Considerable research during the past three decades has provided information on the metabolism and importance of selenium in human nutrition, leading to the establishment of recommended dietary intakes based on amounts required to maximize plasma selenoproteins. More recently, the focus has turned to possible benefits from higher levels of selenium intake in maintaining human health, by protecting against certain types of cancer and cardiovascular disease (CVD), and through the maintenance of a healthy immune system. Genomics is now rapidly advancing our knowledge of functions and requirements for selenium.

11.4.1 Functions of selenium

Selenium exerts its biological effects as a constituent of selenoproteins, of which there are 25 in humans. These selenoproteins are involved in a wide variety of processes in the body, including antioxidant defence and redox metabolism, thyroid metabolism, immune function, reproductive function, and many others, with implications of clinical importance in many diseases such as cancer and autoimmune thyroid disease. The following have been purified and studied:

- glutathione peroxidase (GPx)
  - cytosolic, cellular (GPx1)
  - gastrointestinal (GPx2)
  - plasma (GPx3)

- phospholipid hydroperoxide (GPx4)
- embryonic and olfactory (GPx6)
- selenoprotein P (SEPP)
- iodothyronine 5′-deiodinases (DI1, DI2, DI3)
- thioredoxin reductase (TR1, TR2, TR3)
- also selenophosphate synthetase 2, Sep15 (15 kDa selenoprotein), selenoprotein W, selenoprotein R (methionine-R-sulphoxide reductase; MsrB1), selenoproteins H, I, K, M, N, O, P, S, T, and V.

The selenium is present in all selenoproteins as selenocysteine at the active site. Selenocysteine, the twenty-first amino acid, is inserted into proteins cotranslationally in response to the UGA codon, which, in addition to selenocysteine insertion, functions to terminate protein synthesis.

The first of the selenoproteins to be characterized was GPx, which consists of four identical subunits, each containing selenocysteine at the active site. GPx is present in at least five different forms, all of which use glutathione to catalyse the reduction of hydrogen peroxide and/or phospholipid hyroperoxides. In cells including erythrocytes (GPx1), the gastrointestinal tract (GPx2) and plasma (GPx3), this enzyme may function *in vivo* to remove hydrogen peroxide, thereby preventing the initiation of peroxidation of membranes and oxidative damage. These GPxs may have more specific functions in arachidonic acid metabolism in platelets, microbiocidal activity in leukocytes, immune function, and cancer prevention. GPx1 is one of the selenoproteins more highly sensitive to selenium deficiency and changes in selenium status.

Another selenium-containing enzyme, phospholipid hydroperoxide GPx (GPx4), differs from other GPxs in several ways. It can metabolize phospholipid hydroperoxides in cell membranes, and thus may play a role as an antioxidant in protecting biomembranes. In addition, GPx4 acts as a structural protein, which is required for sperm maturation.

Selenoprotein P (SEPP), a glycoprotein containing multiple selenocysteine residues, has been purified and characterized from rat and human plasma. It is the major selenoprotein in plasma, providing 40–50% of plasma selenium. Its concentration in rat plasma falls to 10% in selenium deficiency and so is a useful biomarker of selenium status. Its function is still unclear, but there is evidence for both an antioxidant role and a transport role in the testis and in the brain.

Three iodothyronine 5'-deiodinases (types 1, 2, and 3) are selenoproteins. These enzymes catalyse the conversion of thyroxine (T_4) to its active metabolite triiodothyronine (T_3). Severe selenium deficiency results in an increase in levels of plasma T_4 and a corresponding decrease in levels of T_3. The interactions of selenium and iodine deficiencies have implications for both human health and livestock production. In humans, selenium deficiency may exacerbate effects of concurrent iodine deficiency.

Another family of selenoproteins is the thioredoxin reductases, NADPH-dependent flavoprotein oxidoreductases that reduce the disulphide of thioredoxin. Activity of thioredoxin reductase declines in selenium deficiency. In humans there are three distinct thioredoxin reductases, which support cell proliferation, antioxidant defence, and redox-regulated signalling cascades and may be involved in spermatogenesis and embryonic development.

Several selenium-containing enzymes have been identified in microorganisms and other selenoproteins have been found in animal tissues, suggesting further functions for selenium.

Selenoprotein W is found in muscle and other tissues and derived its name because it is one of the missing selenoproteins in heart and muscle of lambs suffering from white muscle disease. Its function is still uncertain.

There is growing evidence that mutations or single-nucleotide polymorphisms in selenoproteins most likely affect selenocysteine incorporation efficiency, which in turn may contribute to the aetiology of diseases such as cancer, CVD, and autoimmune diseases.

11.4.2 Metabolism of selenium

Selenoamino acids are the main dietary forms of selenium, with selenium replacing sulphur in selenomethionine in general proteins in plant and animal foods and selenocysteine in selenoenzymes in animal foods. Inorganic forms of selenium, such as selenite and selenate, are used in experimental diets and as supplements.

Absorption Selenium is absorbed mainly from the duodenum. Selenomethionine and methionine share the same active transport mechanism, and selenocysteine probably shares the cysteine transporter. Absorption of inorganic forms such as selenite and selenate is via a passive mechanism. Absorption of selenium is generally high in humans, probably about 80% from most dietary sources; selenomethionine appears to be better absorbed than selenite. Absorption is unaffected by selenium status, suggesting that there is no homeostatic regulation of absorption.

Bioavailability Animal studies show a wide variation in the bioavailability of selenium from different foods. In rats, the bioavailability from mushrooms, tuna, wheat, beef kidney, and Brazil nuts is 5, 57, 83, 97, and 124%, respectively, in comparison with sodium selenite. Human studies also show differences among various forms such as selenate, wheat, and yeast.

Transport Little is known about the transport of selenium in the body, although it appears to be transported bound to plasma proteins: selenomethionine bound to albumin and inorganic selenium to very-low-density lipoproteins. SEPP also appears to be a transport protein, involved particularly in transporting selenium to the brain and testis.

Metabolism and distribution An outline of selenium metabolism is shown in Fig. 11.4. Selenium in animal tissues is present in two main forms: selenocysteine, which is present as the active form of selenium in selenoproteins; and selenomethionine, which is non-specifically incorporated in place of methionine in a variety of proteins, unregulated by the selenium status of the animal.

Selenium levels in tissues are influenced by dietary intake, as reflected in the wide variation in

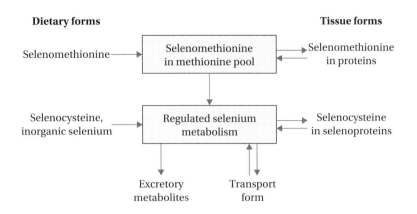

Dietary forms   **Tissue forms**

Fig. 11.4 Outline of selenium metabolism.

Source: Levander, O.A., and Burk, R.F. (1996) Selenium. In: Ziegler, E.E. and Filer, L.J. (eds). *Present knowledge of nutrition*, 7th edn. Washington, DC, ILSI Press, pp. 320–8.

blood selenium concentrations of residents of countries with differing soil selenium levels (Fig. 11.5). The form administered also influences retention of selenium, with selenomethionine more effective in raising blood selenium levels than sodium selenite or selenate. Both inorganic and organic forms of selenium are transformed to selenide. Selenide (the –2 oxidation state) is transformed to selenocysteine on tRNA and the selenocysteinyl residue is incorporated into the active site of selenoproteins by the UGA codon. The non-specific incorporation of selenomethionine into protein contributes to tissue selenium, which is not immediately available for synthesis of selenoproteins, until it is catabolized. Selenoprotein expression is regulated by selenium supply and there is a hierarchy of expression of individual selenoproteins and of retention of selenium in different organs and tissues.

Excretion Urine is the principal route of selenium excretion, followed by faeces, in which it is mainly unabsorbed selenium. Homeostasis of selenium is achieved by regulation of its excretion. Daily urinary excretion is closely associated with plasma selenium

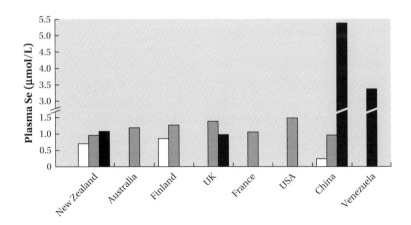

Fig. 11.5 Blood selenium values (µmol/L). New Zealand, pre-1990 (□), 1995–99 (▨), post-2000 (■); Australia, (▨); Finland, pre-1984 (□), post-1984 (▨); UK, pre-1990 (▨), post-1990 (■); France, (▨); USA, (▨); China, low Se (□), medium Se (▨), high Se (■); Venezuela, (■).

and dietary intake and accounts for approximately 50–60% of the total amount excreted. Measurement of plasma renal clearance of selenium shows that New Zealanders appear to have adapted to their low selenium intake by excreting selenium in the urine more sparingly.

Surplus selenium is methylated to methylated selenium metabolites from the common intermediate selenide. 1 β-Methyl seleno-*N*-acetyl-D-galactosamine (selenosugar) is the major urinary metabolite. Trimethylselenonium ion is excreted in response to very high intakes of selenium and may be used as a biological marker for excessive doses.

11.4.3 Deficiency

Interaction between selenium and vitamin E is observed in the aetiology of many deficiency diseases in animals and pure selenium deficiency is, in fact, rare. Thus, selenium deficiency may only occur when low selenium status is linked with an additional stress such as chemical exposure or increased oxidant stress due to vitamin E deficiency. Although residents in some low-selenium areas have low levels of blood selenium and of GPx activity and SEPP, there is little evidence that these are suboptimal or have resulted in changes in other oxidative defence mechanisms. Moreover, people have not shown noticeably improved health when GPx activity is saturated by selenium supplementation. Whether any of the newer functions of selenium are suboptimal in persons with low selenium status is being investigated.

Selenium-responsive diseases in humans: *Keshan disease* An endemic cardiomyopathy occurring in low-selenium areas of China, was reported in 1979 to be responsive to supplementation with sodium selenite. The disease is associated with low selenium intake and low blood and hair levels, and affects mainly children and women of childbearing age. Because some features of Keshan disease (e.g. seasonal variation) cannot be explained solely on the basis of very low selenium status, it is thought likely that a virus was able to cause heart damage in the presence of selenium deficiency, as

has been shown with selenium-deficient mice (Ge and Yang, 1993).

Kashin-Beck disease An endemic osteoarthritis of ankles, knees, wrists, and elbows that occurs during pre-adolescent or adolescent years found in rural areas of Tibet, China, and Siberia has also been associated with severe selenium deficiency, although other factors such as iodine deficiency or presence of mycotoxins on barley may be equally important (Ge and Yang, 1993; Moreno-Reyes *et al.*, 2003).

Selenium deficiency in combination with inadequate iodine status contributes to the pathogenesis of myxodematous cretinism.

Selenium deficiency has been associated with long-term intravenous nutrition, because of previously low levels of selenium in the fluids. Clinical symptoms of cardiomyopathy, muscle pain, and muscular weakness are responsive to selenium supplementation, but are not seen in all patients with extremely low selenium status, such as children on very low selenium synthetic diets for inborn errors of metabolism, indicating that there may be other interacting factors.

11.4.4 Selenium and human health

Selenium and immune function Selenium is essential for optimal function of many aspects of the immune system, influencing both the innate and the acquired immune system, and has a role to play in the defence system of animals against bacteria and other infections, including viral infection. The mechanisms for the involvement of selenium in the immune system are likely to be related to its antioxidant function through the antioxidant selenoproteins GPx, thioredoxin reductases, or SEPP.

Studies of host response to myocarditic and non-myocarditic strains of coxsackievirus B3 in mice showed that selenium deficiency and vitamin E deficiency potentiated cardiotoxicity of myocarditic strains, but in addition, the non-myocarditic strain caused heart lesions in selenium-deficient mice, apparently as a result of a change in the viral genome. This observation is relevant to the aetiology of Keshan disease, which has been attributed in part to an endemic coxsackivirus. Mutational changes as a result of selenium deficiency also enhance the intensity of infection of another RNA virus, influenza A, and the protozoan parasite *Trypanosoma cruzi*.

Selenium and cancer Several lines of scientific enquiry suggest an association of cancer with low levels of selenium in the diet. Evidence for the role of selenium as an anticarcinogenic agent comes from *in vitro* and animal studies that suggest that selenium is protective against tumorigenesis at high levels of intake. Evidence from prospective studies linking low selenium status with increased incidence of cancer at various cancer sites has been conflicting, but the strongest evidence is available for prostate and breast cancer. There have been several intervention trials in humans of the effect of selenium, alone or with other nutrients, on the incidence of cancer or concentrations of biomarkers. Again, the results of these trials are conflicting. The strongest evidence comes from The Nutritional Prevention of Cancer Trial that examined the efficacy of high selenium yeast in preventing skin cancer. There was no effect of selenium on skin cancer, but there was a statistically significant reduction in total cancer (50%) and cancer of the prostate, lung, and colorectum. The effects were strongest in subjects with the lowest selenium status. On the other hand, the more recent Selenium and Vitamin E Cancer Prevention Trial (SELECT) was discontinued early because of a lack of beneficial effect on prostate cancer incidence and an increase in the incidence of diabetes in the selenium group and prostate cancer in the vitamin E group.

The level of selenium intake required for the protective effect appears to be higher than that required to maximize selenoproteins, suggesting that other processes, such as the involvement of anticarcinogenic methylated selenium metabolites such as Se-methyl selenocysteine, might be involved. However, the association of selenium with a reduction in DNA damage and oxidative stress and recent evidence of an effect of selenoprotein polymorphisms on cancer risk suggest that selenoproteins are also involved.

Selenium and cardiovascular disease Lack of dietary selenium has also been implicated in the aetiology of cardiovascular disease, but the evidence is less convincing than for cancer. A meta-analysis of 25 observational studies found a moderate inverse relationship between plasma selenium and coronary heart disease. However, the few clinical trials have found no evidence of selenium supplementation on cardiovascular protection in selenium-replete populations, and this was confirmed in the SELECT trial. In addition, higher selenium status has been shown to be associated with increased total and low-density lipoprotein cholesterol, higher fasting plasma glucose and glycosylated haemoglobin levels, and higher prevalence of diabetes and hypertension. On the other hand, a low level of erythrocyte GPx1 has been shown to be a predictor of cardiovascular events in patients with coronary artery disease. Glutathione peroxidases protect against processes relevant to atherosclerosis, in particular in individuals, such as smokers, at risk from increased oxidant stress. These processes include the inhibition of low-density lipoprotein oxidation.

These confusing observations on the effects of selenium on chronic disease clearly indicate that a U-curve represents the effects of selenium status. Because of the adverse effects of higher-than-recommended selenium intakes—diabetes, hypertension, skin cancer, and hypercholesterolaemia—we should be cautious about recommending selenium supplementation for chronic disease prevention.

11.4.5 Assessment of selenium status

Blood selenium concentration is a useful measure of selenium status and intake, but other tissues are often assessed as well. Plasma or serum selenium reflects short-term status and red cell selenium reflects longer-term status. Toenail selenium is also used, as toenail concentrations provide a stable assessment of longer-term dietary intake, but selenium-containing shampoos restrict the use of hair. Urinary excretion can also be used to assess selenium status, and total dietary intake is estimated as twice the daily urinary excretion.

The close relationship between plasma GPx3 or red cell GPx1 activity and selenium concentrations (Fig. 11.6) is useful for assessment in people with relatively low status, but not once the saturating activity of the enzyme is reached at blood selenium concentrations above 80 µg/L (1.00 µmol/L). SEPP, which accounts for more than 50% of selenium in blood, has been shown to be a reliable marker of selenium status in populations with low-to-moderate selenium status, but like GPx, not with higher selenium status. The conclusions drawn from measurement of one selenoprotein may not apply to all biological functions of selenium because of differences in responses of tissues and these proteins to deficient, adequate, or high levels of selenium.

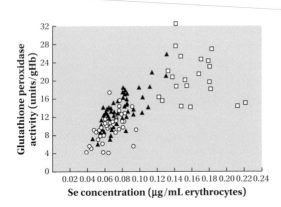

Fig. 11.6 Relationship between selenium concentration of erythrocytes (µg/mL erythrocytes) and glutathione peroxidase (GPx) activity for Otago patients (○), Otago blood donors (▲), and overseas subjects (□) (to convert µg selenium/mL to µmol/L, multiply by 12.66).

Source: Rea, H.M., Thomson, C.D., Campbell, D.R., and Robinson, M.F. (1979) Relation between erythrocyte selenium concentrations and glutathione peroxidase (EC 1.11.1.9.) activities in New Zealand residents and visitors to New Zealand. *Br J Nutr*, **42**, 201–8.

11.4.6 Dietary intake

Food is the major source of selenium, with drinking water contributing little. Dietary intake varies with the geographic source of foods and eating habits of the people. Plant food concentrations reflect selenium content of soils and availability

Table 11.4 Daily dietary intakes and whole blood values of selenium

Country	Selenium intake (µg/day)	Plasma or serum selenium[a] (µmol/L)
China		
Keshan disease area	7–11	0.20–0.30
Non-Keshan disease area	40–120	0.49–1.41
Seleniferous area	750–4990	4.52–6.25
New Zealand		
Before 1990	28–32	0.56–0.87
After 1990	30–60	0.89–1.17
Finland		
Before 1984	25	0.70–1.05
After 1984	67–110	0.92–1.60
Great Britain		
Before 1990	60	1.25–1.52
After 1990	29–39	0.78–1.00
USA	60–220	1.11–1.88
Venezuela	200–350	2.73–3.99

[a]Mean values.

Source: Adapted from Thomson, C.D. (2004) Selenium and iodine intakes and status in New Zealand and Australia. *Br J Nutr*, **91**, 661–72; Combs, G.F. Jr (2001) Selenium in global food systems. *Br J Nutr*, **85**, 517–47.

for uptake, as plants generally do not require selenium for growth; the selenium content of cereals and grains grown in soils poor or rich in selenium may vary 100-fold. However, some plants, such as garlic, mushrooms, and broccoli, have developed the ability to accumulate selenium from the soil and therefore may contain high levels of selenium. Brazil nuts are also exceptionally good sources of selenium, but the content varies greatly, depending on where they are grown. Animal foods vary less because animals have an absolute requirement for selenium, which they must get through feed or supplements. Fish and organ meats are the richest sources, followed by muscle meats, cereals and grains, and dairy products, with fruits and vegetables mostly poor sources. Average daily dietary intakes vary considerably depending on the soil selenium levels (Table 11.4) ranging from about 10 µg selenium in low-soil-selenium areas of China where Keshan disease is endemic, to median intakes in New Zealand of 56 and 39 µg/day for males and females, respectively, and up to over 200 µg or more in seleniferous areas in Venezuela and parts of USA. In 1985, selenium was added to fertilizers in Finland as a way of increasing selenium intake throughout the population, and the daily intake rose from 40 µg to close to 100 µg/day, resulting in a significant increase in serum selenium in healthy individuals of 0.85 µmol/L in 1985 to 1.52 µmol/L in 1989–91. In New Zealand, intakes have increased as a result of increases in selenium concentrations in animal foods due to supplementation of commercial fertilizers and animal feeds and greater consumption of imported foods.

The reason for the reduction in selenium intake in Great Britain is the change from importation of wheat from North America to European wheat.

11.4.7 Requirements and recommended dietary intakes

The minimum requirement to prevent selenium deficiency (20 µg) is based on comparison of intakes in endemic and non-endemic Keshan disease areas of China. However, most countries base their recommended dietary intakes of selenium on estimates of intakes at which saturation of plasma GPx activity occurs, obtained from studies in China and New Zealand. Recommended intakes of the USA and Canada, the UK, and European countries, are summarized in Table 37.2.

Whether optimal health depends upon saturation of GPx activity has yet to be resolved. Recommended dietary intakes of the USA/Canada and most countries are based on desirability of full activity of GPx, whereas a WHO group concluded that only two-thirds of the maximal activity was needed. Several of the other newly discovered selenoproteins might be used as endpoints for determining selenium requirements. However, maximal activity of these proteins occurs at selenium intakes lower than those needed for maximal GPx activity.

Intakes of selenium that may reduce risk of the chronic diseases cancer and CHD are likely to be higher than those for maintenance of maximal selenoprotein levels.

11.4.8 Toxicity

The margin between an adequate and a toxic intake of selenium is quite narrow. Over-exposure or selenosis may occur from consuming high-selenium foods grown in seleniferous areas in Venezuela, Colombia, northern USA, and Enshi county in China. The most common sign of poisoning is loss of hair and nails, but the skin, nervous system, and teeth may also be involved. Garlic odour on the breath is an indication of excessive selenium exposure (from breathing out dimethylselenide). Sensitive biochemical techniques are lacking for selenium toxicity, which is at present diagnosed from hair loss and nail changes. Some effects of selenium toxicity are seen in individuals with dietary intakes as low as 900 µg, and the UIL has been set at 400 µg per day.

Further Reading

1. **Combs, G.F. Jr.** (2001) Selenium in global food systems. *Br J Nutr*, **85**, 517–47.
2. **Ge, K. and Yang, G.** (1993) The epidemiology of selenium deficiency in the etiological study of endemic diseases in China. *Am J Clin Nutr*, **57**, 259S–63S.
3. **Levander, O.A. and Burk, R.F.** (1996) Selenium. In: Ziegler, E.E., and Filer, L.J. (eds). *Present Knowledge of Nutrition*, 7th edn. Washington, DC, ILSI Press, pp. 320–8.
4. **Moreno-Reyes, R., Mattieu, F., Boelaert, M., *et al.** (2003) Selenium and Iodiine supplementation of rural Tibetan children affected by Kashan-Beck osteoartopathy. *Am J Clin Nutr*, **78**, 137–44.
5. **Papp, L.V., Lu, J., Holmgren, A., and Khana, K.K.** (2007) From selenium to selenoproteins: Synthesis, identity, and their role in human health. *Antioxid Redox Signal*, **9**, 775–806.
6. **Rayman, M.P.** (2005) Selenium in cancer prevention: A review of the evidence and mechanism of action. *Proc Nutr Soc*, **64**, 527–54.
7. **Rayman, M.P.** (2009). Selenoproteins and human health: Insights from epidemiological data. *Biochem Biophys Acta*, **1790**, 1533–40.
8. **Rea, H.M., Thomson, C.D., Campbell, D.R., and Robinson, M.F.** (1979) Relation between erythrocyte selenium concentrations and glutathione peroxidase (EC 1.11.1.9.) activities in New Zealand residents and visitors to New Zealand. *Br J Nutr*, **42**, 201–8.
9. **Thomson, C.D.** (2004) Assessment of requirements for selenium and adequacy of selenium status: A review. *Eur J Clin Nutr*, **58**, 391–402.
10. **Thomson, C.D.** (2004) Selenium and iodine intakes and status in New Zealand and Australia. *Br J Nutr*, **91**, 661–72.

11.5 Fluoride
Stewart Truswell

The fluoride iron (F) is generally regarded as a beneficial nutrient at low dosage because intakes of 1–4 mg/day reduce the prevalence of dental caries (decay). Nutritional authorities have until recently hesitated to classify fluoride as an essential nutrient. The dental benefit is not lifesaving. However, many millions of people in the USA, Australia and New Zealand, and parts of other countries—some 400 million worldwide—have fluoride added to their drinking water at the water works, at the controlled level of 1 mg/L (1 ppm). As well as this, most toothpastes contain added fluoride, and dentists periodically paint children's teeth with fluoride solution as a preventive measure against tooth decay.

In 1997, the US Institute of Medicine, in collaboration with Canada, decided to set a recommended intake for fluoride; Australia and New Zealand followed suit in 2005; and in Germany, Austria, and Switzerland 'guiding values' for fluoride have been published in 2001 and 2002.

Natural water supplies commonly range from 0.1 to 5 ppm in fluoride content and in some places (e.g. bore holes) the fluoride concentration is much higher. From many studies of US children, Dean *et al.* (1942) showed an inverse relation between the natural fluoride concentration of communal water supplies in the range of 0–2 ppm (μg/g) fluoride and the prevalence of dental caries (Fig. 11.7). Earlier, a direct association had been found between the fluoride content of water supplies (0–6 ppm) and the occurrence of enamel fluorosis (or mottled enamel), from barely noticeable white flecks affecting a small percentage of the enamel to brown-stained or pitted enamel in the most severe cases (Fig. 11.8). This is a cosmetic effect and milder forms are not readily apparent to the affected individual or casual observer. Figs. 11.7 and 11.8 show

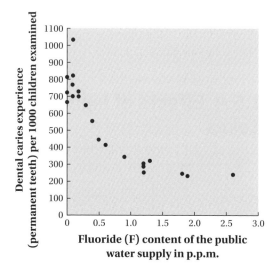

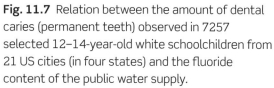

Fig. 11.7 Relation between the amount of dental caries (permanent teeth) observed in 7257 selected 12–14-year-old white schoolchildren from 21 US cities (in four states) and the fluoride content of the public water supply.

Source: Dean, H.T., Arnold, F.A., and Elvove, E. (1942) Domestic water and dental caries. V. Additional studies: experience in 4,425 white children, aged 12 to 14 years, of 13 cities in 4 states. *Pub Health Rep*, **57**, 1155–79.

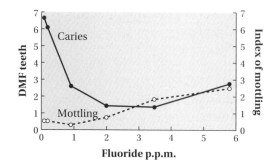

Fig. 11.8 Caries and enamel mottling according to fluoride level in drinking water for UK children aged 12–14 years. DMF, decayed, missing, and filled teeth.

Source: Forrest, J.R. (1956) Caries incidence and enamel defects in areas with different levels of fluoride in the drinking water. *Br Dental J*, **100**, 195–200.

little increase in benefit with water containing fluoride above 1 ppm, while mottling only became apparent above 2 ppm. This concentration therefore offered maximal protection against dental caries with minimal risk of dental fluorosis. Moreover, in communities where the natural water supplies were unusually low in fluoride, less than 0.3 ppm, addition of fluoride or fluoridation of the water supply to achieve 1 ppm has been followed by a remarkable decline in prevalence of dental decay in the children, of up to 60%. Indeed, the impact of fluoridation of water supplies and more recently of toothpastes containing fluoride has been a cost-effective triumph of public health.

11.5.1 Function

Fluoride acts to reduce dental caries in two ways:

1 When ingested by young children while the permanent (second set of) teeth are forming inside the jaw, before they erupt, the blood-borne fluoride combines in the calcium phosphate hydroxyapatite crystals of the enamel, making it more resistant to acid erosion. Erosion of dental enamel by acid, produced by mouth bacteria metabolizing sugars, is the cause of caries. For this fluoride action, young children should either be drinking water with adequate natural or added fluoride or be given fluoride tablets before their permanent teeth erupt.

2 Fluoride also has a post-eruptive action. In solution in the saliva or in contact with the teeth via toothpaste, it inhibits bacterial enzymes that produce acid in plaques on the teeth and it increases remineralization of incipient enamel lesions. This means that fluoride continues to have cariostatic action in adult life.

11.5.2 Metabolism of fluoride

The fluoride ion occurs in water, and both ionic and non-ionic or bound forms occur in food and beverages. Ionic fluoride is rapidly and almost completely absorbed, whereas organic or protein-bound forms are less well absorbed (about 75%), and inorganic bone fluoride as in bone meal even less (<50%). There is a transitory rise in plasma fluoride following fluoride ingestion, after which it returns to about 0.1 ppm. Some fluoride is taken up by the bones and retained for a long time, but most is rapidly excreted in the urine, with small amounts in sweat and faeces. The urinary output gives a good indication of the daily fluoride intake, whereas the bone fluoride content reflects the long-term intake. There is minimal transfer of fluoride across the placenta. Fluoride content of breast milk is little affected by small supplements of fluoride, such as 1.5 mg/day.

11.5.3 Sources of fluoride

Dietary sources Beverages are the principal sources of fluoride but their contribution depends on the fluoride concentration of the water supply. Tea leaves, and hence tea infusions, are also major sources (about 1–2 ppm), depending on the water fluoride content and strength of the infusion. Thus, beverages can give as little as 0.2 mg/day for non-tea drinkers drinking unfluoridated or low fluoride water, and up to 2–4 mg/day or even more for frequent drinkers of strong tea prepared with fluoridated water.

Bottled water The fluoride content of bottled water (and carbonated beverages) depends on that of its source, usually a natural spring, and it may well be absent. If people drink most of their day's water from bottles, they are likely to by-pass the dental benefit of tap water.

Foods contain traces of fluoride, contributing for an adult about 0.5 mg/day; plant foods (1 ppm) generally contain more fluoride than animal foods (0.1 ppm), apart from marine fish (1–3 ppm). The fluoride content of processed food comes mainly from the fluoride content of the water used in processing or in the home. The fluoride content of infant formulas reflects the processing of the powdered formula and also the water used to make it up. Milk formulas usually contain more fluoride than human milk.

Non-dietary sources These include fluoride tablets or drops given mainly to children drinking low-fluoride water during the formation and maturation of teeth, as well as fluoride toothpastes, and fluoride solutions painted on teeth by dentists.

11.5.4 Effects of high intakes

The cosmetic effect of enamel fluorosis occurs when too much is ingested while teeth are forming *during the first 8 years of life*; this can happen from too liberal use of fluoride tablets and/or fluoride toothpastes that can contain as much as 1000 ppm fluoride. Young children are at risk if they regularly swallow large amounts, but toothpastes of lower fluoride content (400 ppm) are now available for them.

The skeleton is affected by chronic high levels of fluoride intake as from long-term drinking water with 20 ppm fluoride. This may cause dense bones and joint abnormalities; this skeletal fluorosis occurs in parts of India, China, and South Africa.

The acute lethal dose of sodium fluoride is 5 g (i.e. 2300 mg). It would be impossible for water containing 1 mg/L to cause this.

Large doses of fluoride have been used in the treatment of osteoporosis, but the bone quality tends to be poor, fractures may increase, and there are doubts about the safety of such treatment.

11.5.5 Fluoride and dental health

The first public water supply to be fluoridated started in Grand Rapids, Michigan in 1945. Hastings in 1954 was first in New Zealand, Canberra and Hobart in Australia 1964. The present world map shows that only in USA, Australia, Colombia, Ireland, Israel, Malaysia, and New Zealand are 80–100% of the population supplied with fluoridated drinking water. Global coverage is estimated at some 380 million. Rates of DMFT (decayed, missing, filled teeth) indicating dental caries fell dramatically in children with water fluoridation.

Yet in other developed countries, in Europe and elsewhere, with only some or no water fluoridated

(10% in the UK), caries rates are also much lower than in earlier generations. The explanation is thought to be fluoride in toothpastes, universal school dental services, and use of topical fluoride by dentists, in some cases fluoride tablets, even fluoridated salt in France and Germany.

While dental caries is controlled in affluent communities it is increasing in poor people in the rest of the world (Bagramian *et al.*, 2009), who cannot afford toothpaste, let alone dentists. A 2006 conference of dental experts from 30 countries 'expressed their deep concern about growing disparities in dental health and the lack of progress in tackling the worldwide burden of tooth decay, particularly in disadvantaged populations'. They called for action to promote dental health by using fluoride.

Water fluoridation has the great advantage of reaching all members of the community, particularly those with poor dental hygiene and no access to dentists. The US Centers for Disease Control and Prevention listed water fluoridation as one of the 10 great public health achievements of the twentieth century. It is endorsed by WHO, the European Academy of Paediatric Dentistry, national dental associations of USA, Canada, Australia, and other countries. When it is proposed that an area's water be fluoridated, a majority of the public usually agree, but people who oppose (similar to those against immunization) tend to be intense. So the decision should ideally be made by the Ministry of Health, not the local Council. Where water is supplied by a private company, objection is because of the (modest) cost to the company—which is very much less than the cost of dental caries to the community.

11.5.6 Recommended dietary intake

Most national and international health organizations recommend a water supply in the range 0.7–1.0 ppm fluoride for temperate climates, using the average local maximum temperature as a predictor of water intake; the lower concentrations are for warmer climates, where more beverages are drunk. The US Institute of Medicine (1997) suggests 'adequate intakes' of fluoride are between 0.5 and 1.0 mg/day for young children from 6 months to 8 years of age, and in adults 4 mg/day in men and 3 mg/day in women. The same amounts are recommended for Australia and New Zealand.

11.5.7 Risks of water fluoridation?

It is widely agreed that fluoridation of drinking water to a level of 1 ppm has no known adverse health effects. There is no good evidence that fluoridated water is associated with allergic reactions or hypersensitivity, sudden infant death syndrome, stomach or intestinal problems, birth defects, Down syndrome, or genetic mutations. No association of cancer with exposure to fluoridated water has been found (Doll and Kinlen, 1977; Smith, 1980).

11.6 Other trace elements
Stewart Truswell

11.6.1 Chromium

Chromium (Cr) has been found in some situations to potentiate the action of insulin. No mammalian enzyme is known that requires chromium. Cr is widely distributed in trace amounts in the food supply. It is poorly absorbed. A small number of cases on long-term total parenteral nutrition developed symptoms—weight loss and high blood glucose that responded to small amounts of chromium salt. Chromium at 10–15 µg/day is now routinely included in the fluids for long-term parenteral nutrition. The Institute of Medicine set the adequate intake (AI) at 25 µg/day for women and 35 µg/day for men.

11.6.2 Manganese

Manganese (Mn) is involved in the formation of bone and in the function of several enzymes, particularly superoxide dismutase and arginase. Mn deficiency can be demonstrated in animals and is a practical problem in the poultry and pig industries. However, the few reports that describe human deficiency features have shortcomings. Tea is a good dietary source. One child on long-term total parenteral nutrition grew poorly and had bone demineralization corrected by manganese supplementation. Manganese at 60–100 µg/day is included in fluids for total parenteral nutrition. The Institute of Medicine set the AI at 5 mg/day for women and 5.5 mg /day for men.

11.6.3 Molybdenum

Molybdenum (Mo) is essential for growing vegetables. In animals, including humans, it is a cofactor (bound to protein) for three enzymes: sulphite oxidase, xanthine oxidase, and aldehyde oxidase. The main case for essentiality of molybdenum is a severe genetic defect that prevents synthesis of sulphite oxidase, but this cannot be corrected by diet. A single case with biochemical features of Mo deficiency occurred in a patient on long-term total parenteral nutrition, corrected with ammonium molybdate. The best dietary source is legumes. Molybdenum is well absorbed. The Institute of Medicine set the RDI at 45 µg/day for men and women.

Further Reading

1. **Bagramian, R.A., Garcia-Godoy, F., and Volpe, A.R.** (2009) The global increase in dental caries. A pending public health crisis. *Am J Dent*, **22**, 3–8.
2. **British Fluoridation Society** (2004) *One in a million: The facts about fluoridation*, 2nd edn. Liverpool, UK, British Fluoridation Society.
3. **Dean, H.T., Arnold, F.A., and Elvove, E.** (1942) Domestic water and dental caries. V. Additional studies: Experience in 4,425 white children, aged 12 to 14 years, of 13 cities in 4 states. *Pub Health Rep*, **57**, 1155–79.
4. **Doll, R. and Kinlen, L.** (1977) Fluoridation of water and cancer mortality in the USA. *Lancet*, **1**, 1300–2.
5. **Forrest, J.R.** (1956) Caries incidence and enamel defects in areas with different levels of fluoride in the drinking water. *Br Dental J*, **100**, 195–200.
6. **Institute of Medicine** (1997) *Dietary reference intakes for calcium, phosphorus, magnesium, vitamin D and fluoride*. Washington, DC, National Academy Press.
7. **McDonagh, M.S., Whiting, P.F., and Wilson, P.M.** (2000) Systematic review of water fluoridation. *BMJ*, **321**, 855–9.
8. **Royal College of Physicians** (1976) *Fluoride, teeth and health*. London, Pitman Medical.
9. **Smith, A.H.** (1980) An examination of the relationship between fluoridation of water and cancer mortality in 20 large US cities. *NZ Med J*, **91**, 413–16.

Useful Websites

 To see topical and scientifically robust updates on nutrition associated with this textbook and web links to many of the journals in the Further Reading sections, please see the dedicated Online Resource Centre at **http://www.oxfordtextbooks.co.uk/orc/mann4e/**

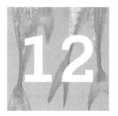

Vitamin A and carotenoids

David I. Thurnham

12.1 History

Vitamin A deficiency has a long history, for it was known to the ancient Egyptians and to Hippocrates. Liver was prescribed for night blindness. More recently, Snell demonstrated in 1880 that cod liver oil was effective in curing not only night blindness but also Bitôt's spots. Poor growth was a common feature of young rats fed on diets of pure protein, starch, sugar, lard, and salts, and McCollum and Davis (1912) reported there was an essential fat-soluble factor in butter, egg yolk, and cod liver oil that would overcome this growth inhibition. Osborn and Mendel reported similar results but it was McCollum and Davis who gave the name 'fat-soluble factor A' to the component in these foods to distinguish it from 'water-soluble factor B' they found in whey, yeast, and rice polishings. Rosenheim and Drummond reported in 1920 that the vitamin A activity in plant foods was related to their content of carotene, a pigment isolated from carrots 100 years earlier. The ultimate confirmation that carotene is the source of plant vitamin A activity came from Thomas Moore in Cambridge in 1957, whose monograph on vitamin A is a classic.

12.2 Units, terminology, nomenclature, and chemical structures

Vitamin A is the generic term used to include retinol and related structures with 20 carbon atoms and the pro-vitamin A carotenoids with 40 carbon atoms. The term 'retinoids' is used for the group of naturally occurring compounds that have a structure similar to retinol as well as others that have been synthesized in the search for new therapeutic compounds.

Pre-formed vitamin A structures include all-*trans* retinol (vitamin A$_1$, alcohol form), all-*trans* retinal (aldehyde form), and 3-dehydroretinol (vitamin A$_2$) (Fig. 12.1). Vitamin A$_2$ is found in freshwater fish. In addition, there are various oxidized forms of retinol with vitamin A activity (e.g. all-*trans* retinoic acid and 9-*cis* retinoic acid, which are important in the genetic control of metabolic functions. The basic unit of activity of vitamin A is the retinol equivalent (RE) by which 1 µg RE is the same as 3.33 IU or 3.5 nmol of retinol. In foods and pharmaceutical preparations, vitamin A$_1$ occurs mainly as vitamin A palmitate, although other esters can also occur. To overcome the need to use different weights if

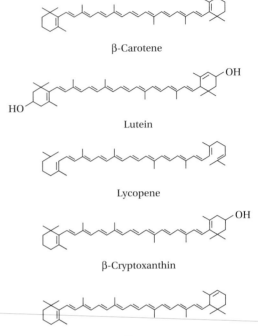

β-Carotene

Lutein

Lycopene

β-Cryptoxanthin

α-Carotene

Fig. 12.2 Carotenoids found commonly in human blood.

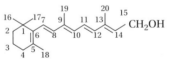

All-*trans* retinol (vitamin A vitamin A$_1$)

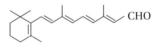

All-*trans* retinal

3-Dehydroretinol (vitamin A$_2$)

All-*trans* retinoic acid

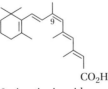

9-*cis* retinoic acid

Fig. 12.1 Structures of the common retinoids.

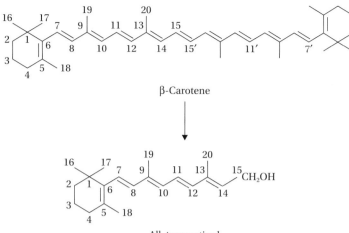

β-Carotene

All-*trans* retinol

Fig. 12.3 β-carotene conversion to retinol.

different esters are present, vitamin A activity is usually expressed as international units (IU).

The common carotenoids found in the blood are shown in Fig. 12.2. Of these only α-carotene, β-carotene, and β-cryptoxanthin are pro-vitamin A carotenoids as they contain at least one β-ionone structure with no functional groups attached. The enzyme required to produce vitamin A_1 from pro-vitamin A carotenes is β-carotene 15,15'-dioxygenase (EC 1.13.11.21) that is predominantly found in the small intestine and the liver. The enzyme is believed to split carotene down the middle of the molecule (Fig. 12.3). β-carotene has two β-ionone structures at each end of the molecule so theoretically should form two molecules of vitamin A_1, whereas all other carotenes have only one β-ionone structure and therefore can only form one molecule of vitamin A_1.

Units of β-carotene are determined by their bio-equivalence to vitamin A_1. Thus on the basis of the recommendations of WHO/FAO (FAO/WHO, 1967), 1 μg RE is equivalent to 1 μg retinol, 6 μg of β-carotene, or 12 μg of carotenoids containing only one β-ionone ring. More recently, the Institute of Medicine (2000) revised the equivalencies of β-carotene and other pro-vitamin A carotenoids to 12 and 24 μg, respectively. IU are not used to quantify carotenes in current literature but older literature does sometimes use them (when 1 μg β-carotene equals 1.67 IU or 1 μg retinol equals 10 IU β-carotene).

12.3 Functions of retinol: physiology, biochemistry, and molecular biology

Retinoic acid supports many of the important functions of vitamin A—cellular differentiation, embryogenesis, synthesis of glycoproteins, immunity, and growth—but it cannot be reduced back to retinol in the body, therefore an animal that is maintained only on retinoic acid will be blind and also fails to reproduce successfully. Only retinol can fully support vision and reproduction.

12.3.1 Vision

Both retinol and retinoic acid are needed to maintain a healthy eye. Retinol is needed for the visual process and one of the earliest signs of vitamin A deficiency is a failure to see in dim light known as night blindness. Impairment of the external surface of the eye in the form of xerosis or Bitôt spots are also early signs of vitamin A deficiency, but are more likely to be due to inadequacy of retinoic acid. The latter is required to maintain the surface epithelium of the eye, and in vitamin A deficiency, tear production is impaired, debris accumulates, and the eye is more vulnerable to bacterial attachment and disease.

The visual process in the retina is dependent on the ability to synthesize 11-*cis* retinal and its behaviour on exposure to light. There are two types of light receptor cell in the retina of the human eye, the rods and the cones. The rods are responsible for seeing at low light intensities, whereas the cones are used for light of higher intensities and colour vision. The chromophore (11-*cis* retinal) is the same in both, but the proteins attached to it are different. In the rods the chromophore is attached to rhodopsin (a guanosine triphosphate (GTP)-binding protein, or G-proteins) while in the cones, there is one of three very similar proteins known as iodopsins. Rhodopsin contains the protein opsin, ethanolamine-containing phospholipid, and the chromophore 11-*cis* retinal linked to interphotoreceptor-binding protein. The basic mechanism of light excitation is common to both systems but has been studied in far more detail in the rods as there are about 100 million rods compared with 3 million cones in the human eye.

The retina of the mammalian eye comprises ten layers and the photoreceptors form the outermost of these, underneath the retinal pigment epithelium. This means that before the process of phototransduction can begin, light has to pass through all nine layers. The chromophore receptors are linked to G-proteins and the latter regulate specific plasma membrane enzymes or, in the case of rhodopsin, ion channels in response to receptor binding. Before light excitation, the chromophore locks the receptor protein opsin by a Schiff-base linkage in its inactive form.

The primary event in visual excitation is the photoisomerization of the 11-*cis* isomer of retinal to its all-*trans* form. The action of a photon of light is converted into the energy of atomic motion and within a few picoseconds a series of intermediates of rhodopsin are formed. The activated rhodopsin is converted through prelumirhodopsin to metarhodopsin and this interacts with transducin (a G-protein),

which ultimately leads to the activation that cleaves cyclic guanosine monophosphate (c-GMP) to guanosine monophosphate (GMP). The changes in c-GMP and GMP lead to the closure of the sodium channel of the rod's outer membrane. Membrane hyperpolarization is then transmitted as an electrical signal to the optic nerve.

The action of light on rhodopsin is to alter its colour from magenta through orange to yellow and ultimately white 'bleached'. In this form it is opsin and unattached to all-*trans* retinal, though the latter is still bound to interstitial retinoid binding protein. The regeneration of 11-*cis* retinal takes place in the retinal pigment epithelium and its re-attachment to opsin generates rhodopsin to commence the cycle again.

12.3.2 Reproduction

Vitamin A deficiency results in infertility in males, while in females there are low rates of conception and high rates of stillbirths. Both retinol and retinoic acid are needed for successful reproduction but the precise roles of the compounds are still not known for certain. β-carotene may also function in reproduction, as it is deposited in substantial amounts in the corpus luteum of the ovaries.

12.3.3 Other functions

Almost all the other functions of vitamin A are under genetic control and are mediated by retinoic acid derivatives. Retinoic acid binds to nuclear receptors and these bind to response elements on specific genes to increase or decrease the specific level of expression of the gene. There are nuclear retinoic acid receptors (RAR) and retinoid X receptors (RXR) and each family has three major subtypes, α, β, and γ. The subtypes are presumed to have different functions because their distribution in cells is different. The nuclear retinoid receptors generally act as hetero-dimers, of which the most common is RAR–RXR. To be active, RAR must bind to retinoic acid (either 9-*cis* or all-*trans*), whereas RXR need not. RXR can bind to 9-*cis* retinoic acid, a synthetic ligand, or it can also form heterodimers with nuclear receptors for triiodothyronine, 1,25-hydroxyvitamin D_3, and the peroxisome proliferator-activated receptor (PPAR) which is probably activated by an essential fatty acid metabolite. These other nuclear receptors are members of a superfamily of nuclear receptors that include the receptors for oestrogen, progesterone, cortisol, and testosterone. When activated, the dimeric nuclear receptors bind to 'response elements' in specific genes to change the level of expression of that gene. In this way vitamin A, through the actions of 9-*cis* and all-*trans* retinoic acid, is an important regulator of gene transcription influencing a great many functions in the body.

Cellular differentiation Cellular differentiation is the series of morphological changes that take place to produce mature epithelia. The outer skin is characterized by keratin-producing cells, whereas the gut is characterized by mucous-secreting tissue containing many goblet cells. Most of the functions of vitamin A in cell differentiation are regulated by retinoic acid. When vitamin A is lacking, keratin-producing cells replace mucous-secreting cells in the intestinal and respiratory tracts. The same process causes the xerosis and drying of the conjunctiva and cornea of the eye.

Embryogenesis Retinoic acid isomers play important roles in embryogenesis through their control of genes linked to development and growth (homeobox genes). Both deficiency and excess can have adverse effects. Implants containing all-*trans* retinoic acid placed in the anterior part of a developing chick limb bud mimic the activity of the naturally occurring zone of polarizing activity. Correct morphological development depends on the concentration of all-*trans* retinoic acid. Experimental evidence and tragedies from overexposure to synthetic retinoids highlight the particular importance of avoiding excess vitamin A during pregnancy.

Synthesis of glycoproteins and glycosaminoglycans (GAGs) Glycoproteins are polypeptides with short chains of carbohydrates. They are important components in mucus. Many glycoproteins on the surface of the cell are receptors for other glycoproteins (e.g. growth factors). GAGs are long, unbranched polysaccharide chains that provide a viscous extracellular matrix on the cell surface. They are important in connective tissue and can provide a passageway for cell migration or lubrication between joints. Retinoids have been shown to be involved in the synthesis of some of these compounds. Sulphate is an important component of several members of the GAG family, e.g. chondroitin sulphate, heparin. A key component in sulphate transfer reactions is adenosine 3'-phosphate-5'-phosphosulphate (PAPS), and all-*trans* retinoic acid has been shown to induce several sulphotransferase enzymes in cellular and animal experiments. Sulphate transfer and incorporation is essential in the synthesis of mucopolysaccharides, hence a lack of vitamin A may contribute to some or all of the features of vitamin A deficiency shown in Box 12.1.

Immunity and host defence Vitamin A is generally believed to be important for resistance to infections—hence the term 'anti-infective vitamin' was coined. Measles is a very serious infection in vitamin A-deficient children and there is a strong protective effect of supplemental vitamin A (Hussey and Klein, 1990). Defining the precise role of vitamin in immune mechanisms is still continuing.

BOX 12.1 Effects produced in vitamin A deficiency by impairment of mucopolysaccharide synthesis

- Reduced wettability of the eye surface
- Reduced tear production contributing to the xerosis (dry and rough) of the eye surface
- Reduced mucous production by mucous membranes with increased susceptibility to bacterial attachment and infection
- Reduced ability to taste through changes in the tastebuds
- Changes in the skin giving rise to follicular keratitis: seen more in adults than children
- Changes in the ground substance of bone, cartilage, and teeth, resulting in defective formation of these substances during growth

Mortality from infections is higher in communities where vitamin A deficiency is found and vitamin A intervention reduces mortality. The importance of mucous production to protect the respiratory tract and bowel from pathogens is well recognized but the mechanism by which the body generates systemic protection against epithelial pathogens is only recently becoming clearer.

Pathogens that infect mucosal surfaces trigger adaptive immune responses by initially interacting with antigen-presenting cells such as dendritic cells. Antigen-loaded dendritic cells interact with antigen-specific B and T-lymphocytes in subepithelial aggregates such as Peyers patches, resulting in proliferation and differentiation of naive T cells into memory/effector T cell subsets, potentially including T helper (Th) 1, 2, and 17 cells. Dendritic cells in the intestine constitutively produce retinoic acid which is not produced by dendritic cells at other sites (Benson *et al.*, 2007). Retinoic acid potentially steers the development of Th cells in the direction of Th2 and Treg subsets (Stephensen *et al.*, 2002). However, the effector functions of mucosal adaptive immunity will only be effective if the IgA-secreting plasma cells, memory B cells, and memory T cells return to the lamina propria underlying the mucosal epithelium in the intestine. Evidence suggests that retinoic acid produced by dendritic cells at the time of antigen presentation promotes the development of specific mucosal cell adhesion molecules, so although lymph from the intestine drains into the vascular system, vascular lymphocytes with the specific adhesion molecules can return 'home' as part of the protective response to pathogens encountered in the intestine (Mora *et al.*, 2008).

Growth Vitamin A influences bone growth by modulating the growth of bones through remodelling. The vitamin is necessary for the normal cycle of growth, maturation, and degeneration of cells in the epiphyseal cartridge. However, in only one study did pre-school children who received extra vitamin A in the condiment monosodium glutamate show higher rates of growth by comparison with children from control villages. In general, observations on the effect of vitamin A supplements on early child growth in areas where vitamin A deficiency is a risk are inconsistent, probably because growth is dependent on many nutrients and just replacing vitamin A in a child's diet may do no more than allow more vitamin A storage, until such time as the correct balance of nutrients in the diet is restored.

Haemopoiesis Vitamin A deficiency in humans and in experimental animals has been consistently associated with anaemia and studies have shown that both vitamin A and iron are required to promote a full haematological response. The role of vitamin A in haemopoiesis is not fully understood, but the anti-inflammatory effects of vitamin A supplements may stimulate re-utilization and absorption of iron indirectly by reducing infection and inflammation (Hess *et al.*, 2005).

12.4 Absorption, distribution, and transport

12.4.1 Digestion

A schematic representation of vitamin A metabolism and role of retinol-binding protein) and transthyretin is given in Fig. 12.4. Vitamin A and its precursors are ingested in the food matrix. Proteolysis in the stomach may release some of the vitamin A and carotenoids from foods. However, to release pro-vitamin A carotenoids from vegetables, they should be thoroughly cooked and masticated, otherwise the carotenoids will remain within the cellulose structures and unavailable for absorption. Released vitamin A and carotenoids aggregate with lipids into globules and pass into the upper part of the small intestine. Here pancreatic lipase and other esterases hydrolyse lipids (triglycerides, etc.), retinyl esters, and any esters of carotenoids. Bile salts assist in emulsifying the contents of the gut lumen and lipid micelles are formed.

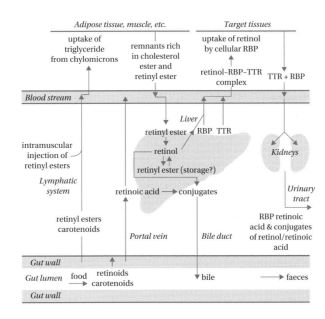

Fig. 12.4 Schematic representation of vitamin A metabolism and role of retinol-binding protein and transthyretin. In the gut wall some β-carotene and retinol is oxidized to all-*trans* retinoic acid, where it may have local activity. Additionally, in target tissues the all-*trans* and 9-*cis* isomers of retinoic acid, are formed from retinol to interact with the retinoic acid receptors (RAR) and retinoid X receptors, respectively, which are found in every cell type (see Section 12.3.3).

12.4.2 Absorption

Retinol Lipid micelles are taken up by the cells lining the intestine and as much as 90% of retinol in foods is absorbed and utilized. The high efficiency of this process may be due to the existence of a specific cellular binding protein (CRBPII) in the mucosal cell that carries the retinol to the enzyme lecithin:retinol acyltransferase (LRAT) and this is the main intestinal enzyme that esterifies retinol and delivers it to the chylomicrons. Very little retinyl ester is absorbed, but hydrolysis of the vitamin A esters in the gut is fairly efficient so more than 50% of the vitamin A in large (pharmaceutical doses) is also absorbed. Within the enterocyte, absorbed retinol is re-esterified to retinol palmitate and, together with triglycerides and other fat-soluble nutrients, is packaged into chylomicrons for transport to the liver.

Carotenoids Carotenoids are also fairly efficiently absorbed at low doses (<5 mg) but the amount absorbed falls off steeply as the dose rises. There are three potential fates for the carotenes absorbed. Some is metabolized by β-carotene 15,15′-dioxygenase to form first retinal, then retinol, and finally retinol palmitate. Some carotene is taken up by the chylomicrons unchanged, while the epithelial cell retains the remainder, which if not converted to retinol is lost through cell turnover in the faeces. The amount of carotene converted to retinol is highly variable in up to 45% of persons. A number of factors may be responsible. Two common nonsynonymous single-nucleotide poor-converter polymorphisms with variant allele frequencies of 42 and 24%, respectively, were recently identified. Carriers of these variant alleles had 32–69% lower ability to convert β-carotene to retinol (Leung *et al.*, 2009). There is also evidence that other carotenoids in the diet like lutein may inhibit conversion of β-carotene to retinol if the molar ratio of lutein: β-carotene is greater than 3:1. β-carotene is then preferentially metabolized in comparison to α-carotene or β-cryptoxanthin.

12.4.3 Transport from the gut to the liver

Retinol esters and carotenoids are transported from the gut, via lymphatic vessels that drain into the jugular vein, with triglyceride in the core of chylomicrons. The chylomicrons circulate around the body on their way to the liver. Most triglycerides are transferred to extrahepatic tissues and most vitamin A is removed from the circulation by the liver's parenchymal cells when the chylomicron remnants (cholesterol esters, retinol palmitate, carotenoids, and other fat-soluble vitamins) reach the liver.

The retinyl esters are hydrolysed in the parenchymal cells and, after meeting any physiological needs, the retinol is transferred to the stellate cells in a process involving retinol-binding protein (RBP). Stellate cells are modified macrophages which comprise 7% of liver cells numbers but only 2% of the volume. Within the stellate cells, the retinol is mainly stored as palmitate (>90%). More than 80% of the total body vitamin A is stored in the liver and some in the kidney. Generally vitamin A in the liver increases with age. On average, a 70-kg man with a liver weighing 1.8 kg would have 150–300 mg of stored vitamin A, enough to last for a year or more of no intake.

12.4.4 Mobilization of vitamin A from the liver and serum transport

Retinol is released from the liver bound to RBP. RBP has a molecular weight of 21 000 and one binding site for retinol. Holo-RBP (the RBP–retinol complex) is released from the liver bound to another protein, transthyretin (TTR). TTR has a molecular weight of 55 000 and was previously known as thyroxine-binding pre-albumin; it also has one binding site, so the whole complex is a 1:1:1 structure. In plasma, 95% of the retinol is bound in the retinol–RBP–TTR complex.

The binding of retinol to RBP confers a number of physiological advantages:

- RBP (and all the vitamin A-binding proteins within the cell) facilitate the transport of a lipid-soluble compound through the aqueous environment of the plasma;
- there is protection of retinol from oxidative damage during transport;
- there is regulation of retinol mobilization;
- there is delivery of retinol to specific sites on the surface of target cells, particularly the eye, where a lack of RBP results in night blindness;
- there is formation of a large molecule as a complex, which is not easily lost from plasma during vasodilatation.

Holo-RBP is taken up by specific cell-surface receptors. Once the retinol is transferred within the cell, the apo-RBP (the free protein) is released from the receptor and can be recycled. Some is excreted by the kidney. Retinol inside the cell is bound to CRBP. Some cells can also take up retinol palmitate from circulating chylomicrons via lipoprotein receptors. Within the cell, the ester is hydrolysed and retinol is bound to CRBP1 for further metabolism.

Inside the cell, retinol is oxidized to retinal and then to all-*trans* retinoic acid by local expression of retinoic acid-synthesizing aldehyde dehydrogenase. Some of the all-*trans* retinoic acid is converted to 9-*cis* retinoic acid. The two forms, all-*trans* and 9-*cis* retinoic acid, interact with the nuclear receptors RAR and RXR, respectively (see Section 12.3.3). The cytochrome P450 enzyme CYP26, which has specific retinoic acid 4-hydroxylase activity, may regulate steady state levels of the active retinoids in target tissues.

Plasma carotenes are transported mainly in the low-density lipoproteins, while the more water-soluble xanthophylls are most concentrated in the high-density lipoproteins. Depletion studies suggest that half-lives of β- and α-carotene and β-cryptoxanthin are <2 weeks, of lycopene is 2–4 weeks, and lutein and zeaxanthin are 4–8 weeks. The shorter half-lives of the pro-vitamin A carotenoids may be evidence of their conversion to vitamin A in the tissues but >80% of retinol synthesis from carotenes takes place in the gut during absorption.

12.4.5 Vitamin A excretion

In a healthy person no vitamin A is excreted per se. Oxidized metabolites can be found in the urine and any conjugated vitamin A products that might be formed by vitamin A excess would be secreted into the bile and then lost in the faeces. During illness, particularly in persons with fever, retinol is lost in the urine, together with RBP, and the amounts can be as high as 500 μg retinol/day.

12.5 Vitamin A deficiency

12.5.1 Experimental deficiencies in animals

In 1928, Green and Mellanby showed that when animals were placed on vitamin A-deficient diets, practically all died with infective lesions. The most useful models for such work are rats and mice, and the chicken is probably the next most useful species. Chickens are also useful to study xanthophyll absorption and metabolism. Viral diseases in the hen provide a useful model to study the influence of infection on both retinol and carotenoid metabolism and interaction with deficiencies.

12.5.2 Experimental human deficiencies

The first important deficiency study in man was the 'Sheffield' study (Hume and Krebs, 1949). Twenty men and three women, conscientious objectors to military service, volunteered to receive a diet containing no vitamin A_1 and <7 μg RE of carotene. By 18 months only three of the volunteers actually showed early signs of vitamin A deficiency but intervention with carefully chosen amounts of retinol or β-carotene in arachis oil, provided the information which established vitamin A requirements in the human adult to reverse signs of vitamin A deficiency to be 750 μg vitamin A1 or 1800 μg β-carotene and the bioequivalence of β-carotene to retinol (6 μg β-carotene ≡ 1 μg retinol). Subsequent depletion/repletion studies by Sauberlich and colleagues provided very similar conclusions in 1974, namely that 1200 μg vitamin A_1 or 2400 μg β-carotene were required to maintain satisfactory serum retinol concentrations.

12.5.3 Natural human deficiencies

For many years, the prevalence of vitamin A deficiency was defined by the number of persons showing signs of xerophthalmia (meaning dry eyes). Using such criteria, Sommer West (1996) estimated that over 40 million children under the age of 6 years have mild to moderate xerophthalmia, 1% go blind annually, and 50–75% of these will die within the year.

Work with vitamin A showed that children at risk of xerophthalmia also have a high risk of infection. The term 'anti-infective vitamin' was re-attached to vitamin A. As techniques to measure plasma retinol concentrations improved, this has been used as the preferred biomarker of vitamin A status and current estimates of vitamin A deficiency in the world are of the order of 500 million. Vitamin A deficiency is a particular problem in groups with the highest vitamin A requirements: infants, preschool children, and pregnant and lactating women. Vitamin A status is commonly assessed in these groups using plasma retinol concentrations. Infection is particularly common in infants and children, and plasma retinol concentrations are depressed by inflammation. So, current estimates of global vitamin A deficiency are probably overestimates. Nevertheless, vitamin A deficiency is a major risk to human health in many parts of Asia, south-east Asia, Africa, Middle Eastern countries, and South and Central America.

12.5.4 Features of deficiency disease in man

Changes in the eye People with marginal vitamin A deficiency become less able to see in dim light. This is 'night blindness' and in communities where vitamin A deficiency exists, there is usually a specific word to describe the condition. The word frequently compares the person's behaviour to that of a chicken. Chickens have no rod cells in their retina and cannot see in the dark. If disturbed after nightfall, they bump into things when moving around. Night blindness correlates with low plasma levels of vitamin A, but note that retinol concentrations depressed by inflammation will not necessarily correlate with night blindness. Night blindness can occur in children and adults.

Another clinical indicator of early or marginal vitamin A deficiency is Bitôt's spots. These are foamy deposits on the surface of the conjunctiva (Fig. 12.5). They are found more frequently in pre- and school-

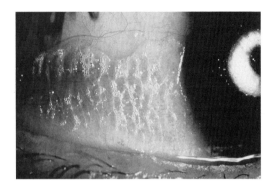

Fig. 12.5 Photograph of a Bitôt's spot.

age children than in adults. Both night-blindness and Bitôt's spots disappear on treatment with vitamin A, with no lasting damage. In prolonged or more severe vitamin A deficiency, a series of changes can take place in the cornea, some of which are irreversible, as summarized in Box 12.2.

Changes to other epithelial tissues The influence of vitamin A on cellular differentiation is

---

BOX 12.2 Stages of xerophthalmia

- Conjunctival xerosis (X1A) consists of one or more patches of dry, non-wettable conjunctiva that has been described as 'emerging like sand banks at a receding tide at the sea-shore' when a child ceases to cry. The condition is due to changes in the epithelium of the conjunctiva and the lack of tear production.
- Bitôt's spots (X1B) are found in association with X1A and are a product of the same condition.
- Corneal xerosis (X2) is an extension of conjunctival xerosis to the cornea. The corneal surface also begins to lose its transparent appearance. A light shone at an angle on the surface of the eye will often reveal the ripple-like surface and irregular reflection of the source of illumination.
- Corneal ulceration (X3A) usually begins first at the edge of the cornea and is characterized by small holes, 1–3 mm in diameter, with steep sides. If treatment with vitamin A is initiated at this stage, it may be possible to reverse the lesion and retain some sight.
- More extensive corneal ulceration (X3B) is characterized by larger defects that result in blindness. In Africa, it is reported that children with measles can develop X3B quickly without the appearance of the intermediate stages.
- Corneal scars (XS) result from the healing of the irreversible changes described above and may appear as white scar-like tissue in the cornea. On the other hand, if the cornea ruptures and the eye contents escape, a shrunken eyeball results.

Source: WHO (1982) *Control of vitamin A deficiency and xerophthalmia*. Report of a Joint WHO/USAID/Helen Keller International/IVACG Meeting. WHO Technical Report Series, No. 672. Geneva, World Health Organization.

reflected in the widespread effects of vitamin A deficiency on other epithelial tissues. Follicular hyperkeratosis seen in vitamin A-deficient adults is due to skin keratinization blocking sebaceous glands with horny plugs, though this may not be a specific vitamin A effect. Vitamin A deficiency also affects the epithelial cell lining of the respiratory, gastrointestinal, and genitourinary tracts, as well as immune cell maturation. The different epithelia lose their characteristic structure and hence specialized function. The tracheal lining, for example, loses the cilia (which sweep foreign material up and out) and in severe cases the columnar epithelium is replaced by squamous epithelium in the intestine, villi are flattened, and mucous glands reduced.

Morbidity and mortality Sommer and colleagues in Indonesia showed that the death rate of children with mild xerophthalmia (night-blindness and Bitôt's spots) was on average four times higher than in those with no xerophthalmia. Meta-analysis of intervention studies with vitamin A in countries where xerophthalmia was occurring showed reduced overall mortality by a highly significant 23%.

Vitamin A and measles One particular infectious disease, measles, is much more severe, with about a 12% fatality rate in communities where xerophthalmia is seen. Even in countries where xerophthalmia does not occur, the benefit of vitamin A treatment in cases of measles is striking. WHO and UNICEF recommend that all children with measles in developing countries should be given a massive dose of vitamin A. It is also advised for severe cases in developed countries.

Nutritional anaemia Human intervention studies with vitamin A have shown that there is a specific effect of vitamin A on haemoglobin synthesis in the absence of additional dietary iron (see Section 12.3.3) (Hess *et al.*, 2005).

12.6 Influence of disease/trauma on plasma retinol concentrations and mobilization of vitamin A from the liver

Infection or inflammation decreases plasma retinol concentrations and reduces mobilization of retinol from liver stores. The effects are part of the acute phase response to stress. RBP is a negative acute phase protein. Stimulation of the acute phase response by infection, surgery, or other stresses induces production of cytokines like interleukin-6 (IL-6) by macrophages that induce a wide variety of responses in the liver and elsewhere in the body. One effect is to reduce transcription of the messenger RNA for RBP synthesis. There is also increased vascular permeability and some plasma retinol moves into extracellular fluid compartments. As much as 500 μg/day of retinol and RBP can be lost in the urine. Fig. 12.6 shows plasma retinol concentrations following surgery.

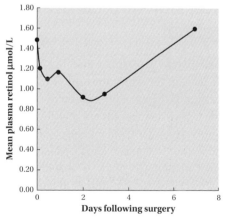

Fig. 12.6 Influence of surgery on plasma retinol concentrations in South African women.

Source: Modified from Louw, J.A., Werbeck, A., Louw, M.E.J., *et al.* (1992) Blood vitamin concentrations during the acute-phase response. *Critical Care Med*, **20**, 934–41.

12.7 Biochemical tests for vitamin A deficiency

The methods of measurement of plasma retinol concentrations to assess vitamin A status are described in Table 12.1. The plasma retinol concentration is the most widely used method of assessing vitamin A status, but it is influenced strongly by age (Fig. 12.7), female sex hormones, and inflammation. Infection or inflammation decrease plasma retinol concentrations and reduce mobilization of retinol from liver stores. These effects can have a major impact on several methods of measurement, viz plasma retinol and RBP concentrations and dose–response tests.

Recently, a method of correcting plasma retinol has been suggested utilizing plasma concentration of two acute-phase proteins, C-reactive protein (CRP) and α1-acid glycoprotein (AGP). CRP is a marker of the early phase of inflammation and is associated with large depressions in plasma retinol concentrations. In contrast, AGP is associated with chronic inflammation or late convalescence when plasma retinol concentrations are less depressed. The use of these two biomarkers enables plasma retinol concentrations to be corrected for the influence of inflammation (Thurnham et al., 2003). In the absence of measurements of inflammation, the presence of β-carotene in plasma is a clue that a low plasma retinol is depressed by inflammation and not poor vitamin A status.

Probably the best (research) method of measuring total body vitamin A reserves is the radioisotope dilution assays. These tests may be more or less unaffected by inflammation, as 3 weeks is allowed for equilibration of the labelled tracer with body stores of vitamin A. This period should allow sufficient time for any inflammation at the time of treatment to subside.

12.8 Functions of carotenoids

12.8.1 Bioavailability and conversion of β-carotene to retinol

Carotenoids are fat-soluble and the presence of adequate fat in the diet at the time of consumption is necessary for optimal absorption of carotenoids. In plant leaves, carotenoids are present within pigment-protein complexes in the cell chloroplasts and an important prerequisite for the satisfactory utilization of plant carotenoids is that the cellulose structure of cell walls is ruptured to release carotenoids into the luminal fluids of the gut. Cooking and chewing assist rupture of the cell walls of leaves during ingestion of food. But in fruit, cell wall structure is usually much weaker than in leaves, and carotenes are found in the lipid droplets in chromoplasts. Hence, carotenoids from fruit are more easily bioavailable than those in leaves.

On the basis of data available to early committees, it was decided that on average only one-third of dietary plant carotene was absorbed. Furthermore, conversion of dietary β-carotene to retinol was also poorly efficient. Even when small amounts of pure β-carotene dissolved in oil (<2 mg) were fed to vitamin A-deficient volunteers, only 50% was converted to retinol. Hence, for many years the assumption was made that 6 μg β-carotene from plant sources was bioequivalent to 1 μg retinol. More recently, work suggested that far less β-carotene was available for absorption. Hence, the Institute of Medicine (2000) decided that the bioequivalence was 12 μg β-carotene in plant food equal to 1 μg retinol (for β-cryptoxanthin and α-carotene, with only one β-ionone ring per molecule the retinol activity equivalent in plant foods is 24:1). However, poorly functioning polymorphisms of the enzyme responsible for converting β-carotene to retinol have recently been found. The prevalence is higher in some populations than others and the

Table 12.1 Measurement of plasma retinol concentrations to assess vitamin A status

Description	Advantages	Disadvantages	Thresholds of adequacy	Alternative tests of vitamin A status
Measurement in fasting plasma or serum	Samples easily obtained and retinol easily quantified	Concentration of retinol depressed by inflammation	Severe risk of deficiency <0.35 μmol/L (<10 μg/dL)	Retinol is also measured as part of the relative dose–response (RDR) test. Both the RDR and modified RDR are also influenced by inflammation
Samples should be protected from light on collection and stored at less than −20°C	HPLC much more widely available	Inflammation more common than vitamin A deficiency	High risk of deficiency <0.7 μmol/L (<20 μg/dL)	Retinol is also used for radioisotope dilution methods
HPLC is best method of analysis		Concentrations of CRP and AGP should be monitored	Possible risk of deficiency in adults <1.05 μmol/L	Milk retinol concentrations are fairly constant in women of different ethnicities (1.75–2.45 μmol/L) and reduced where status is poor
In the absence of inflammation concentrations <0.7 μmol/L indicate low liver stores		Concentrations increased 20–50% by female sex hormones		Presence of β-carotene in plasma is a good proxy indicator of good vitamin A status
Adequacy should always be assessed by comparison with healthy controls of the same age (Fig. 12.7)				
Whole blood can be collected on filter paper, thoroughly dried and stored with dessicant	Easier to transport where cold chain is unavailable. Can be used to measure retinol or RBP	Affected by above and currently (2010) uncertainties still exist about quantitation	Similar to above, but uncertainties still exist	

AGP, α1-acid-glycoprotein, elevated in the later part of infection and usually associated with less depression of retinol or RBP than CRP–in children AGP is more frequently elevated than CRP; CRP, C-reactive protein, elevated in the early part of infection and associated with marked depression of plasma retinol or RBP; RBP, retinol-binding protein.

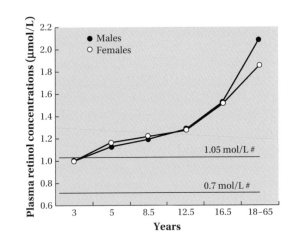

Fig. 12.7 Influence of age on plasma retinol concentrations from three national surveys in Great Britain.#, Thresholds of biochemical deficiency; see blood retinol concentrations in Table 12.1.

Source: Thurnham, D.I., Mburu, A.S.W., Mwaniki, D.L., and de Wagt, A. (2005) Micronutrients in childhood and the influence of subclinical inflammation. *Proc Nutr Soc,* **64**, 502–9.

bioequivalence issue may well have to be re-examined if the prevalence of the poor-converter phenotypes is found to be low in those countries where there is a greater need to convert β-carotene to retinol (Leung *et al.,* 2009).

12.8.2 Macular pigments: lutein, zeaxanthin, and *meso*-zeaxanthin

The retinal epithelium is unique in the human body in containing almost exclusively only the three related xanthophyll carotenoids; zeaxanthin, *meso*-zeaxanthin (MZ), and lutein, the structures of which are presented in Fig. 12.8. They are concentrated in the macula lutea in the centre of the retina and provide its yellow colour. Humans consume 1–3 mg lutein per day and the ratio of lutein to zeaxanthin in the diet is ~5:1. Lutein and zeaxanthin occur in the blood in roughly the same proportions but no MZ is found. The xanthophyll pigments occur widely in vegetables and fruits but MZ is found in only a few foods like shrimp, some fish, and turtle meat. In spite of the amounts of the different xanthophylls in the diet, zeaxanthin and MZ occur in approximately equal amounts in the macula, and their combined concentration exceeds that of lutein. In addition, a binding protein that specifically binds zeaxanthin and MZ and not lutein, has been isolated from optical tissues. This protein may enable the conversion of lutein to MZ in the eye.

Macular pigment optical density (MPOD) is a measure of the pigment density in the macula of

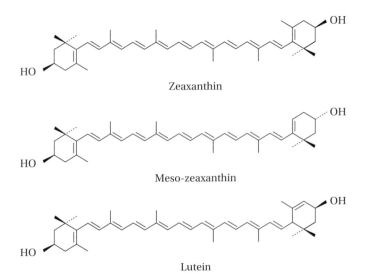

Fig. 12.8 Main macular pigments, showing zeaxanthin, *meso*-zeaxanthin, and lutein.

the eye. The concentration of pigment extracted from the eyes of patients with macula disease at autopsy is lower than that of patients without disease. MPOD can also be measured in living subjects using physiological methods and can be shown to increase following supplementation with xanthophyll supplements and with vegetables like spinach. The increase was particularly rapid with supplements containing MZ (Connolly *et al.*, 2010). Once increased, MPOD remains elevated for several weeks to months after withdrawal of the supplement. Vegetables are the richest source of dietary lutein but lutein and zeaxanthin in eggs yolks are more bioavailable.

Lycopene is the red pigment of tomatoes. It is often the most abundant of the carotenoids in human plasma. Having no β-ionone rings (Fig. 12.2), it is not a pro-vitamin A. It is, however, an antioxidant (as is β-carotene). Early reports of a negative association of tomato sauce consumption and prostate cancer await further substantiation.

12.9 Food sources of vitamin A and carotenoids

In most industrialized countries the predominant dietary source of vitamin A activity is pre-formed vitamin A_1 mainly in the form of retinol palmitate in foods of animal origin. Liver is the richest source of vitamin A but it is also found in milk, butter, cheese, egg yolk, and some fatty fish. Margarine is enriched with vitamin A to levels similar to those in butter. Provitamin A carotenes are also obtained from plant foods, the main ones being dark green leafy vegetables and some yellow- or orange-coloured fruits.

In developing countries, plant sources of vitamin A are predominant in the diet. Certain foods like red palm oil, papayas, mangoes, and carrots are particularly rich in β-carotene and sometime also α-carotene and/or β-cryptoxanthin. Plant sources of vitamin A are often seasonal and fluctuations in vitamin A status in accordance with the season is common in some tropical countries. For example, vitamin A status in West African countries improves with the mango season.

12.10 Recommended intakes

Vitamin A requirements vary with age and the requirement for growth is a major determinant. Thus requirements in infancy and childhood are higher per kg body weight than in adults. Infants are born with almost no stores of vitamin A, so it is critical that new-born infants obtain sufficient vitamin A to meet the needs of growth and a developing immune system as well as to accumulate body stores. Mothers' colostrum and early milk is high in vitamin A and neonatal mortality was significantly less in Nepal and Ghana when infants were breastfed within the first hour after birth. The needs of the infant also increase the vitamin A requirements of lactating mothers. The British (1991) RDIs followed the FAO/WHO (1988) consultation. Some of their RDIs are lower than the more recent North American and Australia/ New Zealand recommendations. They are summarized in Table 12.2.

Table 12.2 Summary of RDIs

	µg retinol equivalents/day
Infants	350–500
1–6 years	400
7–12 years	500
Adolescents	600
Men	600–900
Women	600–900
Pregnant	700–800
Lactating	850, 1100, 1300

12.11 Toxic effects of vitamin A

The most serious toxic effects of vitamin A are teratogenic as a result of overdose during the first trimester of pregnancy. Such effects include spontaneous abortions or foetal abnormalities, including those of the cranium (microcephaly), face (hairlip), heart, kidney, thymus, and central nervous system (deafness and lowered learning ability). Since embryogenesis is under the control of retinoic acid isomers, short-term increases in these compounds are probably responsible. Normal concentrations of plasma retinoic acid are 1–2 nmol/L. In one experiment, large doses of vitamin A (>300 000 IU, >100 mg) given to 10 women caused 10–100-fold increases in plasma retinoic acid concentrations at 4 hours. The same amount of vitamin A given as liver-only increased plasma retinoic acid concentrations 10-fold at 4 hours. Thus, women who are pregnant or who could become pregnant should not be exposed to retinoid therapy either for skin conditions or as supplements. Daily intakes should not exceed 10 000 IU (3 mg RE).

Acute and chronic toxic effects of vitamin A overdose can also occur in all individuals. Very high single doses can cause transient symptoms that may include bulging fontanelles in infants, headaches in older children and adults, and vomiting, diarrhoea, and loss of appetite in all age groups. It is rare for toxicity to occur from ingestion of food sources of vitamin A. When it does, it is usually due to the consumption of a large amount of liver as, for example, in arctic and antarctic explorers who consumed polar bear, seal, or dog liver. In these extreme circumstances additional symptoms included blurred or double vision, vertigo, uncoordinated move-ments, elevated cerebrospinal pressure, and skin exfoliation. Deaths have also occurred.

Single large doses of vitamin A in infancy and childhood have been reported to cause transient toxic effects, but these are usually avoided if the dose is not more than 50 000 IU for infants below 6 months, 100 000 IU between 6 and 12 months, and 200 000 IU for children over 1 year. Doses are not given more frequently than once every 3 months.

Chronic toxicity is induced by consuming for a month or more at least 10 times the recommended daily allowance (e.g. 10 mg RE per day or 33 300 IU). A wide range of symptoms have been reported including headache, bone and muscle pain, ataxia, visual impairment, skin disorders, alopecia, liver toxicity, and hyperlipidaemia. It is usual to find high concentrations of retinol palmitate in the blood (3–8 μmol/L). Normally, retinol palmitate is only found in the blood for 3–4 hours after a meal, in the chylomicron fraction.

High intakes of carotenoids, e.g. from tomato or carrot juice or red palm oil, can lead to hypercarotenaemia and yellow coloration of the skin, especially the palms of the hands or the soles of the feet and the nasolabial folds (not the eyes), but this is not associated with toxic effects. High doses of β-carotene (180 mg/day) are used in the treatment of erythropoietic protoporphyria and have never been found to cause harm. The only worrying effects with carotenoids are prolonged use of high-dose β-carotene in smokers. Doses of 25–30 mg/day were associated with a higher incidence of lung cancer in two large intervention studies.

12.12 Measures to prevent vitamin A deficiency

12.12.1 Using available foods

All nutritional deficiencies are due to a lack of food. Deficiencies rarely occur alone, and the clinical features of deficiencies in a community are those of the most seriously deficient nutrient. In developing countries, vitamin A deficiency is a particular problem because dietary sources of pre-formed vitamin A (animal food products) are expensive and people are reliant on vegetable sources. The bioavailability of carotene in plant food is poor (12.8.1). Fruit carotene is more bioavailable than vegetables but is often seasonal. In many places there is a greater variety of plant foods to overcome seasonal shortages but thorough cooking of vegetables and fat (which improves carotene absorption) optimize bioavailability. Cooking methods are part of the culture of a community and not changed easily, and fat is very often an animal product and in short supply. Where vitamin A deficiencies exist, people need to be made aware of the diversity of foods that can provide vitamin A. Growing mangos, papaya (yellow and orange varieties), red sweet potato, and plantain need to be encouraged, as well as the introduction of chickens for their eggs, and fish where appropriate. As poverty is often the root cause of the lack of food, such schemes will need assistance and take time to be effective. High-dose supplementation of vulnerable groups, food fortification, and introduction of nutrient-enriched foods are short-term measures to rectify specific nutrient deficiencies and some may become part of the long-term solution to vitamin A deficiency.

Prevention—ideally eradication—of vitamin A deficiency is a priority for WHO and UNICEF. The deficiency is widespread and it causes death or blindness in many thousands of young children. Measures of prevention are known, they are safe and practical, and are being generally applied by national governments and NGOs.

12.12.2 Breastfeeding

Infants are born with very little stored vitamin A. They rely on vitamin A in their mothers' milk to supply their needs for growth, immune function, and storage. The colostrum is particularly rich in vitamin A and early introduction of infants to the breast promotes mother–child bonding, more successful breastfeeding, and a continued supply of vitamin A through infancy. Introduction straight after birth has been shown to lower neonatal mortality (Edmond *et al.*, 2006, Mullany *et al.*, 2007).

Delayed introduction is common in some African and Asian countries through cultural taboos, and may play a role in the unacceptably high neonatal mortalities in these continents. Breastfeeding promotion programmes should emphasize early initiation, as well as exclusive breastfeeding.

12.12.3 Massive dosing and supplementation

Massive dosing of communities with vitamin A to overcome vitamin A deficiency was first tried in the 1960s in India. Doses of 200 000–300 000 IU (60–90 mg RE) were given to pre-school children and any children showing side effects were noted. Specific problems included headaches, nausea, vomiting, and bulging fontanelles, but none of the side effects caused permanent damage, and the prevalence of signs like night blindness, Bitôt's spots and xerosis was reduced. Night blindness is cured first. Oral and intramuscular administration of vitamin A dissolved in oil was tested, and oral administration by capsule or spoon was found to be highly effective. Use of the method has extended to many countries and clear benefits in reduced mortality have been demonstrated (see 12.5.4). Currently, recommended treatments are shown in Box 12.3. 200 000 IU vitamin A is given therapeutically to children admitted to hospital with measles, xerophthalmia, or malnutrition.

The high dose for a child provides sufficient vitamin A for a period of 4–6 months, so where vitamin A deficiency is a constant problem, treatment should be provided every 6 months. Women of child-bearing age must not be given high doses

---

BOX 12.3 Massive dosing 6 months apart

- Under 6 months, 50 000 IU orally (15 mg RE)
- 6 months to 1 year, 100 000 IU (30 mg RE)
- Over 1 year, 200 000 IU (60 mg RE)
- Women 1–8 weeks post-partum, 2 × 200 000 IU in separate doses

except immediately post partum. The highest dose for a non-pregnant women is 10 000 IU (3 mg RE) or 1 mg RE daily.

12.12.4 Fortification and enrichment

Fortification is the addition of vitamin A to a widely used food that would not normally contain the vitamin. Enrichment is the addition of vitamin A to a food to replace the vitamin lost during processing. Because vitamin A is lost during storage, the amount of vitamin added should usually be greater than the nominal amount required by legislation or shown on the package. Both processes are introduced where it is decided the community requires extra vitamin A. Margarine has been enriched with vitamin A at a level of the best summer butter (200 IU (60 µg RE) per 100 g) in many European and developing countries. Sugar fortifi-

cation (1.5 mg RE/100 g sugar) has been successful in several Central American countries and it is now being tried in Africa. Oil is also a useful vehicle for fortification, but with all methods the main problem is maintaining quality control of the product. If many manufacturers are involved, the costs of monitoring quality may be prohibitive.

12.12.5 Public health and other indirect methods

Poverty and disease are main factors accompanying vitamin A deficiency in communities throughout Africa, Asia, and South America. Immunization against infections and social improvements to address the issues of poverty, land reform, lack of education, and improvements in agricultural diversity will all help to address the problem of vitamin A deficiency.

12.13 Influence of micronutrient deficiencies and drugs on vitamin A status

12.13.1 Influence of other nutrients on vitamin A status

A balanced and adequate diet is necessary for optimal vitamin A status. Specific deficiencies of protein and zinc, may adversely affect status. Experimental protein deficiency reduces the activity of β-carotene 15,15′-dioxygenase activity, so may impair the conversion of β-carotene to retinal. Absorption of retinol is impaired in kwashiorkor and serum retinol is low. It improves with refeeding before vitamin A is given. Zinc-dependent enzymes convert retinol to retinal, and in one study, night blindness in a group of alcoholics was explained by this. Zinc is also involved in the synthesis of RBP, which is particularly rich in zinc. Plasma retinol concentrations frequently correlate with plasma

α-tocopherol concentrations. Vitamin E may protect retinol from oxidation.

12.13.2 Interactions with drugs

Several drugs are known to affect the absorption of vitamin A, e.g. cholestyramine (antihyperlipaemic), colchicine (antigout), mineral oil (laxative), neomycin (antibiotic which inactivates bile salts), olestra, (anti-obesity), and phytostanols and phytosterols (to lower cholesterol), but unless their use is prolonged over many months, the large liver stores of vitamin A in adults will maintain vitamin A status.

Ethyl alcohol and the female sex hormones can potentially affect vitamin A status. Alcohol abuse results in a striking depletion of hepatic vitamin A. Increased ethanol-oxidizing capacity, as a result of alcohol abuse, may increase the oxidation and loss of retinol from the liver and cause the poor vitamin A status of many alcoholics. In contrast, oestrogen-containing drugs (oral contraceptives, hormone replacement therapy) can have a stimulatory effect on the concentration of plasma retinol.

12.14 Pharmaceutical uses of vitamin A

Several synthetic retinoids influence proliferation and differentiation of the skin epidermis, inhibit keratinization, reduce production of sebum, and influence immune response, especially cell-mediated immunity. These properties have been used in medicine particularly to treat such skin disorders as acne, seborrhoea (overproduction of sebum), and psoriasis (areas covered by profuse silvery scales especially on the elbows, knees, and trunk of the body). One of the more effective drugs is 13-*cis* retinoic acid (isotretinoin, 'Roaccutane'), but even for topical applications, its use is restricted in women of child-bearing age because of the risk of teratogenesis. Topical use of all-*trans* retinoic acid can also reduce wrinkling and hyperpigmentation caused by photo-ageing. All-*trans* retinoic acid and 13-*cis* retinoic acid have been used to treat certain acute myeloid leukaemias (AML), where the retinoids stop proliferation of the cells and induce terminal differentiation to the granulocyte. Unfortunately, there are a number of different AMLs and only a limited number of patients respond.

Further Reading

1. **Benson, M.J., Pino-Lagos, K., Rosemblatt, M., et al.** (2007) All-*trans* retinoic acid mediates enhanced T reg cell growth, differentiation, and gut homing in the face of high levels of co-stimulation. *J Exp Med*, **204**, 1765–74.

2. **Connolly, E.E., Beatty, S., Thurnham, D.I., et al.** (2010) Augmentation of macular pigment following supplementation with all three macular carotenoids: An exploratory study. *Current Eye Research*, **35**, 335–51.

3. **Edmond, K.M., Zandoh, C., Quigley, M.A., et al.** (2006) Delayed breastfeeding initiation increases risk of neonatal mortality. *Pediatrics*, **117**, e380–6.

4. **Hess, S.Y., Thurnham, D.I. and Hurrell, R.F.** (2005) *Influence of provitamin A carotenoids on iron, zinc and vitamin A status*. Washington, International Food Policy Research Institute. Harvest Plus Technical Monographs 6.

5. **Hume, E.M. and Krebs, H.A.** (1949) *Vitamin A requirements of human adults*. A report of the vitamin A sub-committee of the accessory food factors committee. MRC Report No. 264. London, His Majesty's Stationery Office.

6. **Hussey, G.D. and Klein, M.** (1990) A randomized, controlled trial of vitamin A in children with severe measles. *New Engl J Med*, **323**, 160–4.

7. **Leung, W.C., Hessel, S., Méplan, C., et al.** (2009) Two common single nucleotide polymorphisms in the gene encoding beta-carotene 15,15'-monoxygenase alter beta-carotene metabolism in female volunteers. *FASEB J*, **23**, 1041–53.

8. **Louw, J.A., Werbeck, A., Louw, M.E.J., et al.** (1992) Blood vitamin concentrations during the acute-phase response. *Critical Care Med*, **20**, 934–41.

9. **Mora, J.R., Iwata, M., and von Andriano, U.H.** (2008) Vitamin effects on the immune system: Vitamins A and D take centre stage. *Nat Rev Immunol*, **8**, 685–98.

10. **Mullany, L.C., Katz, J., Li, Y.M., et al.** (2007) Breast-feeding patterns, time to initiation, and mortality risk among newborns in southern Nepal. *J Nutr*, **138**, 599–603.

11. **Sommer, A. and West, K.P.** (1996) *Vitamin A deficiency: health, survival and vision.* New York, Oxford University Press.

12. **Stephensen, C.B., Rasooly, R., Jiang, X., *et al.*** (2002) Vitamin A enhances in vitro Th2 development via retinoid X receptor pathway. *J Immunol,* **168**, 4495–503.

13. **Thurnham, D.I., McCabe, G.P., Northrop-Clewes, C.A., *et al.*** (2003) Effect of subclinical infection on plasma retinol concentrations and assessment of prevalence of vitamin A deficiency: Meta-analysis. *Lancet,* **362**, 2052–8.

14. **Thurnham, D.I., Mburu, A.S.W., Mwaniki, D.L., and de Wagt, A.** (2005) Micronutrients in childhood and the influence of subclinical inflammation. *Proc Nutr Soc,* **64**, 502–9.

15. **US Institute of Medicine** (2000) *Dietary reference intakes for vitamin A, vitamin K, arsenic, boron, chromium, copper, iodine, iron, manganese, molybdenum, nickel, silicon, vanadium and zinc.* Washington, National Academic Press, Standing Committee on the Scientific Evaluation of Dietary Intakes, Food and Nutrition Board.

16. **WHO** (1982) *Control of vitamin A deficiency and xerophthalmia.* Report of a Joint WHO/USAID/Helen Keller International/IVACG Meeting. WHO Technical Report Series, No. 672. Geneva, World Health Organization.

Useful Websites

 To see topical and scientifically robust updates on nutrition associated with this textbook and web links to many of the journals in the Further Reading sections, please see the dedicated Online Resource Centre at **http://www.oxfordtextbooks.co.uk/orc/mann4e/**

The International Vitamin A Consultative Group (IVACG) founded in 1976 provided a forum and network for scientists whose work aims at reducing vitamin A deficiency in the world. It has now been replaced by the Micronutrients Forum, but the IVACG's work is still accessible on the web.

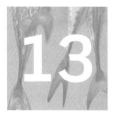

13 The B vitamins

Stewart Truswell

All B vitamins are water-soluble. The water-soluble B vitamin that McCollum differentiated from fat-soluble A in 1915 was later shown to consist of several distinct essential nutrients, though often found in the same foods, like liver and yeast. As they were separately isolated, they were named vitamin B_1, B_2, B_3 at first but some of these were the same as someone else had found in another laboratory and fell by the wayside. So there are now eight well-established vitamins from the original B complex. Most of them are now given their chemical name but B_1 is sometimes still used and B_6 and B_{12} persist in common use.

13.1 Thiamin* (vitamin B_1)

Eijkmann, a Dutch medical officer stationed in Java, discovered around 1897 that a polyneuritis resembling beri beri (which was very common in southeast Asia at that time) could be produced in chickens fed on polished rice. Subsequently, he and his successor, Grijns, showed that this polyneuritis could be cured with rice bran or polishings. This contained B_1, the first of the vitamins to be identified, but it was not until 1936 that R.R. Williams finally elucidated the unusual structure and synthesized thiamin.

*We follow the spelling of the International Union of Nutritional Sciences (no final 'e'). The pharmaceutical sciences still spell it 'thiamine'.

13.1.1 Functions

Thiamin (Fig. 13.1) as the diphosphate (or 'pyrophosphate'), thiamin pyrophosphate (TPP) is a coen-

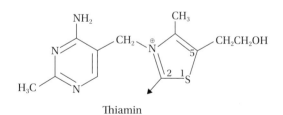

Thiamin

Fig. 13.1 Structure of thiamin.

zyme for the following major decarboxylation steps in carbohydrate metabolism:

1 Pyruvate → acetyl CoA (pyruvate dehydrogenase complex) at the entry to the citric acid cycle. Hence, in thiamin deficiency, pyruvate and lactate accumulate.

2 α-Ketoglutarate → succinyl CoA (α-ketoglutarate dehydrogenase), half-way round the citric acid cycle.

3 Transketolase reactions in the hexose monophosphate shunt, alternative pathway for oxidation of glucose. Hence, in thiamin deficiency, oxidation of glucose is impaired with no alternative route.

4 The second step in catabolism of the branched-chain amino acids, leucine, isoleucine, and valine.

13.1.2 Absorption and metabolism

Thiamin is readily absorbed by active transport at low concentrations in the small intestine and by passive diffusion at high concentrations. Total body content is only 25–30 mg, mostly in the form of TPP in the tissues. There is another coenzyme form, thiamin triphosphate in the brain. Thiamin is excreted both unchanged and as metabolites in the urine. It has a relatively high turnover rate in the body; there is really no store anywhere in the body. On a diet lacking in thiamin, signs of deficiency can occur after only 25–30 days.

13.1.3 Deficiency in animals

Pigeons and chickens are more susceptible than mammals. The characteristic effect is head retraction, called opisthotonus, from neurological dysfunction. In mammals with experimental deficiency there is incoordination of muscle movements, progressing to paralyses, convulsions, and death. The brain is dependent on glucose oxidation for its energy but the decrease in its pyruvate dehydrogenase and

α-ketoglutarate dehydrogenase activities does not seem sufficient to explain the severe neurological dysfunction. Reduced formation of the neurotransmitter, acetylcholine (because acetyl CoA is not being formed), and a role of thiamin triphosphate in nerve transmission are other possible mechanisms.

Loss of appetite, cardiac enlargement, oedema, and increased pyruvate and lactate are also seen.

13.1.4 Deficiency in humans

There are two distinct major deficiency diseases, beri beri and Wernicke–Korsakoff syndrome. They do not usually occur together.

Beri beri is now rare in the countries where it was originally described—Japan, Indonesia, and Malaysia (the name comes from the Singhalese language of Sri Lanka). In Western countries, occasional cases are seen in alcoholics. In *acute* beri beri, there is a high output cardiac failure, with warm extremities, bounding pulse, oedema, and cardiac enlargement. These features appear to be the result of intense vasodilatation from accumulation of pyruvate and lactate in blood and tissues. There are few electrocardiographic abnormalities. Response to thiamin treatment is prompt, with diuresis and usually a full recovery. In *chronic* beri beri, the peripheral nerves are affected, rather than the cardiovascular system. There is inability to lift the foot up (foot drop), loss of sensation in the feet, and absent ankle jerk reflexes.

Wernicke's encephalopathy is usually seen in people who have been drinking alcohol heavily for some weeks and eaten very little. Alcohol requires thiamin for its metabolism and alcoholic beverages do not contain it. Alcohol may also interfere with thiamin absorption. Occasional cases are seen in people on a prolonged fast (such as hunger strikers) or with persistent vomiting (as in Wernicke's first described case). Cases occurred in malnourished soldiers in Japanese prisoner-of-war camps in World War II. Clinically, there is a state of quiet confusion, lowered level of consciousness, and incoordination (fairly non-specific signs in an alcoholic). The characteristic feature is paralysis of one or more of the external movements of the eyes (ophthalmoplegia). This, and the lowered consciousness, respond to injection of thiamin within 2 days, but if treatment is delayed the memory may never recover. The memory disorder that is a sequel of Wernicke's encephalopathy is called Korsakoff's psychosis after the Russian psychologist who first described it. There is an inability to retain new memories and sometimes confabulation.

In people who die of Wernicke–Korsakoff syndrome lesions are found in the mamillary bodies, mid brain, and cerebellum. It is not clear why one deficient person develops beri beri and another develops Wernicke–Korsakoff syndrome and why the two diseases seldom coincide. Possibly, the cardiac disease occurs in people who use their muscles for heavy work and so accumulate large amounts of pyruvate, producing vasodilatation and increasing cardiac work, while encephalopathy is the first manifestation in inactive people.

13.1.5 Biochemical test

Red cell transketolase activity, with and without TPP added *in vitro*, is a good test. But heparinized whole blood must be used, it must be analysed fresh (or specially preserved) and the test will be normal if thiamin treatment has been already started. If the transketolase activity is increased more than 30% in the test tube with added TPP, this indicates at least some degree of biochemical thiamin deficiency. In Wernicke's encephalopathy this 'TPP effect' can be higher than this, around 70% or even 100%. (Note: in this test, reported as 'TPP effect', high values are abnormal.)

13.1.6 Interactions: nutrients

The requirement for thiamin is proportional to the intake of carbohydrates + alcohol + protein. In homogeneous societies, where proportions of fat and carbohydrate do not greatly differ, the thiamin requirement is proportional to the total energy intake.

There are no real stores of thiamin and the body runs out of it after about 3 weeks of starvation. When a malnourished person is given food (that uses thiamin), there is a danger of precipitating Wernicke's encephalopathy, e.g. with an intravenous glucose/water infusion. Thiamin should always be given with refeeding (see Chapter 42).

13.1.7 Food sources

There are no rich food sources of thiamin. The best sources in descending order are wheatgerm, whole wheat and products, yeast and yeast extracts, pulses, nuts, pork, duck, oatmeal, fortified breakfast cereals, cod's roe, and other meats. In many industrial countries (United Kingdom, North America, etc.), bread flour is enriched with thiamin and so are most breakfast cereals. Australia introduced mandatory fortification of bread flour with thiamin in 1991 and it has reduced that country's previously high rate of Wernicke–Korsakoff syndrome. Thiamin is readily destroyed by heat and by sulphite and by thiaminase (present in raw fish).

The recommended dietary intake (RDI) of thiamin is 0.4 mg per 1000 kcal (0.1 mg/kJ), (i.e. about 1.0 mg per day in adults). The toxicity of thiamin is very low.

13.2 Riboflavin

Vitamin B was originally considered to have two components, heat-labile B_1 thiamin) and heat-stable B_2. In the 1930s, it was discovered that a yellow growth factor (riboflavin) in this latter fraction is distinct from the pellagra-preventing substance (niacin).

13.2.1 Structure

Riboflavin or 7,8-dimethyl-10-(1′D-ribityl) isoallaxazine, comprises an alloxazine ring connected to a ribose alcohol—the ribityl side chain is required for full vitamin activity. It is a yellow-green fluorescent compound.

13.2.2 Functions

Riboflavin (Fig. 13.2) is part of two important coenzymes, flavin mononucleotide (FMN) and flavin adenine dinucleotide (FAD), which are oxidizing agents. They participate in flavoproteins in the oxidation chain in mitochondria. They are also cofactors for several enzymes, e.g. NADH dehydrogenase, xanthine oxidase, L-amino acid oxidase, glutathione reductase, L-gulonolactone oxidase, and methylene tetrahydrofolate reductase (MTHFR).

13.2.3 Absorption and metabolism

Absorption is by a specialized carrier system in the proximal small intestine, which is saturated at levels above 25 mg. The vitamin is transported as free riboflavin and FMN or bound to plasma albumin. The body contains only about 1 g of riboflavin, mostly found in the muscle as FAD. Riboflavin is excreted primarily in urine; urinary excretion tends to reflect dietary intake.

13.2.4 Deficiency in animals

The most common effects in animals are cessation of growth, dermatitis, hyperkeratosis, alopecia, and vascularization of the cornea. Abortion or skeletal

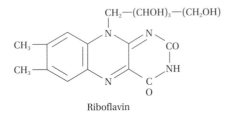

Riboflavin

Fig. 13.2 Structure of riboflavin. Ribitol is the alcohol form of the 5-carbon sugar, ribose. In FMN, two phosphates are attached to the end of the ribitol. In FAD, this is extended further with adenylate (ribose–adenine).

malformations of the fetus may occur. In some species, anaemia, fatty liver, and neurological changes have also been reported.

13.2.5 Deficiency in humans

The clinical symptoms of deficiency—angular stomatitis, cheilosis, atrophy of the tongue papillae, nasolabial dyssebacea, and anaemia—are surprisingly minor, presumably due to the body's ability to conserve riboflavin, and the high affinity of the coenzymes for their respective enzymes. Riboflavin deficiency (ariboflavinosis) is most commonly seen alongside other nutrient deficiencies (e.g. pellagra).

13.2.6 Biochemical tests

1 Erythrocyte glutathione reductase activity (EGRA) coefficient. FAD is cofactor for this enzyme and its activity correlates with riboflavin status.

The activity coefficient (or FAD effect)

$$= \frac{\text{EGRA with added FAD } in\ vitro}{\text{EGRA without FAD } in\ vitro}.$$

Values of < 1.2 are considered to be acceptable, but values of 1.3–1.7 indicate inadequate riboflavin status. However, some doubts have been raised about the validity of the FAD effect, as it is elevated during exercise and pregnancy.

2 Measurement of urinary excretion of riboflavin: non-vitamin flavins (from foods) can be excreted so a high-performance liquid chromatography-fluorometric method should be used to separate the riboflavin. Levels below 100 μg riboflavin/day are low.

13.2.7 Interactions: drugs

Phenothiazine derivatives (e.g. chlorpromazine) and tricyclic antidepressants have similar structures and can interfere with riboflavin metabolism. Reduced riboflavin status is observed in alcoholics, but is due more to decreased dietary intake and absorption, than to a direct effect of alcohol.

13.2.8 Food sources

Riboflavin is present in most foods, although the best sources are milk and milk products, eggs, liver, kidney, yeast extracts, and fortified breakfast cereals. Dairy products contribute significantly to riboflavin intake in Western diets. However, riboflavin is unstable in ultraviolet light, and after milk has been exposed to sunlight for 4 hours, up to 70% of riboflavin is lost.

The RDI for adults is about 1.3 mg/day. The requirement is less in people with small energy intakes and more in those with large energy intakes.

13.2.9 Toxic effects

The toxicity is very low. The gastrointestinal tract cannot absorb more than about 20–25 mg of riboflavin in a single dose.

13.3 Niacin

Niacin (Fig. 13.3) is a generic term for the related compounds that have activity as pellagra-preventing vitamins; the two that occur in foods are nicotinic acid (pyridine 3-carboxylic acid) and its amide, nicotinamide. They have apparently equal vitamin activity. Nicotinic acid is a fairly simple chemical (molecular weight 123) that was known long before its nutritional role was established. It was first isolated as an oxidation product of the natural alkaloid, nicotine, from which its name is derived. But nicotinic acid and amide have very different physiological properties from nicotine (which is α-N-methyl-D-β-pyridyl pyrrolidine).

13.3.1 Functions

Nicotinamide is part of the coenzymes nicotinamide-adenine dinucleotide (NAD) and nicotinamide-adenine-dinucleotide phosphate (NADP), the pyridine nucleotides. NAD has the

structure: adenine–ribose–PO_4–PO_4–ribose–nicotinamide. It plays a central role in metabolism: it functions as the first hydrogen receptor in the electron chain during oxidative phosphorylation in the mitochondria. The pyridine ring of the nicotinamide is the part of the molecule that takes up a hydrogen (NAD $\leftrightarrow$ NADH).

NADP has an extra PO_4 (phosphate) attached to the ribose adjacent to adenine. It has a more specialized function as hydrogen donor in fatty acid synthesis.

13.3.2 Absorption and metabolism

Nicotinic acid and its amide are water-soluble and well absorbed from the stomach and small intestine and are transported in solution in the plasma. Stores of niacin and its coenzymes are only small, and early features of pellagra can occur in human subjects after some 45 days of depletion.

13.3.3 Synthesis from tryptophan

A special feature of niacin is that in most conditions only about half of what is in the body is absorbed as preformed nicotinic acid or amide from the diet. About the same amount is synthesized in the

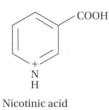

Nicotinic acid

Fig. 13.3 Structure of nicotinic acid (niacin). Nicotinamide is the corresponding amide, with $CONH_2$ in the side chain.

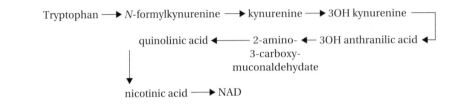

Tryptophan ⟶ *N*-formylkynurenine ⟶ kynurenine ⟶ 3OH kynurenine ⟶

quinolinic acid ⟵ 2-amino- ⟵ 3OH anthranilic acid ⟵
3-carboxy-
muconaldehydate

nicotinic acid ⟶ NAD

Fig. 13.4 Tryptophan conversion to NAD.

liver from tryptophan, the indole amino acid, in a sequence of seven enzyme steps down the kynurenine pathway.

Most tryptophan in the body is used for protein synthesis—it is the least abundant in foods of all the essential amino acids—some also goes to serotonin. The rest goes down the kynurenine pathway (Fig. 13.4). Approximately 60 mg tryptophan has been shown in humans to convert to 1 mg of niacin. The first enzyme in the kynurenine pathway, hepatic tryptophan oxygenase, is under hormonal control, and the amount of niacin formed appears to be increased in pregnancy. It is downregulated when the protein intake is inadequate (Fig. 13.4).

13.3.4 Deficiency in animals

The classic animal model for pellagra is 'black tongue' in dogs. Puppies lose their appetite and have inflamed gums, dark tongue, and diarrhoea with blood. Elvehjem's group at Wisconsin tested different fractions of liver for their ability to cure black tongue and in 1937 found that the 'pellagra-preventing factor' was nicotinamide.

13.3.5 Deficiency in humans

There is one deficiency disease, *pellagra* (the name means 'sour skin' in Italian). The skin is inflamed where it is exposed to sunlight, resembling severe sunburn but the affected skin is sharply demarcated. The skin lesions progress to pigmentation, cracking, and peeling. Often the skin of the neck is involved (Casal's collar) (Fig. 13.5). Students are taught that pellagra is the disease of three Ds: dermatitis, diarrhoea, and delirium or dementia. As well as diarrhoea there is likely to be an inflamed tongue (glossitis). In mild chronic cases, mental symptoms

(the third 'D') are not prominent. It is hard to explain the clinical manifestations by the known biochemical functions of niacin. Because some niacin is formed from tryptophan, pellagra can be cured by giving either niacin or a generous intake of easily assimilated protein.

Pellagra appeared in Europe after maize was introduced as a cereal crop from the new world after 1500, but the Mayas, Aztecs, and indigenous North Americans do not seem to have suffered from pellagra.

There was a major epidemic of pellagra in poor people (share croppers) in the southern states of the USA from around 1905. It was generally thought to be an infectious disease, but Joseph

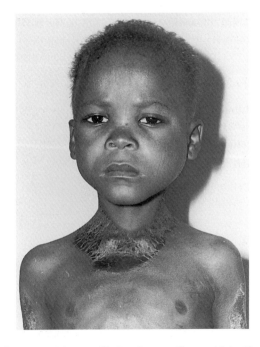

Fig. 13.5 A boy suffering from pellagra. Note the Casal's collar and lesions on outer arms.

Goldberger, investigating for the Federal government between 1914 and 1929, demonstrated by epidemiology and crucial human experiments that it was due to a diet of maize grits and little else. He identified an animal model, black tongue in dogs (rats are not susceptible), cured by yeast in which the pellagra-preventing factor eventually turned out to be nicotinamide, already known in tissue culture biochemistry.

The niacin in cereals is in a complex, 'niacytin', which humans cannot absorb, so that although it appears in food tables (because the complex is split during extraction), it is not biologically available. If subsistence farmers eat a diet predominantly of maize, with few other foods, their niacin has to come from tryptophan in the protein of the cereal. But the protein of maize is deficient in tryptophan, unlike other cereals, so little or no niacin can be made in the body via the kynurenine pathway. All cereals are low in lysine but maize has less tryptophan than wheat and rice. In pre-Columban America, the ground maize was steeped in warm lime water (calcium hydroxide), which liberates the niacin (making it biologically available), and then made into tortillas, flat cakes—as it still is today in Mexico and Guatemala.

Pellagra is rare in developed countries. It occurs in parts of Africa.

13.3.6 Biochemical tests

1 Urinary N'-methylnicotinamide (and/or its 2-pyridone) is the best-known test, but tests that require a 24-hour urine are inconvenient.

2 Red cell NAD concentration.

3 Fasting plasma tryptophan.

13.3.7 Interactions: nutrients

The most important is that tryptophan and hence dietary proteins (except in maize) provide niacin. Tryptophan makes up about 1% of mixed dietary proteins so 6 g protein (60 mg tryptophan) = 1 mg niacin, hence a protein intake of 70 g/day is equivalent to about 12 mg niacin. The niacin requirement is thought to be proportional to the energy expenditure or energy intake.

Two of the enzymes in the kynurenine pathway are vitamin B_6 dependent, so vitamin B_6 deficiency is likely to reduce niacin synthesis from tryptophan.

13.3.8 Food sources

Good sources of preformed niacin, in descending order, are liver and kidney (the richest sources), other meat, poultry, fish, brewer's yeast and yeast extracts, peanuts, bran, pulses, wholemeal wheat, and (surprisingly) coffee, including instant coffee. Other foods that are rich in protein provide tryptophan. If food tables give values for milligram niacin equivalents (NE), this is preformed niacin, mg + (tryptophan ÷ 60). The British food tables (McCance and Widdowson) have separate columns for 'nicotinic acid' and for 'potential nicotinic acid from tryptophan, mg tryptophan ÷ 60'. From this one can see, e.g. that 100 g fresh whole cow's milk provides 0.08 mg preformed niacin but 0.80 mg potential niacin from tryptophan.

The RDI for niacin in adults, expressed as NE is 6.6 mg NE per 1000 kcal (1.6 mg NE per 1000 kJ): in absolute numbers, about 14 mg in women and 16 mg in men.

13.3.9 Pharmacological doses

Well above the nutrient dose, nicotinic acid (but not the amide) produces cutaneous flushing from histamine release, at doses of 100 mg/day or more; it has been used for chilblains. At doses of 3 g/day or more (200 × RDI), nicotinic acid inhibits lipolysis in adipose tissue and lowers plasma triglyceride and cholesterol. It is in the pharmacopoeia as a second-line drug for combined hyperlipidaemia (i.e. high plasma cholesterol plus raised triglycerides). Side effects, as well as flushing, include gastric irritation, impaired glucose tolerance, and disturbed liver function tests.

13.4 Vitamin B$_6$

13.4.1 Structure

Vitamin B$_6$ (Fig. 13.6) occurs in nature in three forms—pyridoxine, pyridoxal, and pyridoxamine—which are interconvertible within the body. Each form (vitamer) also occurs as a phosphorylated compound: the principal one in the body, and in food is pyridoxal 5'-phosphate (PLP).

13.4.2 Functions

The major coenzyme form in the body is PLP. It functions in practically all the reactions involved in amino acid metabolism, including:

1 transaminations, and synthesis of non-essential amino acids;

2 deamination of serine and threonine;

3 metabolism of sulphur-containing amino acids including homocysteine;

4 decarboxylations:

   (a) formation of neurotransmitters adrenalin, nor-adrenalin, serotonin, and γ-amino butyric acid (GABA)

   (b) formation of δ-aminolaevulinic acid, which is the first step in porphyrin synthesis, making haemoglobin

   (c) synthesis of sphingomyelin and phosphatidyl choline (lecithin)

   (d) synthesis of taurine, a conjugator of bile acids and important in eye and brain function

5 kynureninase: for the conversion of tryptophan to niacin. When this reaction is impaired, xan-thurenic acid (major metabolite of 3(OH) kynure-nine) accumulates in the urine, which is used as biochemical marker for B$_6$ status.

However, the role of vitamin B$_6$ is not restricted to protein metabolism. Over half of total body B$_6$ is associated with glycogen phosphorylase enzyme in the muscles, which releases glucose as glucose 1-phosphate from glycogen stores. PLP may also have a role in modulating steroid hormone receptors.

13.4.3 Absorption and metabolism

In the small intestine vitamin B$_6$ is absorbed by passive diffusion, mainly in the unphosphorylated form. Even large doses are well absorbed. The different forms of the vitamin are rapidly converted to pyridoxal in the intestinal cell, by the FMN-requiring enzyme, pyridoxal phosphate oxidase. Pyridoxal is transported in the circulation largely bound to albumin and haemoglobin, and after diffusion into cells, pyridoxal is rephosphorylated by pyridoxal kinase, which maintains it within the cells.

The total body content of vitamin B$_6$ is estimated to be between 50 and 150 mg in adults. Most of this (90%) is tightly bound in tissues. Vitamin B$_6$ in the liver, brain, kidney, spleen, and muscle is bound to protein, which protects it from hydrolysis. The major metabolite of vitamin B$_6$ is 4-pyridoxic acid, which is inactive as a vitamin and excreted in the urine.

13.4.4 Deficiency in animals

Dermatological and neurological changes are commonly observed in animals when vitamin B$_6$ is deficient. In rats, impaired growth, muscular weakness, irritability, dermatitis, anaemia, fatty liver, impaired immune function, hypertension, and insulin insufficiency have all been observed. Neurological changes include convulsions.

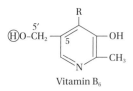

Vitamin B$_6$

Fig. 13.6 Structure of vitamin B$_6$. In pyridoxine, R = CH$_2$OH; in pyridoxal, R = CHO; in pyridoxamine, R = CH$_2$NH$_2$. In coenzyme forms, phosphate replaces the ringed H.

13.4.5 Deficiency in humans

The symptoms of deficiency in humans are general weakness, sleeplessness, peripheral neuropathy, personality changes, dermatitis, cheilosis and glossitis (as in riboflavin deficiency), anaemia, and impaired immunity. Deficiency on its own is rare; it is most often seen with deficiencies of other vitamins, or with protein deficiency. In 1953, a minor epidemic of convulsions in infants in the USA was traced to a milk formula which contained no vitamin B$_6$ because of a manufacturing error. Convulsions in pyridoxine deficiency are probably due to impaired synthesis of γ-aminobutyric acid (GABA), the major inhibitory neurotransmitter in the brain.

13.4.6 Deficiency: secondary

A number of inborn errors of amino acid metabolism may respond to supranutritional doses of pyridoxine. Hyperhomocysteinaemia, a condition which may increase the risk for cardiovascular disease, responds to supplements of folate, vitamin B$_{12}$, and sometimes B$_6$.

Low vitamin B$_6$ status is common in chronic alcoholics, who may have impaired absorption. Acetaldehyde (oxidation product of ethanol) can inhibit the conversion of pyridoxine to PLP.

Pregnant women have a decrease in plasma PLP levels. It is unclear whether this indicates a deficiency or is a normal physiological change.

13.4.7 Biochemical tests

1 Measurement of plasma PLP. Normal levels are above about 30 nmol/L.

2 Increased urinary xanthurenic acid after a load of the amino acid, tryptophan.

3 Activity of erythrocyte alanine aminotransferase, with and without *in vitro* PLP.

4 Urinary 4-pyridoxic acid.

13.4.8 Interactions: other nutrients

High protein intakes increase metabolic demand for vitamin B$_6$.

13.4.9 Interactions: drugs

Isoniazid (used to treat tuberculosis), increases urinary excretion of vitamin B$_6$. Several drugs including cycloserine, gentamicin, penicillamine, L-DOPA, and phenelzine are vitamin B$_6$ antagonists. Some biochemical indices of vitamin B$_6$ state may be abnormal in a proportion of women taking oral contraceptives, but these are indirect indices (e.g. alanine aminotransferase).

13.4.10 Food sources

The vitamin is distributed in a wide range of unprocessed (or lightly processed) foods. Major food sources in the Western diet are meats, whole grain products, vegetables, bananas, and nuts. Refined cereal products such as white bread and white rice are not significant sources of vitamin B$_6$ due to milling losses.

The RDI is 0.02 mg vitamin B$_6$ per gram of protein intake, which works out to about 1.5 mg/day in average adults.

13.4.11 Pharmacological doses

Pharmaceutical preparations, tablets of pyridoxine HCl are indicated for several rare inborn errors of metabolism. They are used for radiation sickness and for premenstrual syndrome. The few controlled trials for the latter condition are unimpressive. Vitamin B$_6$ can contribute to lowering raised plasma homocysteine (though folic acid usually has more effect). Whether it has value in reducing the risk of cardiovascular disease is not clear at present.

13.4.12 Toxic effects

Vitamin B_6 toxicity was first reported in women taking supplements of very large doses of pyridoxine (2000–6000 mg/day). These supplements were taken for premenstrual syndrome or carpal tunnel syndrome and the women developed peripheral neuropathy and lost sensation in their feet. Intakes of supplements down to 200 mg/day ($133 \times$ RDI) have been associated with neuropathy. The upper intake level (UIL) set by the US Institute of Medicine is 100 mg/day. This can only be obtained from supplements. The amount of vitamin B_6 obtainable from foods is far below this.

13.5 Biotin

13.5.1 Functions

Biotin is a coenzyme for several carboxylase enzymes: pyruvate carboxylase (formation of oxaloacetate for the tricarboxylic acid cycle), acetyl CoA (coenzyme A), carboxylase (fatty acid synthesis), propionyl CoA carboxylase (catabolism of odd-chain fatty acids and some amino acids), and 3-methylcrotonyl CoA carboxylase (catabolism of the ketogenic amino acid leucine).

13.5.2 Deficiency: animals and humans

Biotin deficiency is very rare as biotin is found in a wide range of foods, and bacterial production in the large intestine appears to supplement dietary intake. Deficiency can, however, be produced when animals or humans eat large amounts of uncooked egg white, which contains avidin. This tightly binds biotin in the gut, preventing absorption. Avidin is destroyed by heating. 'Egg white injury' (e.g. biotin deficiency) impairs lipid and energy metabolism in animals. It produces seborrhoeic dermatitis, alopecia, and paralysis of the hind limbs in rats and mice.

In humans, cases of biotin deficiency have been associated with a red scaly skin rash (altered fatty acid metabolism may contribute to this skin condition), glossitis, loss of hair, anorexia, depression, and hypercholesterolaemia. Some cases of seborrhoeic dermatitis in young breastfed infants have responded to administration of biotin to the mother. Human milk contains much less biotin than cows' milk. Biotin deficiency has been reported in patients on total parenteral nutrition whose infusions did not contain biotin. The human requirement is estimated to be about 30 µg/day. In experimental human biotin deficiency (feeding egg whites), the biochemical indicators have been reduced urinary biotin and increased 3-hydroxyisovaleric acid (that should normally be metabolized by 3-methylcrotonyl CoA carboxylase).

13.6 Pantothenic acid

Coenzymes often contain unusual structures—unusual in the sense that higher animals have lost the ability to form them and they must be supplied in the diet. For coenzyme A it is pantothenic acid.

13.6.1 Functions

Pantothenic acid is part of coenzyme A (CoA) and acyl carrier protein (ACP). CoA and ACP are both carriers of acyl groups. Acetyl-CoA participates in the tricarboxylic acid cycle in the disposal of carbohydrates and ketogenic amino acids. CoA is also involved in the synthesis of lipids—fatty acids, glycerides, cholesterol, ketone bodies, and sphingosine—and in acylation of proteins. ACP is involved in chain elongation during fatty acid synthesis.

Pantothenic acid is transported primarily in the CoA form by red cells in the blood, and is taken up into cells by a specific carrier protein. The highest concentrations of the vitamin are found in the liver, adrenals, kidney, brain, heart, and testes. Most is in the CoA form.

All tissues are able to synthesize CoA from pantothenic acid. ACP is synthesized from a 4-phosphopantetheine residue transferred from CoA. These metabolically active forms can be degraded to free pantothenic acid, which is the major form of excretion in the urine. Urinary pantothenic acid reflects dietary intake, ranging from 2 to 7 mg/day in adults.

13.6.2 Deficiency: animals

In most species, pantothenic acid deficiency is associated with dermatitis, changes to hair or feathers, anaemia, infertility, irritability, ataxia, paralysis, convulsions, and even death. In rats, a condition called 'bloody whiskers' is caused by release of protoporphyrin via the nose and tear ducts.

13.6.3 Deficiency: humans

Spontaneous human deficiency has never been described. As pantothenic acid is so widely distributed in foods, any dietary deficiency in humans is usually associated with other nutrient deficiencies. The word 'pantothen' means 'from everywhere' (Greek), but highly refined foods do not contain pantothenic acid.

Subjects given the antagonist ω-methylpantothenic acid, developed a deficiency with symptoms of depression, fatigue, insomnia, vomiting, muscle weakness, and a burning sensation in the feet. Changes in glucose tolerance, an increase in insulin sensitivity, postural hypotension, and decreased antibody production were also noted.

During World War II, malnourished prisoners of war in the Far East developed 'burning feet syndrome' which appeared to respond to large doses of Ca-pantothenate, but not to other B complex vitamins.

There is insufficient evidence to derive a requirement figure for pantothenate. The US/Canadian adequate intake is 5 mg/day, based on estimated usual intakes and urinary pantothenate excretion. It must be provided in total parenteral nutrition.

13.7 Folate

Folate is used as the generic name for compounds chemically related to pteroyl glutamic acid, folic acid. Deficiency of folate is quite common in hospital patients, secondary to diseases, especially intestinal, neoplastic, and haematological. Requirements are notably increased in pregnancy. The word 'folic' is from the Latin 'folia' (leaf), coined in 1941 for an early preparation of this vitamin from spinach leaves.

13.7.1 Structure

Folic acid (pteroyl glutamic acid) is the primary vitamin from the chemical point of view, and it is the pharmaceutical form (and used for food fortification) because of its stability. But it is rare (naturally occurring) in foods and in the body. Most folates are in the reduced form, tetrahydrofolate (THF); they also have 1-carbon components (methyl or formyl) attached to nitrogen atom 5 or 10, or bridging between them (5,10-methylene THF) (Fig. 13.7). In addition, they have up to seven glutamic acid residues in a row (at the right in Fig. 13.7).

13.7.2 Functions

Tetrahydrofolate plays an essential role in 1-carbon transfers in the body. It receives 1-carbon radicals from e.g. serine, glycine, histidine, and tryptophan, and donates them at two steps in purine synthesis and one important step in pyrimidine synthesis: insertion of the methyl group in deoxyuridylic acid to form thymidylic acid, the characteristic nucleotide

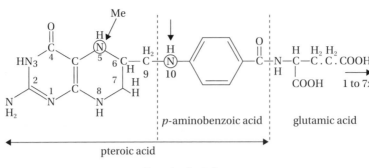

Fig. 13.7 Tetrahydrofolate (pteroyl glutamic acid) monoglutamate: folic acid with extra hydrogens at 5, 6, 7, and 8.

of DNA. The folate derivative involved here is 5,10-methylene THF.

5-Methyl THF cooperates with vitamin B_{12} in the action of methionine synthase, which adds a methyl group to homocysteine and forms methionine and THF (from which 5,10-methylene THF can be formed). When vitamin B_{12} is deficient, folate is trapped as the 5-methyl compound and 5,10-methylene THF is not available to form thymidylate for DNA synthesis (Fig. 13.8).

13.7.3 Absorption and metabolism

Most food folates are in polyglutamate form. These are hydrolysed in the gut by folate conjugase (γ-glutamylhydrolase) and absorbed as monoglutamate. Most food folates are in reduced form as THF. Folic acid is reduced to THF in the process of absorption. Folate is present in plasma mainly as 5-methyl THF. Inside cells it is usually in polyglutamate form. Total body folate has been estimated at about 10 mg, half being in the liver. Very little is excreted in the urine. More is excreted in the bile and about half of this is re-absorbed.

13.7.4 Deficiency in animals

Chicks show reduced growth, anaemia, and impaired feather growth. In guinea-pigs there is a low white blood cell count and growth failure.

13.7.5 Deficiency in humans

Folate is the final anti-megaloblastic substance. In deficiency, the basic abnormality is reduced ability of cells to double their nuclear DNA, in order to divide, because of impaired synthesis of thymidylate.

There is megaloblastic anaemia (cells are enlarged, their nuclei large but with reduced density of chromatin) and similar changes in leukocytes, platelets, and epithelial cells; there is also infertility and may be diarrhoea.

Pure dietary deficiency is seen occasionally. In a previously healthy physician, Victor Herbert, experimental depletion resulted in anaemia after 125 days, with biochemical and histological changes before this. But when there is increased cell proliferation or interference with folate metabolism features of deficiency appear earlier. Secondary deficiency is common in late pregnancy, in alcoholics, in haemolytic anaemias, uraemia, intensive hospital therapy, and people with malabsorption.

13.7.6 Benefits of extra folate

Folate is important at both ends of pregnancy. In late pregnancy megaloblastic anaemia can occur, especially in women in developing countries. This was first described in India by Dr Lucy Wills in 1931 before folic acid was isolated. This anaemia can sometimes be first noticed in the early weeks after childbirth.

In affluent countries too low serum folate and megaloblastic anaemia is possible and is prevented with routine folic acid tablets, sometimes combined with iron.

Neutral tube defects Folic acid supplements have more recently been found to reduce the risk of serious fetal malformations, spinal bifida, and anencephaly, together termed neural tube defects.

In human embryology the neural tube closes at days 24 to 28 after conception and the extra folate must be taken before this (i.e. often before the woman may be sure she is pregnant). In the UK, trial by Medical Research Council Vitamin Study Group (1991), women in several countries who had previously had a baby affected by neural tube defect agreed to take one of four different nutritional supplements periconceptionally, i.e. before as well as during pregnancy. It was found that those taking supplements containing folic acid had 70% fewer deformed babies. Other trials and cohort studies have been supportive. From studies of serum folate of women who were subsequently found to have an abnormal baby, it appears that the neural tube defet is not caused by a deficiency but by a need for extra folate in some women at this time of extra cell division in embryonic development. There is also evidence based on multivitamin use that extra folate reduces the risk of congenital heart defects.

Increased plasma homocysteine Epidemiological evidence accumulated in the 1990s that a raised plasma homocysteine is a risk factor for cardiovascular diseases (chapter 21) and also for the development of dementia (Seshadri et al., 2002). Homocysteine is derived from the aminoacid methionine—it is methionine minus its methyl group—and folic acid supplements increase the activity of methionine synthase, which remethylates homocysteine back to methionine. Extra vitamins B_{12} and B_6 augment this effect.

13.7.7 Folate fortification

Neural tube defect is a very serious deformity and relatively common. With the evidence that folic acid can largely prevent it, there are three options:

1 nutrition education—encourage women aiming to become pregnant to eat more foods with higher folate content;

2 advise such women to take a tablet of 0.4 or 0.5 mg folic acid daily;

3 fortify the national food supply with folic acid.

Option 1 is least efficient. The extra folate has to be taken periconceptionally before the woman is sure she is pregnant. Option 2 will only help woman who are both planning pregnancy and have good health information.

On 1 January 1998 the USA and Canada took the major step of enacting mandatory fortification of all cereal grains (bread, flour, pasta, breakfast cereals, and rice) with folic acid at 140 µg per 100 g of grain food. This was a giant nutrition experiment providing the extra folate needed for pregnancy, but possibly giving the rest of the population more folate than they needed.

Chile and Costa Rica followed North America. Other countries have debated and waited or made smaller moves. In Australia, for example, voluntary folate fortification of certain foods were permitted from 1995 and mandatory fortification of bread flour was introduced in 2009.

In North America, folate intake went up by nearly 200 µg/day, more than had been intended, perhaps from overages added by cereal manufacturers. Serum folate doubled (Jacques et al., 1999) and neural tube defects were roughly halved in North America (Ray, 2004). Homocysteine levels declined (Jacques et al., 1999). There was no change in serum vitamin B_{12} and no masking reported of vitamin B_{12} deficiency.

Have there been other benefits or adverse effects? With increasing pharmaceutical and surgical treatment of cardiovascular diseases (CVD) it is not possible to distinguish any national folic acid effect, and so far the randomized controlled trials of folic acid, with or without vitamin B_{12} and B_6 have not shown significant reduction of CVD. National statistics on incidence of dementia are probably impossible to obtain. There is substantial epidemiological evidence that raised plasma homocysteine predisposes to dementia, but randomized controlled trials with folic acid have yielded mixed results (Durga et al., 2007).

In the big picture there was a small 3-year upswing in the declining tread of incidence of colorectal cancer in both USA and (separately) in Canada (Mason *et al.*, 2007). In one of the trials of folic acid and vitamin B$_{12}$, in Norway (where grain foods are not fortified) those on extra vitamins had developed more cancer (Ebbing *et al.*, 2009). After this colorectal cancer incidence continued down in the USA and is now lower than when folate fortification started.

In the USA, on top of folate fortification of grains about a third of adults take multivitamin supplements that include folic acid so that 5% of older men now consume more than the recommended UIL (see Section 13.7.11). It appears that if people on high folate intakes have very low serum B$_{12}$ they have more severe clinical and biochemical effects of the B$_{12}$ deficiency (Selhub *et al.*, 2009).

Another change that has been observed is that there is now more free folic acid in serum that there was in sera collected before fortification and stored. The significance of this is not clear and it does not seem to affect breast milk.

13.7.8 Interactions

Folate interacts with vitamin B$_{12}$ (see Section 13.8.7). Vitamin C in foods reduces loss of folate in cooking. Several drugs interfere with folate metabolism, most of them by antagonizing dihydrofolate reductase (which converts 2H folate to 4H folate, i.e. THF): methotrexate, aminopterin, amethopterin (used for chemotherapy for cancer), pyrimethamine (antimalarial), cotrimoxazole (antibacterial). Most of the antiepileptic drugs (carbamazepine, phenytoin, valproate) if taken through early pregnancy increase the risk of neural tube defect in the fetus. When they are prescribed, folic acid, at the higher dose of 5 mg/day should be taken periconceptionally.

13.7.9 Genetics

A fairly common single nucleotide polymorphism in the gene for MTHFR, the 667 C → T mutation, affects the activity of this enzyme. Overall, around 10% of people are homozygous for the TT allele (with a range in different communities for 1–20%).

They have reduced activity of MTHFR so that availability of methyl THF, hence THF is lower (Fig. 13.8). They have been found to have lower blood folates (hence higher requirement) and also increased risk of neural tube defects, higher plasma homocysteines, but not more cardiovascular disease.

13.7.10 Biochemical tests

Serum folate reflects recent intake, but not yesterday's. Levels continue upwards for about 3 weeks when intake is moved to a fixed higher level (Truswell and Kounnavong, 1997). Levels below 7 nmol/L (3 ng/mL) reflect deficiency. Since fortification, levels in North America are around 24 nmol/L and higher in those taking supplements. Red cell folate reflects cellular status. It is normally above 225 nmol/L (100 ng/mL).

13.7.11 Recommended intakes

The Institute of Medicine (Food and Nutrition Board and Institute of Medicine, 1998) for USA and Canada recommends (RDI) 400 µg per day of dietary folate equivalents (DFEs) for men and women and for the latter 600 µg/day in pregnancy and 500 µg/day in lactation. The upper level is 1000 µg/day as folic acid or fortified food for adults. Australia and New Zealand followed in 2005 with the same recommendations.

DFEs adjust for better absorption of free folic acid compared with folate naturally in foods (Bailey, 1998). 1 µg of food folate = 0.6 µg of folic acid added to foods or taken with food = 0.5 µg of folic acid supplement taken on an empty stomach.

13.7.12 Food sources

Although the name comes from Latin 'folia' (leaf), and it does occur in leafy vegetables (spinach, broccoli, cabbage, lettuce) folate occurs also in other foods: liver, kidney, beans, beetroot, bran, peanuts, yeast extract, avocadoes, bananas, wholemeal bread, eggs, and some fish. There is even a little folate in beer and tea. In the USA and Canada, all

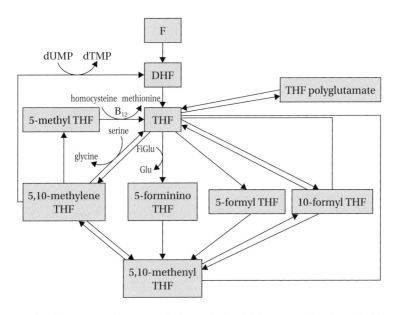

Fig. 13.8 Folate mechanism. Note that 5-methyltetrahydrofolate can only return to the pool for other functions if there is enough vitamin B$_{12}$ for the homocysteine → methionine reaction, which takes up the methyl group. In the reaction of dUMP → dTMP, dTMP is thymidylate, one of the four essential bases of DNA. If there is insufficient 5,10-methylene tetrahydrofolate (the specific cofactor), DNA synthesis is reduced or stops. F, folate; DHF, dihydrofolate; FiGLU, foriminoglutamic acid; THF, tetrahydrofolate.

cereal products have to be fortified with folate. In other countries, voluntary fortification is permitted so that food tables may be out of date in their folate content of foods. Many breakfast cereals and some breads are now fortified with extra folic acid.

Pure folic acid as the supplement is about twice as bioavailable as most food folates. Also the folic acid added in fortifying food is more available than the intrinsic folate in most foods. The US Institute of Medicine proposes the use of DFEs.

Analysis of folate in foods is difficult because of the multiple compounds. Early analyses used microbiological assay, but human cells may not respond to different folate compounds in the same way as bacteria. Some recent methods are based on the major peaks on HPLC (high-performance liquid chromatography). Folate is destroyed in foods by prolonged boiling.

13.7.13 Toxicity

The main concern is that if someone with vitamin B$_{12}$ deficiency (pernicious anaemia) is treated with a fairly high (supranutritional) dose of folic acid (5 mg/day) the anaemia may improve but the biochemical basis for the neurological symptoms of vitamin B$_{12}$ deficiency is not corrected, so correct biochemical diagnosis with serum B$_{12}$ and folate is essential before anyone is treated for anaemia with folic acid. Otherwise, the toxicity of folic acid is low.

13.8 Vitamin B$_{12}$

In the late 1920s it was postulated that human gastric juice contained an 'intrinsic factor' which combined with an 'extrinsic factor' in animal protein foods (notably raw liver) and that the combination would cure a type of anaemia that was until then untreatable, pernicious anaemia. In 1948 the extrinsic factor, vitamin B_{12}, was identified and human intrinsic factor was isolated in the 1960s.

13.8.1 Structure

Vitamin B_{12} or cobalamin is a red compound containing a corrinoid ring (four pyrrole rings) with an atom of cobalt in its centre. It is only synthesized by bacteria. Vitamin B_{12} has the largest molecule of the vitamins, with a molecular weight of 1355. The structure is large and three-dimensional—to view it, refer to a good textbook of biochemistry. Dorothy Hodgkin was awarded the Nobel Prize (Chemistry, 1964) for elucidating vitamin B_{12}'s structure by X-ray-crystallography.

13.8.2 Functions

The coenzyme forms of vitamin B_{12} are methylcobalamin and deoxyadenosylcobalamin. Only two B_{12}-dependent enzymes have been identified in humans: methylmalonyl-CoA mutase (which requires deoxyadenosylcobalamin) and methionine synthase (which requires methylcobalamin).

Methylmalonyl-CoA mutase is involved in the conversion of methylmalonyl-CoA to succinyl-CoA in the catabolism of propionate, in the mitochondria.

Methionine synthase, found in the cytosol, transfers a methyl group from the donor 5-methyl THF to homocysteine to produce methionine (Fig. 13.8). Increased plasma homocysteine, a condition which may increase the risk for vascular disease, responds to supplements of vitamins B_{12}, folate, and B_6.

13.8.3 Absorption and metabolism

Absorption of vitamin B_{12} is by a highly specific mechanism. It first has to be released from its binding to animal proteins in food. This requires pepsin and acid in the stomach. When gastric acid is secreted after a meal, the parietal cells at the same time release the specific glycoprotein, intrinsic fac-

tor (IF). This doesn't attach to vitamin B_{12} until they are both in the duodenum. (While in the stomach, B_{12} is attached to R-binder (haptocorrin) from the saliva, which is digested in the duodenum.) The B_{12}/IF complex passes down the small intestine and in the terminal ileum there are specific receptors for IF. The B_{12}/IF complex is absorbed and after 2–3 hours, vitamin B_{12} appears in the blood stream carried on transcobalamin II (TCII) the main B_{12} transport protein.

Vitamin B_{12} is concentrated, stored in the liver. It is excreted in the bile into the duodenum, where much of it combines with IF (secreted after a meal) and also gets absorbed in the terminal ileum. This enterohepatic cycle helps to conserve the vitamin.

Some anaerobic bacteria in the large intestine can synthesize vitamin B_{12}. But this is formed below the ileal receptor site so it is not likely to be absorbed.

The total body store is estimated to range from only 3–5 mg but enough for several years! Only about 0.2% of total body stores (2–5 µg) are excreted daily. The requirement is only 2 µg/day.

13.8.4 Deficiency in animals

The most common signs of deficiency in animals are lack of growth and reduced food intake. Alterations in lipid metabolism occur—fatty liver, increase in triglycerides, and free fatty acids. In pigs, a mild anaemia is observed. Neurological changes have been observed in monkeys after 3–5 years on a vitamin B_{12}-deficient diet, and in fruit bats after 7 months.

13.8.5 Deficiency in humans

Vegans Very strict vegetarian (vegan) diets containing no fish, poultry, eggs, or dairy products, and without vitamin supplements, contain practically no vitamin B_{12}. Vegans have low circulating levels of vitamin B_{12} but clinical symptoms are surprisingly uncommon. Normal body stores of the vitamin are sufficient to last for 2–5 years. Bacteria in the intestine produce some vitamin B_{12} that might perhaps be absorbed from the caecum, but the bioavailability of such B_{12} is uncertain. However, infants breastfed by strict vegan mothers are at serious risk of impaired neurological development, anaemia, and even severe encephalopathy (Von Shenck *et al.*, 1997). Vegans are advised to take vitamin B_{12} tablets or foods fortified with B_{12} (produced microbiologically, i.e. not from an animal source). But for breastfed vegan infants, vitamin B_{12} supplements are essential.

Pernicious anaemia and vitamin B_{12} neuropathy Inadequate dietary intake is not the usual cause of clinical vitamin B_{12} deficiency. Most common is malabsorption due to an autoimmune atrophy of the gastric mucosa so there is failure to produce IF. Other less common causes include total gastrectomy and disease of the terminal ileum. Severe vitamin B_{12} deficiency from gastric atrophy is called pernicious anaemia because it used to be untreatable. There are two effects of vitamin B_{12} deficiency: megaloblastic anaemia and/or neurological dysfunction. Anaemia usually precedes neurological symptoms, but not always. Anaemia is megaloblastic, so-called because blood cells are characteristically large with reduced nuclear density, and white cells, platelets, and epithelial cells are also affected the same way. Vitamin B_{12} deficiency interrupts normal nuclear division by 'trapping' folate, leading to a reduction in the synthesis of DNA (see Section 13.7). The anaemia is morphologically the same in folate and vitamin B_{12} deficiency. Biochemical tests have to be used to distinguish between them. An injection of $100\,\mu g$/month will successfully treat pernicious anaemia but high oral doses (working by passive absorption) are also used.

The characteristic *neuropathy* of vitamin B_{12} deficiency is subacute combined degeneration of the spinal cord. There is loss of position sense and spastic weakness in the lower limbs due to demyelination of the posterior and lateral (pyramidal) tracts (upper motor neurone). Sometimes the nervous system can be affected in other ways, e.g. with neuropsychiatric disorders. There is not always an accompanying anaemia. Serum vitamin B_{12} is subnormal and symptoms should respond to vitamin B_{12} treatment, though more slowly than the anaemia.

Spinal cord disease is not seen in folate deficiency. The biochemical basis of the pernicious anaemia involves an interaction with folate; the neurological disease does not. The most likely explanation of the neuropathy is impaired methylation of myelin basic protein from deficient methionine synthase.

Subclinical vitamin B_{12} deficiency Pernicious anaemia, being a serious clinical disease has been known since it was first described by Addison in 1894. But in recent years, since serum vitamin B_{12} assays have been generally available, it has been found that subnormal levels of serum B_{12} occur in 10% or more of old people without anaemia in developed countries. Serum methylmalonate is raised; absorption of crystalline vitamin B_{12} is normal. In a proportion of cases, loss of gastric acid and failure to free B_{12} from protein binding in food is the probable cause. Apart from raised homocysteine (a risk factor for cardiovascular disease and dementia), no consistent serious effect has been found. The Institute of Medicine recommends for older people that part of the intake of vitamin B_{12} should be in crystalline form, e.g. fortified food or in multivitamins. Other RDI committees (e.g. Australia and New Zealand) have not yet followed this advice.

13.8.6 Biochemical tests

Serum vitamin B_{12} can be assessed by radioligand-binding assay or microbiological assay. Normal levels range from 200 to 900 pg/mL, ($pg = 10^{-12}$ g) or over 150 pmol/L. Deficiency is indicated by values below this. Concentrations of vitamin B_{12} in serum are exceedingly small; different methods are available. Serum B_{12} results are not always reliable so two other biochemical tests are useful.

Elevated serum or urinary excretion of methylmalonate and raised plasma homocysteine are the other biochemical tests, indicating low B_{12} status. Methylmalonate is more specific because homocysteine is also elevated with folate deficiency. The Schilling test is used to confirm the diagnosis of pernicious anaemia. It measures absorption of oral vitamin B_{12} labelled with radioactive cobalt on two occasions, the first without and the second test with IF.

13.8.7 Interactions: nutrients

In vitamin B_{12} deficiency, 5-methyl THF accumulates due to decreased activity of methionine synthase, thus holding folate in what is termed the 'methyl-folate trap'. The ultimate cause of megaloblastic anaemia is impaired conversion of deoxyuridylic acid to thymidylic acid and so DNA synthesis is impaired, because of lack of 5,10-methylene THF.

13.8.8 Food sources

As vitamin B_{12} is synthesized by microorganisms, the vitamin is only found in bacterially fermented foods, or meat and offal from ruminant animals in which the vitamin is synthesized by ruminal microflora. The richest source of the vitamin is liver. Other sources include shellfish, fish, meat, eggs, milk, cheeses, and yoghurt.

Not all corrinoids exhibit vitamin B_{12} activity. In spirulina—a type of algae often promoted as a source of B_{12} for vegetarians—80% of the corrinoids do not have vitamin B_{12} activity. Up to 30% of the B_{12} in supplement pills may be analogue(s) of B_{12} with little or no activity.

The RDI of vitamin B_{12} is very small: in adults it is 2.5 µg/day.

13.8.9 Toxic effects

Oral intakes of several hundred times the nutritional requirement are safe, as intestinal absorption is specific and limited. Vitamin B_{12} injections (a nice red colour) are used in medicine as a placebo.

Further Reading

Thiamin

1. **Carpenter, K.J.** (2000) *Beri beri, white rice, and vitamin B.* Berkeley, CA, University of California Press.
2. **Truswell, A.S.** (2000) Australian experience with the Wernickle-Korsakoff syndrome. *Addiction*, **95**, 829–31.
3. **Victor, M., Adams R.D., and Collins, G.H.** (1989) *The Wernicke–Korsakoff Syndrome and related neurologic disorders due to alcoholism and malnutrition.* 2nd edn. Philadelphia, PA, FA Davis.

Niacin

1. **Roe, D.A.** (1973) *A plague of corn. The social history of pellagra.* Ithaca and London, Cornell University Press.

Vitamin B_6

1. **Schaumberg, H., Kaplan, J., and Windebank, A.,** *et al*. (1983) Sensory neuropathy from pyridoxine abuse. *N Engl J Med*, **309**, 445–8.

Folate

1. **Bailey, L.B.** (1998) Dietary reference intakes for folate: The debut of dietary folate equivalents. *Nutr Revs*, **56**, 294–9.
2. **Durga, J., Boxtel, M.P.J., Schouten, E.G., Kok, F.J., Jolles, J., Katan, M.B., and Verhoef, P.** (2007) Effect of 3-year folic acid supplementation on cognitive function in older adults in the FACIT trial: A randomized, double blind controlled trial. *Lancet*, **369**, 208–16.
3. **Ebbing, M., Bønaa, K.H., Nygård, O.,** *et al*. (2009) Cancer incidence and mortality after treatment with folic acid and vitamin B-12. *JAMA*, **302**, 2119–26.

4. **Food and Nutrition Board, Institute of Medicine** (1998) *Dietary reference intakes for thiamin, riboflavin, niacin, vitamin B-6, pantothenic acid, biotin and choline.* Washington DC, National Academy Press.

5. **Jacques, P.F., Selhub, J., Boston, A.G., Wilson, P.W.F., and, Rosenberg, I.H.** (1999) The effect of folic acid fortification on plasma folate and total homocysteine concentration. *N Engl J Med,* **340,** 1449–54.

6. **Mason, J.B., Dickstein, A., Jacques, P.F., Haggarty, P., Selhub, J., Dallal, G., and Resenberg, I.H.** (2007) A temporal association between folic acid fortification and an increase in colorectal cancer rates may be illuminating important biological principles: A hypothesis. *Cancer Epidemiol Biomarkers Prev,* **16,** 1325–9.

7. **Medical Research Council Vitamin Study Group** (1991) Prevention of neural tube defects: Results of the MRC vitamin Study Research Group. *Lancet,* **338,** 131–7.

8. **Ray, J.G.** (2004) Folic acid food fortification in Canada. *Nutr Revs,* **62,** 535–9.

9. **Selhub, J., Morris, M.S., Jacques, P.F., and Rosenberg, I.H.** (2009) Folate–vitamin B12 interaction in relation to cognitive impairment, anaemia and biochemical indicators of vitamin B-12 deficiency. *Am J Clin Nutr,* **89** (suppl), 702S–6S.

10. **Seshadri, S., Beiser, A., Selhub, J.,** *et al.* (2002) Plasma homocysteine as a risk factor for dementia and Alzheimer's disease. *N. Engl J Med,* **346,** 476–83.

11. **Truswell, A.S. and Kounnavong. S.** (1997) Quantitative responses of serum folate to increasing intakes of folic acid in healthy women. *Eur J Clin Nutr,* **51,** 839–45.

Vitamin B$_{12}$

1. **Bates, C.J., Schneeds, J., Mishra, G., Prentice, A., and Mansoor, M.A.** (2003) Relationship between methylmalonic acid, homocysteine, vitamin B$_{12}$ intake and status and social-economic indices, in a subset of participants in the British National Diet and Nutrition Survey of people aged 65 y and over. *European J Clin Nutr,* **57,** 349–59.

2. **Von Shenck, U., Bender-Gotze, C., and Koletzo, B.** (1997) Persistence of neurological damage induced by dietary vitamin B$_{12}$ deficiency in infancy. *Archives of Disease in Childhood,* **77,** 137–9.

Useful Websites

To see topical and scientifically robust updates on nutrition associated with this textbook and web links to many of the journals in the Further Reading sections, please see the dedicated Online Resource Centre at **http://www.oxfordtextbooks.co.uk/orc/mann4e/**

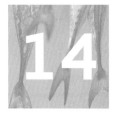

14 Vitamins C and E

Stewart Truswell and Jim Mann

14.1 Vitamin C

Also called ascorbic acid, vitamin C is the antiscorbutic vitamin that prevents scurvy (Latin *scorbutus*).

14.1.1 History

Scurvy became very important after Columbus connected Europe with America (1492). West European explorers and navies ventured ever longer and longer distances in sailing ships that took months to cross oceans and round continents. When Vasco da Gama sailed from Portugal round the Cape of Good Hope in 1490, he lost 60% of his crew of 160 sailors to scurvy. The sailors had food but not vegetables and fruit. It took centuries before the concept was accepted that prolonged lack of certain foods can cause severe illness without people getting thinner.

As early as 1601 Sir James Lancaster had avoided scurvy on an expedition round Africa to Sumatra to buy spices. He gave the sailors lemon juice and put in to ports to buy oranges, etc., but this was an exception. Scurvy was responsible for more deaths at sea than shipwreck, warfare, and all other illnesses combined.

In 1747 James Lind, surgeon on HMS Salisbury performed the first controlled therapeutic trial and cured scurvy in two men with two oranges and a lemon daily; five other treatments had no effect on pairs of sailors in the same sickbay. Captain James Cook sailed to and around the Antipodes on two very long voyages (1768–71 and 1772–75) and returned to England without losing a single sailor from scurvy. He was strict with cleanliness, stopped for fresh vegetables wherever possible and took with him a number of supposed remedies for scurvy, including wort of malt (inexpensive and favoured by the Admiralty), sauerkraut, and small quantities of lemon juice concentrate. Cook himself was not clear which had been the effective preventive.

No official action was taken to prevent scurvy on ships until Dr Gilbert Blane, aristocrat with experience in the 1782 naval war against the French in the West Indies persuaded the Lords of the British Admiralty to issue lemon juice as a daily ration on all navy ships from 1804. This was at the beginning of the Napoleonic war. The much stronger manpower on British ships must have contributed to naval victories like Trafalgar. At one stage West Indian lime replaced Mediterranean lemon juice to save money, but was a less effective preventive (and later shown to contain only a quarter of the vitamin C).

Confusion persisted about prevention of scurvy into the twentieth century, until the antiscorbutic substance was identified and could be quantified in different foods. Scott's tragic South Pole expedition walked 1700 miles under severe conditions with no vitamin C in their rations in 1912.

In 1907 Holst and Frölich in Oslo, Norway had been trying to produce an animal model of beri beri. They found that guinea pigs developed scurvy on a cereal diet with no green food ('one-sided diet'). Common laboratory animals, pigeons, rats, mice, and dogs do not develop scurvy on deficient diets.

A substance, first called hexuronic acid, was isolated from adrenal glands, oranges, and cabbage by Szent-György in 1928. Glen King and Szent-György in 1932 independently showed that it prevents guinea pig scurvy. Vitamins A and B had been identified earlier and Drummond proposed 'vitamin C' for the antiscorbutic vitamin. Its glucose-like structure was worked out by Haworth and Hirst, and ascorbic acid was the first vitamin to be synthesized, by Reichstein (1935). Szent-György and Haworth were awarded Nobel prizes for physiology/medicine and chemistry respectively, both partly for their research on vitamin C.

14.1.2 Deficiency disease

Scurvy in adults is rare today in developed countries and should be diagnosed before the patient is dangerously ill, but recognition of this rare disease requires doctors to be alert to its distinctive features (Box 14.1).

In the old sailing ship days, men with scurvy were listless and weak, with bleeding gums, loss of teeth, foul breath, painful legs, and generalized haemorrhages. Old wounds broke down. Severe cases were fatal, sometimes suddenly.

There are three types of haemorrhage in scurvy: small skin haemorrhages around hyperkeratotic hair follicles with coiled hairs (diagnostic), larger bruises in muscles, and internal haemorrhages, which could be into the brain or pericardium. The spongy bleeding gums have to be distinguished from common gingivitis and do not appear in edentulous people. Most of the features can be explained

---

BOX 14.1 A recent case

A 42-year-old man presented to the emergency department with a 1-month history of lethargy and significant spontaneous bruising and pain over his thighs and bleeding from his gums. There was no known trauma and he had not had any significant bleeding history. His health was otherwise unremarkable.

His social history was significant in that he had severe agoraphobia (extreme fear of public places) and was living with his mother in a retirement village. She had recently been moved to a hostel because of severe dementia. His diet over the past 5 years had consisted almost entirely of sausage rolls, meat pies, wheat cereal, biscuits, peanut butter, chocolate cake, and milk. He had not had any vegetables or fresh fruit in over 5 years and was unable to cook for himself. In recent times his shopping had been done by community-support staff and they had previously tried to encourage a better diet, but he was noncompliant.

On examination, he appeared malnourished and had extreme ecchymoses (bruising) and petechiae (tiny skin haemorrhages) over the lower limbs, and marked gingivitis.

His blood tests on admission showed an undetectable ascorbic acid (vitamin C) level. He had normal electrolytes and renal function but decreased albumin of 29 g/L. His vitamin B12, B1, and folate levels were normal. He was anaemic, with a haemoglobin level of 81 g/L, with normal white cells, platelets, and coagulation studies.

Source: Dean, M.G. (2006) Extensive bruising secondary to scurvy. Intern Med J, **36**, 393.

Two questions

Why did the doctor suspect scurvy, and request plasma vitamin C measurement (not a routine investigation)?

How do you think the patient was treated?

by impaired synthesis (and repair) of collagen and capillary fragility.

In young children Barlow (1894) described infants whose legs were too sore to move. They had lost weight and were anaemic. This was not rickets; it was vitamin C deficiency with haemorrhages under the periosteum of bones or into joints. If the child was too young to have teeth though, there were no bleeding gums. The cause was feeds of condensed or sterilized cows' milk, which lacked any vitamin C (unlike breastfeeding or modern infant formulas).

Experimental vitamin C deficiency was produced in human volunteers in Britain during World War II (supervised by Professor Krebs) and by Hodges *et al.* (1971) in the USA. In the later study the first signs of scurvy appeared after 2–3 months of zero intake. Both studies found that 10 mg of pure ascorbic acid was sufficient to prevent scorbutic features.

14.1.3 Chemistry and biosynthesis

Ascorbic acid is a 6-carbon compound, derived from glucose, but it is $C_6H_8O_6$, not a carbohydrate. It is a weak acid, soluble in water, and a strong reducing agent (antioxidant). X-ray crystallography shows the molecule is flat.

It has two asymmetric carbon atoms, so there are four stero-isomers: L-ascorbic, D-ascorbic, L-isoascorbic and D-isoascorbic. Only the first is antiscorbutic; all four are antioxidants and D-isoascorbic is used for this in food processing.

Vitamin C in solution is unusually sensitive to heat, especially with oxidizing agents, at alkaline pH and in the presence of copper. Care has to be taken, therefore, with vegetables to keep cooking time short, not to add sodium bicarbonate, or use a copper pan.

Biosynthesis For most animals ascorbic acid is not a vitamin: they make what they require from glucose. The steps via glucuronic acid, gulonic acid, and L-gulonolactone are shown in Fig. 14.1. The enzyme for the final step, L-gulonolactone oxidase is lacking only in primates (including man), fruit-eating bats, guinea pigs, and some passerine birds. All these susceptible animals eat fruit as a natural part of their diet.

14.1.4 Functions

Ascorbic acid is a co-factor for eight mammalian enzymes. It is required to convert iron on the enzyme from the ferric state (Fe^{3+}) to ferrous (Fe^{2+}).

The best-established function of vitamin C is its role in synthesis of collagen, the major material in all connective tissue, including bones. Collagen is first synthesized as procollagen polypeptides, rich in proline. Some of the proline and lysine is then hydroxylated post translation. The three hydroxylase enzymes require ascorbate to function. Hydroxyproline is necessary for formation of collagen's triple helix structure. Normal collagen cannot be made in the absence of vitamin C.

The adrenal gland has a very high ascorbate concentration. It plays a role in conversion of dopamine to noradrenaline and is also involved in the effect of ACTH on cortisol production. When ACTH stimulates secretion of cortisol, this is preceded by increased ascorbate in the adrenal vein. Two other organs with very high ascorbate are the pituitary, and the lens of the eye, where it must play a role in preventing photooxidative damage of the transparent lens protein.

Ascorbate is also required for conversion of lysine to carnitine, which transfers long chain fatty acids to the inner mitochondria for conversion to energy by way of β-oxidation. In muscles and the heart, fat is a significant source of energy and function. This can explain muscle weakness in severe scurvy.

White blood cells contain higher concentrations of ascorbate than plasma and lymphocytes appear to have the highest concentration. Detailed mechanisms of how it protects proteins in these cells from free radical damage during phagocytosis are not yet fully elucidated.

14.1.5 Absorption, metabolism, and excretion

Ascorbic acid is absorbed as itself in the small intestine by an active transport mechanism that gets

D-Glucose	D-Glucuronic acid	D-Gulonic acid	L-Gulonic	L-Gulono-lactone		L-Ascorbic acid		dehydro-L-ascorbic acid
*C^{1}HO	*CHO	CH$_2$OH	COOH	O=C⎤		O=C⎤		O=C⎤
HCOH	HCOH	HCOH	HOCH	HOCH		HOC		O=C
HOCH	HOCH	HOCH	HOCH	HOCH ⎦O		HOC ⎦O		O=C ⎦O
HCOH	HCOH	HCOH	HCOH	HC		HC		HC
HCOH	HCOH	HCOH	HOCH	HOCH		HOCH		HOCH
CH$_2$OH	COOH	COOH	*CH$_2$OH	*CH$_2$OH		*C^{6}H$_2$OH		CH$_2$OH

(arrows between D-Glucose → D-Glucuronic acid → D-Gulonic acid "or" L-Gulonic → L-Gulono-lactone; "Gulonolactone oxidase" between L-Gulono-lactone and L-Ascorbic acid; ⇌ between L-Ascorbic acid and dehydro-L-ascorbic acid)

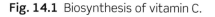

Fig. 14.1 Biosynthesis of vitamin C.

saturated at higher intakes. On ordinary dietary intakes nearly all the vitamin C is absorbed, but above 1 g/day, i.e. with supplements, the law of diminishing returns applies and much of the vitamin is not absorbed.

Ascorbate is carried free in the plasma. Its plasma concentration increases to a plateau of 70 to 80 mmol/L at intakes around 400 mg/day (Levine *et al.*, 1996). Urinary excretion starts before this. This means that if people take more than 500 mg/day, e.g. as supplement, plasma concentration will not increase. Progressively larger proportions are not absorbed and larger proportions are lost in the urine. (Higher plasma ascorbate can only occur if there is renal failure or the vitamin is given intravenously).

In the organs, ascorbate concentrations are higher than in plasma. It is transported into the cells by sodium-dependent vitamin C transporters SVCT1 and SVCT2. When ascorbate is oxidized, the product is dehydroascorbate. In neutrophils this can be taken into the cell with glucose transporters GLUT1 and GLUT3, where it is rapidly reduced to ascorbate by the protein glutaredoxin.

The normal total body pool pf ascorbate is 1500–2500 mg. There are no defined stores.

Ascorbate acid is excreted unchanged in the urine. It is also oxidized reversibly to dehydroascorbatic acid, which is further hydrolysed (irreversibly) to diketogulonic acid, whose metabolic products include oxalic acid.

14.1.6 Interactions

Vitamin C enhances absorption of non-haem iron. It facilitates the conversion of ferric to ferrous iron, which is more soluble. This happens with foods rich in vitamin C.

Smokers have significantly lower serum ascorbate: 40% lower with 20 or more cigarettes/day. This is only partly explained by smokers' lower consumption of fruits and vegetables; radioisotope-labelled ascorbate studies show that the turnover rate is almost doubled. Ascorbate is lost *in vitro* in plasma exposed to cigarette smoke.

Several drugs have been reported to lower plasma ascorbate, including corticosteroids, aspirin, indomethacin, phenylbutazone, and tetracycline.

14.1.7 Biochemical tests

Serum ascorbic acid is the standard laboratory test. Blood taken for measuring vitamin C must be specially preserved with metaphosphoric acid or trichloracetic acid and then frozen if not analysed fresh. Older methods used 2,6-dichlorophenolindophenol for analysis, but this is not completely specific and the method of choice is HPLC with electrochemical detection.

Women have somewhat higher levels than men at the same vitamin C intakes. Serum ascorbate cannot be used to identify people taking very high doses of vitamin C supplements (see Section 14.1.5). Very low levels, between 11 μmol/L and zero are found in scurvy. Leucocyte (buffy layer) ascorbate indicates cell content rather than recent intakes. The expected concentration is higher in mononuclear cells than in neutrophils.

14.1.8 Food sources

Potatoes and brassica vegetables and orange juice are the major contributors in Europe and North America. There is about a 250-fold range in the vitamin C content of fruits (Table 14.1).

Vitamin C is heat labile and lost in cooking or warm holding, whether in the food factory, kitchen, or bain-marie. Alkaline conditions, e.g. sodium bicarbonate and copper containers, accelerate cooking losses. So fresh fruits and salads have more reliable vitamin C than cooked plant foods. Dried fruits have lost their original vitamin C.

In animal foods, there is no vitamin C in usual meats, i.e. muscle, but liver and kidney contain around 10 g/100g (depending on cooking method).

Table 14.1 Ascorbic acid content of foods

Content (mg/100 g edible portion)	Food
<10	Apricot, pear, apple, plum, grape, banana, cherries
10	Potatoes (boiled)
50	Citrus fruit and strawberries
100	Broccoli (raw), parsley, Brussels sprouts (raw), cauliflower (raw), kiwi fruit
200–300	Blackcurrants, guavas, peppers
1250	Rosehips (*Rosa canina*)
1000–2300	Acerola fruit
2300–3150 *mg*	*Terminalia ferdinandiana* (Kakadu plum)

Cows' milk (unwarmed) contains a little, but human milk averages 4 mg vitamin C/100 mL, which is sufficient for the first 6 months of infancy.

14.1.9 Recommended nutrient intakes

Some Expert Committees (see Chapter 37), FAO/WHO, UK, and Australia/New Zealand, recommend 40–45 mg/day for adults as sufficient to prevent scurvy (10 mg/day), with generous safety factors, including for smokers. USA/Canada and Germany/Austria/Switzerland recommend 90–100 mg vitamin C/day as the amount to achieve saturation of white blood cells* without wastage from urinary secretion.

Average vitamin C intakes from food in the 2000–01 Diet and Nutrition Survey of British Adults were 83 mg in men and 81 mg/day in women. Intakes are higher in the USA and Australia. In Australia (1995) intakes were 116 mg in men and 98 mg in women. In addition, a minority of people consume extra vitamin C as such in multivitamin supplements.

Nutrient recommendations are for healthy people and based on physiological research. In sickness, more vitamin C may be desirable (see Box 14.2). Serum or leucocyte ascorbate have been reported low with trauma and during recovery from surgery (which involves a big increase in collagen synthesis) and in people with severe infections.

14.1.10 Toxic effects

The US Institute of Medicine (2000) set the upper intake level for adults at 2000 mg/day. The more recent Australian/New Zealand committee were not able to set a definite upper level but considered 1000 mg/day would be a prudent limit.

Urinary oxalate stones Ascorbic acid is partly metabolized to oxalic acid, which is a common ingredient of urinary tract stones (it is not only derived from ascorbate). For years this was

*Cells saturate with vitamin C at lower intakes than plasma; there is active transport into cells.

considered a serious side effect of vitamin C supplements, but more recently it was found that (a) an important proportion of the oxalate found in urine from people taking vitamin C tablets is formed from chemical change after the urine has been passed and (b) in the large Harvard Health Professional cohort (over 45 000) those who suffered urinary tract stones had not had higher vitamin C intakes (Curham *et al.*, 1996).

Iron absorption Because ascorbic acid increases absorption of non-haem iron, people with haemochromatosis (see Chapter 10) or with the gene for it should be advised to avoid vitamin C supplements.

BOX 14.2 Case study: does extra vitamin C have health benefits?

The problem is the intake distance between prevention of scurvy and a possible optimal intake. As ascorbate is concentrated in immune reactive cells and in the adrenal, pituitary, and anterior eye, it is reasonable to suppose that more than enough to prevent scurvy may help achieve optimal immune function, response to stress, and prevention of cataract. The antioxidant function was stressed in health education until randomized controlled trials with vitamin C or E proved very disappointing. The British MRC/BHF trial in over 20 000 people did not find any benefit in total mortality, coronary heart disease, strokes, or cancer mortality in those who took 250 mg/day vitamin C plus vitamin E and β-carotene (Heart Protection Study Collaborative Group, 2002). Cohort studies such as EPIC-Norfolk have shown an inverse relation of plasma ascorbate and deaths from all causes of cardiovascular diseases (Khaw *et al.*, 2001), but the authors think it more likely that plasma vitamin C is a marker for intake of fruits and vegetables, which contain mixtures of potentially protective substances.

Ascorbic acid is secreted in the gastric juice and can reduce formation of nitrosamines, which are carcinogenic. An international panel made a thorough review of all the epidemiological evidence about diet and cancer in 1997 for the World Cancer Research Foundation. They concluded that vitamin C 'possibly' protected against stomach cancer. This extensive review was repeated in 2007 with stricter evidence-based criteria, and now vitamin C has largely disappeared from the conclusion tables. For oesophagus cancer, 'foods containing vitamin C' are probably protective; for stomach cancer, 'non-starchy vegetables, allium vegetables, and fruits are probably protective' (i.e. vitamin C is not specifically named).

There is still a popular belief that if you take vitamin C tablets they will prevent colds. Randomized controlled trials to prove this are easy to organize; many have been done and the findings have nearly all shown no reduced incidence of colds; they may possibly be of shorter duration (Truswell, 1986; Douglas *et al.*, 2001).

There have been several reports of low plasma ascorbate in people with diabetes. Doctors in the diabetic clinic might justifiably advise more fruit and vegetables (or small doses of vitamin C tablets).

With cataract, the largest cohort study found that women who took vitamin C tablets in the long term had a significantly lower incidence of cataract operations (Hankinson *et al.*, 1992). There remains the possibility of confounding, e.g. people who take vitamin supplements may use sunglasses.

Convalescence after a major illness, surgery, or trauma and old people with poor appetite, especially if bedsores threaten, are situations where intake is close to the EAR or requirements may be increased. Such patients should be encouraged or helped to increase their vitamin C intake, by eating more fruit or vegetables: if they cannot manage this, with 100 mg vitamin C tablets.

Vitamin C tablets are provided by the pharmaceutical industry at doses of 50, 100, 250, 500, and 1000 mg partly as sodium ascorbate. Indications in prescribers guides are 'general well being, antioxidant, colds, flu, assist wound healing'. It seems very unlikely that there could be any possible benefit from doses above 500 mg/day, because plasma ascorbate is tightly controlled and cannot be pushed higher with oral administration, as Levine *et al.* (1996) showed.

Further Reading

1. **Curham, G.C., Willett, W.C., Rimm, E.B., and Stampfer, M.J.** (1996) A prospective study of the intake of vitamins C and B6, and the risk of kidney stones in men. *J Ural*, **755**, 1847–51.
2. **Dean, M.G.** (2006) Extensive bruising secondary to scurvy. *Intern Med J*, **36**, 393.
3. **Douglas, R.M., Chalker, E.B., and Treacy, B.** (2001) Vitamin C for preventing and treating the common cold (Cochrane Review). In: The Cochrane Library 3, 2001. Oxford Update Software.
4. **Hankinson, S.E., Stampfer, M.J., Seddon. M.J., et al.** (1992) Nutrient intake and cataract extraction in women: A prospective study. *BMJ*, **305**, 335–9.
5. **Heart protection Study Collaborative Group** (2002) MRC/BHF Heart Protection Study of antioxidant vitamin supplementation in 20,536 high-risk individuals: A randomized placebo-controlled trial. *Lancet*, **360**, 23–33.
6. **Hodges, R.E., Hood, J., Canham, J.E., Sauberlich, H.E., and Barker, E.M.** (1971) Clinical manifestation of ascorbic acid deficiency in man. *Am J Clin Nutr*, **24**, 432–43.
7. **Khaw, K-T., Bingham, S., Welch, A., Luber, R., Wareham, N., Oakes, S., and Day, N.** (2001) Relation between plasma ascorbic acid and mortality in men and women in EPIC-Norfolk prospective study: A prospective population study. *Lancet*, **357**, 657–63.
8. **Levine, M.** (1986) New concepts in the biology and biochemistry of ascorbic acid. *N Engl J Med*, **314**, 892–902.
9. **Levine. M., Cowry-Cantilena, C., Wang, Y., et al.** (1996) Vitamin C pharmacokinetics in healthy volunteers: Evidence for a recommended dietary allowance. *Proc Nat Acad Sci*, **193**, 3704–9.
10. **Levine, M., Wang, Y., and Morrow, J.** (2001) A new recommended dietary allowance for healthy young women. *Proc Nat Acad Sci*, **98**, 9842–6.
11. **Padayatty, S.J. and Levine, M.** (2001) New insights into the physiology and pharmacology of vitamin C. *Canadian Medical Assn Journal* **164**, 353–6.
12. **Truswell, A.S.** (1986) Ascorbic acid. *N Engl J Med*, **315**, 709.

14.2 Vitamin E

14.2.1 History

In 1922 two researchers, Evans and Bishop, found that a lipid-soluble factor was essential for reproduction in rats. Fetal resorption occurred when female rats were fed on a diet including rancid fats, but was found to be preventable by the addition to the diet of wheatgerm, dried alfalfa leaves, or fresh lettuce. This lipid-soluble factor was named vitamin E and, because of its role in reproduction, tocopherol (from the Greek: to bring forth offspring, the 'ol' indicates the alcohol in its structure). The vitamin was isolated and chemical structure identified in the 1930s.

14.2.2 Sources, structure, and bioavailability

Vegetable oils (especially wheat germ oil), nuts, sweet potatoes, and, to a variable extent, other vegetables and fruits are the richest dietary sources of vitamin E. There are eight naturally occurring forms of vitamin E: four tocopherols and four tocotrienols. All forms consist of a chromanol ring with an isoprenoid 16-carbon side chain, saturated in the case of tocopherols and unsaturated in the case of tocotrienols. The α, β, γ, and δ forms of the tocopherols and tocotrienols differ with regard to the position and number of the methyl groups (Fig. 14.2).

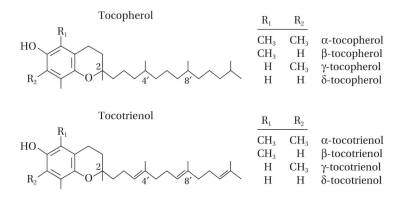

Fig. 14.2 Structure of tocopherols and tocotrienols.

Furthermore, there are potentially eight stereo-isomers for each of the vitamin E compounds. Tocopherols occur in foods as the free alcohols and tocotrienols as free alcohols and esters. Acetate and succinate esters are used by the pharmaceutical industry since they are more stable.

Biological activity of these compounds is expressed by comparing potency in an animal model system with the potency of a synthetic tocopherol (all-*rac*-a-tocopherol acetate), the activity of which is set at 1.00 IU/mg. The most potent naturally occurring form of vitamin E is 2R,4′R,8′R-α-tocopherol. The vitamin E content of the diet is typically expressed as α-tocopherol equivalents (α-TE), where 1 α-TE is the activity of 1 mg RRR-α-tocopherol. The eight stereoisomers of α-tocopherol (known collectively as all-*rac*-α-tocopherol), when considered as a group, have relatively high biological activity and make the major contribution to the vitamin E content of the diet. The β, γ, and δ tocopherols and the entire group of tocotrienols make a relatively small contribution to total vitamin E activity.

14.2.3 Functions

Vitamin E is one of the body's principal antioxidants. Free radicals are generated as the body's cells use oxygen as an energy source. Free radicals react with the polyunsaturated fatty acids of cell membranes and protein in a process known as lipid peroxidation, which can influence and impair membrane fluidity and function. Oxidation of apolipoprotein B results in the accumulation of oxidized low-density lipoprotein in the arterial walls, thus promoting the development of atherosclerotic plaques and increasing the risk of cardiovascular disease. Free radical damage plays a role in other disease processes including cancer, arthritis, and cataracts.

Vitamin E is able to neutralize free radicals by transferring an electron from the hydroxyl group on the chromanol ring to the free radicals, thus making it less reactive. Following this transfer, the remaining vitamin E (now α-tocopheroxyl radical) has an impaired electron, which can become permanently inactivated by reacting with another free radical or it can react with vitamin C or glutathione and be regenerated to active vitamin E. Although there are several other important antioxidant systems and there are close relationships between these and vitamin E, vitamin E appears to have a uniquely important role in preventing the peroxidation of the polyunsaturated fatty acids of cell membranes.

A range of additional functions of vitamin E, independent of its antioxidant properties has been reported. α-tocopherol has a role in modulating gene transcription, inhibits platelet aggregation and vascular smooth muscle proliferation, and may have a further signalling role in the immune system.

14.2.4 Absorption, transport, and metabolism

Vitamin E is, like other dietary lipids, absorbed in micelles into the cells lining the small intestine. Absorption is fairly efficient; generally at least half of the dietary intake is absorbed, but the proportion is reduced at the high intake levels associated with pharmacological doses and in any situation where absorption of fat is reduced.

In the mucosal cells, all forms of tocopherols and tocotrienols present in the diet are incorporated into chylomicrons, which are broken down to chylomicron remnants by the action of lipoprotein lipase. Most are transported to the liver where α-tocopherol, especially RRR α-tocopherol, binds to liver α-tocopherol transport protein and is then exported in very-low-density lipoprotein to various tissues, especially to those organs with a high fatty acid content (e.g. liver, brain, and adipose tissue). Most of the other stereoisomers which do not bind well to α-tocopherol transport protein are metabolized in the liver and excreted in bile. The preferential binding of RRR α-tocopherol to the transport protein, incorporating into very-low-density lipoprotein (VLDL) and transport to the tissues explain its high biological activity.

There is some transfer of vitamin E directly to adipose tissue and muscle via chylomicron remnants which do not reach the liver. Generally little vitamin E is released from adipose tissue. However, in experimentally depleted subjects, plasma tocopherol levels do not fall for many months because under such circumstances vitamin E is released from the substantial tissue reserves.

14.2.5 Deficiency states

Soon after the first discovery by Evans and Bishop, deficiency of the lipid-soluble factor was found in experimental animals to be associated with other conditions, including sterility in male rats and muscle wasting in guinea pigs and rabbits. No symptoms or signs of experimental vitamin E deficiency have been found in humans and deficiency appears not to be a problem, even among people consuming relatively poor diets. However, vitamin E status is low in the newborn due to poor placental transfer, and premature infants are given vitamin E. Furthermore, deficiency in some uncommon clinical situations shows that vitamin E is an essential nutrient for humans. Children with rare inherited conditions (congenital abetalipoproteinaemia, familial isolated vitamin E deficiency) have exceptionally low or undetectable levels of plasma vitamin E, resulting in vitamin E not reaching the tissues. Patients with these conditions develop a range of severe neurological signs which are similar to those seen with vitamin E depletion associated with severe chronic malabsorption of fat, which occurs in diseases such as cystic fibrosis and cholecystatic liver disease. These conditions require treatment with very high doses of vitamin E, which can halt progression and may result in improvement of the neurological signs. If vitamin E deficiency is detected and treated at the early stage these neurological consequences can be avoided.

14.2.6 Assessment of vitamin E status

Vitamin E status is typically assessed by measuring plasma vitamin E, of which over 90% is generally α-tocopherol. The reference range is 12–30 μmol/L. Because raised levels of plasma lipoproteins are associated with high levels of vitamin E, vitamin E status is also often expressed per unit of plasma cholesterol, an index of greater than 2.0 μmmol/mmol cholesterol regarded as an indication of adequate status.

14.2.7 Recommended nutrient intakes

Because clinical deficiency of vitamin E is so rare in humans, even when diets are poor, recommended intakes are somewhat arbitrary. Average requirements are considered to be around 10–12 mg of α-tocopherol equivalents per day, which is relatively easy to achieve, given the high content of polyunsaturated oils. Since, at least in theory, vitamin E requirements are increased if intake of polyunsaturated fats is high, requirements are sometimes expressed in terms of amount of the fatty acids in the diet, a ratio of 0.4 mg α-tocopherol/g polyunsaturated fat intake is considered to be an adequate intake of vitamin E.

The antioxidant properties of vitamin E and the findings of some prospective studies have led to the suggestion that intakes higher than physiological requirements might protect against heart disease, some cancers, and other chronic diseases. However, most randomized controlled trials and systematic literature reviews have not confirmed these earlier suggestions (see Chapter 21) and supplementation at exceptionally high intakes may cause harm. Thus despite very low toxicity up to intakes of around 3000 µg or more/day, there is no justification for recommending extremely high doses as preventive or therapeutic measures. The Institute of Medicine in the USA has suggested an adult upper limit of 1000 mg/day for adults. Some 40 years ago, it was suggested that 'Vitamin E is one of those embarrassing vitamins that have been identified, isolated and synthesized by physiologists and biochemists and then handed to the medical profession with the suggestion that a use should be found for it, without any satisfactory evidence to show that human beings are ever deficient of it or even that it is a necessary nutrient for man.' (Davidson and Passmore, 1969). While it does appear to be an essential nutrient for humans, its role is still not fully understood.

Further Reading

1. **Brigelius-Flohe, R., Kelly, F.J., Salonen, J.T., Neuzil, J., Zingg, J.-M., and Azzi, A.** (2002) The European perspective on vitamin E: Current knowledge and future research. *Am J Clin Nutr*, **76**, 703–16.
2. **Davidson, S. and Passmore, R.** (1969) *Human nutrition and dietetics*. Baltimore, Williams & Wilkins.
3. **Horwitt, M.K.** (1960) Vitamin E and lipid metabolism in man. *Am J Clin Nutr*, **8**, 451–61.
4. **Kayden, H.T. and Traber, M.G.** (1993) Absorption, lipoprotein transport, and regulation of plasma concentrations of vitamin E in humans. *J Lipid Res*, **34**, 345–58.
5. **Leth, T. and Sondergaard, H.** (1977) Biological activity of vitamin E compounds and natural materials by the resorption-gestation test, and chemical determination of the vitamin E activity in foods and feeds. *J Nutr*, **107**, 2236–43.
6. **Meydani, M.** (1995) Vitamin E. *Lancet*, **345**, 170–5.
7. **Traber, M.G. and Arai, H.** (1999) Molecular mechanisms of vitamin E transport. *Ann Rev Nutr*, **19**, 343–55.

Useful Websites

To see topical and scientifically robust updates on nutrition associated with this textbook and web links to many of the journals in the Further Reading sections, please see the dedicated Online Resource Centre at **http://www.oxfordtextbooks.co.uk/orc/mann4e/**

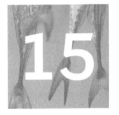

Vitamins D and K

Stewart Truswell

15.1 Vitamin D

15.1.1 History

In the first step towards identifying individual vitamins, E.V. McCollum at the University of Wisconsin postulated (1915) two essential dietary factors as well as macronutrients and minerals—'fat-soluble A' and 'water-soluble B'. Fat-soluble A prevented growth failure and the eye disease xerophthalmia in animals fed purified diets. In 1919, Edward Mellanby in London found that some fats would cure experimental dietary rickets in puppies kept indoors but others would not. Cod liver oil was very active against the bone disease rickets and against xerophthalmia (Chapter 12), but when heated, with oxygen bubbled through, its antixerophthalmia activity was lost, but not its antirachitic (antirickets) activity, and McCollum realized in 1922 that there were two nutritional factors in cod liver oil. He designated the antirachitic factor vitamin D because 'water-soluble C' had been proposed for the antiscorbutic (antiscurvy) factor in 1919. Meanwhile, Harriette Chick, a British scientist, proved that rickets in children in Vienna after World War I could be cured either by cod liver oil or by exposure to an ultraviolet (UV) light lamp. Pure vitamin D_2 was first obtained by irradiating ergosterol with UV light in 1927. Its chemical structure was established by A. Windaus in Germany and F. Askew in England in 1932. In 1936, Windaus published the structure of vitamin D_3, the natural form of the vitamin made by UV light in the skin and present in cod liver oil.

15.1.2 Chemistry and metabolism

Vitamin D_3, cholecalciferol, is derived by the effect of UVB irradiation (wavelength 290–315 nm) on 7-dehydrocholesterol (cholesterol with a double bond at carbon 7), a minor companion of cholesterol, in the skin. There is a rearrangement of the molecule, with opening of the B ring of the steroid nucleus (Fig. 15.1). Cholecalciferol is the naturally occurring form of the vitamin in man and animals, for example, in cod liver oil, fatty fish, butter, and animal liver.

Vitamin D_2 is derived from ergosterol (a fungal sterol) by irradiating it with UV light via the same sequence of chemical changes and is called ergocalciferol. It is used as a pharmaceutical (also called calciferol) and in some of the foods fortified with vitamin D (e.g. milk in North America, margarine). Ergosterol and ergocalciferol differ from 7-dehydrocholesterol and cholecalciferol only in having an extra double bond at carbon 22 and a methyl group at carbon 24 in the side chain (Fig. 15.1). The original vitamin D_1 turned out to be an impure mixture of sterols. Using the older quantitative unit for

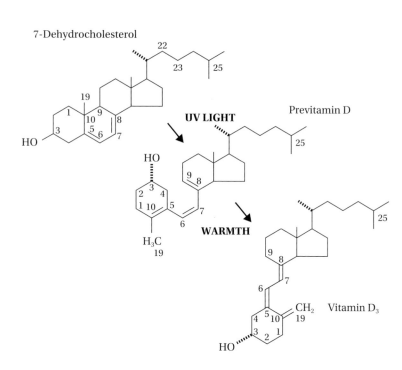

Fig. 15.1 Formation of vitamin D3 in the skin. 7-Dehydrocholesterol is present in the skin as a minor companion of cholesterol. Under the influence of short-wavelength UV light (290–315 nm) from sunlight, the B ring of the sterol opens to form a secosterol, previtamin D3. The first step takes place rapidly. The second stage is a rearrangement of the secosterol to make vitamin D3 (cholecalciferol). It takes place more slowly, under the influence of warmth.

vitamin D, one international unit (IU) = 0.025 µg of cholecalciferol (so 1 µg = 40 IU).

In the tropical and subtropical regions of the world, enough vitamin D is made in the skin to meet the body's needs (unless people are housebound or completely covered). Since cholecalciferol is formed in one organ of the body (the skin) and transported by the blood to act on other organs (the bones, gut, kidneys), it can be called a hormone. However, when people live in high latitudes, are covered with clothes, spend nearly all their time indoors, and the sky is polluted with smoke, there is insufficient UV exposure in the winter to make enough vitamin D in the skin. Dietary intake is required, so that the cholecalciferol present in a few foods and the ergocalciferol in fortified foods assume the role of a vitamin.

Inside the body, vitamin D itself is not active until it has been chemically modified (hydroxylated) twice. The first clue to this was the observation of a lag period of 8 hours before one could see an effect of administered vitamin D in experimental animals. Vitamin D, whether of cutaneous origin or absorbed (D_3 or D_2), is carried in the plasma on a specific α_2-globulin, vitamin D-binding protein. In liver microsomes, the end of the side chain is hydroxylated to form 25-hydroxy-vitamin D (25(OH)D). This compound has a more stable concentration in the blood than that of vitamin D, which rises temporarily as some is absorbed or synthesized in the skin.

25(OH)D is still not the active metabolite. It has to have a third hydroxyl (OH) group put on at carbon 1. This is done by an enzyme, 1α-hydroxylase, in the kidneys (in the mitochondria of the proximal convoluted tubule) to make 1,25-dihydroxy-vitamin D (1,25(OH)$_2$D), also called calcitriol (Fig. 15.2). The plasma concentration of 1,25(OH)$_2$D is about one thousand times smaller than that of 25(OH)D. The activity of renal 1α-hydroxylase is tightly controlled, so the rate of production of 1,25(OH)$_2$D is increased

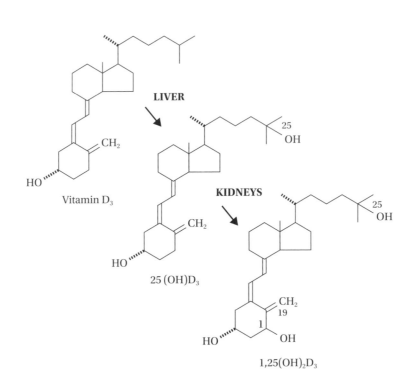

Fig. 15.2 Activation of vitamin D. In the liver parenchymal cells, vitamin D_3 (or D_2) is hydroxylated to 25-hydroxy-vitamin D (25(OH)D), which circulates in the blood. A small proportion of the available 25(OH)D is further hydroxylated by a specific 25(OH)D-1α-hydroxylase in the kidneys to the active form, 1,25(OH)$_2$ vitamin D. During pregnancy, some 1α-hydroxylation also takes place in the placenta.

by any fall in plasma calcium or rise in parathyroid hormone level.

1,25(OH)$_2$D is one of the three hormones that normally act together to maintain the extracellular calcium concentration constant; the other two are parathormone and calcitonin (see Chapter 9). There are about 30 other known metabolites of vitamin D, probably all inactive.

1,25(OH)$_2$D acts in a similar manner to steroid hormones. There is a specific vitamin D receptor (VDR) protein in the cell nucleus, which has great affinity for 1,25(OH)$_2$D. It also has a DNA-binding domain. This receptor, when activated, switches on the gene that induces synthesis of a calcium-transport protein (calbindin) in the epithelium of the small intestine. VDR has actually been found in a range of tissues (see Section 15.1.6) but normally has its main effect in the small intestinal epithelium and the cells in bone, osteoblasts (that form new bone), and osteoclasts (that break bone down).

Less vitamin D is made in the skin of dark-skinned people than white-skinned people because the melanin in skin absorbs UV light. Old people also make less vitamin D after exposure to short-wave UV light; their skin contains less of the starting material, 7-dehydrocholesterol. Vitamin D taken by mouth is digested and absorbed, then transported from the upper small intestine on chylomicrons, like other lipids. Like other lipids, its absorption can be impaired in chronic biliary or intestinal disease with malabsorption. Excretion of vitamin D is in the bile, principally as more polar metabolites.

15.1.3 Deficiency diseases

In *rickets*, there is reduced calcification of the growing ends (epiphyses) of bones. Thick seams of uncalcified osteoid cartilage are seen histologically. Rickets only occurs in young people, whose bones are still growing. *Osteomalacia* is the corresponding decalcifying bone disease in adults, whose epiphyses have fused so that the bones are no longer growing. Bone density is reduced. This is because the bones contain less calcium: the ratio of calcium to organic bone is reduced. Rickets can occur in premature infants and in children in northern Britain (especially of Asian origin). Surprisingly, rickets and osteomalacia can also occur in the tropics in dark-skinned children and women usually staying indoors and fully covered when outdoors. In affluent countries, osteomalacia is possible in elderly people confined indoors. Malabsorption increases the risk. Muscular weakness and susceptibility to infections in rickets or osteomalacia may reflect roles for VDR in the muscles and the immune system. In chronic kidney failure, 1α-hydroxylation is impaired. Renal osteomalacia does not respond to vitamin D (or sunlight), only to administration of $1,25(OH)_2D$ (pharmaceutical name calcitriol) or to $1\alpha(OH)D$ (pharmaceutical name alphacalcidol). This shows the critical importance of 1α-hydroxylation to normal vitamin D function.

15.1.4 Biochemical tests of vitamin D status

Plasma calcium and phosphate levels fall in severe vitamin D-deficient states. Plasma alkaline phosphatase (the isoenzyme originating in bone) is increased in mild as well as in severe rickets and osteomalacia. It can be elevated in some other bone diseases and does not directly indicate vitamin D status. This is best assessed by assaying plasma $25(OH)D$ levels, and it can be seen how the concentration goes down in population samples at the end of the winter in those temperate countries that have little vitamin D fortification. In 7437 British-born people measured at age 45 years, 16% had $25(OH)D$ levels below 25 nmol/L in winter and spring. Only 3% were this low in summer and autumn. Levels below 25 nmol/L indicate deficiency; 25–50 nmol/L is low or borderline; over 50 nmol/L is normal. In the alternative units (divide by 2.6), this normal level is 20 ng/mL. Plasma $1,25(OH)_2D$ can also be measured but is a specialized investigation.

15.1.5 Osteoporosis as well as osteomalacia

It used to be thought that vitamin D deficiency causes osteomalacia, not osteoporosis. (In osteoporosis, total bone is reduced—organic as well as calcium.) Now that vitamin D status can be quantified with serum $25(OH)D$, it is becoming clear that as levels fall below 50 nmol/L there are compensatory secondary increases of parathyroid hormone and increased mobilization of bone. Some long-term prevention trials in older people using vitamin D (with or without calcium supplements) have shown delayed development of osteoporosis and fewer fractures.

15.1.6 Other possible roles for vitamin D beyond bones

Vitamin D is an unusual vitamin: its biological actions are still being discovered! The vitamin D receptor is expressed in many different cell nuclei and $1,25(OH)_2D$ has been shown in *in vitro* and animal experiments to control more than 200 genes (Holick, 2007). Clues to possible non-bone actions of vitamin D are diseases more common at high latitude, with low winter sun. There is also suggestive experimental or case–control epidemiological evidence that vitamin D may help protect against some cancers, multiple sclerosis, tuberculosis, hypertension, and diabetes, particularly type 1.

Randomized controlled prevention trials are needed before we can be more positive about these actions. It seems unlikely, at present, that vitamin D will be valuable for treating those conditions, except psoriasis, which has long been known to improve in the summer. Ointments containing $1,25(OH)_2D$ or derivatives are now standard treatment for this skin condition. Obese people have lower serum $25(OH)D$. This is, of course, not causative. Their excess adipose tissue sequesters vitamin D intake (from skin or ingested), so there is less $25(OH)D$ in plasma than in normal-weight people.

15.1.7 Food sources

Fish liver oils (e.g. cod and halibut) and some fish and marine animal's livers are rich sources. Moderate sources are fatty fish (herring, sardine, salmon, etc.), margarines (which in most countries are fortified with vitamin D), infant milk formulas, eggs, red meat, and liver. Milk is fortified with vitamin D in North America and Scandinavia. Human milk contains little vitamin D (moderate exposure to sunlight is good for babies).

15.1.8 Interactions

Long-term use of anticonvulsants (e.g. for epilepsy), by inducing liver microsomes, increases metabolic losses of vitamin D. Glucocorticoids (e.g. prednisone) inhibit vitamin D-dependent intestinal calcium absorption; patients on long-term steroids may benefit from additional vitamin D to maintain plasma 25(OH)D in the mid-normal range (above 50 nmol/L).

15.1.9 Recommended nutrient intake

The US Institute of Medicine estimates adequate intakes (AI) of vitamin D for those with no sun-mediated synthesis in the skin. For ages 0–50 years (including pregnancy and lactation), the AI is 5 µg/day, for 51–70 years 10 µg/day, and over 70 years of age 15 µg/day. Older people make less vitamin D in their skin and also tend to avoid sun exposure and use UV light-blocking sunscreen. If they are house-bound and cannot get in the sun, they probably need vitamin D supplements because most diets provide under 5 µg vitamin D/day unless the milk is fortified. There is not enough UV light at the latitude of Boston (42° N) in the winter months to make adequate vitamin D. Vegans who avoid milk and fish are at risk of subclinical vitamin D deficiency if they live at high latitudes.

15.1.10 Toxicity

Exposure of the skin to sunlight, if excessive, causes sunburn and brings up the plasma 25(OH)D level if it was low, but does not lead to vitamin D toxicity because with excessive UV light, previtamin D_3 (7-dehydrocholesterol) is photoisomerized to biologically inert products (lumisterol and tachysterol). Vitamin D_3 is also photodegraded if it is not taken inside the body by vitamin D-binding protein. However, with oral intake, the margin between the upper limit of the nutritional dose and the lower limit of the toxic dose is quite narrow. Overdosage causes raised plasma calcium (hypercalcaemia), with thirst, anorexia, raised plasma levels of 25(OH)D, and risk of calcification of soft tissues and of urinary calcium stones. Infants are most at risk of hypervitaminosis D; a few children have developed hypercalcaemia on intakes of only 50 µg/day. The upper level of 50 µg (2000 IU) per day for adults set by the US Institute of Medicine in 1997 has been shown to be unnecessarily cautious (Vieth *et al.*, 2007). In some conditions, people are unusually sensitive to vitamin D (e.g. in sarcoidosis and a rare condition in infants with elfin facial appearance, Williams syndrome).

15.2 Vitamin K

15.2.1 History

The name 'vitamin K' was proposed by Henrik Dam of Denmark in 1935. K was the next letter of the alphabet not already used for a vitamin at that time. It is also the first letter of the German word *koagulation*, which refers to its best-known function. While investigating the essentiality of cholesterol in the diet of chickens (their eggs, of course, are rich in cholesterol), Dam fed them rations from which the lipid had been extracted with organic solvents. They developed haemorrhages and their blood was slow to clot. This bleeding tendency could be corrected with alfalfa or with decayed fishmeal. The alfalfa was soon shown to provide vitamin K_1; bacteria in the fishmeal were responsible for producing vitamin K_2.

15.2.2 Chemistry

H.J. Almquist solved the chemical search in 1939, reporting that a lipid from the sheath of tubercle bacilli, phthiocol, had vitamin K activity (Fig. 15.3A). Vitamin K_1 and the K_2 series are all based on this 2-methyl-3-hydroxy-1,4-naphthoquinone. They have side chains in place of the 3-hydroxyl group. In vitamin K_1 (phylloquinone), the side chain is a 20-carbon terpenoid alcohol (four-fifths of the phytol side chain of chlorophyll) (Fig. 15.3B). It is found in green leaves.

Vitamin K_2 comprises a family of compounds, called menaquinones, whose side chain consists of repeated (5-carbon) isoprene units, from 1 to 14 of them (Fig. 15.3C). Depending on the number of isoprene units, they are referred to as MK1–MK14. The menaquinones are synthesized by several bacterial species (*Bacteriodes*, *Enterobacteria*, etc.), some of which occur naturally in the large intestine of animals, including humans.

15.2.3 Functions

In the liver, vitamin K promotes the synthesis of a special amino acid with three carboxylic acid groups, γ-carboxyglutamic acid (Gla) (Fig. 15.4). The enzyme responsible for putting another carboxylic acid on to glutamic acid requires vitamin K as a cofactor.

Gla is an essential part of four of the coagulation factors, all proteins: prothrombin (factor II) and factors VII, IX and X. Factors II and VII contain 10 Gla

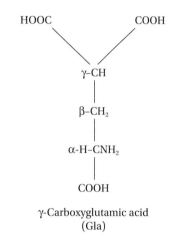

γ-Carboxyglutamic acid
(Gla)

Fig. 15.4 γ-Carboxyglutamic acid (Gla).

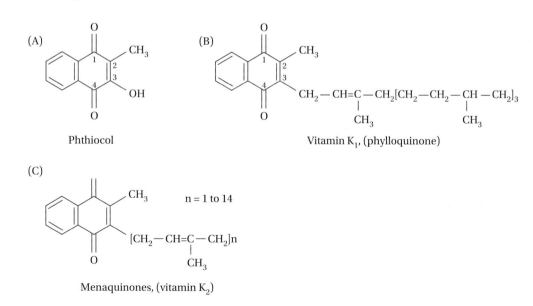

Phthiocol

Vitamin K_1, (phylloquinone)

Menaquinones, (vitamin K_2)

Fig. 15.3 Structures of (A) phthiocol, (B) phylloquinone (vitamin K_1), and (C) menaquinones (vitamin K_2).

residues per molecule; factors IX and X each contain 12. The Gla residues confer on these coagulation proteins the capacity to bind to phospolipid surfaces in the presence of calcium ions.

Five other Gla-containing and vitamin K-dependent proteins were discovered more recently. Proteins C, S, and Z all have anticoagulant activities. They seem to act to limit clot formation. In bone are osteocalcin and MGP (matrix Gla protein). Osteocalcin can be assayed in plasma.

Vitamin K, being fat-soluble, requires bile for its absorption. It is transported in the plasma on triglyceride-rich lipoproteins. Analysis of vitamin K in tissues has been difficult because the several compounds are present in very tiny (nanomolar) amounts. In adult liver, there is not only vitamin K_1 derived from green leaves in the diet, but also significant amounts of menaquinones (K_2), some presumably synthesized by anaerobic bacteria in the large intestine and absorbed. MK-4 is apparently derived from phylloquinone (K_1).

15.2.4 Deficiency disease

In vitamin K deficiency, there is a bleeding disorder, characterized by low plasma prothrombin activity (hypoprothrombinaemia). Vitamin K deficiency can occur in obstetric or paediatric practice, in surgical patients, and in medical patients.

For most people in developed countries, the first injection of their life is vitamin K_1 given intramuscularly straight after birth to prevent haemorrhagic disease of the newborn. This is to prevent the small risk of haemorrhage in the first days after birth because vitamin K, like other fat-soluble vitamins, is poorly transported across the placenta from the mother's blood; the gut of the newborn is sterile (there are no resident bacteria, so no vitamin K_2); it is some days before bacteria colonize the large intestine, and human milk has a low concentration of vitamin K (K_1).

In surgical practice, vitamin K status is critical in obstructive jaundice, whereby bile cannot flow into the small intestine so that vitamin K_1 is not absorbed. It is, of course, very dangerous to operate on someone with a coagulation defect, so before surgery on

the bile duct, the prothrombin activity must be checked and vitamin K_1 given as a precaution. Vitamin K deficiency also occurs in patients with malabsorption, and sometimes following prolonged use of broad-spectrum antibiotics by mouth (which can destroy the colonic bacteria). In serious liver disease, the coagulation factors may not be adequately synthesized, but this is because of poor liver function, rather than vitamin K deficiency.

In internal medicine, the most common cause of vitamin K deficiency is the use of anticoagulant drugs, given to prevent clotting in veins: warfarin and dicoumarol, which owe their therapeutic action to blocking one of the enzymes that recycle vitamin K in the liver.

Dosage is controlled by following the prothrombin time in patients' blood. This is usually expressed as international normalized ratio, which adjusts for the thromboplastin used in the test. This is the usual way to make the diagnosis of vitamin K deficiency, because plasma concentrations of K1 are minute. A more specific method is to measure under γ-carboxylated prothrombin.

There are reports of low circulating vitamin K in elderly patients with femoral neck fractures or spinal crush fractures, suggesting that suboptimal vitamin K status may play a role in osteoporosis, presumably because osteocalcin is not made adequately.

15.2.5 Dietary sources

Vitamin K_1 is present in dark-green leaves eaten as foods. Some contain more than others. It is associated with the photosynthetic tissues. Kale, spinach, brussels sprouts, broccoli, parsley, coriander, endive, mint, mustard greens, cabbage, and lettuce are good sources (in descending order). Other good sources are some vegetable oils (soybean and canola). Small amounts are present in beef liver, apples, and green tea, and there is some vitamin K_2 in cheese and fermented soybeans.

There are no experimentally derived reference values yet for vitamin K, but it is agreed that 1 μg/kg body weight is a safe and adequate intake (i.e. around 80 μg/day in men and 65 μg/day in women). Bone Gla protein may be more sensitive to low intakes than the Gla haemostatic proteins. Usual adult intakes are variously estimated at 60–200 µg/day.

No application has been devised for supernutritional doses of vitamin K_1, but even milligram doses by mouth have not been found toxic. However, the synthetic water-soluble pharmaceutical with vitamin K activity, menadione, can cause haemolytic anaemia and jaundice in newborn babies. It is now obsolete, superseded by vitamin K_1.

Further Reading

Vitamin D

1. **Bischoff-Ferrari, H.A., Willett, W.C., Wong, J.B., Giovannucci, E., Dietrich, T., and Dawson-Hughes, T.** (2005) Fracture prevention with vitamin D supplementation. A meta-analysis of randomized controlled trials. *J Am Med Assoc*, **293**, 2257–64.
2. **Diamond, T.H., Eisman, J.A., Mason, R.S.,** *et al*. (2005) Vitamin D and adult bone health in Australia and New Zealand: A position statement. *Med J Aust*, **183**, 281–3.
3. **Food and Nutrition Board, Institute of Medicine** (1997) *Dietary reference intakes for calcium, phosphorus, magnesium, vitamin D and fluoride*. Washington, DC, National Academy Press.
4. **Fraser, D.R.** (1995) Vitamin D. *Lancet*, **345**, 104–7.
5. **Holick, M.F.** (2007) Vitamin D deficiency. *N Engl J Med*, **357**: 266–81.
6. **Hyppönen, E. and Power, C.** (2007) Hypovitaminosis D in British adults at age 45: Nationwide cohort study of dietary and lifestyle predictors. *Am J Clin Nutr* **85**: 860–6.
7. **MacLaughlin, J. and Holick, M.F.** (1985) Ageing decreases the capacity of human skin to produce vitamin D_3. *J Clin Invest*, **76**, 1536–8.
8. **van Amerongen, B.M., Dijstra, C.D., Lips, P., and Polman, C.H.** (2004) Multiple sclerosis and vitamin D: An update. *Eur J Clin Nutr*, **58**, 1095–109.
9. **Vieth, R; Bischoff-Ferrari, H.A., Boucher, B.J.,** *et al*. (2007) The urgent need to recommend an intake of vitamin D that is effective. *Am J Clin Nutr* **85**: 649–50.

Vitamin K

1. **Booth, S.L., Sadowski, J.A., Weikrauch, J.L., and Ferland, G.** (1998) Vitamin K (phylloquinone) content of foods: A provisional table. *J Food Comp Anal*, **6**, 109–20.
2. **Duggan, P., Cashman, K.D., Flynn, A., Bolton-Smith, C., and Kiely, M.** (2004) Phylloquinone (vitamin K_1) intakes and food sources in 18–64-year old Irish adults. *Br J Nutr*, **92**, 151–8.
3. **Feskanich, D., Weber, P., Willett, W.C., Rockett, H., Booth, S.L., and Colditz, G.A.** (1999) Vitamin K intake and hip fractures in women: A prospective study. *Am J Clin Nutr*, **69**, 74–9.
4. **Johnson, M.A.** (2005) Influence of vitamin K on anticoagulant therapy depends on vitamin K status and the source and chemical forms of vitamin K. *Nutr Rev*, **63**, 91–7.
5. **Suttie, J.W.** (1995) The importance of menaquinones in human nutrition. *Ann Rev Nutr*, **15**, 399–417.

Useful Websites

 To see topical and scientifically robust updates on nutrition associated with this textbook and web links to many of the journals in the Further Reading sections, please see the dedicated Online Resource Centre at **http://www.oxfordtextbooks.co.uk/orc/mann4e/**

16 Other biologically active substances in plant foods: phytochemicals

Bernhard Watzl and Claus Leitzmann

Plants contain a wide range of secondary metabolites of low-molecular weight that, in the broadest sense, are biologically active molecules that have evolved in the interaction between the plant and its environment, including ultraviolet light. When plant foods are consumed, a diverse range of secondary plant metabolites is ingested. In the past, emphasis was placed on secondary metabolites as natural toxicants that are present in plant foods (i.e. glycoalkaloids in potatoes and tomatoes, cyanogenic glycosides in cassava) and their potential hazardous effects on humans. However, for the past two decades there has been increasing recognition of the health benefits of consuming diets rich in vegetables and fruits. Therefore, a resurgence of interest in secondary plant metabolites has evolved due to the epidemiological evidence that has demonstrated a protective effect of vegetable and fruit intake against chronic illnesses such as cardiovascular disease and cancer.

Primary plant metabolites are substances that mainly contribute to energy metabolism and to the structure of the plant cell, i.e. carbohydrates including dietary fibre, proteins, and fats. Secondary plant metabolites are non-nutritive dietary components (excluding vitamins) that have been referred to as *phytochemicals*. Secondary plant metabolites have various functions in the plant such as serving as a defence against destructive weeds, insects, and microorganisms, as growth regulators and as pigments. They are essential for the plant's interactions with its environment. Chemically, these secondary plant metabolites are quite diverse compounds and are found only in minute amounts in contrast to the primary plant metabolites. Secondary plant metabolites have potential pharmacological effects on humans, a thought that was already discussed in the 1950s. More recently, nutrition scientists have systematically begun to investigate the health-promoting effects of these plant substances.

The total number of naturally occurring phytochemicals is not known. Present assumptions vary from 60 000 to 100 000 substances. With a mixed diet, around 1.5 g of secondary plant metabolites are ingested daily. On a vegetarian diet regimen, the intake of secondary plant metabolites can be distinctly higher.

Phytochemicals can have beneficial as well as detrimental health effects. Until a few years ago, they were merely seen under the aspect of toxicity and some were described as antinutritive, or even toxic, metabolites because they restrict the availability of nutrients and increase the permeability of the intestinal wall. However, under the usual conditions of food consumption, nearly all natural components—with a few exceptions such as solanine—are harmless. Many phytochemicals that were previously regarded as having health-adverse effects may have a variety of health-promoting effects. This is exemplified by protease inhibitors in legumes and glucosinolates of various *Cruciferae* species.

In the following, the health-promoting potential of phytochemicals is illustrated on the basis of experimental findings of their biological activity. The evidence found in epidemiological studies helps to estimate the importance that phytochemicals may have for human health.

16.1 Classification of phytochemicals

Phytochemicals are classified according to their chemical structure and their functional characteristics. The main groups of phytochemicals and their physiological effects show their great diversity (Table 16.1).

16.1.1 Carotenoids

Carotenoids are widespread phytochemicals in fruits and vegetables and one of their main functions in plants is to provide the red and yellow pigments

Table 16.1 Classification of phytochemicals and their main effects

Phytochemical	Evidence for the following effects:								
	A	B	C	D	E	F	G	H	I
Carotenoids	X		X		X			X	
Phytosterols	X							X	
Saponins	X	X			X			X	
Glucosinolates	X	X						X	
Polyphenols	X	X	X	X	X	X	X		X
Protease inhibitors	X		X						X
Monoterpenes	X	X						X	
Phyto-oestrogens	X		X		X				
Sulphides	X	X	X	X	X	X	X	X	

A = anticarcinogenic
B = antimicrobial
C = antioxidative
D = antithrombotic
E = immunomodulatory properties

F = anti-inflammatory
G = influence on blood pressure
H = cholesterol-lowering effect
I = modulate blood glucose levels

Source: Modified from Watzl, B. and Leitzmann, C. (2005) *Bioaktive Substanzen in Lebensmitteln*. 3rd edn. Stuttgart, Hippokrates.

essential for photosynthesis. They can be divided into oxygen-free and oxygen-containing (xanthophylls) carotenoids. Of the about 700 natural carotenoids, only around 40–50 are of significance in human nutrition. Depending on the carotenoid structure, several carotenoids possess provitamin A activity (Chapter 12). Human serum mainly contains the oxygen-free carotenoids α- and β-carotene, lycopene as well as the xanthophylls lutein, zeaxanthin, and β-cryptoxanthin in varying proportions, depending on the individual diet. β-carotene accounts for 15–30%. Oxygen-free and oxygen-containing carotenoids differ mainly in their thermal stability. β-carotene in carrots and lycopene in tomatoes, for example, are heat stable; xanthophylls (mainly in green vegetables) are sensitive to thermal processing. The total daily intake of carotenoids on a Western diet is about 6 mg. The absorption of carotenoids differs between raw and heat-treated vegetables and fruits (Table 16.2).

16.1.2 Phytosterols

Phytosterols such as β-sitosterol, stigmasterol, and campesterol are mainly found in plant seeds, nuts, and oils. Chemically, phytosterols differ from cholesterol by an additional side chain only. The daily phytosterol intake amounts to 100–500 mg. In humans absorption of phytosterols is low (0–10%) compared to the >40% for cholesterol. Absorbed phytosterols in the enterocytes are actively transported back to the intestinal lumen, contributing to the low bioavailability of phytosterols. The cholesterol-lowering effect of phytosterols (see Chapter 21) has been known since the 1950s and is, in part, due to their property to inhibit cholesterol absorption. This activity of phytosterols resulted in the generation of one of the first functional foods, a margarine enriched with phytosterol or phytostanol.

16.1.3 Saponins

Saponins are bitter-tasting, surface-active compounds that form complexes with proteins and lipids, such as cholesterol. Saponins are particularly abundant in legumes. The daily intake of saponins may be higher than 200 mg, depending on the dietary habits, but usually averages around 15 mg/day. Saponins have a low absorption rate (Table 16.2) and therefore are primarily active in the intestinal tract. Due to their haemolytic properties, saponins were solely considered to be detrimental to health. In studies conducted with humans, however, this could not be confirmed.

16.1.4 Glucosinolates

Glucosinolates (thioglucosides) are found in food plants belonging to the family of cruciferae. Their degradation products contribute to the typical flavour of mustard, horseradish, and broccoli. In these plants, glucosinolates are associated with but sterically separated from the enzyme myrosinase. Mechanical damage of the plant tissue (cutting, chewing) eliminates the sterical separation between the enzyme and its substrates. Myrosinase then hydrolyses the glucosinolate to its active metabolites: isothiocyanates, thiocyanates, and indoles. Heating of cabbage reduces its glucosinolate content by 30–60% and inactivates its myrosinase activity. However, microbial myrosinase activity in the large intestine contributes to glucosinolate

Table 16.2 Absorption of phytochemicals in humans

Absorption		
High (>15%)	Medium (3–15%)	Low (<3%)
Carotenoids*	Phytosterols	Carotenoids**
Glucosinolates	Phenolic acids	Saponins
Flavonoids***	Protease inhibitors	Anthocyanins
Phyto-oestrogens		Flavones
Monoterpenes		
Sulphides		

*From heat-treated food; **From raw food;
***Flavonoids excluding anthocyanins and flavones.

degradation. The total daily intake of glucosinolates is in the range of 10–50 mg. With vegetarian diets, the total daily intake can be as high as 100 mg. The glucosinolate metabolites, such as isothiocyanates, are completely absorbed in the small intestine (Table 16.2). An isothiocyanate that has been intensely studied is sulphoraphane, which has an anticarcinogenic effect and induces antioxidant responses (Table 16.1).

16.1.5 Polyphenols

The term polyphenol is used for all substances that are made up of phenol derivatives. Polyphenols mainly include phenolic acids (including hydroxy-cinnamic acids) and flavonoids (including flavonols, flavones, flavanols, flavanones, and anthocyanins; Fig. 16.1). Polyphenols normally occur bound to sugars and are rarely found as aglycones in plant

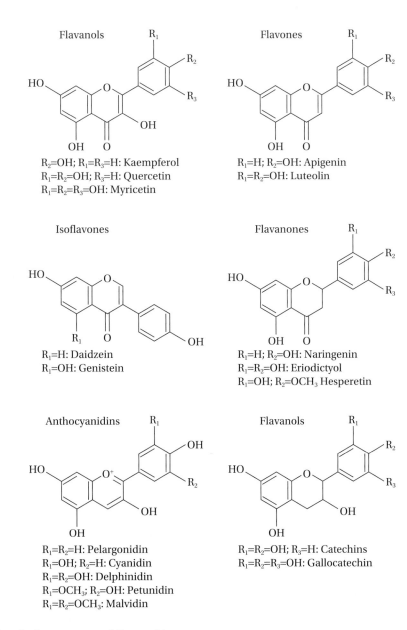

Flavanols

R_2=OH; R_1=R_3=H: Kaempferol
R_1=R_2=OH; R_3=H: Quercetin
R_1=R_2=R_3=OH: Myricetin

Flavones

R_1=H; R_2=OH: Apigenin
R_1=R_2=OH: Luteolin

Isoflavones

R_1=H: Daidzein
R_1=OH: Genistein

Flavanones

R_1=H; R_2=OH: Naringenin
R_1=R_2=OH: Eriodictyol
R_1=OH; R_2=OCH$_3$ Hesperetin

Anthocyanidins

R_1=R_2=H: Pelargonidin
R_1=OH; R_2=H: Cyanidin
R_1=R_2=OH: Delphinidin
R_1=OCH$_3$; R_2=OH: Petunidin
R_1=R_2=OCH$_3$: Malvidin

Flavanols

R_1=R_2=OH; R_3=H: Catechins
R_1=R_2=R_3=OH: Gallocatechin

Fig. 16.1 Chemical structures of flavonoids.

foods. Besides monomeric flavonoids, oligomeric flavonoids (with two or more linked molecules) such as the flavanols (procyanidins) occur in red wine, tea, dark chocolate, and apples. Fresh vegetables contain up to 0.1% polyphenols located almost exclusively in the outer layer of fruits (e.g. apple skin) and vegetables (green leaves of lettuce). The flavonoid content of green leafy vegetables is highest with increasing ripeness. Field-grown vegetables have a higher flavonoid content than greenhouse produce. The most commonly found flavonoid is the flavonol quercetin, with a daily intake of about 25 mg. Recent findings suggest that some flavonoids, such as quercetin, can be absorbed by humans in quantities relevant to human health, while other flavonoids such as the anthocyanins are hardly absorbed (Table 16.2). Polyphenols exert a variety of physiological effects (Table 16.1).

16.1.6 Protease inhibitors

Protease inhibitors are found especially in plant seeds (legumes, grains). Dependent on the mammalian species, protease inhibitors in the gut hamper the activity of endogenous proteases, such as trypsin. In response, the organism reacts with an increased synthesis of digestive enzymes. Humans synthesize a specific trypsin form, among others, which is resistant to protease inhibitors. Cooking significantly reduces the activity of protease inhibitors. Protease inhibitor intake averages about 300 mg daily. The protease inhibitor intake of vegetarians with a diet high in grains and legumes can be considerably higher. Absorbed protease inhibitors can be detected in various tissues in biologically active form.

16.1.7 Monoterpenes

Active substances in herbs and spices such as menthol (peppermint), carvone (caraway seeds), and limonene (citrus oil) are examples of monoterpenes in food. The average daily intake of monoterpenes is up to 200 mg. Due to their fat solubility monoterpenes display a high degree of bioavailability in humans (Table 16.2). Limonene has been studied in animal models as an anticarcinogen and has been undergoing preliminary trials in cancer patients.

16.1.8 Phyto-oestrogens

Phyto-oestrogens are plant components that bind to mammalian oestrogen receptors and have effects similar to those of endogenous oestrogens. Isoflavones and lignans, chemically both polyphenols, are the two major groups of the phyto-oestrogens in plant foods. Phyto-oestrogens have only about 0.1% of the efficacy that human oestrogens exhibit; however, their concentration in body fluids and tissues may be 100- to 10 000-fold higher. Therefore, phyto-oestrogens can act both as oestrogens and anti-oestrogens, depending on the amount and concentration of endogenous oestrogens. Isoflavones are almost exclusively found in soybeans and soybean products. Lignans are present in higher concentrations in flax seeds and whole grain products. The major isoflavones in soy are the glycosides of genistein and daidzein. With traditional Asian diets and vegetarian diets, the phyto-oestrogen intake is high (15–40 mg/day), but Western diets provide little phyto-oestrogens (<2 mg/day). Phyto-oestrogens have a high absorption rate resulting in blood concentrations associated with various *in-vitro* and *in-vivo* effects (Tables 16.1 and 16.2).

16.1.9 Sulphides

The sulphides among secondary plant metabolites include all organosulphur compounds of garlic and other bulbous plants. The main active substance of garlic is oxidized diallyl disulphide or allicin. Damage to the tissue in the garlic clove leads to the release of the enzyme alliinase which produces allicin from the basic compound, alliin or S-allylcysteine sulphoxide.

16.1.10 Other phytochemicals

Apart from the secondary plant metabolites listed above, there are further phytochemicals that do not fit in the categories above. Lectins, for example, are present in legumes and grain products. They may have blood glucose-lowering effects. Other examples are glucarates, phthalides, chlorophyll, and tocotrienols, as well as phytic acid.

16.2 Physiological effects of phytochemicals

The following is a short overview of the major effects of phytochemicals. For detailed information and references see Watzl and Leitzmann (2005), Liu (2004) as well as Kris-Etherton *et al.* (2004).

16.2.1 Anticarcinogenic effects

Cancer is the second-most frequent cause of death in industrialized countries. Nutrition is the major exogenous factor that modulates cancer risk and contributes to about one-third of all types of cancer. There are dietary factors that may promote carcinogenesis, but also others that may lower cancer risk. Evidence from epidemiological and animal experimental studies as well as information from biomarker and mechanistic studies indicate that a higher intake of vegetables and fruits is associated with a lower risk of various types of cancer. For all classes of phytochemicals occurring in vegetables and fruits, anti-cancer effects have been described. Based on the potential cancer-preventative activity of plant foods, it has been recommended to increase the consumption of vegetables and fruits to at least five servings per day.

Phytochemicals may interfere and inhibit carcinogenesis at almost any stage in the multistep process: tumour initiation, promotion, and progression (Fig. 16.2). Knowledge of anticarcinogenic effects of vegetables and fruits, and of isolated phytochemicals, has been obtained from different experimental systems (*in vitro*, animal, human). Animal experiments yield direct information about the extent of suppression of spontaneous and chemically induced tumours by ingestion of certain plant foods or isolated phytochemicals (dose–effect studies). However, human studies, especially epidemiological, intervention, and biomarker-related studies are of particular relevance.

Carcinogens (e.g. nitrosamines) are usually ingested in their inactive form. Their endogenous activation by phase I enzymes (e.g. cytochrome P-450-dependent monooxygenases) is a prerequisite for the interaction with the DNA and genotoxic activity. Phase II enzymes (e.g. glutathione S-transferase, GST) usually detoxify activated carcinogens. In general, phytochemicals (glucosinolates, polyphenols, monoterpenes, sulphides) can inhibit carcinogenesis by inhibiting phase I enzymes and inducing phase II enzymes in cell cultures and in animal experiments, thereby acting as blocking agents (Fig. 16.2). In this manner, the risk of DNA damage and tumour initiation is reduced. For example, the isothiocyanate sulphoraphane that can be isolated from broccoli activates the phase II detoxifying enzyme quinone reductase in cell culture systems. In human studies, 300 g Brussels sprouts/day led to increased levels of alpha-GST (phase II enzyme) in male subjects, but not in female subjects.

Recent data on genetic polymorphisms in humans contribute to a better understanding of the cancer-preventative activity of phytochemicals and of vegetables and fruits. According to new studies, the potential effects of phytochemicals such as carotenoids and isothiocyanates on cancer prevention, for example, depend highly on GST genotypes. In subjects with deletions of certain GST isotypes, a high intake of these phytochemicals was associated with a lower cancer risk.

An influence on hormone metabolism has been demonstrated by phyto-oestrogens. This is an example of cancer-suppressive activities of phytochemicals during tumour promotion and progression (Fig. 16.2). Animal experiments have shown

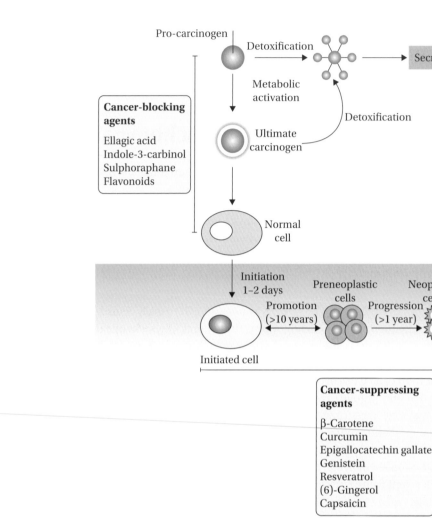

Fig. 16.2 Dietary phytochemicals that block or suppress multistage carcinogenesis.

Source: Surh, Y.J. (2003) Cancer chemoprevention with dietary phytochemicals. *Nature Rev Cancer*, **3**, 768–80.

that phyto-oestrogens and the glucosinolate metabolite indole-3-carbinol influence oestrogen metabolism in such a manner that oestrogens known for their low-promoting tumour-growth properties are produced (i.e. catechol oestrogen). Furthermore, phyto-oestrogens induce the synthesis of the sex hormone-binding globulin (SHBG) in the human liver, leading to an increase of oestrogens bound to this transport protein, making them less active. In prospective studies, however, phyto-oestrogens were not associated with lower cancer risk. Genistein, an isoflavone

and phyto-oestrogen present in soybeans that can be detected in humans after soybean consumption, inhibits the growth of blood vessels *in vitro*, possibly having an effect on the growth and metastasis of tumours.

A further point of attack for anticarcinogenic phytochemicals is the regulation of cell growth (proliferation) and programmed cell death (apoptosis). Tumour cells distinguish themselves by a distorted regulation of cell proliferation and apoptosis. Phytochemicals such as isothiocyanates and carotenoids could intervene in such a twisted regulation by modulating the endogenous formation of cell growth-promoting substances and the process of intracellular signal transduction.

16.2.2 Antioxidative effects

The pathogenesis of cancer and cardiovascular diseases has been associated with the presence of reactive oxygen molecules and free radicals. The human body is equipped with several protective mechanisms against these reactive substances, including enzyme systems, superoxide dismutase, and glutathione peroxidase, as well as endogenous antioxidants (uric acid, glutathione, α-lipoic acid, coenzyme Q_{10}). Essential nutrients with antioxidant activity include vitamins E and C. Additionally, phytochemicals (carotenoids, polyphenols, phyto-oestrogens, and sulphides) exhibit antioxidative effects.

Certain carotenoids such as β-carotene, lycopene, and canthaxanthin provide effective protection against singlet oxygen or oxygen radicals *in vitro*. However, human studies have failed to demonstrate an antioxidative effect of carotenoid supplements in well-nourished individuals. Of all antioxidants in plant foods, polyphenols *in vitro* have the highest potential in terms of quantity and effect. While most human studies could not demonstrate an antioxidative effect of polyphenols *in vivo*, recent studies using dark chocolate or tea showed an effect on plasma antioxidant capacity of polyphenol-rich foods.

Certain fruit and vegetable species influence the level of naturally occuring oxidative DNA damage. For example, the daily consumption of apples or Brussel sprouts over a 3–4 week period led to a significant decrease of oxidative DNA damage as assessed in blood lymphocytes or urine (reduced excretion of 8-oxo-7,8-dihydro-2-deoxyguanosine). Essential nutrients with antioxidative potential (vitamins C and E) are ingested in amounts of around 100 mg/day. In contrast, the daily ingested amount of phytochemicals with antioxidant potential may exceed 1 g. This emphasizes the potential physiological importance of phytochemicals as antioxidants and as agents for other mechanisms that reduce the risk of chronic diseases by consumption of vegetables and fruits.

16.2.3 Immunomodulatory effects

The immune system, primarily responsible for the defence against pathogens and transformed cells, is also involved in pathophysiological processes that lead to cancer and cardiovascular disease. Adequate nutrition is the basis for an optimally functioning immune system. Of special importance in this respect are total energy intake, quantity and quality of fats, and certain micronutrients.

Immunomodulatory activities of phytochemicals are a further mechanism through which plant foods may reduce disease risk. The immunomodulatory effects of phytochemicals have so far only been investigated to a very small extent, except for carotenoids. The stimulating effects of various carotenoids and carotenoid-rich foods on the immune system have been demonstrated in numerous animal experiments and human intervention studies.

Flavonoids, in contrast to the carotenoids, have been almost exclusively studied *in vitro*. Most studies demonstrate immunosuppressive activity of the flavonoids. Recent human studies suggest that dietary flavonoids can inhibit the inflammatory processes which are associated with obesity. Saponins, sulphides, phyto-oestrogens, and phytic acid show immunomodulatory effects. As human studies with pure phytochemicals are lacking, with the exception of certain carotenoids, the evaluation of their immunomodulatory effects in humans is not yet possible. For some phytochemicals, however, such an effect seems likely.

16.2.4 Antimicrobial effects

Vegetables, fruits, and spices have been used to treat infections since antiquity. The discovery of sulphonamides and microbial antibiotics and their successful use in treating infections resulted in a decline of interest in antimicrobial constituents in food. Only recently is there a renewed interest in plant foods with antimicrobial effects.

Earlier studies clearly verified the antimicrobial action of sulphides from bulbous plants. Recent studies also demonstrated an inhibitory effect of garlic sulphides against *Helicobacter pylori in vitro*. Eliminating allicin from garlic prevented this effect. The glucosinolate metabolites isothiocyanate and thiocyanate have likewise been shown to have antimicrobial activity. They are present in bacteriostatic concentrations in the urinary tract after consumption of garden cress, nasturtium, and horseradish roots. However, the consumption of these plants alone will not lead to successful therapy.

In naturopathy, some berries such as cranberries and blueberries are frequently used for the prevention and therapy of infectious diseases. Data from several human intervention studies indicate that the daily intake of 300 mL of cranberry juice as well as of other berries significantly reduces the risk of urinary tract infections, mainly in women. Juice consumption increased the intake of polyphenols (procyanidins) that inhibit the adherence of infectious bacteria to the urinary tract epithelium.

16.2.5 Cholesterol-lowering effects

Phytosterols, saponins, sulphides, flavonoids, and lycopene have been found to lower serum cholesterol levels in both animal experiments and in clinical studies. The extent to which cholesterol levels are reduced depends on the cholesterol and fat content of the diet. The minimal effective dose of phytosterol is 1 g/day, while 170–440 mg/day is consumed in a typical Western diet. Margarines enriched with the esters of phytosterol or phytostanol provide 1.5–3.0 g/day, resulting in a 10–15% reduction of low-density lipoprotein cholesterol (see Chapter 21).

Although the cholesterol-lowering effect of phytochemicals has been known for over 50 years, the underlying mechanism is still not clear. Several mechanisms may be responsible for this. Saponins

bind to primary bile acids in the gut and form micelles. These micelles are too large to pass the intestinal wall, thus leading to reduced absorption of bile acid and, in turn, to their excretion. As a consequence, an increased synthesis of primary bile acids in the liver from the endogenous cholesterol pool is initiated, leading to a decrease of the serum cholesterol level. Phytosterols probably also retard cholesterol absorption by driving cholesterol out of the micelles that normally help to absorb cholesterol from the gut.

Phytochemicals can also inhibit key enzymes of the cholesterol synthesis in the liver. Of these key enzymes, the most important is 3-hydroxy-3-methylglutaryl-CoA-reductase, which is inhibited by monoterpenes and sulphides in animals.

16.2.6 Phytochemicals affecting drug metabolism

Phytochemicals in grapefruit juice interact with the metabolism of a variety of drugs. Drinking a single glass of grapefruit juice before administration of these drugs can severely affect drug bioavailability and pharmacokinetics of the drug. The mechanism for this effect is the post-transcriptional inhibition of the cytochrome P-450 3A4 enzyme in the small intestine, without affecting the same enzyme system in the large intestine or in the liver. This results in a reduction of pre-systemic metabolism of the drug followed by enhanced drug effects. A further mechanism could be the inhibition of a transporter system (P-glycoprotein) that normally carries drugs from the enterocyte back to the small intestinal lumen. Human experimental data suggest that furanocoumarins contribute to this grapefruit effect.

Other health-promoting effects of phytochemicals include regulation of blood pressure, blood glucose level and blood coagulation and inhibition of inflammatory processes (Table 16.1). Further, carotenoids may be involved in the prevention of macular degeneration in the retina as well as other diseases of the eye (see Chapter 12).

16.3 Epidemiological evidence for the protective effects of vegetables, fruits, whole grains, and phytochemicals

A number of epidemiological studies analysed by the World Cancer Research Fund, the American Institute for Cancer Research, and the International Agency for Research on Cancer of the WHO suggests that a high intake of plant foods is inversely associated with the risk for some cancers. While the outcome of recent prospective cohort studies was less supportive for a general cancer-protective effect, overall the totality of evidence still suggests that constituents in plant foods protect against cancer. In addition, data from prospective studies analysing associations at the level of phytochemical intakes and cancer risk suggest that phytochemicals are related to the reduction of cancer risk. As well as evidence about cancer, a number of prospective cohort studies have reported a reduction of risk of cardiovascular disease by 30% in subjects consuming high amounts of vegetables, fruits, and whole grains compared to subjects with a low intake. Similar trends for the intake of specific phytochemicals in prospective as well as in human intervention studies were observed. For example, the increased intake of specific flavonoids reduced blood pressure in human intervention studies.

With the present state of knowledge, it is hard to differentiate to what degree the various components in plant foods (essential nutrients, dietary fibre, and phytochemicals) contribute to the observed reduction in disease risk. Human intervention studies are needed to prove that the health-promoting effects of plant foods observed in epidemiological studies are causally related to the intake of phytochemicals.

Conclusions

Present knowledge of the effects of phytochemicals allows us to conclude that these non-nutritive dietary compounds of plant foods can have health-promoting effects. Phytochemicals, along with vitamins, minerals, trace elements, fatty acids, and dietary fibre, are responsible for the protective effects of vegetables and fruits, nuts, whole grains, and legumes against cancer and cardiovascular disease. Clearly, there is no evidence that a single phytochemical is especially effective in the prevention of cancer or cardiovascular disease. The most protective effect is observed when a high number of different phytochemicals is consumed with plant foods, which presumably exerts cumulative or synergistic effects. For many phytochemicals, detection methods in foods and body fluids have been established. Although the determination of phytochemicals in terms of content, bioavailability, and biokinetics is now possible, only key phytochemicals of the individual classes have been carefully studied. Further epidemiological and experimental studies should elucidate the links between the ingestion of certain phytochemicals and the incidence of specific disease, including mechanisms of protection. In short-term intervention studies, biomarkers need to be identified that yield indications for long-term preventative effects of phytochemicals in humans.

The toxic potential of phytochemicals is negligible, as long as consumption habits are restricted to whole food and avoid extracts or isolates from food. So far no adverse effects of phytochemicals as part of wholesome foods have been reported, even in subjects on predominately vegetarian diets.

Nutritional recommendations do not need to be modified in the light of the latest understanding of the health benefits of phytochemicals. Recommended dietary allowances for certain plant foods for prevention or therapy of certain diseases cannot be given at this point in time. However, most nutritional recommendations include an increase in the consumption of plant-derived foods (to five a day) based on epidemiological evidence that phytochemicals have beneficial effects on the health and wellbeing of humans. In summary:

- Plant foods contain phytochemicals of different chemical classes.

- Intake of dietary phytochemicals modulates physiological processes in humans.

- A high dietary intake of phytochemicals with vegetables, fruits, nuts, legumes, and whole grains is associated with a reduced risk for cardiovascular disease and other diseases.

Further Reading

1. **Adlercreutz, H.** (2007) Lignans and human health. *Crit Rev Clin Lab Sci*, **44**, 483–525.
2. **Chun, O.K., Chung, S.J., and Song, W.O.** (2007) Estimated dietary flavonoid intake and major food sources of U.S. adults. *J Nutr*, **137**, 1244–52.
3. **Dauchet, L., Amouyel, P., Hercberg, S., et al.** (2006) Fruit and vegetable consumption and risk of coronary heart disease: A meta-analysis of cohort studies. *J Nutr*, **136**, 2588–93.
4. **Jones, P.J.H. and AbuMweis, S.** (2009) Phytosterols as functional food ingredients: Linkages to cardiovascular disease and cancer. *Curr Opin Clin Nutr Metab Care*, **12**, 147–51.
5. **Kris-Etherton, P.M., Lefevre, M., Beecher, G.R., et al.** (2004) Bioactive compounds in foods: Their role in the prevention of cardiovascular disease and cancer nutrition and health-research methodologies for establishing biological function: The antioxidant and anti-inflammatory effects of flavonoids on atherosclerosis. *Annu Rev Nutr*, **24**, 511–38.
6. **Liu, R.H.** (2004) Potential synergy of phytochemicals in cancer prevention: Mechanism of action. *J Nutr*, **134**, 3479S–85S.
7. **Manach, C., Williamson, G., Morand, C., et al.** (2005) Bioavailability and bioefficacy of polyphenols in humans. I. Review of 97 bioavailability studies, and II. Review of 93 intervention studies. *Am J Clin Nutr*, **81** (supp 1), 230S–42S and 243S–55S.
8. **Paine, M.F., Widmer, W.W., Hart, H.L., et al.** (2006) A furanocoumarin-free grapefruit juice establishes furanocoumarins as the mediators of the grapefruit juice-felodipine interaction. *Am J Clin Nutr*, **83**, 1097–105.
9. **Shi, J., Arunasalam, K., Yeung, D., et al.** (2004) Saponins from edible legumes: Chemistry, processing, and health benefits. *J Med Food*, **7**, 67–78.
10. **Silaste, M.L., Alfthan, G., Aro, A., Kesäniemi, Y.A., and Hörkkö, S.** (2007) Tomato juice decreases LDL cholesterol levels and increases LDL resistance to oxidation. *Br J Nutr*, **98**, 1251–8.
11. **Surh, Y.J.** (2003) Cancer chemoprevention with dietary phytochemicals. *Nature Rev Cancer*, **3**, 768–80.
12. **Verkerk, R., Schreiner, M., Krumbein, A., et al.** (2009) Glucosinolates in *Brassica* vegetables: The influence of the food supply chain on intake, bioavailability and human health. *Mol Nutr Food Res*, **53**, S219–65.
13. **Watzl, B. and Leitzmann, C.** (2005) *Bioaktive Substanzen in Lebensmitteln*. 3rd edn. Stuttgart, Hippokrates.
14. **World Cancer Research Fund/American Institute for Cancer Research** (2007) *Food, nutrition, physical activity, and the prevention of cancer: A global perspective.* 2nd edn. Washington, DC, AICR.

Useful Websites

To see topical and scientifically robust updates on nutrition associated with this textbook and web links to many of the journals in the Further Reading sections, please see the dedicated Online Resource Centre at **http://www.oxfordtextbooks.co.uk/orc/mann4e/**

Part 3

Nutrition-related disorders

17 Overweight and obesity

Stephan Rössner

Overweight and obesity are very common conditions in developed societies, and are becoming more common in developing countries and those in transition. Indeed, the increased prevalence of these disorders in many societies and countries has been accompanied by an increased risk of many associated diseases, health disorders, and premature mortality. The complications of obesity also have a profound health economic effect.

17.1 Definitions and measurements

Obesity is a condition in which the fat stores are excessive for an individual's height, weight, gender, and race to an extent that produces adverse health outcomes. Several measures for assessing and defining adiposity exist (Box 17.1). In clinical practice and epidemiological research, obesity is most often defined in terms of the body mass index (BMI), a measure that gives a reasonable approximation of adiposity. BMI is derived by dividing an individual's weight in kilograms by height in metres squared (kg/m^2). Adults with a BMI between 25 and 29.9 kg/m^2 are categorized as overweight, and those with a BMI greater than 30 kg/m^2 are categorized as obese (Table 17.1). In the aged or the very fit and muscular, the BMI definitions given above are not as useful as

> **BOX 17.1** Techniques for measuring adiposity
>
> - Body mass index (BMI)
> - Waist circumference
> - Waist/hip ratio
> - Skinfold thickness
> - Hydrodensitometry (underwater weighing)
> - Air displacement
> - Bioelectrical impedance
> - Dual-energy X-ray absorptiometry (DEXA)
> - Computerized tomography (CT)
> - Nuclear magnetic resonance spectroscopy

Table 17.1 Recommended definition of obesity according to WHO (2000) for European populations and WHO (Western Pacific Region) /IOTF (2000) for Asian populations

Classification	BMI (kg/m²)		Risk of comorbidities
	Caucasian	Asian	
Underweight	<18.5	<18.5	Low (but risk of other clinical problems increased)
Normal range	18.5–24.9	18.5–22.9	Average
Overweight	≥25.0	≥23.0	
Pre-obese	25–29.9	23.0–24.9	Mildly increased
Obese	≥30.0	≥25.0	
Class I	30.0–34.9	25.0–29.9	Moderate
Class II	35.0–39.9	≥30.0	High
Class III	≥40.0		Very high

an obesity measure. Furthermore, in children, BMI can only be used if corrected for age, and special charts are used to assess overweight and obesity up to age 18 (see Chapter 34).

BMI cut-offs were based on mainly American epidemiological studies that showed a steady increase in risk of the consequences of obesity (see Section 17.8) as BMI increased above 25. These studies were initially based on life insurance data, which may not be truly representative of the population as a whole. However, the association between increasing BMI and total mortality has recently been confirmed in a pooled data set involving 1.46 million white adults, aged 19–84 years participating in 19 prospective studies. All-cause mortality was lowest with a BMI of 20.0–24.9 (de Gonzalez *et al.* (2010)). In several other ethnic groups, the proportions of adipose tissue and lean body mass for a given BMI may differ from that which might be predicted from studies in those of European descent. Some Asian populations (notably those from the Indian subcontinent and China) tend to have a greater fat mass (which is also more likely to be centrally distributed) and less lean body mass for a given BMI than Europeans. Therefore, the Western Pacific Region of the World

Health Organization (WHO) and the International Obesity Taskforce (IOTF) have suggested different cut-off points for Asian adults. A BMI between 23 and 24.9 kg/m² is categorized as overweight or 'at risk' and a BMI over 25 kg/m² is categorized as obesity (Table 17.1). This range has been accepted by Japan, while other Asian countries are still considering appropriate action points. People of Polynesian descent have more lean body mass than Europeans for a given BMI. However, because they appear to have a strong predisposition to developing diabetes and other comorbidities of obesity, it may not be appropriate to recommend a different range from that used for Europeans.

The site of the increased fat tissue is important in identifying individuals at increased risk of obesity-related disease. In particular, excess abdominal (visceral) adipose tissue is associated with considerable risk of cardiovascular disease and metabolic disorders such as diabetes, dyslipidaemia, and the metabolic syndrome (see Section 17.8 and Chapter 23). Therefore, it is important to measure abdominal fat. Scanning techniques (e.g. DEXA, CT) are used for research purposes but in clinical practice and epidemiological research, measuring waist circumference provides a satisfactory surrogate measure of abdominal obesity. Measurements >102 cm in men and >88 cm in women indicate a greatly increased risk of metabolic disease. Measurements >94 cm in men and >80 cm in women suggest an increased risk. Those of Asian extraction tend to have more abdominal fat and it has been suggested that waist circumferences >90 cm in men and >80 cm in women signify increased risk in Asians. The waist, or abdominal circumference, is measured by placing a non-stretchable measuring tape in a horizontal plane around the abdomen at the level midway between the iliac crest and the lowest rib margin in the mid-axillary lines. Clothing from around the waist should be removed to ensure correct positioning of the tape and the measurement is made at a normal minimal respiration. The waist (W) to hip (H) ratio (W/H ratio) can also be used as a measure of abdominal adiposity. (The hips are measured around the maximal protrusion of the buttocks). A W/H ratio of >0.8 in women and >0.9 in men suggests abdominal obesity.

Underwater weighing is now rarely used, but BodPod, measuring air rather than water displacement in a closed box is an option, mainly for research purposes. Skinfold thickness measured at several sites is associated with a high level of observer error unless the observers have been formally trained. Skinfold is, however, an appropriate measure in determining underweight. The remaining methods (Box 17.1) are more costly and are used predominantly for research purposes, though several of the more elaborate techniques are becoming more widely available and are increasingly being used in a clinical setting.

17.2 Prevalence

Obesity and overweight are very common and affect all regions in the world, despite the many public health interventions that have been implemented over the past several decades. The basal metabolic rate decreases with age as obesity increases. Typically BMI increases by about one unit per decade after age 20 years. In the developed world, prevalence is greater amongst lower socioeconomic groups than amongst the more affluent. Obesity prevalence has been increasing steadily in most countries over the past few decades. Examples of prevalence data for some countries are illustrated in Fig. 17.1 and

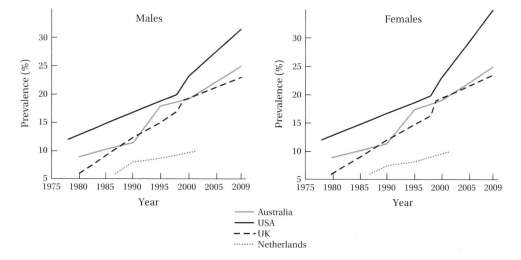

Fig. 17.1 Changing obesity prevalence rates in four countries.

Table 17.2 Global prevalence of adult obesity

	Country	Year of data collection	Survey sample size	Age category	Male (%)		Female (%)	
					Overweight % (BMI 25–29.9)	Obesity % (BMI 30+)	Overweight % (BMI 25–29.9)	Obesity % (BMI 30+)
Europe	England	2009	4100	16+	43.7	22.1	32.8	23.9
	France	2006	3115	18–74	41	16.1	23.8	17.6
	Netherlands	1998–2002	3691	20–59	43.5	10.4	28.5	10.1
	Scotland	2008	4115	16+	41.4	24.9	33.1	26.5
	Sweden	2002	1032	25–64	43.5	14.8	26.6	11.0
Africa	Seychelles	2004	1255	25–64	37	14.7	33	34.2
	Kenya	2009		15–49			17.9	7.2
	Cameroon	2003	9454	15+	21.6	6.5	28.6	19.5
SE Asia	India	2005/6	177523	15–49	8	1.3	9.8	2.8
	Thailand	2004		18+	17.7	4.7	25.2	9.1
	Indonesia	2000	20593	20+	10.2	1.3	17.4	4.5
Western Pacific	Australia	2008	16601	18+	42.1	25.6	30.9	24
	New Zealand	2006/7	12488	≥15	40.7	24.7	29.4	26
	Nauru	2004	2254	15–64	26.5	55.7	21.8	60.5
	Japan	2000	15000	20+	24.5	2.3	17.8	3.4
	China	2002	221,044	18+	16.7	2.4	15.4	3.4
Eastern Mediterranean	Egypt	2008	11258	15–49	34.3	18.2	28.3	39.5
	Lebanon	1998–2002	2846	25–64		36.3		38.3
	Saudi Arabia	1995–2000	17223	30+	42.4	26.4	31.8	44.0
	Pakistan	1990–1994	8972	15+	8.5	4	11.3	7.3
Americas	USA	2007/8	5555	20+	40.1	32.2	28.6	35.5
	Canada	2004	12428	18+	42.0	22.9	30.2	23.2
	Brazil	2003		20+	32.2	8.9	26.9	13.1
	Chile	2003	3619	17+	43.2	19.6	32.7	29.3
	Paraguay	1991–1992	1606	20–74	41.6	22.9	36.1	35.7

Source: Selected country data provided by International Association for the Study of Obesity (IASO) (last updated October 2011).

Table 17.2. Global prevalence data are continuously updated by the International Association for the Study of Obesity (IASO), found at the IASO (www. iaso.org) and WHO (http://apps.who.int/bmi/ index.jsp) websites.

Obesity is very prevalent in the East Mediterranean region, with almost half of Egyptian women being classified as obese. Alarming statistics have been reported from some African countries and amongst the indigenous people of the South Pacific. For example, 44% of the black female population in the Cape Peninsula in South Africa were found to be obese using current criteria. This is in contrast to Ethiopia, where only 0.7% of the population is obese. In Tonga, 70% of women and 47% of men were found to be obese. South Asian countries appear to have the lowest overall rates.

Overweight is far more common than obesity. Interestingly, in many countries men have higher rates of overweight than women, despite similar or higher rates of obesity amongst women. For example, in Australia, 42% of adult males and 31% of adult females are overweight, whereas about a quarter of all adults are obese. In China, 17% of men and 15% of women are overweight, using BMI cut-offs more appropriate for European populations. Given the observation that Asian populations may have a greater degree of adiposity than Europeans for any given BMI (Table 17.1), it seems likely that the degree of adiposity and associated disorders may have been underestimated in some Asian countries.

17.3 Perceptions

Perceptions of body size differ from country to country and influence public health and clinical approaches to the management of obesity. In most Western countries, those who are obese are perceived poorly by the community and health professionals, and the individuals themselves often have low self-esteem. The common failures in treatment programmes are often due to unrealistic expectations. Women try to lose weight for appearance and health.

In contrast, men generally do not present for weight control or treatment, unless persuaded to do so as a result of a comorbidity associated with obesity. In some cultures (e.g. Polynesian), overweight and obesity may still be regarded as desirable attributes. Ironically, in countries with very high AIDS prevalence, an obese body suggests freedom from that infection and hence health. Parents often underestimate the extent to which their children are overweight.

17.4 Genetics of obesity

Although the rapid increase in obesity prevalence cannot be explained by genetic factors, they nevertheless play an important role in determining weight gain and obesity. For example, Stunkard *et al.* showed in an adoption study published in 1986 that the weight of adults adopted as children was related to the weight of their biological parents, rather than the weight of their adopting family. In addition, Bouchard's classical overfeeding studies from the 1990s involving twins demonstrated a strong genetic component in the amount of weight gained with the same amount of overfeeding. Adoption, twin, and family studies indicate that adiposity is highly heritable. However, families share environments as well as genes and the estimated genetic and shared environment contribution to BMI ranges between 60% and 84%.

Several hundred genes are involved in body weight regulation. Only a few single gene mutations that cause obesity have been discovered. Some of the genes are listed in Box 17.2. These monogenic causes of obesity are extremely uncommon and usually involve mechanisms

BOX 17.2 Examples of single genes, mutations of which may be associated with massive obesity

Melanocortin-4 receptor
Leptin
Leptin receptor
Pro-opiomelanocortin
Prohormone convertase 1

associated with energy homeostasis (e.g. appetite regulation). Such single-gene mutations are typically associated with massive obesity. In addition, pleiotropic syndromes such as Prader–Willi syndrome (PWS), where obesity is a clinical feature, have also been described, and they are often associated with mental retardation, organ abnormalities, and dysmorphism. The molecular mechanisms by which these genes act to produce obesity are not clear.

17.5 Adipocyte factors

Traditionally thought of as an inert mass acting as a reservoir for energy storage, adipose tissue is now known to be an active endocrine organ playing key roles in energy and metabolism homeostasis. This dynamic organ exerts its effects via endocrine, paracrine, and autocrine functions, secreting hormones and cytokines (adipokines) that influence the body's energy, and immune and autonomic systems. Some consequences of changing patterns of adipocyte hormone secretion following weight gain and weight loss are illustrated in Fig. 17.2.

Several novel adipocyte-related proteins have fuelled research interest into the adipocyte (fat cell). Two of the adipocyte hormones, leptin and adiponectin, are discussed briefly below. For a discussion of the many other hormones and proteins associated with the adipocyte, the reader is referred to recent reviews (see Further reading).

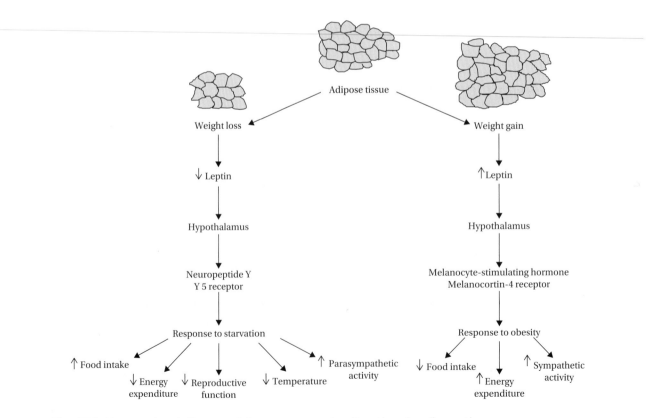

Fig. 17.2 Hormonal and other regulatory responses to alterations in adipose tissue mass.

17.5.1 Leptin

Leptin is a polypeptide protein produced by adipocytes and secreted in direct proportion to adipose tissue mass and the individual's nutritional status. Leptin levels are high in obese individuals and low in lean people, with females tending to have higher leptin levels than men. More leptin is secreted from subcutaneous than from visceral adipose tissue. When adults lose weight, leptin levels fall. Leptin's main actions are on energy balance (intake and expenditure) predominantly acting via central hypothalamic pathways, with some effects on peripheral tissues such as muscle. In adolescents, increasing leptin may act as a signal of adequate fat stores to initiate puberty and for fertility. Low leptin levels signal fat depletion. Secretion of leptin is influenced by many factors, such as glucose metabolism (insulin), inflammation (tumour necrosis factor-α (TNF-α)), and steroid pathways (glucocorticoids and oestrogens), indicating leptin's complex interactions with several physiological systems. Deficiency of leptin results in hyperphagia, decreased energy expenditure, and severe obesity. In those extremely rare cases where primary leptin deficiency exists, treatment with leptin results in a reduction in energy intake and weight loss.

17.5.2 Adiponectin

Adiponectin, a polypeptide secreted exclusively by adipocytes, circulates at high concentrations in the bloodstream. Adiponectin is inversely associated with adipose tissue mass, and among the obese, levels of adiponectin are reduced. In addition, inflammatory and insulin-resistant states and coronary heart disease are associated with decreased adiponectin levels. Acting on the liver, muscle, and blood vessels, adiponectin exerts a wide range of effects that include insulin sensitization, anti-inflammatory effects by antagonizing pro-inflammatory cytokines such as TNF-α, and anti-atherogenic properties by decreasing monocyte adhesion and smooth muscle proliferation in vessel walls. Weight loss and improvement in insulin sensitivity are associated with increasing levels of adiponectin.

17.6 Energy balance

Weight stability implies a balance between energy intake (food and beverages consumed) and energy expenditure (calories expended). Despite energy balance oscillating from meal to meal and from day to day, under normal conditions there are no persistent changes in body stores. It is in fact amazing that a body with an intake of 40–50 tonnes of food over a lifespan can maintain a reasonably stable body weight, indicating that long-term weight regulation is extremely well balanced. However, when such a balance is positive for longer periods, body weight will increase. Human eating behaviour is influenced by many factors including hunger and appetite, social influences, palatability of food, and mood. This is balanced by energy expenditure, which includes basal metabolic rate, dietary thermogenesis (meal-induced heat production) and physical activity (see Chapter 6).

Energy homeostasis involves complex mechanisms that exist centrally (brain) and peripherally (adipose tissue and gut). Appetite and ensuing food intake may be initiated by physiological factors, such as hunger and thirst, but also by environmental factors and biochemical interactions. Environmental factors include cultural and psychological influences and olfactory and visual stimuli. The biochemical interactions that control appetite occur principally in the arcuate nucleus of the hypothalamus in response to peripheral stimuli.

The so-called satiety cascade describes the extremely complex interaction, following food intake in response to hunger signals (Fig. 17.3). Following *hunger*, *satiation* is initiated after food intake towards the latter part of a meal, bringing it to an end, followed by *satiety*. This sensation keeps us satisfied between meals, until with time the next

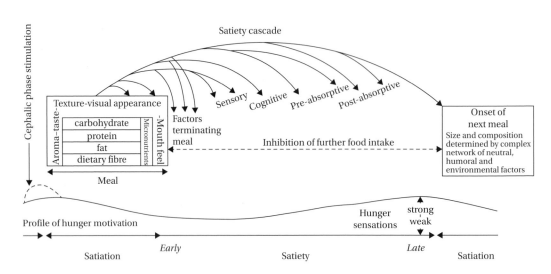

Fig. 17.3 Post-prandial satiety cascade involving mechanical social, hormonal, and neuronal regulatory functions.

Source: Blundell J. (1991) Pharmacological approaches to appetite suppression. *Trends Pharmacol Sci*, **12**, 147–57.

hunger feeling develops. The appetite-stimulating pathway is situated in the ventromedial part of arcuate nucleus. Decreased leptin levels activate neurones that express two neuropeptides that increase appetite: neuropeptide Y (NPY) and agouti-related protein (AGRP). Ghrelin, secreted by the stomach during fasting, also stimulates the neurones that express NPY and AGRP. The central appetite-suppressing pathway is situated in the dorsolateral part of the arcuate nucleus. This pathway is stimulated by leptin and insulin via the expression of melanocortins and corticotrophins.

Cholecystokinin (CCK) and peptide YY (PYY) are gut-derived factors that are released after eating and also stimulate the appetite suppression pathway. Thus, leptin, which circulates in proportion to adipose tissue mass, may be regarded as a long-term signal to appetite control, whereas insu-

lin, CCK, and PYY are more acute responses to meal ingestion. In theory, these complex biochemical interactions should ensure energy balance and weight stability. However, psychological factors, and the presentation and energy density of food (high fat, high sugar, and their combination) may override the control mechanisms and lead to weight gain. It is important to appreciate that a very small daily excess of energy may lead to a large accumulation of fat over a prolonged period. For example, a daily excess provided by three lumps of sugar with coffee or tea (about 40 kcal, so small that it cannot be measured in a laboratory calorimeter) would, if not counterbalanced, lead to a 2–3 kg weight gain over a year. On the other hand, a daily walk of only few minutes may produce a similarly small but negative effect on energy balance to maintain weight control.

17.7 Environmental and lifestyle factors

In addition to the genetic factors underlying overweight and obesity, environmental and lifestyle factors are important determinants of the current obesity epidemic. Obesity rates have increased

over the past several decades (see Section 17.2), while the gene pool has been stable. The potential for environmental factors to overpower genetic effects is well illustrated by two groups of genetically similar Pima Indians. Those living on social support in reservations in Arizona in the USA do little physical activity and consume much energy-dense food. They have exceptionally high rates of obesity and comorbidities. Their distant relatives following their traditional subsistence lifestyles in mountainous areas of Mexico have low rates of obesity and associated diseases. The same phenomenon has been described in other ethnic groups with similar changes in life style. Transition from traditional to more Western ways of life (increased food energy density and a sedentary lifestyle) seems to help explain the relatively rapid increase in obesity rates.

17.7.1 Food intake

Individuals who are overweight or obese tend to underestimate their total energy consumption, sometimes by as much as 50%, and then report what they regard as socially acceptable. It has also been reported that food waste has increased in recent years. Thus national statistics regarding energy consumption based on individual reporting or national production data are not particularly reliable. In a number of countries it appears that total mean individual intake energy may have declined, despite the increase in BMI levels. This suggests that a decline in activity must also play an important role in the increasing rates of obesity. It seems unlikely that the increased prevalence of obesity is entirely explained by a reduction in energy output and that an increase in intake must in some way contribute to the excess accumulation of body fat. Precise methods for measuring energy intake cannot be easily used in epidemiological studies. Therefore, the nature of the food consumed has been the focus of more recent research. Foods, food groups, and nutrients are more easily measured than total energy intake. The WHO/FAO Expert Consultation on Diet, Nutrition, and the Prevention of Chronic Diseases (TR 916) has identified a number of lifestyle-related factors that are considered to promote or protect against excessive weight gain (Table 17.3). A high intake of energy-dense foods (which are typically also micronutrient poor) is considered promotive and a high intake of non-starch polysaccharide is considered to be protective. Energy-dense foods are high in fat, free sugars, and starches and may be more easily overconsumed than other foods, since satiety signals are weak and set in later. Trials that have covertly manipulated energy density have established that passive overconsumption over time can lead to excessive intakes of total energy. High intakes of sugars, sweetened soft drinks, and fruit juices are also regarded as probable causal factors contributing to overweight and obesity. Sugar in soft drinks seems to be associated with lower satiety signals and to lead to energy overconsumption.

The environment may provide a range of societal determinants that alter food intake and contribute to excessive intake. For example, heavy marketing of energy-dense foods is likely to increase the risk, whereas a home and school environment that supports appropriate food choices will probably be associated with a decreased risk. Also, foods high in fat and sugar tend to be cheap and are easier to transport over long distances than fruit and vegetables and so may be more readily purchased by those in lower socioeconomic situations.

17.7.2 Physical inactivity

Low levels of voluntary and incidental activity are important factors in weight gain. This may result from changes in lifestyle, ageing, or disease (such as arthritis, which restricts mobility, or respiratory or cardiovascular disease, which reduce exercise capacity). Also, urbanization, affluence, and modernization of lifestyle have resulted in changes to exercise amount and pattern. The modern lifestyle relies more on technology and the incidental activities of daily living have been reduced. The prevalence of obesity in children can be related directly to hours of television viewed. Television watching may result in obesity because of reduced activity, reduced resting metabolic rate while viewing, excessive food intake during periods of inactivity, or because of inappropriate food selection resulting from television marketing. It has been shown that NEAT (Non-Exercise Activity Thermogenesis) is an important and hitherto overlooked component of

Table 17.3 Summary of strength of evidence of factors that might promote or protect against weight gain and obesity

Evidence	Decreased risk	No relationship	Increased risk
Convincing	Regular physical activity High dietary intake of non-starch polysaccharide		Sedentary lifestyles High intake of energy-dense, micronutrient-poor foods
Probable	Home and school environments that support healthy food choices for children Breastfeeding		Heavy marketing of energy-dense foods and fast-food outlets High intake of sugar-sweetened soft drinks and fruit juices Adverse socioeconomic conditions*
Possible	Low glycaemic index foods	Protein content of the diet	Large portions High proportion of food prepared outside the home (developed countries) 'Rigid restraint/periodic disinhibition' eating patterns
Insufficient	Eating freqency		Alcohol

*Especially for women in developed countries.

Source: Adapted from WHO/FAO (2003) *Diet, nutrition and the prevention of chronic diseases*. Report of a Joint WHO/FAO Expert Consultation, Technical Report Series 916, Geneva, World Health Organization..

energy expenditure. NEAT indicates the small but still measurable energy expenditure that comes from non-planned locomotion, such as standing, talking, moving around in an office. Even laughter has been found to increase energy expenditure in a measurable way. Studies are underway where school classes, offices, etc. are built around locomotion instead of sedentary behaviour.

17.7.3 Other factors

Other possible factors in the aetiology of overweight and obesity include cessation of smoking (a 1–4 kg weight gain is common), pregnancy, or initiation of treatment with some medications, particularly some antidiabetic, antiepileptic, and antipsychotic medications (Box 17.3). Hormonal alterations are often blamed as the cause of obesity, but in reality such diseases rarely produce more than minimal weight increase. The weight gain associated with

BOX 17.3 Medications associated with weight gain

- Diabetes management
  - Insulin
  - Sulphonylureas
  - Thiazolidinediones
- Steroids
- Antipsychotic medications (including newer antipsychotics)
- Antidepressants
- Lithium
- Antiepileptics
  - Valproate
- Beta-blockers
- Antihistamines
- AIDS medication (abdominal fat increase)

- Hypothyroidism
- Acromegaly
- Cushing's syndrome
- Polycystic ovarian syndrome
- Hyperprolactinaemia
- Insulin resistance

Table 17.4 'Overlooked' non-genetic factors related to the increase in the prevalence of obesity

- More thermoneutral homes
- Increasing age of first pregnancy
- Iatrogenic effects of drugs
- Endocrine disrupting pollutants
- Viruses
- Intestinal bacteria
- Altitude
- Reduced non-exercise activity thermogenesis
- Decreased rates of smoking
- Reduced sleep
- Intrauterine effects

endocrine conditions (Box 17.4) is usually of the order of 5–10 kg. Type 2 diabetes mellitus is often associated with obesity; about 80% of such patients have weight problems.

Although nobody disputes that the laws of thermogenesis apply in body weight regulation, a number of additional potential factors, possibly explaining the development of overweight, have been proposed. They are summarized in Table 17.4 and further underscore the complexity of body weight regulation. Again, each of these alternatives may have a small contribution to a positive energy balance, but over longer periods of time may become relevant contributors.

17.8 Clinical consequences of obesity

There is no doubt regarding the adverse health consequences of obesity, with some of these listed in Box 17.5. Being overweight is associated with a modest increase in risk of the conditions discussed below and the risks increase with the degree of obesity, so that for those with a BMI >30 kg/m^2, total mortality rates are approximately two times greater than for those with a BMI in the healthy range. These data are based on Caucasian populations, and the risks of metabolic disease may be much greater in Asians. In addition, the distribution of obesity is an important determinant of the health risks associated with obesity. The metabolic complications of obesity, listed in the box, are associated with increased visceral fat, even if the BMI is within the desirable range.

While weight reduction is associated with a reduction in the various risks, the evidence that life can actually be prolonged by intentional weight loss has now been confirmed in a number of clinical trials, in particular with bariatric surgery as the means of achieving and maintaining weight loss.

17.8.1 Metabolic and hormonal consequences

Secondary dyslipidaemias are common in those who are obese, and especially in those with abdominal obesity. These dyslipidaemias are characterized by moderately raised levels of very-low-density lipoproteins (VLDLs), raised triglycerides, and low levels of high-density lipoprotein (HDL) cholesterol and atypical low-density lipoprotein (LDL) particles, which tend to be smaller and denser than usual. LDL levels may also be raised. Abnormalities of carbohydrate metabolism, manifesting as insulin resistance,

BOX 17.5 Consequences of obesity

- *Metabolic*:
  Insulin resistance, impaired glucose tolerance and type 2 diabetes
  Dyslipidaemia
  - Increased VLDL, triglyceride, increased LDL cholesterol
  - Reduced HDL cholesterol
  - Increased apo B lipoprotein (small dense molecules)
  Non-alcoholic fatty liver disease (NAFLD) leading to non-alcoholic steatohepatitis (NASH)
  Gallstones
  Polycystic ovarian syndrome/infertility in women
  Gout

- *Cardiovascular*:
  Hypertension
  Coronary heart disease
  Varicose veins
  Peripheral oedema

- *Cancer*:
  Breast, endometrium
  Prostate
  Kidney
  Pancreas
  Colon

- *Mechanical*:
  Osteoarthritis
  Spinal complications
  Obstructive sleep apnoea

- *Social*:
  Low self-esteem, depression
  Adverse judgement by society

- *Other*:
  Increased anaesthetic risk
  Increased risk of fractures
  Dementia, Alzheimer's disease

impaired glucose tolerance (IGT) and often type 2 diabetes, are associated with central adiposity, as are elevated liver transaminases. In the absence of excess alcohol consumption, the latter suggests the diagnosis of non-alcoholic fatty liver disease (NAFLD), later leading to non-alcoholic steatohepatitis (NASH). This condition is associated with increasing rates of liver cirrhosis. This clustering of metabolic abnormalities along with hypertension, which is associated with central obesity is often referred to as the metabolic syndrome, and while the precise mechanism is not understood, insulin resistance is believed to play an important role (see Chapter 23).

The prevalence of gallstones increases with increasing age and weight. Polycystic ovarian syndrome and associated decreased fertility are associated with obesity. Of note, many of those women undergoing *in vitro* fertilization programmes are overweight or obese and with weight loss the success of such programmes increases substantially, as does the likelihood of a natural pregnancy. Caesarean sections are about twice as common in obese women giving birth than in those of normal weight.

17.8.2 Cardiovascular consequences

Obesity is an important risk factor for the development of cardiovascular disease. In part, this may be due to the constellation of metabolic and other abnormalities associated with the metabolic syndrome (see Chapter 21). Obesity particularly increases the risk of coronary heart disease in those younger than 50. Varicose veins and peripheral oedema occur more commonly in obese than normal-weight individuals and cardiac abnormalities such as cor pulmonale and lymphoedema may occur with gross obesity.

17.8.3 Obesity-associated cancer

Recent studies have emphasized that several cancers are strongly associated with obesity (see Chapter 22). It is possible to understand this association in tumours that are hormone-dependent (breast, endometrium, and prostate), given the hormonal function of adipose tissue. Cancers of the entire intestinal tract are also associated with obesity, and could be associated with the fact that with increased food intake more toxic products and bile also pass through the gastrointestinal tract, inducing cellular changes. It is less easy to explain the overrepresentation of cancers of the kidney and brain or melanoma.

17.8.4 Mechanical consequences

Osteoarthritis of both the weight-bearing and non-weight-bearing joints (e.g. in the hands) is more common in obesity. Obstructive sleep apnoea is common among obese individuals, especially in men. They often report symptoms such as snoring, stopping breathing during sleep (apnoea), morning headache, daytime sleepiness, and difficulty in mental concentration. These symptoms can be successfully treated with weight loss and/or continuous positive airways pressure (CPAP) administered by a nasal mask during sleep.

17.8.5 Social consequences

Obese people, particularly those who have made many unsuccessful attempts to lose weight, often have low self-esteem. Obesity or its medical consequences may prevent individuals from doing many activities that they enjoy, resulting in impairment of quality of life. Obese children are often teased at school or feel socially isolated. In some societies, there is a poor perception of obesity by the community at large and obese individuals may experience discrimination in various forms, including reduced employment opportunities. This does not apply to all societies. In many Polynesian and some African countries, being overweight or obese is still regarded as a desirable state, although there is evidence to suggest that the younger generation may be adopting more Western views of body image.

17.9 Management

17.9.1 Whom to treat?

Given the high prevalence of overweight and obesity in many countries, individualized care for all would place an unsustainable burden on health care resources. Public health approaches (see Section 17.10) to reduce the risks of becoming overweight or obese are a priority. Some overweight and obese individuals succeed in losing weight and maintain weight loss without the help of health professionals. The text which follows applies to those who seek advice from doctors, dietitians, and other health professionals.

For the healthy overweight or obese individuals with no family history of diabetes and heart disease, societal attempts to reduce the 'obesogenicity' of the environment combined with simple dietary advice and encouragement to increase activity will facilitate weight loss and may suffice. However, it is important to provide ongoing encouragement and follow-up to ensure that lifestyle changes are sustained. This long-term approach for weight loss maintenance is often neglected.

For those with a BMI >27 kg/m² and abdominal adiposity, the metabolic syndrome, or other medical complications, and all those with BMI >30 kg/m², both intensive dietary advice (if possible from a dietitian or nutritionist) and medical supervision (to decide whether adjunctive treatment is required if there is no weight loss with diet and increased activity alone) are necessary (Table 17.5). In Asians, because of the greater risk and higher prevalence of metabolic diseases at lower BMIs, active intervention for overweight should be considered even earlier.

17.9.2 Basic interventions

At the outset, it is important to for patients to appreciate that weight-loss therapy involves appreciable

Table 17.5 Possible approaches to the management of overweight and obesity. General dietary and exercise advice are given to all groups and specialist dietary advice should be available for all those with BMI >30 kg/m²

BMI (kg/m²)	Intervention				
	General dietary and exercise advice	Specialist dietary advice and medical assessment	VLCDs (initial)	Pharmacotherapy	Surgery
25.0–29.9 High risk*	Required	Required			
30.0–34.9 High risk*		Required Required	Consider Consider	Consider	
35.0–39.9 High risk*		Required Required	Consider Useful	Consider Consider	Consider
40+		Required	Useful	Consider	Consider

*Individuals at high risk for a given BMI are those with high waist circumference and the presence of comorbidities (e.g. type 2 diabetes, impaired glucose intolerance, coronary heart disease, sleep apnea, polycystic ovary syndrome, dyslipidaemia).

lifestyle changes that have to be maintained long term. There are two phases of therapy, active weight loss and weight maintenance. The basic interventions involve a change in eating and exercise habits and such changes invariably involve behaviour modification. It is important to set achievable goals for each individual, and these should extend beyond the number of kilograms to be lost (Table 17.6). Goals should include one short-term approach (e.g. manage weight control the week before Christmas) and one long-term approach (e.g. lose enough weight to go off diabetes medication). Weight loss should be planned in stages. Goals should be recorded and discussed at subsequent visits, and the attaining of goals acknowledged. Patients should be aware that even a modest weight loss (of the order of 5–10% of original weight) results in clinically important benefits (Box 17.6). Non-caloric rewards should be planned when targets have been reached.

An 'eating plan' rather than a 'diet' is recommended. Eating plans should be realistic and designed so that they can be sustained in the long-term. Most overweight and obese people will be aware that there are different dietary approaches to

Table 17.6 Goals of obesity therapy

- Weight loss—set realistic targets, in stages
- Change in body shape and size (less abdominal fat)
- Control of associated disorders:
  - impaired carbohydrate metabolism (diabetes, impaired glucose tolerance)
  - dyslipidaemia
  - hypertension
  - sleep apnoea
  - arthritis
  - polycystic ovary syndrome
- Improved mobility
- Reduction in medications
- Improved cardiovascular fitness
- Psychological and social factors
- Individual goals:
  - fitting into clothes
  - need for, or ability to have, necessary operation reduction in pain
  - Improved self-esteem

weight loss and that many diet books are available. The Atkins, Zone, South Beach, Low GI (glycaemic index) and CSIRO approaches, and various Mediterranean and low-fat diets (Box 17.7) have been best sellers. Regardless of which eating plan is to be implemented, patients need to understand and accept that weight loss only occurs when energy intake is less than energy output. Reducing energy intake is principally achieved by consuming smaller portions and reducing energy-dense foods. The latter are high in fat and sugars and the combination of the two increases palatability and thereby the risk of overconsumption. Increasing carbohydrate-containing foods rich in non-starch polysaccharides (dietary fibre) promotes satiety, as do high-protein foods, and an increase of either in the diet may help weight loss. These principles constitute the conventional approach to weight loss. Several of the novel approaches to weight loss rely to some extent on the satiating effects of protein (Zone, South Beach, CSIRO, Atkin, Mediterranean diets), though the novelty and prescriptive nature of some may also account for the reduced energy intakes.

The ketosis associated with very high intakes of fat recommended in the Atkins approach and the very-low-calorie (or energy) diets (VLCD or VLED) may result in nausea. However, the ketonaemia in itself seems to reduce appetite. Several of these approaches result in enhanced weight loss during the early phase of adoption but by 1 year there appears to be little difference between these 'new' and the 'conventional' approaches using low-fat, low-energy-dense foods and less total energy. While the newer high-fat and high-protein approaches do not appear to be associated in the short term with adverse effects on cardiovascular risk factors, no long-term follow-up

Dietary approach	Nutritional characteristics
Low fat/high carbohydrate	High in fibre-rich carbohydrate Low glycaemic index foods emphasized Relatively high protein
Moderate to low carbohydrate: Zone CSIRO Scarsdale South Beach Mediterranean	Variable amounts of CHO from low to moderate, typically low GI Unsaturated fat emphasized
High fat: Atkins	High fat, high protein, very low carbohydrate

studies of safety or efficacy have been undertaken. Studies up to 2 years show that the only determinant of long-term success is negative energy balance, however achieved. On the other hand, most of these studies demonstrate that subjects under study never lose as much as anticipated, suggesting that low compliance is the key issue.

Recently, call centres and internet-based programmes have been developed. They are difficult to evaluate because of low compliance, but are extremely cost-effective. In many countries now, most people do have access to a computer.

Medical and nutrition authorities tend to endorse both relatively high-carbohydrate and high-protein dietary approaches provided other nutritional requiremets are met. However, it is essential to have an individualized approach for each patient. For example, there is little point in recommending a high-fibre, high-carbohydrate diet to a man with an occupation involving intense physical activity and accustomed to large meat meals. Far more effective would be to reduce portion size and ensure lean meat intake, with some small changes to food choices. 'Calorie counting' may be useful for some patients who require highly prescriptive advice to achieve weight loss. However, for well-motivated people, ensuring appropriate food choices, with quantitative advice regarding particularly energy-dense foods or with regard to fat and free sugars, is usually sufficient. A programme should not be initiated in times when the patient has other distracting commitments. Nobody can change job, partner, location and at the same time focus on weight loss. It is obviously essential to ensure that energy-reduced diets are nutritionally adequate in all respects. Encouraging a variety of foods from the different food groups will usually ensure this and make the diet more enjoyable.

Not all obese and overweight people have an excessive caloric intake all the time. They may be binge eaters, overeating periodically. Such binges tend to be produced by emotional problems or stress and be the cause of regaining weight after satisfactory loss. Patients can be helped to recognize stress cues and learn alternative ways of dealing with them. Alcohol may be an important source of extra energy intake, particularly in some overweight and obese men, and this needs to be considered in their programme. The use of low-alcohol beers is often a good starting point.

Exercise—or rather any physical activity—is an important part of any programme. In itself it may not produce major weight loss, but it helps to alter body composition favourably, reducing fat mass and increasing muscle mass. It also increases mobility, induces a feeling of wellbeing, and improves the metabolic and clinical comorbidities of obesity. For the obese and overweight, low-intensity but prolonged exercise produces these changes, even if cardiovascular fitness is not achieved. Increasing the total 'volume' of activity (volume = time × frequency × intensity) should be emphasized. One way of doing this is by increasing 'incidental activity' (or taking the active choice) wherever possible; it may involve using the stairs, walking to the shops, and even such small changes as not using the television remote control. This so-called non-exercise activity thermogenesis (NEAT) creates energy expenditure that can be measured over a day and significantly increases energy output.

Increasing exercise to a sufficient extent to achieve cardiovascular fitness confers additional benefit, regardless of BMI. An individual with a high degree of cardiovascular fitness will be at lower risk than someone with the same BMI who does not have this greater level of fitness ('fat but fit'). Weight loss reduces the cardiovascular risk even more.

Behaviour modification (see Chapter 38) is an integral and important part of therapy and it is essential to prevent regain of weight by aiming to change habits in the long term. The techniques used include the keeping of food and exercise logs, cognitive restructuring (removing the guilt from eating), awareness and changing of habits, and improving self-esteem. Such therapy may be given to individuals or in groups. Several handbooks are available (see Chapter 38).

17.9.3 Adjunctive therapies

If lifestyle interventions alone do not achieve the set goals, it is necessary to consider whether any additional adjunctive therapies are required. Very-low-calorie (or energy) diets may be of particular use in initating weight loss in obese individuals, especially when comorbities are present. Drug therapy may be considered in those who are markedly obese or when the comorbidities of obesity have developed, when there has been no weight loss, or inadequate loss, after 12 weeks on a lifestyle programme.

Very-low-calorie (or energy) diets (VLCD or VLED)

VLCD or VLED, which provide between 400 and 800 calories per day, are largely protein-based with essential fatty acids, vitamins, and minerals and very little carbohydrate. They are effective at producing rapid and early weight loss in the very obese but the weight loss at longer-term follow-up may not be greater than that achieved by following a standard programme. However, they have been shown to produce weight loss that can be sustained for 4–5 years when used for 2–3 months to replace two meals a day and then replacing one or two meals daily. They are of particular use when rapid weight reduction is needed for medical reasons (e.g. preoperatively, to relieve pain, to treat sleep apnea). When consumed as replacements for all meals for more than 3 weeks, VLCDs should only be used under medical (or nutritionist) supervision. Common side effects include tiredness (or euphoria), constipation, extreme cold, and loss of hair, which can generally be managed and are reversible. Some potential dangers, including cardiac arrhythmias, electrolyte abnormalities, gallstones, and gout, are in practice infrequent. Particular care should be taken when VLCDs are used by those on multiple medications, especially insulin or sulphonylureas, when there is a greater risk of hypoglycaemic reactions. Reducing the dosage of these agents when the VLCDs are commenced and monitoring blood sugar levels thereafter is necessary. Many patients can adjust their medication themselves by monitoring their blood sugar levels more frequently. VLCDs are generally administered as outpatient care as part of a programme that includes exercise and behaviour modification, regular follow-up, and preparation for the reintroduction of normal eating. Their use should be followed by a period of intensive education regarding the lifestyle changes necessary to maintain weight loss.

Pharmacotherapy

The development of antiobesity drugs has been a great disappointment. For most diseases more and better drugs have been developed over time. For obesity pharmacotherapy the opposite has happened, and several potentially promising drugs have been removed from the markets because of major side effects which only emerged after fairly prolonged use. Dexfenfluramine, sibutramine, and rimonabant are examples of such drugs.

Orlistat

Orlistat is an intestinal lipase inhibitor. By this action, it reduces fat absorption by 30%. Treatment with orlistat can produce an extra 70% weight loss over that achieved by an intensive lifestyle programme alone. It is associated with reductions in cholesterol over that to be expected with weight loss, falls in blood pressure, and serum triglycerides, and improvement of insulin sensitivity. Glycaemic control is improved in those who have already developed diabetes. The major so-called side effects of this drug are gastrointestinal but result from the mode of action of the drug. With adherence to a low-fat diet such side effects are minimal. In theory, absorption of fat-soluble vitamins might be compromised with long-term usage, but levels of these vitamins remain in the normal range even after 4 years of treatment. Generally, these vitamins are supplemented if a long-term course of treatment is contemplated. The standard dose of orlistat is 120 mg three times daily.

Other drugs

In those who are depressed, the SSRI antidepressant drugs (e.g. fluoxetine) may temporarily assist weight reduction. Metformin when used in people with diabetes may result in some weight loss. The antiepileptic drug topiramate may be effective, despite not necessarily being licensed for this purpose, but its use is limited by side effects. Dexfenfluramine was initially used on its own, then combined with phentermine in the so-called 'Redux' programme in the USA. Several severe clinical events associated with valvular heart disease followed and the combination was eventually banned.

The immediate future of pharmacotherapy in obesity is uncertain. Following the rimonabant withdrawal, there has been little further research on cannabinoid blockers. Combinations of drugs, acting simultaneously on the brain and the gut may have potential in the future. Leptin, CCK, and PYY are examples of endogenous hormones to which agonists or antagonists would seem to be natural targets for drug development, which so far has not been successful.

Surgery Bariatric surgery is the most effective for severe obesity. In conjunction with a lifestyle programme and regular follow-up, substantial weight loss (20–30 kg) has been maintained for >12 years. This weight loss is associated with resolution of many of the associated disorders, particularly type 2 diabetes. However, whereas glycaemic control persists, hypertension often recurs despite weight maintenance. The operations are laparoscopic variations of the gastric bypass but the far less invasive gastric banding (an inflatable band inserted laparoscopically) is still in use. The procedures generally result in a combination of mechanical and malabsorbtive effects. The side effects of surgery are due to the restriction surgery places on eating, and large meals or some particular foods may cause vomiting. There are also potential problems with band slippage, or ulceration at the site of the bypass operation, but these are rare in the hands of an experienced surgeon. Still, reoperations may be necessary. Those who have had bariatric surgery need to have regular continuous nutritional follow-up consultations to ensure appropriate nutrient intake.

Bariatric surgery may be considered in those with grade 2 obesity (BMI >35 kg/m^2) who have associated diseases and all those with BMI >40 kg/m^2. Whether it should be used in subjects with lower BMIs or in very obese children is still under discussion.

17.9.4 Maintenance therapy

The planned maintenance phase is critical to all weight-reduction programmes. This may consist of regular reinforcement visits and regular weigh-ins, as well as the continued application of behaviour modification principles and techniques. Group therapy in which patients support each other is often a cost-effective way to run maintenance programmes. Even when weight loss is achieved, the predisposing factors remain and so does the propensity for weight regain. Weight regain should be identified early so that appropriate treatment may be reintroduced. Intensive logging of food intake and behaviour may help to increase awareness. Repeated short booster courses of VLCDs (for 2–4 weeks every 6 months or so) should be considered. As with 'diets' intended to achieve weight loss, there have been claims that some dietary patterns have advantages over others in facilitating weight maintenance following weight loss. In particular, it has been suggested that relatively high-protein diets with moderate intakes of low glycaemic index carbohydrate may be most appropriate. While studies of 6–12 months' duration do suggest some advantages over higher carbohydrate diets, there is little evidence from longer-term studies that macronutrient distribution is an important determinant of weight outcome or indicators of comorbidities of obesity, especially when the carbohydrates are derived from whole grains, vegetables, and fruits, high in fibre, and have a low glycaemic index. Energy balance and personal preference are the key determinants, and a number of different dietary patterns are acceptable.

Weight-reduction programmes are often run by commercial organizations, but general practitioners working in conjunction with dietitians, physiotherapists, and exercise physiologists, and other specialists, have a particularly important role to play because they know their patients and are trusted. Programmes run by dietitians (and/or other health professionals) in the context of general practice can be particularly effective. Recently call centres or internet-based programmes have been developed. The overall effect may be modest, but these tools are extremely cost-effective and can be used anywhere and around the clock.

17.10 Prevention of obesity

The rapidly increasing prevalence of overweight and obesity in many countries and the difficulties involved in achieving and maintaining satisfactory weight loss in those who are already obese mean that preventative approaches offer the only meaningful long-term solution to halting and reversing the worldwide epidemic of obesity. Many approaches have been tried to date, but no country has been able to convincingly reverse the escalating rates in the population as a whole. However, the fact that there is now less overweight in those of higher socioeconomic status in some Western societies shows that despite the role of genetic factors, obesity is partially preventable. Several clinical trials suggest that increased physical activity in children and reduced consumption of sugary drinks may slow the rate of excessive weight gain. Although there is still uncertainly whether obesity has been prevented in adults, several studies indicate more success in children.

Targeted preventative programmes need to be developed and evaluated. For children, the most appropriate first step is to ensure that some planned physical activity is done each day at school and that there is a correct approach to nutrition and eating in the curriculum and school canteen. Lack of time and cost seem to be the justification for rejection of this approach by schools or education authorities. In order to make major inroads into the obesity epidemic, further environmental changes will also be necessary. These will require changes in attitudes and political will, especially since overweight is more of a problem in lower socioeconomic classes.

Facilities for physical activities are required in both urban and rural environments. Appropriate food choices must be available at reasonable cost. Advertising of energy-dense food and drinks to children should be restricted. Taxation of 'junk food' has been discussed, as well as the opposite—subsidizing of healthy foods. The development of programmes that aim to prevent excessive weight gain in children and adults and that are appropriate for specific groups must be one of the most important challenges for preventative medicine in both affluent and developing countries. Reducing the obesogenic environment will not only help to stem the tide of the obesity epidemic and its consequences, but will facilitate weight reduction in those who are already overweight and obese.

Further Reading

1. **Blundell J.** (1991) Pharmacological approaches to appetite suppression. *Trends Pharmacol Sci*, **12**, 147–57.
2. **Blundell, J.E., Lawton, C.L., Cotton, J.R., and Macdiarmid, J.I.** (1996) Control of human appetite: implications for the intake of dietary fat. *Annu Rev Nutr*, **17**, 285–319.
3. **Bouchard, C., Tremblay, A., Després, J.-P., et al**. (1990) The response to long-term over-feeding in identical twins. *N Engl J Med*, **322**, 1477–82.
4. **Bray, G.A. and Popkin, B.M.** (1998) Dietary fat intake does affect obesity! *Am J Clin Nutr*, **68**, 1157–73.
5. **Cole, T.J., Bellizzi, M.C., Flegal, K.M., and Dietz, W.C.** (2000) Establishing a standard definition for child overweight and obesity worldwide: International survey. *BMJ*, **320**, 1240–3.
6. **De Gonzalez, A.B., Hartge, P., Cerhan, J.R., et al**. (2010) Body-mass index and mortality among 1.46 million white adults. *N Engl J Med*, **363**, 2211–19.
7. **Delzenne, N., Blundell, J., Brouns, F., et al**. (2010) Gastrointestinal targets of appetite regulation in humans. *Obes Rev*, **11**, 234–506.

8. **Elfhag, K. and Rössner, S.** (2005) Who succeeds in maintaining weight loss? A conceptual review of factors associated with weight loss maintenance and weight regain. *Obes Rev*, **6**, 67–85.

9. **Hession, M., Rolland, C., Kulkarni, U., Wise A., and Broom, J.** (2009) Systematic review of randomized controlled trials of low-carbohydrate vs. low-fat/low-calorie diets in the management of obesity and its comorbidities. *Obes Rev*, **10**, 36–50.

10. **Kos, K. and Wilding, J.P.** (2009) Adipokines: Emerging theraupeutic targets. *Curr Opin Investig Drugs*, **10**, 1061–8.

11. **Melin, I., Karlstrom, B., Berglund, L., Zamfir, M., and Rössner, S.** (2005) Education and supervision of health care professionals to initiate, implement and improve management of obesity. *Patient Educ Couns*, **58**, 127–36.

12. **Sjöström, L., Gummesson, A., Sjöström, C.D., *et al.*** (2009) Swedish Obese Subjects Study. Effects of bariatric surgery on cancer incidence in obese patients in Sweden (Swedish Obese Subjects Study): A prospective, controlled intervention trial. *Lancet Oncol*, **10**, 653–62.

13. **Stern, L., Iqbal, N., Seshadri, P., *et al.*** (2004) The effects of low-carbohydrate versus conventional weight loss diets in severely obese adults: One-year followup of a randomized trial. *Ann Intern Med*, **140**, 778–85.

14. **Stunkard, A.J., Sorensen, T.I., Hanis, C., *et al.*** (1986) An adoption study of human obesity. *N Engl J Med*, **314**, 193–8.

15. **Taylor, R.W., Brooking, L., Williams S.M., *et al.*** (2010). Body mass index and waist circumference cutoffs to define obesity in indigenous New Zealanders. *Am J Clin Nutr*, **92**, 390–7.

16. **Van der Mark, M., Jonasson, J., Svensson, M., Linné, Y., Rössner, S., and Trolle Lagerros, Y.** (2009) Older members perform better in an internet-based behavioral weight loss program compared to younger members. *Obes Facts*, **2**, 74–9.

17. **WHO** (2000) *Obesity: Preventing and managing the global epidemic*. Report of a WHO consultation. Technical Report Series 894. Geneva, World Health Organization.

18. **WHO /FAO** (2003) *Diet, nutrition and the prevention of chronic diseases*. Report of a Joint WHO/FAO Expert Consultation, Technical Report Series 916, Geneva, World Health Organization.

19. **York, D.A., Rössner, S., Caterson, I., *et al.*** (2004) Prevention Conference VII: Obesity, a worldwide epidemic related to heart disease and stroke: Group I: Worldwide demographics of obesity. *Circulation*, **110**, 463–70.

Useful Websites

To see topical and scientifically robust updates on nutrition associated with this textbook and web links to many of the journals in the Further Reading sections, please see the dedicated Online Resource Centre at **http://www.oxfordtextbooks.co.uk/orc/mann4e/**

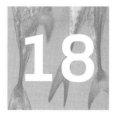

18 The challenge of the chronic diseases epidemic for science and society

Phil James and Neville Rigby

18.1 The impact of chronic diseases and their relationship to diet

The term 'chronic diseases' usually refers to the adult conditions of cardiovascular disease, cancers, diabetes, and obesity. The non-communicable diseases (NCDs) include mental illnesses, respiratory diseases, and many other conditions, which are not traditionally considered to relate to nutritional problems.

Sixty per cent of all deaths in the world are caused by NCDs, and cardiovascular diseases are the principal causes of premature death (now calculated from a global, standard-age, specific life expectancy) and disability in the world. Nine million people die from NCDs every year before they reach their sixtieth birthday. Eighty per cent of all cardiovascular deaths now occur in low- and lower middle-income countries and nearly half of these are in adults of working age (Table 18.1). Cardiovascular

diseases and cancers have been the principal causes of death in the developed world for many years and have a major impact on both the overwhelmed health services and the economy of many lower-income countries. Indeed, 40% of families in south-east Asia are in catastrophic debt because of medical expenses.

Fig. 18.1 shows the global deaths attributable to the 19 leading risk factors. Smoking is of great importance, but the major effects of nutrition and physical inactivity on many of the other risk factors make diet-induced or -related diseases the biggest contributor to premature death in the world.

The detailed analysis of the relative importance of each nutritional factor in determining the development of a particular risk factor is difficult to calculate, but Table 18.2 gives an estimate of the possible

Table 18.1 WHO analyses of the leading causes of death by country income group (2004 data collated in 2008)

	Disease or injury	Deaths (millions)	Deaths (%)		Disease or injury	Deaths (millions)	Deaths (%)
	World				**Low-income countries[a]**		
1	Ischemic heart disease	7.2	12.2	1	Lower respiratory infections[a]	2.9	11.2
2	Cerebrovascular disease	5.7	9.7	2	Ischaemic heart disease	2.5	9.4
3	Lower respiratory infections	4.2	7.1	3	Diarrhoeal diseases	1.8	6.9
4	COPD	10	5.1	4	HIV/AIDS	1.5	5.7
5	Diarrheal diseases.	2.2	3.7	5	Cerebrovascular disease	1.5	5.6
6	HIV/AIDS	2.0	3.5	6	COPD	0.9	3.6
7	Tuberculosis	1.5	2.5	7	Tuberculosis	0.9	3.5
8	Trachea, bronchus, lung cancers	1.3	2.3	8	Neonatal infections[b]	0.9	3.4
9	Road traffic accidents	1.3	2.2	9	Malaria	0.9	3.3
10	Prematurity and low birth weight	1.2	2.0	10	Prematurity and low birth weight	0.8	3.2
	Middle-income countries				**High-income countries**		
1	Cerebrovascular disease	3.5	14.2	1	Ischaemic heart disease	1.3	16.3
2	Ischaemic heart disease	3.4	13.9	2	Cerebrovascular disease	0.8	9.3
3	COPD	1.8	7.4	3	Trachea, bronchus, lung cancers	0.5	5.9
4	Lower respiratory infections	0.9	3.8	4	Lower respiratory infections	0.3	3.8
5	Trachea, bronchus, lung cancers	0.7	2.9	5	COPD[a]	0.3	3.5
6	Road traffic accidents	0.7	2.8	6	Alzheimer and other dementias	0.3	3.4
7	Hypertensive heart disease	0.6	2.5	7	Colon and rectum cancers	0.3	3.3
8	Stomach cancer	0.5	2.2	8	Diabetes mellitus	0.2	2.8
9	Tuberculosis	0.5	2.2	9	Breast cancer	0.2	2.0
10	Diabetes mellitus	0.5	2.1	10	Stomach cancer	0.1	1.8

[a]Countries grouped by gross national income per capita–low income ($825 or less), high income ($ 10 066 or more).
[b]This category also includes other non-infectious causes arising in the perinatal period, which are responsible for about 20% of deaths shown in this category.

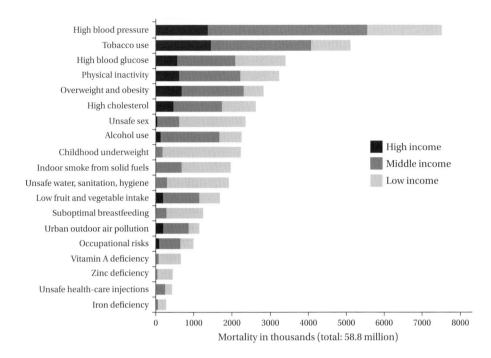

Fig. 18.1 WHO 2009 analyses of deaths attributed to 19 leading risk factors by country income level. For simplicity these analyses are presented in terms of total mortality, whereas the disability-adjusted life years lost (DALYs) analyses relate both to the years of life lost (YLL) compared to a WHO-calculated global standard life expectancy appropriate for each age and to the number of years lost from disability (YLD) incurred by diseases before the projected global standard for mortality. The YLD incurred by adult chronic diseases is usually far greater than the YLL.

Source: WHO (2009) *Global health risks: Mortality and burden of disease attributable to selected major risks.* Geneva, World Health Organization.

Table 18.2 The relative merits of dietary change and weight loss in determining blood pressure in normal and hypertensive adults

	Systolic BP change (mmHg)		Diastolic BP change (mmHg)	
	Normotensives	Hypertensives	Normotensives	Hypertensives
Increase fruit and vegetable by 200 g/day*	−0.8	−7.2	−0.3	−2.8
Reduce fat intake by 10% energy*	−2.7	−4.1	−1.8	−2.6
Reduce salt from 10 g/day to 4 g/day*	−1.6	−7.6	Average: 3.5	
Total weight-independent dietary benefit*	−7.1	−11.5	Average: 4.5	
Increased free sugars intake of 145 g/day	+6.9		+5.3	
Reduce weight by 10 kg or 10%	Average: 6.1 for 10% loss		Average: 3.7 for 10 kg loss	

*The basis for these analyses is set out by Haslam, D.W., and James, W.P. (2005) Obesity. *Lancet*, 366, 1197–209.

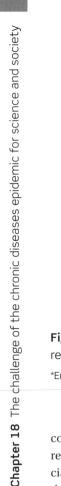

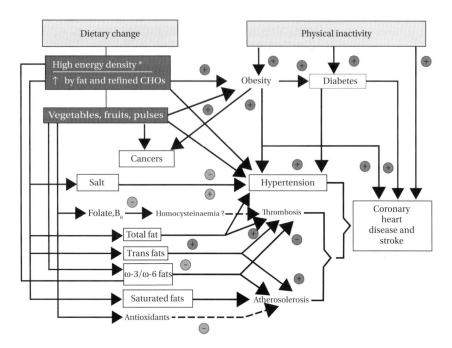

Fig. 18.2 The interaction of dietary factors and physical inactivity in causing amplifying (+) or reducing (-) chronic diseases.

*Energy density reduced by water-holding bulky foods, e.g. tubers, cereals, vegetables, fruits, pulses. CHOs, carbohydrates.

contributors to high blood pressure. When people reduce weight, this can have a substantial, beneficial effect in lowering blood pressure, but part of the fall reflects the direct impact of dietary changes such as reduced fat and increased fruit and vegetable intakes, which are used to induce the weight loss. The relative effects of different dietary factors are calculated from short-term studies in adults, but there seem to be other longer-term effects of diet on blood pressure, starting with inappropriate fetal nutrition, which may establish the lifelong trends in blood pressure or the magnitude to which the child and adult's blood pressure responds to

diet. Early exposure of infants to high-salt diets seems to programme a child to greater increases in their future blood pressure and perhaps a greater sensitivity to some nutritional factors. Thus, the classic INTERSALT studies showed that in some very isolated societies, where salt intakes are very low, blood pressures do not rise with age and hypertension is almost unknown. The subjects tend, however, also to be thin, on low-fat diets, and with ample vegetable and fruit intakes—three conditions that help to reduce blood pressure. Fig. 18.2 sets out a range of nutritional factors that contribute to the chronic diseases.

18.2 Optimum intakes of nutrients

The original Seven Country studies on the relationship of coronary heart disease to environmental factors showed that high blood pressure, high total

serum cholesterol levels, and smoking were the three biggest risk factors. However, in Japan in the 1950s, men smoked heavily and had the highest blood pressures of all seven countries, but, with the Grecian islands the lowest rates of coronary heart disease. Their high blood pressure was explained by their extraordinarily high salt intakes, amounting to 20–30 g/day compared with the goal of less than 5 g/day, but their low rate of coronary heart disease was explained by their very low saturated fat intakes in an average total fat intake of only 14%, and therefore very low blood cholesterol levels. Similar findings in China in the 1980s showed that with total fat intakes varying from 4% to 24% (average 14%), the correspondingly low saturated fat intakes induced very low cholesterol levels in the blood, and coronary heart disease rates were also exceptionally low and in proportion to the cholesterol concentrations at levels down to 3 mmol/L. These low levels were never observed in Western studies, where total fat intakes were >40% energy, saturated fat intakes >20%, and blood cholesterol levels >6 mmol/L. So again the low blood cholesterol levels were the main determinant of the low risk of coronary heart disease, despite the high blood pressures of the Chinese and the high smoking rates in men. Since then, it has become clear that smoking and high blood pressure amplify the atherosclerotic and thrombotic processes, but these are primarily caused by diet-induced alterations in blood lipids. The lipid changes are therefore the permissive factor that allows the other risk factors to become so important. The latest data from intervention trials to lower cholesterol levels with the use of statin drugs suggest that the lower the cholesterol levels the better, and the data are now beginning to reproduce the pre-existing data from Asia about optimum cholesterol levels and therefore the optimum saturated and total fat intake levels. Thus, the first classical 1982 World Health Organization (WHO) report on the prevention of coronary heart disease set the total fat intake goals at 20–30% energy and saturated fat intakes at <10%, simply because with exceptionally high intakes of fat in US and European diets the experts could not bring themselves to really consider fat levels of 15% with negligible saturated fat intakes as the optimum—they therefore presented, in practice, intermediate targets.

Currently, the average blood pressures of populations in almost all countries of the world are high because salt has been such a sought-after condiment for millennia: huge trade routes were developed for the commodity, which had proven so useful for food preservation as well as for making food more attractive. The word 'salary' comes from the practice of paying Roman soldiers with salt. The salt receptors in the tongue explain the human drive for a rare commodity during our evolution and the same applies to the sugar-responsive sweet-taste receptor and the newly discovered essential fatty acid receptor. So as societies transfer from their rural environments and become more affluent, their serum cholesterol, body weights, and blood pressures rise as they gain easier access to dietary fats, sugars, and salty foods. These foods are relatively easy to store compared with the problem of transporting vegetables and fruit from the countryside. This 'nutritional transition' continues to affect hundreds of millions in countries such as China, India, Indonesia, and many African and Latin American countries.

Although cardiovascular disease and cancers are now the major causes of death in most countries, there has also been a remarkable rise in both obesity and type 2 diabetes in the past 20 years. There are now more than 1.5 billion people who are overweight or obese globally, with more obese in the developing countries than in the developed world. Excess weight gain amplifies insulin resistance and precipitates the development of type 2 diabetes. Both these conditions increase the risks of cardiovascular disease, but in the West, the rates of stroke and coronary heart disease have been until recently going down, despite obesity and diabetes rates rapidly increasing. This is explained by the progressive fall in blood cholesterol levels in these societies over the past 30 years as dietary saturated and *trans* fatty acids were replaced by mainly ω-6 polyunsaturated fats. The monounsaturated and polyunsaturated fats still, unfortunately, promote obesity by virtue of increasing dietary energy density and therefore type 2 diabetes is also induced, even if the dietary fat changes have advantageous effects on the atherosclerotic and thrombotic processes.

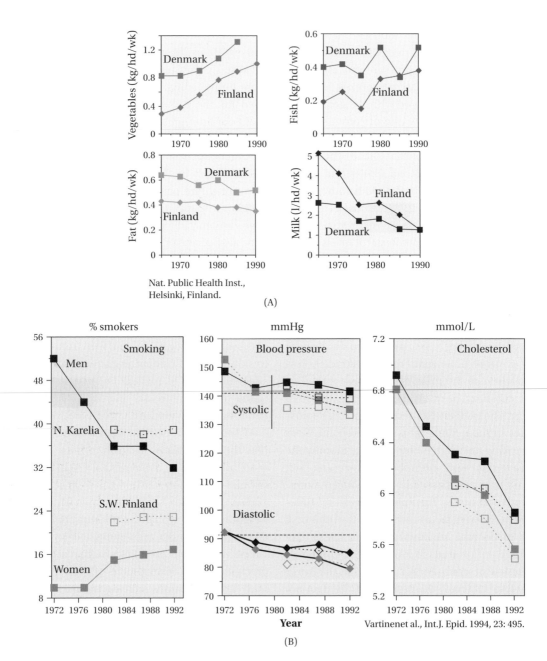

Fig. 18.3 (A) Changing dietary patterns (in kg per head per week) in Finland in response to public health measures. (B) Changing average population cardiovascular risk factors in Finnish men and women aged 30–39 years in response to dietary change before intensive use of drugs for high blood pressure and before statin use for high cholesterol levels. (C) Falling death rates from coronary heart disease in Finnish men aged 35–64 years in both North Karelia, where the first public health measures were taken, and then in Finland as a whole.

Source: (A) National Public Health Institute, Helsinki, Finland. (B) Vartiainen, E., Puska, P., Jousilahti, P., Korhonen, H.J., Tuomilehto, J., and Nissinen, A. (1994) Twenty-year trends in coronary risk factors in North Karelia and in other areas of Finland. *Int J Epidemiol*, **23**, 495–504. (C) Statistics Finland.

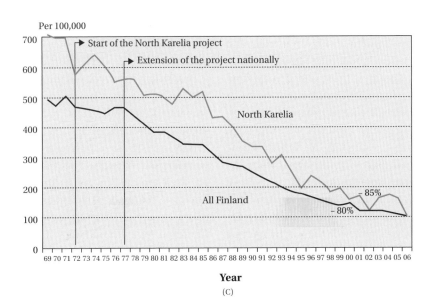

Fig. 18.3 *(Continued)*

18.3 The global nutritional transition

The diet changes markedly as a population's wealth increases. Animal foods and sugar intakes rise with a fall in unprocessed cereal and vegetable intakes. In Asia, rheumatic heart disease is still a problem, but haemorrhagic strokes, precipitated by salt-induced high blood pressures, are the dominant causes of cardiovascular disease and premature death. Then, as oil imports (e.g. palm oil) increase, body weight, and blood cholesterol levels also rise, with ischaemic stroke and coronary artery disease now emerging as major problems, together with breast, colon, and prostate cancers.

Western countries slowly began to respond to the nutritional transition in the 1960s with public health measures including changes in catering, school, food processing, and agriculture policies aimed at combating the epidemic of coronary heart disease, as shown in Finland in Fig. 18.3. To understand why lower-income countries are now experiencing the same chronic diseases epidemic as seen in the Western world 50 years ago, one needs to understand why diets have been changing so rapidly. The story goes back about 100 years.

18.4 The cycle of global nutrition transitions: the discovery of vitamins and national survival

A hundred years ago, nutrition was exciting and at the centre of a huge public debate in the UK because it had become evident that the poor living in cities were chronically unwell, anaemic, and far smaller and thinner than their forebears who had lived in the countryside.

Then the Nobelist Gowland Hopkins described strange accessory food factors as crucial to growth, needing to be added to the list of what were thought to be the vital amines already discovered and needed for the avoidance of such diseases as pellagra. These scientific discoveries of the 'vitamins' were important because they proved to be essential dietary factors in special feeding experiments on both animals and children. Thus, when groups of stunted children were given milk, they grew taller, and thin children became heavier when given extra butter or sugar (Fig. 18.4). The Carnegie data on urban poverty, collected by another Nobelist Boyd Orr, were crucial in persuading Winston Churchill, as British Prime Minister in the early part of World War II when the German submarines were destroying the majority of ships carrying food from the colonies, that food rationing had to be based on the new scientific principles if Germany was not to win the war by starving the British into defeat. Churchill also insisted that pregnant and lactating women, as well as children, had extra milk, orange juice, and cod liver oil; he also decreed that all children should have a good meal at school to ensure their wellbeing and limit the work of their mothers, now recruited into the war effort. Thus, the recent ground-breaking animal experiments, the controlled feeding trials in children, and the detailed national epidemiological surveys of the nutritional state of poor families all contributed to

major government policies affecting health and social policies—and also now to national security and even survival policies during the war.

The British survived, and the national experiment was hailed as a great success and the world became convinced that milk, meat, butter, and sugar were dietary guarantees of a good protein and energy supply, as well as containing a multitude of special vitamins and minerals. Thus, the world put a priority on their production as a fundamental issue of national security. Vast subsidies, guaranteed prices, and a variety of schemes including the European Common Agricultural Policy (CAP) were started to nurture the farming community with the aim of producing far more cheaply the luxury foods of meat, milk and butter, and plentiful, purified sugar, previously only readily available for the rich. A cheap food policy, approved by all concerned nutritionists, would allow even the disadvantaged and poor to eat and grow well.

All other Western authorities emphasized the importance of a balanced diet with a variety of foods and the message that 'a little bit of what you fancy

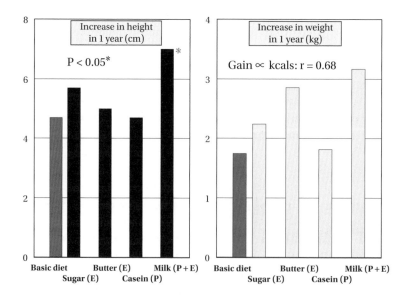

Fig. 18.4 The response of stunted children to food supplements containing energy (E) either with or without additional protein (P).

Source: Recalculated by Celia Petty (PhD, London, 1987) from Corry Mann, H.C. (1926) Diets for boys during the school years. *MRC Sep Rep Series* 105. London, HMSO.

does you good' took hold. Originally after the Second World War, great efforts were needed to make food taste interesting and varied so children and adults delighted in the new luxury foods of different cakes, biscuits, sweets, trifles, chocolates and fizzy pop drinks. These rare products were soon consumed weekly and then daily; with ice cream becoming routine.

Chapter 21 describes the underlying basis for the epidemic of heart disease that became the principal cause of death in the Western world during the 1950s with the resurgence of ever-more-intensive agriculture and the development of a much stronger food industry. Animal fat intakes rose as meat, cream, butter, and milk consumption were promoted by government, the farming community, and many in the nutritional community. Nutritionists joined forces with the food industry to advise them on the new opportunities to develop suitable energy-packed products, with snacks being seen as another way of ensuring adequate intakes in children and those workers who were physically very active. Most nutritionists were then perplexed when Keys and his colleagues in the Seven Country Study showed that the higher the saturated fat intake, the greater the incidence and death rates from coronary heart disease in a community. Since Keys, Hegsted and others had already demonstrated in tightly controlled month-long feeding studies that the response in serum cholesterol, although varying individually, could be predicted from the nature of the dietary fatty acids, it became clear that the nutritional messages needed to change, with a new emphasis on the crude assessment of the polyunsaturated/saturated ratio in the dietary fat. Only relatively recently is it accepted that it is important in policy making to distinguish between *trans* fats, different saturated fatty acids, and the relative importance of ω-3 and ω-6 unsaturated fatty acids.

18.5 The emergence of a powerful farming and food industry: local food becomes global food

Post-war nutritionists were no longer seen to be involved in particularly exciting research because the principal problems had apparently been solved by the national policy experiments during and after the Second World War! Now the real challenge was how best to cope with the huge numbers of children suffering from kwashiorkor and other forms of malnutrition in the developing world. Protein deficiency seemed to fit with previous concepts of essential food ingredients, so a controversy started about the so-called 'protein gap' in so many 'developing countries' where, with the exception of centres in India, the Lebanon, Uganda, South Africa, Mexico, Chile, and Jamaica, there were few nutritionists undertaking fundamental research with modern techniques. The top nutritionists linked their work to the earlier pre-war concepts and recognized that these undernourished children would do better if the poor countries followed the West's example and fed children more milk, meat, butter, and other forms of energy, and that agriculture should be developed on Western lines.

Animal nutritionists came to dominate the nutritional world because cheap meat, butter, and milk were national priorities. It was then shown that feeding ruminants such as cows and sheep with cereals rather than grass allowed them to grow far faster, producing more milk and meat cheaply. Thus, cereal growing for animals rather than for humans became the top agricultural priority. Vegetable oil production was also favoured because this would prove a marvellous source of energy for both human and animal feeding. Thus, new agriculture policies were set across the world with huge agriculture budgets for subsidizing the farmers; those in the new European Community (EC) accounted for nearly the total EC budget. Networks of special national agricultural institutes and extra international institutes funded through the United Nations system and referred to as the Consultative Group on International Agricultural Research (CGIAR) dominated government (and particularly agricultural ministry) thinking across the world. In 2008, the total farming subsidies still amounted in the Organisation for Economic Co-operation and Development (OECD) countries to US$ 265 billion annually, and were almost a third of the total farmers' income. Some countries now provide negligible support, e.g. New Zealand, whereas Korean, Norwegian, and Swiss governments subsidize 64–69% of farm incomes.

The food industry also blossomed because the war-time experience had shown that housewives could manage to bring up their children as well as being in the workforce if they were able to buy more convenience and readily cooked meals that used processed ingredients. The national economy benefited enormously from mobilizing the female workforce, so the food industry was a crucial contributor to governments' economic policies.

The power of the food industry then grew remarkably; it is now the biggest manufacturer in the European Union, accounting for 13% of total manufacturing turnover. As intense competition developed, it was possible with good air and ship transport systems and standard cultivation, harvesting, and storage systems to provide quality guaranteed products throughout the year for wealthy societies. African and Latin American governments as well as other developing countries were then manoeuvered by powerful food companies into producing foods for export and consumption within days of collecting. So there is now no such thing as a seasonal cycle in food availability because the crops can be grown in different parts of the world throughout the year and shipped or air freighted into the rich countries. Only in the past 3 years have there been remarkable changes in thinking: current agricultural practices in terms of tractor use for planting, seeding, spraying, and harvesting are all, together with fertilizer production, totally dependent on the price of oil, which is rising steadily and predicted to rise to very high levels over the next 5–10 years. Already food price increases have sparked major riots in many parts of the world with policy makers still thinking simply in terms of cereal and oil production, rather than the real nutritional needs of a rapidly expanding world population.

18.6 Profitability in the food industry: manipulating the price, availability, and marketing of products as the determinants of societal intakes

The food industry has had to develop under the same commercial pressures as any other business— they have to make more money and bigger profits each year to be distributed to the owners or shareholders. Thus, there are constant food wars as companies compete for market share. Box 18.1 lists some recent strategies for persuading consumers to buy their products. The price of the food is a critical issue. Indeed, food prices are a crucial part of governments' inflation analyses and social policies. They are also critical for the poorer consumers, since they use 80–100% of their income on food in the poorest developing world, whereas in the developed world this proportion has been steadily dropping for years. In the UK, it is 7% for the richest tenth of the population compared with 15% for the poorest. However, the poorest have much less to spend and still focus on price when buying food; economists for years have calculated the 'price elasticity' of different foods, which shows how intakes fall when prices rise. Thus, in the annual review of the European CAP pricing policies for milk, butter, meat, and sugar, they used to juggle the subsidies and price guarantees to farmers in order to change the price of the foods in the market place. This then allowed an increase or decrease in the mountains of

BOX 18.1 Fifteen strategies to improve profitability in the food industry, often to the disadvantage of health

1 Design foods to appeal to the palate by reducing bulk and ensuring fat, sugar, and salt sufficient for maximum impact on primary taste buds.

2 Engage new flavour specialists to identify the thousands of flavours in a food or drink, which contribute to activating specific olfactory receptors, through molecular techniques. Identify which flavours lock into cerebral pleasure responses using novel brain-imaging techniques, taking account of genetic diversity of the population's receptors, sex differences in responses, and the combination effects of other ingredients, e.g. alcohol if the desired target is increased alcohol consumption in young women.

3 Reduce prices paid to farmers.

4 Offer larger portion sizes for 'value' where ingredient costs are small and fixed costs of production and distribution the same: the consumer purchases a larger portion but the manufacture gets a much bigger profit.

5 Provide ready-to-eat meals, e.g. hamburgers, fried chicken, and pizzas: sell for immediate consumption with maximum convenience.

6 Provide food in ready-to-eat or -drink cartons for 'take away'. (Develop the market concept of eating and drinking on the move because distracted purchasers will eat and buy more.)

7 Increase the availability of outlets for purchase, e.g. in vending machines, specialist shops (e.g. coffee, hamburger) and other specialist outlets where populations congregate, e.g. in town centres.

8 Build 'brand value' by intensive marketing using famous popular figures, e.g. football stars.

9 Target children, preferably below the age of five when particularly amenable to image building and acceptance of all messages. Employ child psychologists to gear messages to bypass parents and increase the 'pester power' of children to overcome parental resistance.

10 Extend the variety of marketing approaches: TV advertising is progressively less important: place foods and drinks as routine scenes in soap operas, boost internet marketing, and use 'viral marketing', where key children are paid to receive and pass on text messages on mobile phones.

11 Take over school food and drink supplies and give schools a minor profit share to encourage removal of alterative water and food sources at school.

12 Fundamental new drive on the developing world with huge investments dominating economic and social policy thinking of the recipient countries: get in early and establish market dominance, especially in major societies, e.g. China, India, Indonesia, Brazil, Nigeria, Mexico.

13 Employ media-friendly nutritional experts to sanction ideas based on values of pleasure and quality of food for maximum individual choice in a 'balanced diet'; use economic influence to access ministers and prime ministers; consider inducements.

14 Target opponents' scientific or personal credentials if they criticize new developments and oppose non-governmental organizations (NGOs) involved in public health.

frozen foods, which had originally been kept for national emergencies. Changes in the consumption of these foods by the population could be very accurately predicted if the price was changed.

The food industry has got around the problem of raising prices by reducing their costs through a number of mechanisms, including merging and acquiring new businesses, closing factories, mechanizing for mass production, using as few employees as possible, focusing on a relatively small number of branded goods, and buying up small competitors to remove them from the market place.

Apart from the price of foods and convenience pre-prepared meals, the other factors profoundly affecting food purchases are the ready availability of a variety of foods so that consumers can gain easy access to them at any time. Then there is the marketing of foods. The food industry manipulates portion size to make foods appear cheaper and they also pay supermarkets to have their products placed at particular points and shelf heights in the supermarkets to promote sales. Local councils, schools, and work sites are also offered special deals to ensure that their products are immediately available. Thus, one hamburger chain suggests 4 minutes as the appropriate maximum time for anybody to have to drive to get to their outlet within any reasonably sized town in the USA, and soft-drink companies ensure there is an outlet and advertising of their products in every reasonably sized village throughout the world. Marketing is also directed to the most susceptible and responsive groups, such as young children. Commercial interests therefore now routinely target young children before they are able to discriminate marketing from general information and try to manipulate the educative processes by providing schools with teaching materials that have the companies' products as suitable examples.

To keep the rising expectations of company profits (when, biologically, children and adults in the affluent world cannot eat any more food), the Western food companies now have to take over the food system of the developing world—as their highest priorities. They promise prime ministers and policy makers huge investments to establish soft-drink and fast-food factories, and often provide financial and other inducements to ensure the deals are agreed. Some indication of the power of the food industry is shown in Box 18.2. While the food companies have become powerful, so too have the supermarkets—now, individually, they also often have a greater turnover than many countries. Thus, the biggest, Wal-Mart, a US-based company operating in 10 countries, had annual retail sales of US$ 405 billion in 2010; in most affluent countries >70% of food sales are through a small number of huge supermarkets. This then gives major food companies a major negotiating power for influenc-

ing consumers and governments throughout the world. They also control what farming communities earn and produce. The most rapidly expanding Western supermarkets are now in most middle-income countries, where their sales are already growing far faster than in the West. This then explains the huge and overwhelming epidemic of chronic diseases in developing countries.

> **BOX 18.2** Analysis of the power of the industry
>
> 1 The global food advertising budget is probably over $100 billion—more than the total income of 70% of the world's countries.
>
> 2 The food industry spends 500 times more on promoting high-energy-density Western diets than the total governmental prevention budget on promoting good nutrition.
>
> 3 Food advertising accounts for half of all adverts on children's TV; 75% are for high-energy, low-nutrient foods without voluntary or regulatory restrictions.
>
> 4 Transitional economies (e.g. Eastern Europe) find 60% of foreign investment is for sugar, confectionary and soft drinks—10 times the investment in vegetable and fruit production. Processed foods are now the global priority; Asia targeted by soft drink firms.

18.6.1 Implications for prevention

The massive global epidemic of obesity, type 2 diabetes, and other chronic diseases is guaranteed to continue unless the nutritional world focuses on the prime drivers affecting the food system and recognizes that individuals have to be very well educated, affluent, and motivated to create their own 'nutritional microculture' when they live in what is now termed 'a toxic obesogenic environment'. Traditionally, nutritionists are trained to expect that patients or individuals given advice will act upon it, and therefore they can be made responsible for their own nutritional wellbeing. It is, however, exceptionally difficult for even discerning consumers to understand current food labels because they are set out for the benefit of regulators and analysts who can readily understand the sodium or fat content/100 g of a product. Consumers, however, cannot work out how to limit their fat or saturated fat intake given the usual advice, for example, about limiting total fat to <30% and saturated fat to <10% energy, when almost nobody knows what their own energy needs are. Many surveys show that a traffic-light signalling system is much preferred by the public, but such systems are opposed by many food industries, who lobbied the EU Parliament in November 2010 to prevent their introduction. Unfortunately, some nutritionists persist with the crude concept that there are only 'good' or 'bad' diets not foods, while the food companies now promote their own version of good healthy foods or 'functional foods' at premium prices! When the more responsible nutritionists insist on a food having an appropriate nutritional profile (e.g. with the food being low in total fat, saturated fat, sugars, and salt) before any health claim is made, this is resisted intensively by the food industrial consortia using tactics analogous to those used by the tobacco industry—confusing policy makers with spurious claims, targeting personally the nutritional critics of their marketing strategies, and rewarding some industry-friendly nutritionists who dispute the nutritional evidence. Many of the prominent nutritionists of the world are now targeted to ensure they do not create trouble for the marketing of major food brands.

Nutritional education has now been shown to be a hopelessly inadequate approach for dealing with the population's public health problems. This means that nutritionists are going to have to learn completely different approaches involving policy making and a changed role for themselves in society if they are really going to help the population, as distinct from individual patients. The huge environmental and industrial pressures to eat the wrong foods and remain physically inactive are overwhelming most people's desire to remain healthy, so a new outlook by nutritionists is now

needed. The current inducements to sit while working or watching entertainment and a huge range of gadgets, mechanical aids, cars, and computers are all based on industrial interests which benefit from children and adults being inactive. Evidence suggests that we therefore need huge environmental measures to induce spontaneous physical activity. At lower activity levels the nutritional quality of the normal diet needs to be higher and the energy density lower than traditionally found in Western societies. Clearly, economic and other policy methods analogous to those involved in the control of tobacco and alcohol will be required to limit the intense promotion of nutrient-poor, energy-dense foods.

Summary

Finally there is an increasing tendency to assume that soon we will be able to identify by gene scanning those individuals who merit specific dietary advice or interventions while allowing the rest of the population to eat their current diets. Many different genes are now being identified as increasing the risk of hypertension, obesity, dyslipidaemia, diabetes, and the responses to particular dietary sensitivities, e.g. sodium. However, there are very few situations in which a singe gene identifies individuals with a potentially modifiable risk factor or preventable disease state, e.g. familial hypercholesterolaemia, familial polyposis coli. In the vast majority of clinical situations, a disease or risk factor results from an interaction between many genes and environmental factors, so that identification of most high-risk individuals by genetic testing is not feasible. Rose showed decades ago that one gains greater benefit from reducing the average cholesterol or blood pressure level of the whole population rather than only concentrating on the high-risk group. This is simply because the identified very-high-risk individuals are a small minority, whereas the majority of the populations of the world are now at an increased risk of cardiovascular disease, obesity, and hypertension because of modest increases in several risk factors. Thus even small improvements in risk factors in the population at large translate into a large population benefit, Only an orchestrated public health approach aimed at achieving major changes in diet and physical activity patterns has any hope of reversing these NCDs, which have now achieved epidemic proportions worldwide.

Further Reading

1. **Alwan, A., Maclean, D.R., and Riley, L.M.**, et al. (2010). *Monitoring and surveillance of chronic non-communicable diseases: Progress and capacity in high-burden countries. Lancet*, **376**, 1861–8.
2. **Corry Mann, H.C.** (1926) Diets for boys during the school years. *MRC Sep Rep Series* 105. London, HMSO.
3. **Haslam, D.W. and James, W.P.** (2005) *Obesity. Lancet*, **366**, 1197–209. (Review.)
4. **James, W.P.T., Norum, K., Smitasiri, S.,** et al. (2000) *Ending malnutrition by 2020: An agenda for change in the millennium. Final Report to the ACC/SCN by the Commission on the Nutrition Challenges of the 21st Century. Food Nutr Bull*, **21** (Suppl. 3), 1–88.
5. **Johansson, L., Drevon, C.A., and Bjorneboe, G.-E.** (1996) *The Norwegian diet during the last hundred years in relation to coronary heart disease. Eur J Clin Nutr*, **50**, 277–83.
6. **Lang, T. and Heasman, M.** (2004) *Food wars: The global battle for mouths, minds and markets.* London, Earthscan.
7. **Monteiro, C.** (2010) The big issue is ultra-processing [commentary]. *World Nutrition*, **1**, 6, 237–69.
8. **Popkin, B.** (2009). What can public health nutritionists do to curb the epidemic of nutrition-related noncommunicable disease? *Nutrition Reviews*, **67**(Suppl. 1), S79–82.
9. **Schlosser, E.** (2001) *Fast food nation. The dark side of the all-American meal.* London, Allen Lane/ Penguin Press.
10. **Stuckler, D.** (2008). Population causes and consequences of leading chronic diseases: A comparative analysis of prevailing explanations. *Milbank Q*, **86**, 273–326.
11. **USDA** (2010) Global food markets. Washington, DC, US Department of Agriculture. http://www.ers.usda.gov/Briefing/GlobalFoodMarkets/.
12. **Vartiainen, E., Puska, P., Jousilahti, P., Korhonen, H.J., Tuomilehto, J., and Nissinen, A.** (1994) Twenty-year trends in coronary risk factors in north Karelia and in other areas of Finland. *Int J Epidemiol*, **23**, 495–504.
13. **WHO** (2003) *Diet, nutrition and the prevention of chronic diseases.* Report of a Joint WHO/FAO Expert Consultation. WHO Technical Report Series No. 916. Geneva: World Health Organization.
14. **WHO** (2009) *Global health risks: Mortality and burden of disease attributable to selected major risks.* Geneva, World Health Organization. http://www.who.int/healthinfo/global_burden_disease/GlobalHealthRisks_report_full.pdf (accessed 12 December 2010).

Useful Websites

To see topical and scientifically robust updates on nutrition associated with this textbook and web links to many of the journals in the Further Reading sections, please see the dedicated Online Resource Centre at **http://www.oxfordtextbooks.co.uk/orc/mann4e/**

19 Protein-energy malnutrition

Stewart Truswell

People, young or old, who eat less food than they usually eat and need, lose body weight; the deficit of energy (or calories) in the diet is made up by drawing on the body's energy reserves: first fat, later muscle. The weight loss is carbon dioxide (breathed out) and water (excreted) from oxidation of fat:

$$2\left(C_{55}H_{106}O_6\right) + 157O_2 \rightarrow 110CO_2 + 106H_2O + heat.$$

(This representative fat molecule is a triglyceride with oleic (18:1), linoleic (18:2), and palmitic (16:1) acids). This is undernutrition (Box 19.1).

> ### BOX 19.1 Definitions of malnutrition
>
> - Undernutrition is depletion of energy (calories).
> - Malnutrition is serious depletion of any of the essential nutrients (other than energy).
> - Fasting is voluntary abstention from food.
> - Starvation is involuntary lack of food.
> - Famine is severe food shortage of a whole community.
> - Wasting is loss of substance, especially muscle (from insufficient food, disuse, or disease).

Undernutrition can be mild or severe, beneficial (in someone who was obese), or dangerous.

The loss of weight is a manifestation of energy depletion. Essential nutrients, protein and micronutrients, are likely to be depleted at the same time, but some micronutrients have large stores in the body, and requirements of some others are lower when energy intake is reduced. In children, who have higher protein requirements than adults, important depletion of protein is likely to accompany serious undernutrition.

Protein depletion can affect the body in two different ways:

1 *In somatic protein depletion*, the loss of tissue shows as general wasting of muscles, which together contain the largest amount of the body's protein.

- *In visceral protein depletion*, the brunt of the protein loss is borne by the liver, pancreas, and gut. This is the less common type of protein malnutrition and nutritional scientists still do not fully agree why it occurs.

Protein-energy malnutrition (PEM) occurs in three situations:

1 in young children in poor communities, usually in developing countries;

2 in adults, even in affluent countries, due to severe illness (hospital malnutrition);

3 in people of all ages in a famine.

19.1 Protein-energy malnutrition in young children

There are two forms of severe PEM: marasmus and kwashiorkor.

19.1.1 Nutritional marasmus

Nutritional marasmus is the common form; it is starvation in an infant or young child. (The word is from the Greek, 'marasmos', meaning 'wasting'.) The child is very thin. Weight is less than 60% of the median reference weight-for-age and there is marked wasting (Fig. 19.1). There is no oedema.

There is loss of almost all the adipose tissue and (to a smaller extent), wasting of the voluntary muscles. Growth has stopped and it has taken weeks of inadequate feeding for a child to become very wasted like this. The cause is a diet very low in total energy, that is, not enough food, for example,

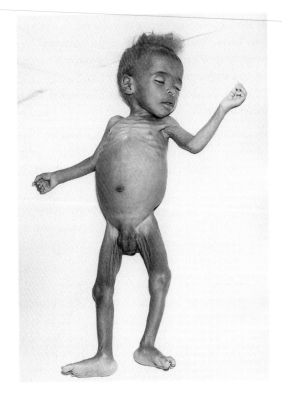

Fig. 19.1 Marasmus.

early weaning from the breast on to dilute food, because of poverty or ignorance. Poor food hygiene leads to gastroenteritis, diarrhoea, and vomiting. This leads to poor appetite, so more dilute feeds are given. Further depletion in turn leads to intestinal atrophy and more susceptibility to diarrhoea.

Not enough food implies not enough protein because most foods contain some protein. It is most unlikely that a child not getting enough food would still be eating a protein-rich food, since such foods are expensive. With negative energy balance the major fuel to maintain life is free fatty acids, drawn from the adipose tissue. Blood glucose needed for tissues that can only metabolize glucose (brain, red blood cells) is maintained by gluconeogenesis of glucogenic amino acids (e.g. alanine) drawn from the body's proteins, usually the muscles, sometimes the viscera. Although energy depletion predominates in marasmus, there is inevitably insufficient protein intake and loss of protein inside the body.

Inside the body the heart, brain, liver, and kidneys are least wasted but in advanced cases the heart becomes atrophied (wasted) and brain weight is reduced. There is increased mobilization of free fatty acids from adipose tissue, with ketosis (increased concentration of 3(OH) butyrate and acetoacetate). The blood glucose may be subnormal. The basal metabolic rate goes down; an increased proportion of triiodothyronine is in the inactive rT3 form. Plasma insulin is low and leptin is low.

Infections which are only a temporary nuisance in well-nourished children become life-threatening in children with severe PEM. Their bodies are not capable of producing the usual responses to common bacterial infections, pyrexia, and increased white blood cells (leucocytosis). Cell-mediated immunity, the main defence against viruses and tuberculosis, is impaired. Pathogenic bacteria in the intestines can more easily gain access to the blood circulation (Table 19.1).

Table 19.1 Classification of malnutrition

	Moderate	Severe
Symmetrical oedema	No	Yes (ie kwashiorkor)
Weight-for-height (length)	–2 to –3 SD of reference (70–79%), wasting	<3 SD below reference (–70%), severe wasting (i.e. marasmus)
Height-for-age	–2 to –3 SD of reference (85–89%), stunting	<3 SD below reference (<85%), severe stunting

*–2 to –3 SD below reference also called Z score –2 to –3.
'Reference' is WHO reference weight-for-height (length) and height-for-age.

Source: WHO (1999) *Management of severe malnutrition: a manual for physicians and other senior health workers*. Geneva, World Health Organization.

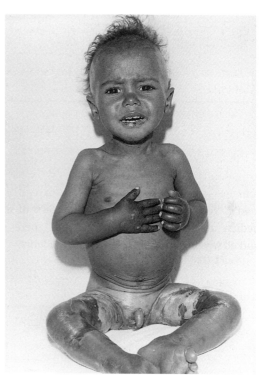

Fig 19.2 Kwashiorkor.

19.1.2 Kwashiorkor

Marasmus has been known for centuries; but the other type of severe PEM (Table 19.1), kwashiorkor, was not generally recognized until the 1950s. The classic description was by Cecily Williams in the *Lancet* in 1935. She wrote from Accra, Ghana and gave the syndrome the name that the mothers used there, in the Ga language.

Typically, a child with kwashiorkor (Fig. 19.2) develops oedema, which is generalized. The child is miserable, withdrawn, obviously ill, and will not eat. Changes can be seen in the skin: there are areas of pigmentation which are symmetrical in distribution, most commonly in the nappy area (Fig 19.2). The skin later shows cracks and the superficial layer peels off. The hair is thinned and discoloured, blond or red or grey, instead of black. There is diarrhoea. Inside the body, the liver is enlarged and its parenchymal cells contain numerous fat droplets. The

protein in the liver is reduced and two of the main features of kwashiorkor can be explained by failure of the liver to make two important (export) plasma proteins. Failure to synthesize albumin and the consequent very low plasma albumin may, because of low plasma osmotic pressure, at least partly explain the oedema. Failure to synthesize very-low-density lipoproteins, and inability to transport fat out of the liver to the periphery explains the accumulation of fat in the liver. There is an abnormal and characteristic pattern of amino acids in plasma (Table 19.2).

Kwashiorkor develops more quickly than marasmus. One day the oedema appears and the mother seeks medical help—though changes in skin and hair must have been developing over a longer period. The child with kwashiorkor is not necessarily underweight. The original meaning of kwashiorkor is 'the deposed child' or 'first second'. Mothers in Accra thought that this was the illness a child can get when a second baby follows and displaces the first one from the breast.

Table 19.2 Biochemical findings in kwashiorkor compared to marasmus (on admission to hospital)

	Kwashiorkor	Marasmus
Plasma albumin	Very low	Usually normal range
Plasma amino acids	Reduced branch chain and tryosine	More normal
Serum amylase	Very low	Normal/low normal
Plasma (total) cholesterol	Very low	Normal/low normal
Plasma free fatty acids	Increased	Increased
Plasma growth hormone	Raised	Not as high
Red cell glutathione	Low	Normal
Fasting blood glucose	Low-normal	Low
T lymphocytes	Low	Low
Plasma retinol	Low	Low
Somatomedin-C (IGF-1)	Low	Not as low
Plasma transferrin	Very low	Low normal
Plasma urea	Low	Not as low
Plasma urate	Low	Raised
Plasma zinc	Low	Not as low

There are two schools of thought on the cause of kwashiorkor. The question is why is there an acute depletion of protein from the liver and other viscera rather than from the muscles in these cases of PEM?

The original theory is that the child who develops kwashiorkor has been fed on a diet moderately adequate in carbohydrate but very low in protein so that there is a relative deficiency of protein to energy (i.e. protein malnutrition), whereas the diet that leads to marasmus is low in both energy and protein. Researchers who disagree with this classical theory argue that in their experience dietary histories are indistinguishable between children with kwashiorkor and children with marasmus. Something else must explain the visceral protein depletion—'dysadaptation', mycotoxins, or free radical damage have been suggested. A practical trial of antioxidants in over 2000 pre-school children in Malawi failed to prevent kwashiorkor (Ciliberto et al., 2005).

Individual dietary histories are not likely to be scientifically reliable from the carer(s) of a child who has become severely malnourished. Kwashiorkor children are not necessarily underweight (energy-deficient). Their very low blood and urinary urea levels indicate low protein intakes. Cure of kwashiorkor has been initiated with a diet consisting only of casein, dextrose, and salts. Kwashiorkor occurs in countries where the staple diets for weaned children have very low protein/energy ratios (e.g. cassava, plantains, sweet potato, or refined maize). Whitehead et al. (1997) made observations comparing children in The Gambia, where the usual form of severe PEM is marasmus, with children in Uganda, where kwashiorkor occurs. Ugandan children grew more in weight and height and had more subcutaneous fat but lower plasma albumin concentrations. They had higher plasma insulin levels and lower plasma cortisols. Protein/energy ratios of their food were lower. Whitehead suggests that on a very low protein diet, but with adequate carbohydrate, the carbohydrate stimulates insulin, which is known to favour deposition of amino acids in muscles. On a very-low-protein diet amino acids are in short supply, so muscle proteins can only be maintained at the expense of the liver (and other viscera). The liver is stimulated by infection to put much of its protein synthetic effort into making 'acute phase' plasma proteins that should help to fight the infection. Syndromes resembling kwashiorkor can be produced in monkeys on a diet of cassava with added sugar, and in young rats on a 5% protein ration.

19.1.3 The spectrum of severe protein-energy malnutrition

Kwashiorkor and marasmus are distinct diseases, but in communities where both occur cases of severe PEM often have some features of both (e.g. they are very underweight and also have skin or hair changes). This is marasmic kwashiorkor.

The Spanish name for PEM, *syndrome policaren-cial infantile,* means the polynutritional deficiency of infants. In severely malnourished cases there must be deficiencies of micronutrients, notably vitamin A, with risk of xerophthalmia and potassium from diarrhoea, which contributes to the oedema. Niacin deficiency (where maize is the staple) may contribute to the skin lesions and zinc deficiency further weakens immune response to infections.

Malnourished children have diarrhoea. An infection has probably precipitated the severe illness. These children stand infections poorly; measles is especially lethal. In parts of Africa HIV infection underlies a proportion of malnourished children.

19.1.4 Management of severe malnutrition

Children who are severely wasted or have generalized oedema should be admitted to hospital, where they can be treated and fed day and night. Complications need medical treatment. The nutritional management is similar for marasmus and kwashiorkor. 'Take it slowly' is the established principle for refeeding severely malnourished children and adults. Management is in these stages (WHO, 1999):

1 *Treatment of acute complications*: correction of dehydration and/or electrolyte disturbance and/or very low blood glucose and/or low body temperature (hypothermia) and start of treatment for infections. Nearly all severely malnourished children have bacterial infections, though they may not show fever or leucocytosis. All should receive broad spectrum antibacterial treatment. The fluid given to rehydrate malnourished children should contain less sodium and more potassium than the standard UNICEF oral rehydration solution. ReSoMal contains, per litre of water, only 45 mmol sodium, but 40 mmol potassium, more glucose, and some magnesium and zinc.

2 *Initiation of cure*: refeeding, gradually working up the energy and protein intake and giving multivitamin drops and potassium, magnesium, and zinc supplements. Children with kwashiorkor have poor appetites. They have to be handfed, with frequent feeds, preferably in the lap of their mother or a nurse they know. To start refeeding the standard 'formula' is F75 recommended by WHO, which provides 75 kcal and 1 g protein/100 mL. This is given for the first few days, in small amounts which add up to around 100 mL/kg/day. Although the child is malnourished, energy and protein must be limited to avoid metabolic stress.

When the child is starting to recover, F100 is introduced, which contains 100 kcal and 2.9 g protein/100 mL (12% protein and 53% fat). This can be given to satiety. F75 and F100 are available as powders that can be reconstituted with water. They contain dried skimmed milk, sugar, vegetable oil, mineral mix, and vitamin mix. Details of the formula can vary in different centres.

3 *Nutritional rehabilitation*: after about 3 weeks the child should be obviously better, with oedema cleared and mentally bright with good appetite, yet still below the reference weight-for-height. At this stage, catch-up growth should occur if the child is well looked after and given nutritious combinations of local familiar foods. If the child has been in hospital they may be able to go on to a nutrition rehabilitation unit if one is available in the area. Sooner or later they will go home. It is unlikely that the home of a malnourished child is well resourced with nourishing food. At this stage, locally produced ready-to-use (therapeutic) food (RUTF) is being increasingly useful for rehabilitation of children recovering from severe malnutrition and also to manage children with moderately severe malnutrition, so that they do not require

expensive (and often distant) hospital treatment (Box 19.2).

RUTF is being increasingly used in the 21st century in areas with extensive malnutrition. A typical example is 'Plumpy Nut'™, made of peanut butter, milk powder, vegetable oil, sugar, vitamin, and minerals and packed in air-tight sachets. They are pastes that the child can eat as solid food. They have very low water activity, resist bacterial contamination so can be stored, and do not have to be cooked. Their nutrient content approximates to the water-based WHO's F100. The main difference is the peanut butter in RUTF. Allergic reactions appear to be very rare in malnourished children.

There are several different names for RUTFs. Some are commercial products, some made locally. They are provided by NGOs, charities, food aid, and/or the countries' health services. They should be treated as medicines and not shared with other family members.

BOX 19.2 Prognosis of children with PEM

Even in well-equipped hospitals, the death rate of children with severe PEM is around 20%. Prognosis is worse for cases with kwashiorkor or HIV infection. Are there lasting effects in those who survive? Follow-up biopsies after kwashiorkor have shown that the liver returns to normal; the fatty change does not progress to cirrhosis (unlike that in alcoholics). In marasmic children, who have become severely wasted in the first 2 years of life, growth of the head (circumference easily measured), is retarded so the brain must be smaller than normal, and such children may subsequently have impaired intelligence unless they are fortunate thereafter and brought up in an excellent environment.

19.2 Mild to moderate protein-energy malnutrition

For every florid case of marasmus or kwashiorkor, there must be 7–10 children in the community with mild to moderate PEM. Like an iceberg, there is more malnutrition below the surface and not easily recognized. Mothers often do not realize that their child is malnourished because he or she is similar in size and vitality to many of the same age in an impoverished neighbourhood. Most children with mild to moderate PEM can be detected, however, by their weight-for-age, which is less than 80% of the international standard (Table 19.1). Such children are either wasted, with subnormal weight-for-height/length or *stunted* (nutritional dwarfism), with subnormal height-for-age (but not wasted), or both. Wasted children have used up body fat, and some muscle, to maintain their fuel supply. Stunted children have adapted in a different way, by stopping or slowing their growth. Reference tables (or graphs) are available from the World Health Organization (WHO) for weight-for-age, height/ length-for-age, and weight-for-height for prepubertal children (see Chapter 34).

In many developing countries, around 2% of preschool children have severe PEM and 20% (in some places more) have mild to moderate PEM. The importance of this mild to moderate PEM is that affected children are growing up smaller than their genetic potential and have increased susceptibility to severe gastroenteritis and respiratory infections. Mild to moderate PEM is a major underlying reason why the 1–5 year mortality in poorer developing countries is 30–60 times higher than in Europe, North America, or Australasia. Nine of the 10 countries with highest 1–5 year mortality (270–204 per 1000 in 2006) are in Africa and one is Afghanistan. Deaths are recorded as due to pneumonia, diarrhoea, and malaria (Black *et al.*, 2010) but micro and macro-analysis indicate that poor nutrition is the underlying cause of 35 to 50% of these deaths (Bejan *et al.*, 2008; Black *et al.*, 2008).

19.3 Prevention of protein-energy malnutrition

Kwashiorkor most often occurs in the second year of life; marasmus mostly in the first year. Kwashiorkor is more amenable to the medical model of education, for example, education of mothers about the need for protein foods for weaned children and encouraging their provision at the political level. Marasmus is a more intractable problem, bound up with poverty, the status and education of women, lack of contraceptive resources, and poor sanitation. UNICEF has achieved reductions in rates of PEM with four simple measures: represented by GOBI (Box 19.3). Rates of immunization are now 80% or more across the world. Measles and tuberculosis immunizations are particularly valuable. In many developing countries, there are extensive programmes for (large dose) vitamin A supplements to be given at the same time (see Chapter 12).

BOX 19.3 UNICEFs inexpensive measures to prevent PEM

G *for growth monitoring.* The mother keeps the simple weight-for-age chart in a cellophane envelope and brings the child to a maternal and child health clinic regularly for weighing and advice.

O *for oral rehydration.* The UNICEF ORS formula (NaCl 3.5 g, NaHCO$_3$ 2.5 g, KCl 1.5 g, glucose 20 g in clean water to 1 litre) is saving many lives from gastroenteritis.

B for breastfeeding. This has overwhelming advantages for a baby in a poor community with no facilities for hygiene. It should be continued as long as possible while solid foods are added. Additional foods, which should be prepared from locally available foods, are not usually needed before 6 months of age.

I *for immunization.* For a few dollars, a child can be protected against measles, diphtheria, pertussis, tetanus, tuberculosis, poliomyelitis, etc., infections that predispose to and aggravate malnutrition.

19.4 Famine

The worst famines in recent times have been in areas torn by civil war. The hostilities greatly hamper communication of early warning and confirmation of the severity of the food shortage and transport of relief food into the area.

When there is not enough food for an entire community, children stop growing and children and adults lose weight. Starving people feel cold and weak and crave for food. Subcutaneous fat disappears and muscles waste. Pulse is slow and blood pressure low. The abdomen is distended; diarrhoea is common. Infections are to be expected, especially gastrointestinal infections, pneumonia, tuberculosis, and typhus.

The problem in a famine is not so much loss of food as loss of ability to obtain it. People have to sell all their assets in the attempt to buy food. The community's social and economic structures break down.

Aid professionals in relief operations should expect to have a mainly administrative and organizational role. It is impossible to give most time to treatment of a few very sick individuals. Therapeutic feeding is not an effective use of resources. Field workers have three options for distributions of food where supplies are insufficient to provide the minimum requirements of 1900 kcal (7.9 mJ)/day: (i) where community and family structure are still intact and community representatives can be identified, let the community decide how the limited food is to be distributed; (ii) where community structures have been disrupted, distribute food selectively to those assessed to be at the highest risk of mortality; or (iii) the third alternative is equitable distribution of the same basic ration to all members of the affected population, with selection of particularly vulnerable members. The standard food aid rations usually consist of cereals, legumes, and some oil. If the cereal is whole grain, milling equipment is necessary. Milk powder is used for malnourished children. Provision of clean water is a priority. Care must be taken that the population gets the critical micronutrients, which are not the same in different areas and situations, e.g. vitamin C, potassium.

In emergency feeding situations, micronutrient powders are distributed for people and children to add to their food when they eat it. 'Sprinkles' and 'Mix Me' contain in one dose the recommended nutrient intakes of vitamins and minerals iron, zinc, iodine, and selenium.

To assess the degree of undernutrition in individuals two measures are commonly used: mid-upper arm circumference (MUAC) and weight-for-height in children or body mass index (BMI, kg/m^2) in adults. MUAC is obviously quicker and tape measures can be given to several workers. Weight and height are slower to measure. In children, low MUAC tends to select younger children as malnourished and miss older children with low weight-for-height (or BMI). In adults, MUAC and BMI appear to correlate fairly well. A MUAC of 220 mm in men or 210 mm in women corresponds approximately to a critical BMI of 16 kg/m^2. As a general rule, moderate starvation = weight-for-height 80–71% of reference (in children), BMI of 18–16 kg/m^2 (in adults); severe starvation = weight-for-height $\leq$ 70% of reference (in children) or BMI $\leq$ 15.7 kg/m^2 (in adults).

The clinical photographs in this chapter were kindly provided by Professor J.D.L. Hansen of Cape Town.

Further Reading

Five major books have been written (in English) on PEM of children, the first in 1954. The two most recent are by Suskind and Lewinter-Suskind (1990) and by Waterlow (1992)(see below).

1. **Ashworth, A., Chopra, M., McCoy, D., et al.** (2004) WHO guidelines for management of severe malnutrition in rural South African hospitals: Effect on case fatality and the influence of operational factors. *Lancet,* **363,** 1110–15.
2. **Bejan, P., Mohammed, S., Mwangi, I., et al.** (2008) Fraction of all hospital admissions and deaths attributable to malnutrition among children in rural Kenya. *Am J Clin Nutr* **88,** 1626–31.
3. **Black, R.E., Allen, L.H., Bhutta, Z.A., et al.** (2008) Maternal and child undernutrition: Global and regional exposures and health consequences. *Lancet,* **371,** 243–60.
4. **Black, R.E., Cousens, S., Johnson, H.L., et al.** (2010) Global, regional and national causes of child mortality in 2008: A systematic analysis. *Lancet,* **375,** 1969–87.
5. **Bhutta, Z.A.** (2009) Addressing severe acute malnutrition where it matters. *Lancet,* **374,** 94–6.
6. **Ciliberto, J.H., Ciliberto, M., Briend, A., Ashorn, P., Bier, D., and, Manary, M.** (2005) Antioxidant supplementation for the prevention of kwashiorkor in Malawian children: Randomised, doubled blind, placebo controlled trial. *BMJ,* **330,** 1109–11.
7. **Collins, S., Dent, N., Binns, P., Bahwere, P., Sadler, K., and Hallam, A.** (2006) Management of acute severe malnutrition in children. *Lancet,* **368,** 1992–2000.
8. **Diop, E.H.I., Dossou, N.I., Ndour, M.M., Briend, A., and Wade, S.** (2003) Comparison of the efficacy of a solid ready-to-use food and a liquid, milk-based diet for the rehabilitation of severly malnourished children: A randomized trial. *Am J Clin Nutr* **78,** 302–7.
9. **Suskind, R.M. and Lewinter-Suskind, L.** (1990) *The malnourished child.* New York, Raven Press.
10. **Waterlow, J.C.** (1992) *Protein-energy malnutrition.* London, Edward Arnold.

11. **Whithead, R.G., Coward, W.A., Lunn, P.G., *et al.*** (1997) A comparison of the pathogenesis of protein energy malnutrition in Uganda and the Gambia. *Trans R Soc Trop Med Hyg* **71**, 189–95.

12. **WHO** (1999) *Management of severe malnutrition: A manual for physicians and other senior health workers.* Geneva, World Health Organization.

Useful Websites

To see topical and scientifically robust updates on nutrition associated with this textbook and web links to many of the journals in the Further Reading sections, please see the dedicated Online Resource Centre at **http://www.oxfordtextbooks.co.uk/orc/mann4e/**

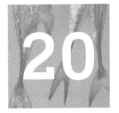

20 Nutritional crises

M. Alain Mourey and Jennifer McMahon

A nutritional crisis can be said to occur when an individual or a population group is unable to maintain the 'feeding process'—they are unable to access adequate supplies of food or are unable to consume or utilize sufficient nutrients. Any nutritional crisis has two phases: a *preliminary phase*, during which a crisis may be averted by adaptation, utilization of reserves, or other defence mechanisms (governments sometimes suppress information relating to an impending crisis and prevent such news from reaching the international community), and an *acute phase*, during which protective mechanisms fail, household and societal systems disintegrate, and the 'feeding process' breaks down, resulting in hunger and ultimately nutritional inadequacy, before the starvation associated with famine can be seen. Identification of the preliminary phase represents a major challenge to local and national governments and humanitarian organizations, since there may be opportunities to facilitate interventions that have the potential to halt progression to the acute phase. The progression to a crisis is usually when the event (generally referred to as a phenomenon) affects a vulnerable group or population (Fig. 20.1). A single event such as an isolated drought episode in an arid setting is unlikely to pose a serious threat because the population is accustomed to responding with adaptive mechanisms to recurrent, and therefore familiar, phenomena. However, several drought episodes in rapid succession are likely to deplete adaptive mechanisms and enhance the vulnerability of the population.

20.1 Causes of nutritional crises

Events (phenomena) causing crises are either human (war, economic, social, cultural, accidents, and illness, or inappropriate farming practice) or environmental (geophysical: earthquakes, volcanic eruption, tidal waves; climatic variation: drought, floods, hurricanes, erosion; nonhuman predators: insects, birds, rodents, parasites, diseases).

20.1.1 Human phenomena

Political War is a major trigger of nutritional crises. Looting, destruction, danger, restrictions on access and movement, population displacements, confinement, occupation, terror and harassment, seizure of goods, embargoes and conscription: all

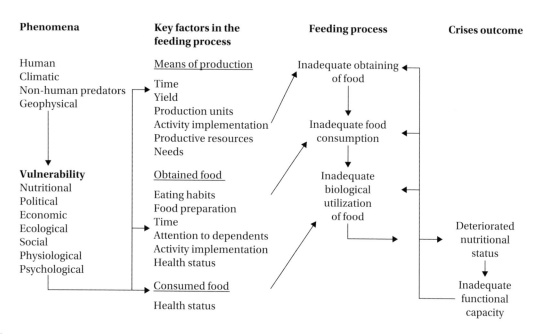

| Phenomena | Key factors in the feeding process | Feeding process | Crises outcome |

Fig. 20.1 Progression of events leading to a nutritional crisis.

undermine household economy and food security. Displacement of populations may result in epidemics of infectious disease with direct consequences to consumption and utilization of food, further reducing production potential.

Economic Increased levels of poverty and restricted choices by families can result from such activities as speculation by market traders, and power struggles by an elite group, whereby shortages develop and prices of essential commodities rise. Likewise, farmers may be forced to sell produce to those who trade outside their region, or even abroad, also leading to reduced local availability or excessive prices, particularly if harvest yields are poor. Any devaluation of currency can have devastating effects on pensioners and others living on fixed incomes. Following currency devaluation and price inflation in Abkhazia (the western region of Georgia), pensioners were in a desperate position when the price of bread increased approximately 10 000-fold.

Deterioration in economic stability will also result when small domestic economies become dependent on new agricultural practices and costly imports.

Compared with traditional crops, hybrid or genetically modified seeds require annual purchases, appreciably greater use of fertilizers and pesticides, and often controlled irrigation. A community in Angola would almost certainly have experienced a nutritional crisis without humanitarian aid in 1999 as it became isolated due to war and was dependent on such seeds and related inputs, which were no longer obtainable.

Misguided economic development policies may result in environmental deterioration—erosion, desertification, soil salinity, deforestation, resource depletion and pollution—from excessive exploitation. This in turn contributes to a rural exodus towards urban centres, resulting in the impoverishment of both migrants and residents who remain in the areas (as it is usually the decision maker and the fit who migrate).

Social In the more affluent communities and countries the increase in population has been accompanied by both industrial and agricultural development and a service sector, shifting the concern to the adverse environmental consequences created. However, in the developing world, population growth results in competition for resources, increasing the risk for conflict, adding to the disintegration of the social fabric, allowing an introduction of misguided development policies, and contributing to a deterioration of the environment, all increasing the risk of a nutritional crisis.

Cultural While social phenomena can occur in any society, cultural phenomena are specific to communities. For example, the belligerent nature of Somali clans led to suppression and looting of those without strong family affiliations and perceived wealth. This individualistic behaviour led to one of the twentieth century's most devastating famines. Such behaviour is acquired, and is thus eminently cultural. Some weaning and infant-feeding practices also have serious consequences for the consumption and biological utilization of food. For instance, the Baganda children of Uganda are weaned from maternal milk by a sudden shift to mostly starchy food, which is low in protein and other nutrients, and poor in energy. In addition, they lose the immune protection of breastfeeding, while the weaning food exposes them to new forms of bacterial contamination. Thus, their appetite is satiated without their nutritional requirements being met. Infective illness compounds the problem, and severe malnutrition frequently results (see Section 19.1).

Accidents and illnesses Accidents can cause massive pollution, such as the mercury poisoning in Minamata, Japan, the toxic gas and chemical leak in Bhopal, India, and the nuclear explosion in Chernobyl, Ukraine. They can contaminate entire regions, making them uninhabitable for large population groups. Workplace and traffic accidents and illness affect individuals and households to an extent that may predispose to nutritional crises, especially in societies with limited support systems.

Inappropriate farming practices Inappropriate farming practices, including over-farming, may also contribute to an adverse environmental impact, including erosion, desertification, drought, and pollution.

20.1.2 Environmental phenomena

20.1.2.1 Geophysical

Hurricanes, earthquakes, volcanic eruptions, and tidal waves These climatic phenomena are invariably of short duration but may predispose to nutritional crises by destroying crops, devastating arable land, and displacing communities from their homes and properties to areas where they must depend on international agencies or on others who are barely in a position to feed themselves.

20.1.2.2 Climatic

Drought Especially when combined with war, drought may have devastating consequences. This has been seen in recent times in Ethiopia, Angola, Mozambique, Somalia, and Sudan. An isolated drought episode in a country prone to yearly variation in rainfall rarely results in a nutritional crisis because the population may be able to implement tried and tested adaptive mechanisms. However, pendulum variations, in which relatively humid years and dry spells may last for around 5 years (as occurs in southern Africa) or as long as 10–18 years (as in the Sahel), and permanent climatic changes are of far greater concern. Climatic changes have occurred as natural phenomena over time and it is unclear whether the apparent increase in drought in many countries in recent years is as a result of such an occurrence or whether environmental overexploitation (particularly by deforestation) and global warming are responsible. However, regardless of the cause, there is no doubt that persistent drought is resulting in devastating consequences in many parts of Africa. In the totally arid areas of northern Mali, for example, pools lined with shell residues provided a supply of permanent water until 1972. Since then, because of the severity of drought, they have dried up completely. Angola and Mozambique were countries that seldom experienced drought, but since the late 1980s and early 1990s, consecutive drought years have been relatively common-place. In Angola and Ethiopia, endemic malaria is occurring at higher altitudes than previously, indicating rising temperatures.

Floods Flooding principally leads to a crisis situa-tion when it occurs during the main planting sea-son, when it follows a drought, when repeated flooding occurs, and when the geographic and polit-ical environment preclude efficient action. Like droughts, floods may be natural climatic phenom-ena or may be a consequence of human activity, especially deforestation.

20.1.3 Nonhuman predators

Plagues of locusts, caterpillars, and other insects and birds can devastate crops. Insects and rodents can attack stored harvests. Epidemics of infectious disease have the potential to precipitate a nutri-tional crisis, by not only reducing the capacity of sick individuals to produce or secure food, but may deci-mate herds, from which a population group may secure its nutritional inputs (i.e., rinderpest in cat-tle). Severe infections reaching epidemic propor-tions will also slow the economy of a region and perhaps a country.

20.2 Vulnerability

The phenomena described in Section 20.1 are most likely to result in nutritional crises when affecting vulnerable groups. Equally vulnerabili-ties increase susceptibility to the causal phenom-ena, especially since several of the phenomena are closely associated with the range of factors increasing any vulnerability.

20.2.1 Nutritional vulnerability

Young children, pregnant and lactating women, the elderly, and the ill are universally regarded as vulner-able. It is these groups that are likely to be the first to show evidence of any breakdown of the feeding process—the difficulty in obtaining food (Box 20.1), the failure to consume adequate and appropriate food (Box 20.2), or the inadequate biological utiliza-tion of food (Box 20.3).

20.2.2 Political vulnerability

Political instability is not only associated with the risk of conflict, repression, and discrimination, but can hinder adaptive mechanisms needed to arrest the development of a crisis. When there is political instability, there is often inadequate transportation and communication services, plus a disregard for human rights, affecting all but a privileged few.

20.2.3 Economic vulnerability

Communities and populations are economically vulnerable whenever food production, the attain-able yield and subsequent access to food is hampered, whether the cause is a natural or human phenomena.

20.3 Pathology of nutritional crises

Famine represents the acute phase of a nutritional crisis; however, it is noteworthy that famine is a relatively rare event when one considers how often the famine process is initiated. The immediate causes of famine can be summarized (Box 20.4). The severity of a famine depends on the level of

BOX 20.1 Difficulties in obtaining food may result from:

- Poor health, affecting functional capacity
- Low food availability within the society resulting in price rises of essential commodities
- Insufficient economic production at household level (indicating an inadequate economic performance)
- Losses before and after harvest
- Loss of reserves through excessive sale, consumption, or looting
- Impoverishment from the use of reserves to cover essential needs
- Any increase in time to find or produce food
- Climate change influencing harvests, hunting, collecting, and fishing activities
- Disturbances in market forces from shortages, infrastructural damage, and/or transport disruptions
- Government favouring certain communities and regions, and neglecting others.

BOX 20.2 Failure to consume adequate and appropriate food results from:

- Inability to obtain sufficient food
- Disturbed eating habits from changes in availability of food products, the time available for preparation and sharing of food, and weaning practices
- Lack of means and/or knowledge to care for dependents when circumstances change and any imposed measures are unfamiliar or impossible to apply
- Lack of adequate health care and exposure to infectious diseases when living conditions change
- Health problems affecting food consumption (most often anorexia).

BOX 20.3 Inability to utilize food results from:

- Reduced and inadequate food consumption
- Gastrointestinal pathology associated with reduced digestion, and absorption of nutrients
- Infectious disease having an impact on metabolism and nutrient requirements.

food insufficiency, its duration, and the persistence of the cause of the famine.

Each famine situation is different, but the effect on household economy is the same and can be summarized through the four stages (there does tend to be some overlap between the stages):

1 *Adaptation* Households modify their activities to maximize economic output and productive activities. Reserves may be used to preserve normal life.

2 *Impoverishment* There is an increase in activities usually found loathsome or demeaning; the sale or exchange of nonproductive items, termination of reserves, spending limited to the absolute minimum, strict control of food consumption, and increase in access and use of social support networks. Seeds and means of production are preserved in order to maximize chances of recuperation. Food restriction may result in early signs of nutritional inadequacy.

> **BOX 20.4** Immediate causes of famine (one or more may apply)
>
> - Household food production is insufficient or nonexistent.
> - Foraging, hunting or fishing activities are insufficient or nonexistent.
> - Household means to buy food in the market are insufficient because of inadequate supply or high price.
> - No food in market place following infrastructure destruction, problems of security, or isolation.
> - Local mutual aid and social aid systems are exhausted or nonexistent.
> - National support systems against famine are insufficient, neglected, nonfunctioning, or nonexistent.
> - International support has not been given to humanitarian agencies to help feed the population.
> - Humanitarian agencies are unable to access.

3 *Decapitalization* Households exploit all possible means of income generation, by sale or exchange of their remaining items and productive assets. Further food restrictions are initiated, resulting in more advanced nutritional inadequacies and reduced functional capacity. Social services can no longer cope, and social norms disintegrate alongside economic degradation. Individuals struggle to remain alive, at whatever cost.

4 *Hunger and exhaustion* This stage represents the full-blown picture of famine. All reserves are exhausted, and mortality from malnutrition and infectious diseases reaches epidemic proportions.

The extent to which households and communities recover from famine depends upon the stage at which the famine is alleviated by outside intervention or reversal of causal phenomena or aggravating factors.

Increasingly, humanitarian agencies and the donor community are attempting to intervene early. For example, when the International Committee of the Red Cross (ICRC) realized early in 2010, that the condition of the herds in Niger were deteriorating, it immediately started a programme aimed at decreasing the size of herds, slaughtering the sickest and weakest animals whilst vaccinating, and treating and feeding the remaining ones, so that they could survive until the next rainy season. The ICRC gave a cash compensation for the animals slaughtered, allowing their owners to buy food, until general food distribution could be implemented. When conditions return again to normal, the ICRC will continue its support in order to decrease the vulnerability of the pastoralists.

20.4 Diagnosing a crisis: the need for surveys

Frequently when a nutritional crisis occurs, there is a call from local and international media, local authorities, and the world at large for instant humanitarian assistance. While the situation is often dire, it is imperative to undertake a full evaluation and develop a logical plan of action before implementing an appropriate programme. Ideally, surveys should be undertaken prior to the development of the acute phase of the crisis, since it may be possible for the full consequence of the causal phenomena to be averted.

The purpose of the initial survey is not only to define the extent of the problem and to determine both the immediate and future needs of the affected groups, but also the causal phenomena responsible for the existing or impending crisis. Although standard information will be required, the strategies to obtain the necessary information will need to be adapted to individual circumstances.

Ideally, a multidisciplinary team should gather the information with expertise in nutrition, public health, water, and shelter and, from the relevant economic sector, an agronomist for a subsistence agricultural population and an economist for urban or war-affected economies, such as existed after the break-up of Yugoslavia.

20.4.1 Identification of existing or potential problems

The steps to be followed may appear obvious, but if they are not followed, there will be an inappropriate response. Once the affected regions and populations have been identified, a range of quantitative and qualitative information is required, especially as it relates to the most vulnerable sections of the affected population (Box 20.5). The nutritional status of the population must be defined, and the extent to which this can be formally assessed depends upon circumstances.

In order to determine the extent of support that will be required to maintain the 'feeding process', it is necessary to make a quantitative assessment of the remaining food stocks and the expected agricultural production. To this is added a qualitative assessment of what might be available from forage activities, exchange, and purchase, taking into account the changed circumstances (how are the current circumstances compared to average year?). For example, in normal circumstances, forage activities may produce nuts and fish of high nutritive value, but in a crisis may only produce green leaves and wild grains of limited nutritive value. Likewise, in good times, home-brewed beer and gathered firewood may generate income or provide items for exchange, but, during a crisis others may be attempting similar activities

---

BOX 20.5 Summary of initial survey (with methods to obtain the required information)

1 Geographic localization of the affected area (*maps and views in cross-section*).

2 Identification of the population groups affected by the crisis.

For each population, undertake and determine:

3 Subdivision of each group to economic classes (poor, average, rich), an economic profile for each class (number and types of economic activity), both in usual times and at the time of the survey (*functional classification; proportional piling*).

4 Assess the relative importance and proportion of activity for each economic class in the economy: when the situation is normal; when the situation is the worst they remember; when the situation is the best they remember; and the situation at the time of the survey; incorporating food consumption, both qualitatively and quantitatively, and the general system of social obligation in different situations (*proportional piling and study of food consumption*).

5 Minimum economic resources for economic self-sufficiency in usual times (*household economy models with budget equilibrium*).

6 Usual means of adaptation or modification to normal variations in the economy and climate (*proportional piling and seasonal calendars*).

7 Methods that might be employed to alleviate particular crises.

8 Stages of the famine process, including assessment of nutritional status (*model of household activities; anthropometry; evaluation of nutritional resources*).

9 Causes of the present situation (*diagrams of events; graphical representation of market prices; income/exchange rates*).

10 Events that could ameliorate or worsen the situation.

11 Problems faced by the population (*class in order of priority*).

12 Requirements for aid (*class in order of priority*).

13 Programme required to deliver aid (*identify all actions, Strengths, Weaknesses, Opportunities, Threats (SWOT) analysis, decision-making tree*).

and their value is thus reduced. For those who rely habitually, or during a crisis, on food purchase for family needs, the extent to which available income can meet food costs must be established. In general, when as much as 80% of available income is required for food purchase, a critical phase has been reached. Although the gap between means and needs is difficult to assess, such information is essential.

In addition to assessing the absolute severity of the crisis, it is important to discover how the situation differs from 'normal'. Access to food (quality as well as quantity), food preparation, distribution within the family, and means of distributing the food need to be compared. It is also important to establish how the population or high-risk groups have coped with comparable problems in the past. Box 20.6 gives an example of the initial assessment of a crisis in Irian Jaya.

This crisis was linked to the severity of the 1997 El Nino (drought and frost killing sweet potato crops) and the villagers being prevented from leaving their villages by the Indonesian Army. Sweet potato vines were provided to the affected villages with the assistance of an Indonesian agricultural specialist. This, combined with normal climatic conditions and the ability to freely move, led to an amelioration of conditions.

Working through the list of phenomena with a potential to interact with vulnerability and precipitate the acute phase of the crisis is an integral part of the initial survey, and it is an essential prerequisite to determining the solution. For example, if in a subsistence agricultural zone the cause of the famine is drought, one might expect the harvest after the next rainy season to relieve the problem, and this might require only temporary food assistance. However, if the famine is a result of armed conflict, prolonged support and intensive negotiation with military authorities may be necessary. Table 20.1 summarizes the phenomena that influenced access to food, the difficulties encountered, and the responses made during the course of the prolonged famine in southern Sudan. Despite the wide-ranging and desperate responses made by the population to the phenomena, the stage was reached when outside aid offered the only means of survival.

BOX 20.6 Initial assessment of the 1997 crisis in Irian Jaya

In 1997, rumours circulated that El Nino would lead to an unprecedented drought in Irian Jaya, leading to a risk of famine. The signal led to a preliminary survey. The approach to the situation consisted of documenting the climate, the mode of living of the inhabitants, and the factors that could influence progress of the survey. The nutritionist in the survey team learned that, despite the drought, it rained heavily in some places and field conditions were extremely difficult with village access almost impossible without helicopter. The population lived essentially on sweet potato and forage. There were almost no health posts, malaria was rampant, and communication with the local people required translators. Initial preparation involved obtaining as much local information as possible, including information on the cultivation and nutritional value of sweet potatoes. Such preliminary data gathering helped to define the logistical constraints should an assistance programme prove necessary. Once in the field, the rumours of the drought and the famine were confirmed, despite not being able to verify the effects directly on the affected population. The surveying nutritionist believed that, despite the drought being well established, it was necessary to verify the effects on the population as the people are well known for their resilience and abilities to forage, hunt, and fish. In the first village visited, it was clear that the population already had signs of severe malnutrition. Thus, the approach was changed. Levels of malnutrition were measured and a state of famine due to drought declared. Visits to the agricultural areas confirmed the virtual absence of production due to drought. General poor health resulting from malaria, chest infections, and diarrhoea, which were exacerbated by the reappearance of rain and cold, aggravated the situation. The situation could only be relieved by humanitarian aid.

Table 20.1 Access to food (in order of importance), phenomena, and difficulties encountered and the responses made in the course of the famine in a region in southern Sudan

Access to food	Phenomena and difficulties	Population responses
Milk from the herd (normal access)	– Attacks against the cattle herd in 1991–1992 – Seasonal migration	– Agriculture – Fishing – Forage for wild resources – Marriage – Salaried employment – Social obligations
Cattle sales for sorghum purchase (normal access) Agriculture (seasonal activity, normally marginal)	– War between 1989 and 1994 – Drought in 1993 – Destruction by insects in 1993 and 1994 – Lack of tools and seeds – Seasonal factors – Forced displacement between 1988 and 1992	– Agriculture – Salaried employment – Fishing – Forage for wild resources – Salaried employment – Social obligations
Fishing (seasonal activity, normally marginal)	– Drought in 1993 – Lack of equipment – Seasonal factors – Forced displacement between 1988 and 1992	– Forage for wild resources – Salaried employment – Social obligations – Reduction in food consumption
Forage for wild resources (seasonal activity, normally marginal)	– Drought in 1993 – Seasonal factors – Competition for natural resources	– Salaried employment – Social obligations – Reduction in food consumption
Salaried employment (activity undertaken only in cases of necessity)	– More workers than work available – Insecurity impedes access to work – Unable to fulfil employers' requirement	– Social obligations – Reduction in food consumption
Social obligations (reciprocal assistance)	– Poor overall economic situation for the community – Relationships breakdown	– Reduction in food consumption – Humanitarian aid in 1993
Humanitarian aid (occasional, irregular, rather rare)	– Political constraints in 1994 – Season access factors – Donor fatigue in 1994	– Reduction in food consumption

Table 20.1 *(Continued)*

Access to food	Phenomena and difficulties	Population responses
Reduction in food consumption (response to the crisis situation)	– Physiological reserves already made poor	– No more response possible – Significantly increased mortality

It is hoped change for the tribes of South Sudan will be seen in the near future, following the cessation of fighting and associated increased access to market, and the ability to travel throughout the region.

20.4.2 In-depth survey, continuing surveillance, and evaluation

An action plan is generally developed after the initial survey. However, there is often need for more in-depth information to ensure the most appropriate level and type of support. This includes consideration of any possible untoward effects of the intervention, obtaining a better understanding of relevant cultural issues (specifically those related to food) and identification of the vulnerable groups. One of the principal lessons learned by the International Federation of Red Cross and Red Crescent societies (IFRC/RC) post the 2004 Indian Ocean tsunami (and one used to develop the response to the 2010 Haiti earthquake) was the importance of planning for recovery early in the evaluation and development of an action plan. Much useful information is often obtained from discussion with community leaders and affected individuals, and thus the recovery and development phase should be addressed at this time. Once any plan has been implemented, ongoing surveillance is essential, as is a final evaluation to ensure that lessons learned can inform future interventions and that resources have been appropriately utilized. An example of this are the lessons learned by the IFRC/RC and explained in Box 20.7.

BOX 20.7 Lessons learned from the 2004 tsunami

1 Each institution needs strong leadership to continually acknowledge the importance of sustainable recovery when planning its disaster assistance (to think beyond the 'here and now' of the relief phase, to create holistic programmes integrating the re-establishment of essential services, permanent housing reconstruction, and livelihood restoration).

2 To link relief, recovery, and development from the beginning of a disaster operation required consultation with communities, governments, and partners (a needs assessment with communities carried out in the early days concurrently with a relief operation, to avoid 'white elephant' projects or funds being diverted to lower priority projects).

3 Accountability to beneficiaries and communities can be achieved by placing them at the centre of any programming, by including them in design, implementation, and programme monitoring (e.g. vulnerable households identified by community volunteers reviewing each and every household according to agreed criteria and allocating a point-score; as was done in the Maldives).

(Continued)

BOX 20.7 Lessons learned from the 2004 tsunami (*Continued*)

4 Disaster preparedness and risk reduction integral to rebuilding safer and more resilient communities (communities do their own risk mapping and develop plans and skills to build resilience and take care of themselves), reducing risk of 'white elephant' projects (e.g. a housing project with low occupancy).

5 Partnership with other organization aid in meeting the full range of community needs, especially with expertise and capacity.

6 Accountability to donors through effective monitoring, evaluation, and reporting must be planned for and resourced from the beginning. If not, there is a risk of donor dissatisfaction, possible loss of confidence, and subsequent loss of future support.

7 Even during large-scale recovery programmes, capacity building of host National Societies must be sustainable, and focused on the areas prioritized by them.

8 Coordination can only be effective on both strategic and operational levels if there are sufficient resources and roles are clearly defined. Important to avoid ad hoc arrangements to not have confusion or impede effective coordination.

9 To Identify risks, monitoring the situation as it develops, and adopting risk mitigation strategies in the midst of rapidly changing environments is essential to minimize financial and legal exposure.

10 A pool of trained personnel to deploy to emergencies is essential. Insufficient experienced and qualified staff to support activities results in poor performance, poor decision-making, inefficiencies, disputes, and grievances.

Source: International Federation of Red Cross and Red Crescent Societies (2009) *Tsunami five year progress report 2004–2009*; Personal communication from Mr Jerry Talbot, former Head of Tsunami Operations for the IFRC/RC.

20.5 Planning the emergency intervention

Box 20.8 lists the eight stages of the development of an emergency intervention plan. In defining priorities, the two most important factors are ensuring the protection of individual rights and providing assistance for survival, if the population is no longer self-sufficient in productive activities. This may involve general food distributions, rehabilitational feeding programmes, selective feeding programmes, and nutrition education. It is at this point that recovery and development, in consultation with the community, is initiated. Once priorities have been established, it is important that these are followed, regardless of the logistical or security constraints. Every effort must be made to overcome the difficulties because 'second- best' strategies are seldom successful. The protection of rights to access food are an integral component of Protocols of the Geneva Conventions, the Declaration of International Human Rights, and the International Covenant on Economic, Social and Cultural Rights.

The implementation plan includes the development of detailed work plans that include the activities, the resources, and the means of mobilizing them according to the defined priorities and objectives. It includes coordination with others politically involved in providing relief, including local authorities, and the roles and responsibilities of personnel, security, and such details as lodging for personnel. At the outset, it is necessary not only to establish the means for adjustment if surveillance and evaluation demonstrate that this is necessary, but also the terms of disengagement (total or partial). The terms and methods of withdrawal also need to be considered if an intervention is made obsolete by a change in the situation, be it a deteriorating political situation, adverse effects resulting from the intervention, or other logistical issues resulting in an untenable situation.

BOX 20.8 Planning an emergency intervention programme

1 Define the priorities, ensuring protection of human rights and assistance necessary for survival.

2 Define the objectives
Statement of the problem, including who and how many will benefit, and time required for stated outcome.

3 A plan of activities and resources
Qualitative and quantitative plan, including human resources, material, logistics, and financial requirements in order of priority.

4 Plan mobilizing resources
Includes finding required personnel, material, the approach to donors, and time period in which resources can be obtained.

5 Plan of the tasks
Implementation, including the roles and responsibilities of the personnel, the logistic chain, a calendar of activities, administration for personnel (lodging, regulations, and security), work plans, and coordination with others involved.

Surveillance includes methods to identify key indicators and persons responsible for surveillance and reports methods and timing.

6 Plan to evaluate the intervention's impact, including measuring against identified key indicators, and who is responsible.

7 Awareness of the possibility of adjustment to intervention if necessary.

8 Plan for disengagement
This includes a calendar for withdrawal, use of remaining resources, and follow-up after withdrawal.

20.6 Nutrition-related programmes in the management of a crisis

20.6.1 General food distribution

Ideally, a general food distribution to families or households is implemented before a famine situation fully develops, to avoid a crisis and preserve the way of life. However, it is usually a means to provide macronutrients and some micronutrients to a population already in a famine situation in order to prevent further deterioration, or, in the early recuperative phase to facilitate recovery to a level where the individual is able to function adequately. A general food distribution is usually accompanied by programmes that provide water, shelter (especially in the case of displaced populations), health services, and appropriate opportunities to restore the economy. A general food assistance depends more on a population's capacity to procure food than the nutritional status, as inappropriate food assistance may prolong a crisis and can lead to what has been described as 'assistance syndrome', avoided with good evaluation and detailed planning (see Sections 20.4 and 20.5).

Distribution rations can be made to households or groups by a humanitarian organization (the preferred method) or by giving the food to a community for redistribution amongst its members. Rations may be given either as bulk food items to be taken home, survival rations, or prepared meals for immediate consumption. Survival rations are based on the average nutritional needs of a population, with appropriate quantities provided for each household. A complete ration theoretically provides all necessary macronutrients and micronutrients. In reality, there is often a need to supplement this in some way from local sources (e.g. foraging). However, it is essential that rations provide food in acceptable forms. For predominantly agricultural populations, this is relatively easy because cereals and legumes can be distributed in dried form. The situation is far more complex for groups who traditionally consume tubers and bananas, pastoralists, or those who rely on fish. Diversity is essential in the foods provided in order to avoid deficiencies.

Food rations are based on energy requirements (Table 20.2) and typically contain a principal energy source (usually a cereal), a concentrated energy source (e.g. oil enriched with vitamin A), a protein source (legumes, tinned fish or meat, dried fish), iodized salt, complementary food to provide micronutrients or micronutrient tablets, and spices, condiments, tea, coffee, and sugar.

Rations that form part of a general food distribution may need to be augmented in certain situations. Where nutritional rehabilitation is required, an appreciable increase in both energy and protein is necessary. If grain, which needs to be milled, is provided (rather than cereal flour), the inevitable loss of energy and nutrients needs to be taken into account, as does the cost of milling. However, grain is often preferred over flour because it travels and stores better and it is cheaper. Flour, on the other hand, can be consumed immediately, can be fortified, and is regarded as preferable in dire situations when an immediate source of energy and micronutrients is required. Theft can be a major problem that prevents food aid from reaching the target group, and humanitarian organizations are often

Table 20.2 Reference rations based on average weight by age group, gender, and level of physical activity

WHO 1			WHO 2		
Age (years)	%*	Energy needs (kcal (kJ))	Age (years)	%*	Energy needs (kcal (kJ))
0–1	3	820 (3290)	0–4	12.37	1290 (5390)
2–3	9	1360 (5680)	5–9	11.69	1860 (7770)
4–6	8.7	1830 (7650)	10–14	10.53	2210 (9240)
7–9	8.5	2190 (9150)	15–19	9.54	2420 (10 120)
10–14 M	6.3	2800 (11 700)	20–59	48.63	2230 (9320)
10–14 F	6.2	2450 (10 240)	60+	7.24	1890 (7900)
Adults M	29.2	3000 (12 540)	Pregnant (suppl)	2.4	285 (1190)
Adults F	26.2	2200 (9200)	Lactating (suppl)	2.6	500 (2090)
Pregnant	1.5	2550 (10 660)			
Lactating	1.4	2750 (11 490)			
Average		**2350** (9820)			**2080** (8690)

*Approximate proportion of age group in the population.
WHO 1—Basic ration for a developing country. The population is considered to be moderately active, with an average weight of 65 kg for men and 55 kg for women. This ration is used by the International Committee of the Red Cross rounded to 2400 kcal/person/day.
WHO 2—Reference ration for a developing country. The population is considered to be lightly active, with average weights of 60 kg and 52 kg for men and women. This ration is used by the WHO, the World Food Programme, and the High Commission for Refugees. In practice, the absolute minimum ration of 1900 kcal/person/day is usually distributed.
F, female; M, male; suppl, supplemental.
Energy requirements should be increased with reductions in the ambient temperature or with increased requirements for physical activity.

faced with finding ways to ensure that armed groups, sometimes government agencies, do not redirect the aid for their own purposes.

Putting in place a general food distribution, in practice, involves creating a beneficiary population and establishing good relations with the population and their traditional authorities, starting from the moment of the initial survey. If the general food assistance is to be provided to households rather than the community or local government, there needs to be a population census and the provision of distribution cards that provide access to the assistance programme. Recipients need to understand the process by which the food distribution will take place. Explanation regarding place, frequency, quantity, and control of distribution is essential to avoid frustration, cheating, and misunderstanding. Firmness and reliability relating to procedures ensures respect of the population and authorities, and helps to guarantee security in conflict zones. It also facilitates the logistical chain and is important vis-á-vis donors, media, and political authorities.

Complementary rations A complementary ration can be considered if a population is not self-sufficient in acquiring food and/or it is too dangerous to complete all activities to acquire sufficient food. The complementary ration furnishes the foodstuffs unable to be found (partially or totally), or is of replacement value to allow continued survival. While the concept of complementary rations is straightforward, the principles involved in planning and implementing a programme involve a process that is similar to that required for a general food distribution.

Targeting a population Targeting a beneficiary population for general food assistance reduces wastage by not assisting those who have no real need. Targeting can be geographical or can be of specific households within communities. Although it can be difficult to find objective criteria to differentiate between the extremely poor and the very poor, targeting too far may also be dangerous because those who do not qualify for inclusion in the programme may be resentful and may retali-

ate. It can also be important to target a host community, to ensure the displaced people under their care will be well accepted, integrated, and helped. Protocols as described for a general food distribution are required.

Feeding kitchens Feeding kitchens may be required to meet the food needs of a population if a beneficiary population has no means of cooking their own meals, or security situations prevent carrying food items to homes. They may also be required in institutions. Community kitchens provide the same energy and protein requirements as would a general food ration and they require the census and control mechanisms described earlier.

20.6.2 Rehabilitational feeding

Rehabilitational feeding is necessary to treat severe malnutrition and specific deficiencies, which almost invariably occur in a famine situation. The purpose is to identify such individuals and restore them to a satisfactory nutritional status to permit survival in their natural environment, even if this involves dependence on other humanitarian programmes. If the target population is concentrated in an area, it is conceptually relatively easy to establish a rehabilitational centre, although invariably there are logistical difficulties to overcome to ensure security, an uninterrupted supply line of medications and provisions, and adequate supplies of water. If, on the other hand, the population is a nomadic one, it may be impossible to implement a rehabilitation programme.

Ideally, a rehabilitation programme involves rehydration, correction of electrolyte imbalance, and treatment of infections before refeeding and nutritional rehabilitation (see Section 19.1.4). Surveillance should continue once the patient has returned 'home' so that corrective measures can be resumed in the event of a relapse.

Detailed methods to achieve rehabilitation can be found in handbooks published by the International Committee of the Red Cross, Médicins Sans Frontières, and the WHO. An example from the

Planalto of Angola describes the two main means for achieving nutritional rehabilitation and the required parallel programmes (Box 20.9).

20.6.3 Supplementary feeding programmes

Supplementary feeding programmes involve distribution of a food supplement to individuals or groups considered vulnerable, in order to prevent deterioration in nutritional status. Conceptually it is a hybrid measure, somewhere in between a small general food assistance and the provision of a partial nutritional rehabilitation centre. Because what little food distributed is often further redistributed by the beneficiary, it is generally not a particularly appropriate or successful measure and is usually implemented when there are insufficient resources for general food assistance.

BOX 20.9 Nutritional programmes required to relieve a crisis in Angola

In late 1993, a nutritional evaluation on the Planalto of Angola revealed a drought situation exacerbated by inaccessibility to other areas as a result of on-going conflict, with no access to work or means of food procurement.

Increasing mortality associated with severe malnutrition required rapid intervention. The closure of road access by landmines left an airlift as the only means for logistical supply. A 3000-metric-tonne per month supply pipeline capacity required the setting of priorities. While bulk food items were assembled for distribution, a census of the population was undertaken, rehabilitational feeding centres established (a total of five for the young severely malnourished), with 18 community kitchens (to provide energy and essential nutrients ensuring rehabilitation for those able to eat sufficient bulk food to achieve adequate weight gain), water supplies protected, and provision of medicines to medical facilities and vaccination programmes initiated.

Once monthly general food assistance was meeting the food needs of the population, and nutritional rehabilitation and health programmes functioning, non-food (blankets, soap, and kitchen sets) and agricultural distributions (seeds and tools) were undertaken at appropriate seasonal interludes.

Disengagement of activities in this instance was precipitated by military activity. However, a resumption of nutrition programmes was unnecessary, as nutrition rehabilitation had been achieved and a deterioration in status was not expected following a satisfactory harvest and the re-opening of road transport routes to the coast facilitating trade. However, a programme of continued surveillance with random cluster surveys measuring nutritional status and following food access ensured adequate monitoring.

In this case, the full range of approaches was required to deliver an adequate food supply to 600 000 beneficiaries and the daily rehabilitation of 21 000 people to reduce mortality. Cooperation and collaboration between the implementing agencies enabled survival of the population.

Recommended Reading

1. **Mourey, A.** (2008) *Nutrition manual for humanitarian action*. Geneva, Comité International de la Croix-Rouge (CICR).

Further Reading

1. **De Ville de Goyet, C.** (1978) *The management of nutritional emergencies in large populations*. Geneva, World Health Organization.
2. **FAO/WHO/UN** (1985) *Energy and protein requirements*. Report of a Joint FAO/WHO/UNU Expert Consultation. Technical Report Series 724. Geneva, World Health Organization.

3. **International Federation of Red Cross and Red Crescent Societies** (2009) *Tsunami five-year progress report 2004–2009:* Chapter 6 Learning lessons. http://www.ifrc.org/Global/Publications/disasters/tsunami/IFRC-Tsunami-5Yrs-Report-Final-Web.pdf.

4. **MSF** (1995) *Nutrition guidelines.* Paris: Médicins Sans Frontières.

5. **Pratt, B., and Boyden, J.** (1985) *The field director's handbook. An Oxfam manual for development workers.* London, Oxfam.

6. **Shoham, J.** (1995) *Emergency supplementary feeding programmes. Good practice review 2. Relief and rehabilitation network.* London, Overseas Development Institute.

7. **Sphere Project** (1998) *Humanitarian charter and minimum standards in disaster response.* A programme of The Steering Committee for Humanitarian Response and InterAction with VOICE, ICRC, ICVA. Geneva, The Sphere Project.

8. **UNICEF** (1986) *Assisting in emergencies. A resource handbook for UNICEF field staff.* New York, United Nation Children's Fund.

9. **WFP/UNHCR** (1997) *Guidelines for estimating food and nutritional needs in emergencies.* World Food Programme and United Nations High Commissioner for Refugees.

10. **WHO** (1999) *Management of severe malnutrition: A manual for physicians and other senior health workers.* Geneva, World Health Organization.

11. **WHO** (2000) *The management of nutrition in major emergencies.* Geneva, World Health Organization.

Useful Websites

To see topical and scientifically robust updates on nutrition associated with this textbook and web links to many of the journals in the Further Reading sections, please see the dedicated Online Resource Centre at **http://www.oxfordtextbooks.co.uk/orc/mann4e/**

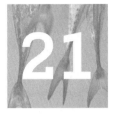

21 Cardiovascular diseases

Jim Mann and Alexandra Chisholm

Cardiovascular disease includes coronary heart disease (CHD), also referred to as coronary artery disease or ischaemic heart disease, cerebrovascular disease or stroke, and peripheral arterial disease. A similar pathological process underlies each of these three groups of conditions which affect the heart, the brain, and peripheral arteries. Inappropriate nutrition has most consistently been linked with CHD, and this chapter deals primarily with CHD and those risk factors for the disease which are influenced by diet.

Coronary heart disease

CHD is a common condition in most affluent and some developing societies. In most industrialized countries, it is the single most common cause of death, often accounting for around one-third of all deaths. In addition, each year there are about as many non-fatal cases as there are deaths. A high proportion of the health-care budget in these countries is spent treating CHD and its consequences. Genetic as well as nutritional factors contribute to the aetiology of the condition, but lifestyle modification is undoubtedly the most effective means of reducing CHD risk in high-risk populations and individuals. Dietary modification is also important in the treatment of people who have already developed CHD.

21.1 Pathological and clinical aspects

The basic pathological lesion underlying CHD is the atheromatous plaque, which bulges on the inside of one or more of the coronary arteries that supply blood to the heart muscle (myocardium). In addition, a superimposed thrombus or clot may further occlude the artery (Fig. 21.1). A variety of cells

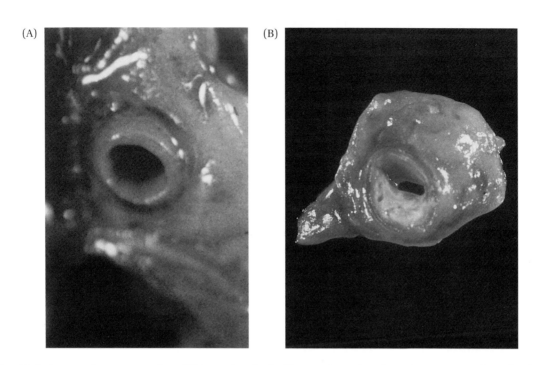

Fig. 21.1 A normal coronary artery (A) is contrasted with an artery showing atheromatous deposits (B).

and lipids are involved in the pathogenesis of the atherosclerotic plaque and the arterial thrombus, including lipoproteins, cholesterol, triglycerides, platelets, monocytes, endothelial cells, fibroblasts, and smooth muscle cells. Nutrition can influence the development of CHD by modifying either atherogenesis or thrombogenesis or both these processes. Two readily identifiable clinical conditions result from these pathological processes:

1 *Angina pectoris* is characterized by pain in the centre of the chest, which is brought on by exertion or stress, and which may radiate down the left arm or to the neck. It results from a reduction or temporary block to the blood flow through the coronary artery to the heart muscle. The pain usually passes with rest and seldom lasts for more than 15 minutes.

2 *Coronary thrombosis* or *myocardial infarction* results from total occlusion of the artery, which causes infarction or death of some of the heart muscle cells and is associated with prolonged, and usually excruciating, central chest pain. The terms coronary thrombosis and myocardial infarction are used to describe the same clinical condition, although they really describe its two distinct pathological processes.

21.2 Epidemiological aspects

Most of the available epidemiological data relate to mortality rates but, where available, it seems that there are comparable trends in rates for nonfatal disease. There are marked international differences in CHD mortality rates (Fig. 21.2). Overall rates are higher in men than women, though as women age, CHD contributes a greater proportion of total mortality. Mortality rates are more than seven times higher in some Eastern European countries than they are in Japan and within Europe, and there is an almost

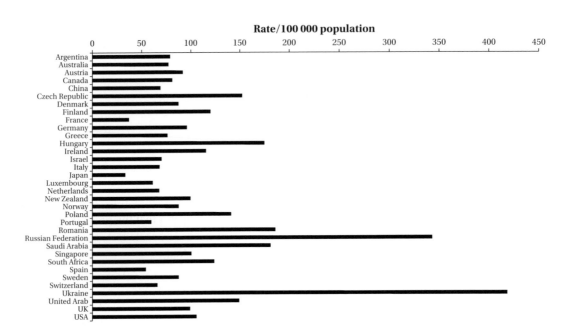

Fig. 21.2 International differences in estimated ischaemic heart disease death rates. League table for 2002: mortality in men and women aged 40–69 years.

Source: WHO (2002) *Death and DALY estimates.* Geneva, World Health Organization.

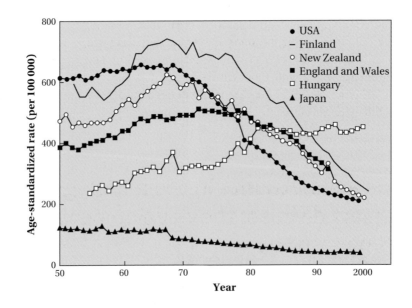

Fig. 21.3 Trends in age-standardized coronary heart disease mortality rates in men aged 40–69 years, in six countries from 1950 to 2000.

Source: Modified from Beaglehole, R. (1999) International trends in coronary heart disease mortality and incidence rates. *J Cardiovasc Risk*, **6**, 63–8.

threefold difference between France, Spain, and Portugal on the one hand and some of the more northern countries such as Scotland, Northern Ireland, and Finland. The experience of migrants and changing rates in various countries suggest that environmental and behavioural differences account for much of the variation between countries. People who have migrated from a low-risk country (e.g. Japan) to a relatively high-risk country (e.g. the USA) tend to have rates approaching the host country. There is also some evidence for the reverse: Finns living in Sweden have appreciably lower rates than those in their country of origin. In the UK, where CHD rates are higher in Scotland and Northern Ireland than in England, CHD risk depends upon country of residence at the time of death, rather than country of birth.

Some examples of the rapidly changing rates (increases as well as decreases) are shown in Fig. 21.3. Some of the most striking changes have been the increase in many European countries, North America, Australia, and New Zealand during the third quarter of the twentieth century. Then, in the fourth quarter, rates declined appreciably in those countries but increased strikingly in most countries of Eastern Europe. In general, a decline has occurred in those countries where the attempt to reduce cardiovascular risk factors has been most active, and excellent facilities are available for treating acute cardiovascular events. The situation is particularly complex in some countries where afflu-

ence and poverty coexist and which are said to be in a state of nutrition transition. In such countries, (e.g. India, South Africa), CHD rates are high amongst the relatively affluent and those rapidly accumulating wealth, whereas diseases of undernutrition remain prevalent amongst the poor and underprivileged. This situation is the reverse of what has been observed in more affluent societies, where the socioeconomically disadvantaged have higher CHD rates than better-educated, more affluent groups in the community. The most recent available data suggest that the previously observed decline in rates in some relatively affluent countries has now been halted.

Projections suggest that CHD will become an increasingly important health issue in developing countries and that the majority of cases and deaths worldwide will be in developing rather than developed countries. The changes that have occurred are compatible with lifestyle changes that have occurred in these countries, but given the complex interactions between various lifestyle attributes that may influence CHD rates, it is very difficult from such data to disentangle individual effects. This may be done using more sophisticated epidemiological and experimental approaches discussed later. The observation that changes in CHD rates have occurred over relatively short time periods encourages the belief that CHD is largely preventable. The hope is to reduce morbidity and mortality from CHD in those who are in the prime of life.

21.3 Foods and nutrients in the aetiology of coronary heart disease: the development of the diet–heart hypothesis

Early studies investigating the role of dietary factors in the causation of CHD involved correlating national dietary intakes (based on food balance data) with CHD death rates (mortality) in countries with varying rates or with changes in CHD mortality over time in individual countries. Positive associa-

tions between CHD death rate (age-standardized) and saturated fat, sucrose, animal protein, and coffee consumption and negative correlations with flour (and other foods rich in complex carbohydrates) and vegetables are some of the most clearly described. However, both food balance data and mortality statistics can be unreliable. Studies that measure food intake of individuals and relate this information about food and nutrients to accurately recorded information regarding CHD events and mortality are much more reliable.

It was the pioneering Seven Country study that was started around half a century ago, coordinated by Ancel Keys and colleagues, which gave credence to the suggestion that nutrition plays an important role in determining risk of CHD. Food consumption of people in 16 defined cohorts in seven countries, selected because of their widely varying rates of CHD, was related to subsequent CHD incidence. The strongest correlation was observed between CHD and percentage of energy derived from saturated fat (Fig. 21.4). Weak inverse associations (suggesting protective effects) were found with percentages of energy from mono- and polyunsaturated fat and CHD. Total fat did not correlate with CHD, and of the other well-known risk factors for CHD (see Section 21.4); only plasma (total) cholesterol and blood pressure appeared to explain part of the geographic variation in the frequency of this condition. These observations led to the suggestion that nutrition-related factors may be particularly important in determining whether countries are likely to have high CHD rates and that the diet–heart disease link was principally mediated via an effect of saturated fat on plasma cholesterol, which in turn increased the risk of CHD. The Seven Country study also provided evidence that the degree of risk conferred by other lifestyle factors is strongly influenced by nutrition-related factors: the relationship between cigarette smoking and CHD was found to be much more powerful in those countries where saturated fat intake and mean plasma cholesterol levels were high (e.g. in the USA and northern European countries) than in southern Europe and Japan, where saturated fat intake and cholesterol levels were lower.

More recently, prospective cohort studies have examined the relationship between foods and nutrients and the subsequent development of CHD within a single population. In addition to the problems associated with the long-term follow up of tens of thousands of individuals, there are particular difficulties associated with attempting to establish nutritional causes of disease from cohort studies: no methods for measuring dietary intake are fully reliable, and a single assessment does not necessarily provide a truly representative indication of lifelong, or even long-term, dietary practices. Some more recent studies have assessed dietary intake using more sophisticated food frequency questionnaires administered several times during the follow-up period and have used biological markers as surrogate measures of dietary intake (e.g. plasma levels of antioxidants; fatty acid composition of red cells, platelets, or adipose tissue as indicators of the nature of dietary fat).

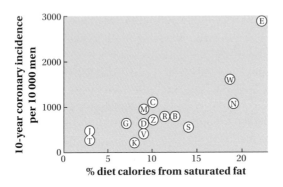

Fig. 21.4 Association between CHD and percentage energy derived from saturated fatty acids in the Seven Country study. Letters on the graph indicate the location of the cohorts in the seven countries: B, Belgrade; C, Crevalcore; D, Dalmatia; E, East Finland; G, Corfu; J, Ushibuka; K, Crete; M, Montegiorgio; N, Zutphen; R, Rome railroad; S, Slavonia T, Tanushimaru; V, Velika Krsna; W, West Finland; Z, Zrenjanin.

Source: Keys, A. (1980). *Seven countries: A multivarate analysis of death and coronary heart disease.* Massachusetts, Harvard University Press.

Among the best-known and most meticulous of the prospective studies have been those undertaken by the Harvard group, led by Willett, and based on follow-up of huge cohorts of female nurses and male health professionals. These studies are impressive because of their size and excellent retention rates, the detailed and validated food frequency questionnaires from which intakes of foods and nutrients are computed, and the sophisticated statistical analyses

Table 21.1 Age-adjusted relative risk of coronary heart disease according to quintile of intake of certain foods or nutrients

Study population	Relative risk according to quintile of intake					*P* for trend
	1	**2**	**3**	**4**	**5**	
43 757 male health professionals (40–75 years) (Rimm *et al.*, 1996)	Total dietary fibre 1.00	0.97	0.91	0.87	0.59	< 0.001
75 521 female nurses (38–63 years) (Liu *et al.*, 2000)	Wholegrain consumption 1.00	0.87	0.82	0.72	0.67	< 0.001
87 245 female nurses (34–59 years) (Stampfer and Rimm, 1995)	Total vitamin E intake 1.00	0.90	1.00	0.68	0.59	< 0.001
39 910 male health professionals (40–75 years) (Rimm *et al.*, 1996)	Carotene intake 1.00	0.93	0.93	0.86	0.71	0.02

that have examined the effects of potential confounding by other factors related to CHD. The Harvard and other longitudinal studies have suggested several foods and nutrients that may be protective against CHD: fish, wholegrain cereals, fruits and vegetables, nuts, garlic, moderate intakes of red wine and some other alcoholic drinks, antioxidant nutrients, nonstarch polysaccharides (dietary fibre), folic acid and several long-chain unsaturated fatty acids—C18:2, ω-6; C18:3, ω-3; C20:5, ω-3—and three that might increase risk, dietary cholesterol, *trans*-unsaturated fatty acids, and coffee. Many of these associations between foods, foodgroups, nutrients, and disease have been further examined in systematic reviews and meta-analyses. Some examples of the studies in which these associations have been demonstrated are given in Table 21.1 and an example of a meta-analysis is shown in Fig. 21.5.

It should be noted that, even in longitudinal studies where dietary intake has been carefully measured and endpoints accurately assessed, it may be extremely difficult to determine whether any demonstrated association is causal. The fact that a recent meta-analysis of prospective studies found no evidence that dietary saturated fat was associated with an increased risk of CHD or stroke illustrates the need to examine the effects of foods and nutrients on cardiovascular risk factors (see Section 21.4) and in intervention trials (see Section 21.5) before drawing conclusions about their causal role. Whether or not a risk factor is causally related to CHD and modification is likely to reduce risk depends upon the totality of evidence, not just the findings from one type of study.

21.4 Cardiovascular risk factors and their nutritional determinants

Attempts to explain the pathological process underlying CHD and to identify individuals at risk suggest

that there is no single cause of the disease. An understanding of the characteristics that put individuals at

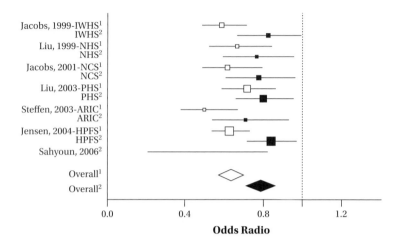

Fig. 21.5 Odds ratios of incident cardiovascular disease, comparing high versus low wholegrain intake. ARIC, Atherosclerosis Risk in Communities; HPFS, Health Professionals' Follow-up Study; IWHS, Iowa Women's Health Study; NCS, Norwegian County Study; NHS, Nurses' Health Study; PHS, Physicians' Health Study; 1, demographic-adjusted model; 2, demographic + risk factor-adjusted model.

Source: Mellen, P.B., Walsh, T.F., and Herrington, D.M. (2008) Wholegrain intake and cardiovascular disease: A meta-analysis. *Nutr Met Cardiovasc Dis* **18**, 283–90.

particular risk of developing CHD provides a useful background against which to examine in more detail the role of diet in the aetiology. The term 'risk factor' is used to describe features of lifestyle and behaviour, as well as physical and biochemical attributes that predict an increased likelihood of developing CHD. Potential risk factors are often identified when comparisons are made between people who have developed CHD and healthy controls (case–control studies) and are confirmed by cohort (prospective) studies in which these factors are measured in a large group of apparently healthy people who are then followed to see if they develop the disease or not at some future date. The presence, absence, or degree of each factor can then be related to the risk of developing CHD. Table 21.2 lists most of the important risk factors for CHD that have been identified in this way. When more than one risk factor is present, the effect is synergistic; that is, the overall increase in risk of CHD is greater than might be expected from simply adding together the risk associated with each. The irreversible psychosocial and geographic factors, as well as cigarette smoking and physical activity, are reviewed in textbooks of medicine and epidemiology. This chapter concentrates

on potentially reversible factors that have been shown to be influenced by diet in controlled studies in humans.

21.4.1 Dyslipidaemia

Altered levels of blood lipids and lipoproteins (see Chapter 4) may place individuals at increased risk of CHD in three ways. First, a relatively small proportion of people have an exceptionally high risk because of a clearly inherited increase of plasma lipids and lipoproteins. Second, a large number of people (perhaps as many as half the adult population in high-risk countries) have a slight to moderately increased risk because their blood lipids are higher than desirable as a result of an interaction between polygenic (many genes involved) and lifestyle-related factors. They are described as having 'polygenic' or 'common' hyperlipidaemia. Third, some people are also at increased CHD risk because of low levels of high-density lipoprotein (HDL). Some people may have altered lipid levels secondary to other medical conditions. Table 21.3 provides a classification of the most frequently occurring forms of dyslipidaemia.

Table 21.2 Risk factors for coronary heart disease

Irreversible	• Masculine gender
	• Increasing age
	• Genetic traits, including monogenic and polygenic disorders of lipid metabolism
	• Body build
Potentially reversible	• Cigarette smoking
	• Dyslipidaemia: increased levels of cholesterol, triglyceride, low-density and very-low-density lipoprotein, and apolipoprotein B; low levels of high-density lipoprotein; atypical lipoproteins
	• Oxidizability of low-density lipoprotein
	• Obesity, especially when associated with high waist circumference or waist/hip ratio
	• Hypertension
	• Physical inactivity
	• Diabetes, hyperglycaemia, and insulin resistance
	• Increased thrombosis: increased haemostatic factors and enhanced platelet aggregation
	• High levels of homocysteine
	• High levels of inflammatory markers (e.g. CRP, IL-6, TNFα)
	• Impaired fetal nutrition
Psychosocial	• Stressful situations
	• Coronary-prone behaviour patterns: type A behaviour
Geographic	• Climate and season: cold weather
	• Soft drinking water

CRP, C-reactive protein; IL, interleukin; TNF, tumour necrosis factor.

Familial hypercholesterolaemia Familial hypercholesterolaemia, a dominantly inherited condition, is the most common of the clearly inherited lipid disorders. It results from mutations in the LDL receptor gene and is characterized by markedly raised levels of total and low-density lipoprotein (LDL) cholesterol, cholesterol deposits (xanthomas) in the tendons, and, if untreated, a very high risk of premature coronary heart disease. *Familial combined hyperlipidaemia* is often diagnosed when appreciably raised levels of cholesterol and triglyceride, LDL and VLDL, and sometimes low levels of HDL occur in families in which premature coronary heart disease is a frequent occurrence. The mode of inheritance and mechanisms are not clearly understood. *Polygenic hypercholesterolaemia* is the presumed diagnosis in people with raised lipid levels who are not diagnosed as having a clearly defined genetic disorder. There is no agreed level of total or LDL cholesterol above which the condition is diagnosed, as the

Table 21.3 Frequently occurring forms of dyslipidaemia

	Atherosclerosis risk	Inheritance	Relative prevalence	Lipid abnormalities
Familial hypercholesterolaemia	+++	Dominant	++	LDL ↑↑↑ Cholesterol typically 9–11 mmol/L in heterozygotes
Familial combined hyperlipidaemia	++	Uncertain	+	LDL ↑↑↑ VLDL ↑↑ HDL possibly ↓
Polygenic hypercholesterolaemia	++	Polygenic	++++	LDL ↑ VLDL possibly ↑ HDL possibly ↓
Severe hypertriglyceridaemia	Uncertain (associated with pancreatitis)	Uncertain (usually secondary)	Uncommon	VLDL ↑↑ Chylomicrons possibly ↑

↑, raised; ↑↑, markedly raised; ↓, lowered; +, relatively low prevalence; ++++, extremely high prevalence; VLDL, very-low-density lipoproteins; HDL, high-density lipoproteins; LDL, low-density lipoproteins. *Hyperlipidaemia* may be secondary to diabetes, obesity, hypothyroidism drugs, liver disease, and alcohol excess.

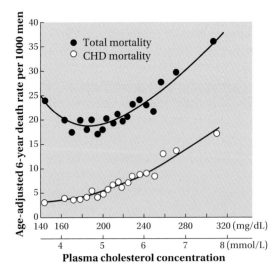

Fig. 21.6 Within-population relationship between plasma cholesterol and CHD and total mortality.

Source: Martin, M.J., Hulley, S.B., Browner, W.S., et al. (1986) Serum cholesterol, blood pressure, and mortality: implications from a cohort of 361,662 men. *Lancet*, **2**, 933–6.

association between cholesterol and CHD is characterized by a gradient of risk (Fig. 21.6).

The levels of total and LDL cholesterol are determined by an interaction between the genes involved and dietary factors. The saturated fatty acids myristic, palmitic, and, to a lesser extent, lauric acids are associated with substantial increases in total and LDL cholesterol when compared with isocaloric intakes of carbohydrate or unsaturated fatty acids, other than those with a trans configuration. ω6-Polyunsaturated fatty acids, especially linoleic acid (C18:2, ω-6) on the other hand have cholesterol-lowering properties.

Hypertriglyceridaemia
Hypertriglyceridaemia is a less clearly defined risk factor for CHD. People who have had myocardial infarctions tend to have higher levels of triglycerides and VLDL than controls, and this association is confirmed by prospective studies. Raised triglycerides and VLDL are commonly seen in people with polygenic hypercholesterolaemia, or familial combined hyperlipidaemia and the metabolic syndrome (see Chapter 23), and may be a

particularly important determinant of cardiovascular disease in people with diabetes. Markedly raised levels are most frequently seen as a consequence of uncontrolled diabetes or alcohol excess in predisposed individuals, but is occasionally seen as an isolated inherited lipid disorder. High intakes of sugars and fibre-depleted starch foods are associated with raised triglycerides and VLDL. Overweight and obese people tend to have high levels.

Reduced high-density lipoprotein concentrations

There has been considerable interest in plasma HDL as a protective factor. Women have higher levels of HDL than men and a lower risk of CHD. An attempt to aggregate the findings of four large US studies suggests that an increase of 1 mg/100 mL (0.026 mmol/L) HDL cholesterol is associated with a 2–3% reduction in CHD. Low HDL levels may also be a feature of polygenic hypercholesterolaemia, familial combined hyperlipidaemia, the metabolic syndrome, and type 2 diabetes. HDL levels are reduced in heavy cigarette smokers and by high intakes of *trans*-unsaturated fatty acids. Nutritional determinants of lipids and lipoproteins are considered in more detail in Section 4.3.4.

21.4.2 Thrombogenesis

Factors that increase the tendency to thrombosis (either as a result of increased platelet aggregation or a high level of coagulability of blood) have received less attention than those influencing lipids and lipoproteins. They are more difficult to study and much of the relevant research is based on *in vitro* tests, which may not correspond to what goes on inside the body. One clue to the potential for dietary factors to enhance or reduce the tendency for platelets to aggregate stems from observations made on the Eskimo people (Inuits) of Greenland. They have low rates of CHD and reduced platelet aggregation compared with Western nations, despite high intakes of total fat. However, this fat comes largely from marine foods rich in ω3 fatty acids (eicosapentaenoate, C20:5, and docosahexaenoate, C22:6), which form the antiaggregatory prostanoid PGI_3. Platelet aggregation is largely controlled by a balance between the proaggregatory compound thromboxane A_2 (synthesized from arachidonic acid released from the platelet membrane after injury to the blood vessel wall) and the antiaggregatory substance prostacyclin PGI_2 (also synthesized from arachidonic acid in the endothelial cells of the arterial wall). C20:5 and C22:6 inhibit conversion of arachidonic acid to thromboxane A_2 as well as facilitate the production of the additional antiaggregatory substance PGI_3 (Fig. 21.7). Polyunsaturated fatty acids of the ω6 series may also reduce platelet aggregation by providing the series 1 prostanoid PGE_1, which is also antiaggregatory. Oleic acid may also act as a inhibitor of platelet aggregation, though the effect is less than for polyunsaturated fatty acids.

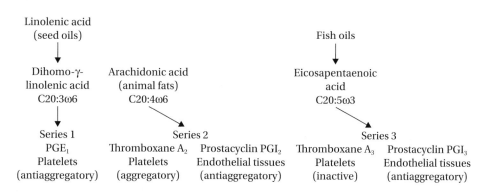

Fig. 21.7 Prostanoids formed from different fatty acids.

Source: Ulbricht, T.L.V. and Southgate, D.A.T. (1991) Coronary heart disease: Seven dietary factors. *Lancet*, **338**, 985–92.

Although there have been studies of the antithrombogenic effect of polyunsaturated fatty acids in humans, the thrombogenic effect of saturated fatty acids has been more extensively studied in laboratory animals. The findings are consistent: the longer-chain saturated fatty acids (C14:0, C16:0, and C18:0) all appear to accelerate thrombosis. One mechanism may be via inhibition of antiaggregatory prostacyclin, but stearic acid (C18:0), which appears not to raise LDL, may promote thrombosis by increasing fibrinogen levels.

Dietary factors may also influence thrombogenesis via an effect on the *coagulation system*. The physiological function of coagulation is to secure haemostasis after an injury. Thrombin is produced, which enables the conversion of soluble fibrinogen to insoluble fibrin. Several prospective studies suggest that factors involved in the coagulation system (notably factor VII and fibrinogen) are important predictors of CHD. Too high a level of coagulability might predispose to thrombosis. High levels of fibrinogen are associated with obesity, cigarette smoking, and perhaps also high intakes of stearic acid. Factor VII is associated to a greater extent with dietary factors: increasing dietary fat can increase levels within 24 hours. Levels of a range of clotting factors, including factor VII, are lower in populations and groups eating a low-fat, high-polyunsaturated/saturated-ratio, high-fibre diet, and individuals changing to such a diet show reduction in these factors. Levels of another prothrombotic agent, plasminogen activator inhibitor-1 (PAI-1), are reduced on low-glycaemic-index diets.

21.4.3 Diabetes, hyperglycaemia, and insulin resistance

Many studies have shown that people with diabetes and prediabetes have an increased risk of CHD. Genetic factors play important roles in the aetiology of type 2 diabetes, but nutrition-related factors, especially those contributing to body fatness, the main determinant of type 2, are also important. Nutritional determinants of type 2 diabetes are discussed further in Chapter 23.

21.4.4 Hypertension

Increasing levels of both systolic and diastolic blood pressure are associated with increased rates of CHD, strokes (cerebral vascular disease), and peripheral vascular disease. Worldwide, high blood pressure has been ranked as the leading risk factor contributing to death (7.5 million, or nearly 13% of all recorded deaths in adults in 2004) and amongst high-income countries high blood pressure ranked second only to tobacco use as the leading cause of death, accounting for nearly 17% of deaths.

Sodium (salt) Over 30 years ago, Dahl drew attention to the correlation between salt intake and prevalence of hypertension in populations. This and other similar studies were flawed by methodological difficulties associated with measuring salt intake and blood pressure. Also, the association may not be causal because increased salt intake is associated with greater acculturation and many other lifestyle-related attributes of a 'Western' diet could explain the link with CHD. The best available method for assessing sodium intake is 24-hour urinary sodium excretion. This method and standardized blood pressure measurements were used in the Intersalt study, which collected data on 10 000 people in 32 countries. The results suggested that a reduction in sodium intake of 100 mmol/day would be expected to result in differences of approximately 10 mmHg in systolic blood pressure and 6 mmHg in diastolic blood pressure over a 30-year period. Meta-analyses of published observational studies and randomized controlled trials of sodium restriction have demonstrated broadly comparable results. A Cochrane review based on a meta-analysis of randomized controlled trials demonstrated for adults that a rather more modest average reduction in sodium intake by at least 40 mmol/day would lead to an average reduction in blood pressure of 5/3 mmHg for hypertensives and 2/1 mmHg in normotensive adults. If this were to be achieved at a population level, stroke deaths might be expected to reduce by about 14% and CHD deaths by 9% in adults with hypertension and 6% and 4%, respectively, in those with normal blood pressure. Data from Japan, where salt intakes and blood pressure levels have traditionally been high, suggest that a nationwide salt reduction campaign was associated with a reduction in blood pressure levels and an 80% decrease in mortality from stroke.

Several mechanisms have been suggested to explain the association between salt intake and blood pressure, including reduced urinary sodium excretion and fluid retention by some individuals, increased sympathetic nervous system activity, and impaired baroreflex function and alterations of ion transport in vascular smooth muscle. The heterogeneity in the response of individuals to sodium restriction suggests the possible existence of a group of hyper-responders, but there is as yet no simple test by which such individuals might be identified.

Potassium In the Intersalt study, urinary potassium excretion—an assumed indicator of intake—was negatively related to blood pressure. A pooled analysis of a number of intervention trials suggests that potassium supplementation might reduce blood pressure in both normotensive and hypertensive people by an average of 6/3 mmHg. However, several limitations reduce the likely effectiveness of increasing potassium intake as an important means of treating hypertension. The effect of potassium appears to be relatively small when compared with a reduction in sodium intake. The amount of potassium required to reduce blood pressure is relatively high, so that supplements rather than dietary modification would be necessary to achieve appreciable blood pressure lowering. Naturally occurring foods do not contain sufficient potassium to provide the increase in intake achieved in the trials—between 50 and 140 mmol potassium per day.

Body weight Obese people have higher blood pressures than lean people and if they lose weight their blood pressure falls, even if usual salt intake is maintained on the calorie-restricted diet. Raised blood pressure is particularly associated with obesity that is centrally rather than peripherally distributed. The Intersalt study showed a highly significant correlation between body mass index as an index of obesity and blood pressure. An Australian study showed, in a clinical trial setting, that dietary weight reduction (mean loss of 7.4 kg) compared favourably with a standard β-blocker drug, metoprolol, in the treatment of mild hypertension. Furthermore, diet was associated with an improvement in the lipid profile, which was not seen with the drug.

Calcium Intracellular calcium is an important determinant of arteriolar tone, and some claims have been made that increased calcium intake can reduce blood pressure. However, two meta-analyses summarizing the results of more than 20 trials showed that intakes of 1000 mg or more of calcium per day have only a trivial effect on blood pressure levels. Calcium supplements or a high-calcium diet might be useful in a very small number of hypertensive patients who have low serum calcium levels or increased plasma parathyroid levels.

Combining dietary factors It is conceivable that combining the effects of the various nutrients that appear to influence blood pressure levels will have a far greater effect than altering a single nutrient. A series of trials, known as the DASH (Dietary Approaches to Stop Hypertension) trials have examined the potential of modifying foods, other than restricting salt intake, to reduce blood pressure levels. The most striking effect was seen in a diet characterized by high amounts of fruit and vegetables, low-fat dairy products to ensure low intakes of saturated fats and cholesterol, low sodium content, and sufficient amounts of other nutrient-rich foods that contain minerals known to have a blood pressure-lowering effect, including calcium, potassium, and magnesium. Fig. 21.8 illustrates that with intermediate or high sodium intakes there were marked differences between the DASH and control diets. Even at the lowest level of sodium intake, addition of the other components of the DASH diet can produce additional blood pressure-lowering. These effects are comparable with those resulting from some blood pressure-lowering medications. A vegetarian diet is also associated with lower levels of blood pressure than a typical Western omnivores' diet. Both the vegetarian diet and the combination diet of the DASH trial have many nutritional attributes that

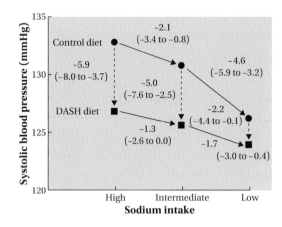

Fig. 21.8 The effect on systolic blood pressure with a control diet when sodium is reduced (●) and on the DASH diet with similar reductions in sodium (■). Differences between DASH and control diets are significant at each level of sodium intake but smallest when sodium intake is low (1.5 g/day).

Source: Sacks, F.M., Svetkey, L.P., Vollmer, W.M., *et al.* (2001) Effects on blood pressure of reduced dietary sodium and the Dietary Approaches to Stop Hypertension (DASH) Diet. *N Eng J Med*, **344**, 3–10.

could be contributing to the blood pressure-lowering effect, and it is probably impossible as well as clinically unhelpful to attempt to disentangle which have the greatest effect.

Alcohol In epidemiological studies, blood pressure increases progressively when reported alcohol intake increases above three drinks per day. Several intervention studies have shown that reduction of alcohol intake can produce an appreciable reduction in blood pressure amongst hypertensive heavy drinkers. For example, one double-blind study showed that replacing standard beer (5% alcohol) with a reduced-alcohol beer (0.9% alcohol) produced a reduction in alcohol intake from 450 to 64 mL/week and a significant fall in blood pressure.

Other factors Small and inconsistent inverse associations have been reported between blood pressure and polyunsaturated fatty acids, magnesium, protein, and dietary fibre. A small positive association with caffeine has also been reported.

21.4.5 Obesity

Obesity is a major risk factor for CHD. While increasing body mass index shows a modest and graded association with myocardial infarction, increasing waist circumference and waist/hip ratio show a more striking relationship. The effect is not surprising given the association between excess adiposity (especially when centrally distributed) and several other risk factors, notably dyslipidaemia, hypertension, raised levels of inflammatory markers, insulin resistance, and type 2 diabetes. Weight loss corrects most of the clinical and metabolic derangements seen in overweight and obese individuals (see Chapter 17).

21.4.6 Inflammatory markers

Inflammation is acknowledged as a process that can appreciably increase cardiovascular risk to the extent that high-sensitivity C-reactive protein (CRP) is regarded as a useful risk indicator. Raised levels of other inflammatory markers (e.g. interleukin 6 and tumour necrosis factor α) may also be associated with increased risk. Information regarding the extent to which nutritional factors can influence the inflammatory response is limited. However, diets very low in fat have been shown to reduce levels of high-sensitivity CRP. Moderately high intakes of ω-3 fatty acids may also reduce the inflammatory response.

21.4.7 Impaired fetal nutrition

Barker and colleagues in Southampton observed some time ago that low-birthweight babies, especially those who tended to gain weight rapidly in early life, were more prone than those of normal weight to a range of clinical and metabolic abnormalities (including obesity, hypertension, dyslipidaemia, insulin resistance) that predispose to the increased risk of CHD and diabetes in later life. The fetal origins (Barker) hypothesis suggests that maternal malnutrition at critical stages of fetal development leads to intrauterine growth retardation, including decreased pancreatic islet β cells, decreased number of nephrons, insulin resistance, and a range of other abnormalities that may not be associated with later chronic diseases if the child remains in a relatively deprived nutritional environment. However, problems are proposed to occur if the malnourished fetus is born into conditions of adequate nutrition or overnutrition and rapid catch-up growth occurs. Much debate and research centres around the explanation for the observation, but the hypothesis has been offered as an explanation for the massive increase in cardiovascular disease and type 2 diabetes that has occurred with increasing affluence in some developing countries. The main message to be taken from this research at this stage is the importance of adequate and appropriate nutrition for women of childbearing age. There is insufficient evidence to recommend altering current advice regarding infant feeding practices (see Chapter 33).

21.4.8 Raised plasma homocysteine levels

Patients with inborn errors of homocysteine metabolism have very high levels of plasma homocysteine, homocysteinuria, and a high risk of cardiovascular disease. It has also been found that in the general population there is a gradient of CHD risk associated with increasing levels of plasma homocysteine, i.e. homocysteine is an independent risk factor for CHD. Experimental evidence suggests that homocysteine damages the endothelium of coronary arteries. Interest in this relatively newly identified risk factor centres around the fact that folic acid and vitamins B_6 and B_{12} can reduce raised homocysteine levels. However, there is no evidence from randomized controlled trials that reducing homocysteine levels can reduce clinical CHD.

21.5 Clinical trials of dietary modification

Ideally, evidence from epidemiological and experimental studies should be further examined in randomized controlled trials involving clinical endpoints. Such trials have the potential to firmly establish causal links between individual foods and nutrients and CHD and to determine the extent to which dietary modification may be expected to reduce risk of CHD. Conceptually they do not differ from trials which examine the effects of dietary manipulation on risk factors, but in order to reliably study clinical endpoints thousands rather than tens of participants are required, with a follow-up period of many years rather than weeks or months. All the relevant trials were undertaken during the second half of the twentieth century.

The early trials all attempted to lower cholesterol levels, usually by increasing the polyunsaturated/saturated (P/S) ratio, i.e. they were single-factor intervention trials. The more recent trials have involved multifactorial interventions, including dietary change intended to improve all nutrition-related risk indicators, as well as attempts to modify other risk factors that are not diet-related (e.g. cigarette smoking). Some trials have involved nutrient supplements generally in very large doses rather than altering food intake. Dietary intervention trials have been undertaken in people with and without evidence of CHD at the time the trial was started (i.e. secondary and primary prevention trials). The difficulties and cost involved in undertaking such trials are considerable, and it is hardly surprising that many were underpowered and generated less than conclusive results. Several of the landmark trials are summarized in Table 21.4. Unfortunately, it is inappropriate to aggregate the results of the trials in a meta-analysis in view of the wide range of

Table 21.4 Results of selected intervention trials (confidence intervals are given in parentheses)

Trial	No. of subjects	Experimental (E) & Control diets (C)	% reduction in cholesterol	Odds ratios (experimental vs control)		Comments
				Total mortality	Fatal and nonfatal CHD	
Veterans Administration (Dayton et al., 1969)	846 males, 55–89 years	ω-6 PUFA replaced much of the SAFA in C so that P/S = 2 in (E) Total fat in both: 40%	13	0.98 (0.83–1.15)	0.77[+]	• 8-year duration • Daily main meal provided • Double-blind conditions • Increased non-CHD mortality in (E) but low power
Oslo (Hjermann et al., 1981)	1232 males, cholesterol 7.5–9.8	A Total and SAFA markedly reduced, replaced by fibre-rich fruit, vegetables, and wholegrains in (E)	13	0.64 (0.37–1.12)	0.56[+]	Smoking intervention included, but 60% CHD reduction attributed to cholesterol reduction
DART (Burr et al, 1989)		Randomized to receive or not receive advice on each of three dietary factors: fat, fish, increased cereal fibre				
Fat advice	2033 MI survivors	Fat reduction, increase in P/S in (E)	3.5	0.98 (0.77–1.26)	0.92	Absence of cholesterol changes with fat reduction suggests poor compliance. Also no effect for cereal fibre
Fish advice	2033 MI survivors	At least two weekly portions of fatty fish in (E)	Negligible	0.74 (0.57–0.93)	0.85[+]	

Lyons Heart (de Lorgeril et al., 1994)	605 clinical CHD	Mediterranean-type diet (E) and ω-3 supplemented margarine (E)	Negligible	0.30 (0.11–0.82)	0.24†	Small and underpowered explains wide confidence intervals
GISSI Prevenzione (1999) ω-3 fatty acids	2836 MI survivors	Supplementation with EPA and DHA or vitamin E in (E)	NA	0.80 (0.67–0.94)	0.80†	
Vitamin E	2830 MI survivors	Vitamin E 300 g in (E)	NA	0.86 (0.72–1.02)	0.88	
HOPE (2000)	1511 high CVD risk	Supplementation with 400 iu Vit E in (E)	NA	1.00 (0.89–1.13)	1.05	Vit E was one arm of a trial which also included ACE inhibitor Ramipril

NA, not available; SAFA, saturated fatty acid; P/S, ratio of polyunsaturated to saturated fatty acids.

†Statistically significant.

ACE, angiotensin-converting enzyme; CVD, cardiovascular disease; DART, Diet and Reinfarction Trial; DHA, docosahexaenoic acid; GISSI, Gruppo Italiano per lo Studio della Sopravvivenza nell'Infarto miocardico; HOPE, Heart Outcomes Prevention Evaluation; MI, myocardial infarction; NA, not available; P/S, ratio of polyunsaturated to saturated fatty acids; PUFA, polyunsaturated fatty acids; SFA, saturated fatty acid.

interventions that were employed. Nevertheless an overall perspective of the trials enables some important conclusions to be drawn. Most of the trials had cholesterol-lowering as the primary aim and of great importance is the convincing evidence that cholesterol lowering by dietary means reduces coronary events in the context of both primary and secondary prevention. Indeed, there is a clear dose–response effect which mirrors the findings of observational epidemiological studies and trials of pharmaceutical reduction of cholesterol by statin drugs, that each 1% of cholesterol lowering achieved is associated with a 2–3% reduction in coronary events.

No conclusions can be drawn regarding the optimal dietary approach to cholesterol lowering. This was successfully achieved in the Veterans Administration study by substantially reducing saturated fatty acids and replacing them with ω-6 polyunsaturated fatty acids (chiefly linoleic acid (C18:2, ω-6), whereas in the Oslo trial a reduction in total and saturated fat was accompanied by an increase in fruit, vegetables, and wholegrain cereals.

Two trials provide some support for the suggestion that dietary modification has the potential to reduce cardiovascular risk by means other than cholesterol lowering. The DART and GISSI trials achieved appreciable reductions in cardiovascular mortality with minimal change in cholesterol, presumably because the increase in C20:5, ω-3 and C22:6, ω-3 in the fish or fish oil supplements resulted in reduced tendency to thrombosis or perhaps reduced the risk of dysrythmias. The Lyons Heart study has been much quoted as demonstrating the appreciable benefit conferred by a Mediterranean-type diet and its many potentially protective cardio-protective components, including decreased intakes of total and saturated fatty acids and increased intakes of oleic and α-linolenic acid and fruits, vegetables, and wholegrains, which would have increased intakes of antioxidant nutrients as well as dietary fibre. Somewhat surprisingly there was little change in cholesterol, but it should be noted that the study is relatively small, with the estimates of risk reduction consequently subject to wide confidence intervals.

The trials of nutrient supplements have generally been disappointing, apart perhaps from the GISSI-Prevenzione study, which suggests potential benefit of supplementation with modest amounts of fish oils. The HOPE study and a meta-analysis based on it and several others provide convincing evidence for the absence of a benefit of supplemental vitamin E for high-risk individuals. There is no clear explanation as to why the vitamin E and other antioxidant nutrient supplementation trials have been largely negative, despite strong suggestions of benefit from epidemiological data. The most likely explanations would seem to be either that a longer time frame might be necessary in order to demonstrate benefit or that a blend of these nutrients, in proportions similar to those found in foods, might be required to produce benefit, rather than a pharmacological dose of a single antioxidant nutrient. It is conceivable that confounding may have explained the association between vitamin E and CHD in the epidemiological studies. Trials of folic acid supplementation aimed at reducing homocysteine levels have similarly been unable to confirm reduction of cardiovascular risk.

21.6 Foods and nutrients as causes of coronary heart disease: strength of evidence

The epidemiological evidence discussed above has generated a large number of associations between foods and nutrients, and CHD and experimental studies in humans and animals have identified nutritional determinants of risk factors. WHO/FAO Expert Consultations (2003, 2009) considered the strength of evidence for all of the putative lifestyle-related variables and categorized them as being

Table 21.5 Summary of strength of evidence on lifestyle factors and risk of developing cardiovascular diseases

Evidence	Decreased risk	No relationship	Increased risk
Convincing	Regular physical activity Linoleic acid[a] Fish and fish oils (EPA and DHA) Vegetables and fruits (including berries) Potassium Low to moderate alcohol intake (for coronary heart disease)	Vitamin E supplements	Myristic and palmitic acids[a,b,c] *trans*-fatty acids High sodium intake Overweight High alcohol intake (for stroke)
Probable	α-Linolenic acid Oleic acid[c] NSP (dietary fibre) [c] Wholegrain cereals[c] Nuts (unsalted) Plant sterols/stanols Folate	Stearic acid	Dietary cholesterol Unfiltered boiled coffee
Possible	Flavonoids Soy products		Fats rich in lauric acid Impaired fetal nutrition β-Carotene supplements
Insufficient	Calcium Magnesium Vitamin C		Carbohydrates[b] Iron

[a]Convincing evidence that replacing saturated fatty acids (C12–C16) with polyunsaturated fatty acids decreases CHD risk.

[b]Probable evidence that replacing saturated fatty acids largely with sugars and rapidly digested starches has no benefit on CHD and may increase the risk of CHD.

[c]Insufficient *direct* evidence that replacing saturated fatty acids with either monounsaturated fatty acids or wholegrain carbohydrates decreases CHD, but *indirect* evidence suggests that this might be the case.

EPA, eicosapentaenoic acid; DHA, docosahexaenoic acid; NSP, non-starch polysaccharides.

Source: Modified from WHO/FAO (2009) Fats and fatty acids in human nutrition. Proceedings of the Joint FAO/WHO Expert Consultation. November 10–14, 2008. Geneva, Switzerland. *Ann Nutr Metab*, **55**, 5–300.

convincingly, probably, or possibly causally related to cardiovascular disease, taking into account all available evidence. For some, the evidence was regarded as insufficient (Table 21.5). Associations graded as convincing or probable were deemed to be sufficient to translate into recommendations. Most of these associations have been discussed in the preceding sections and in Chapter 4, but are reviewed briefly below to justify the evidence gradings and resultant recommendations.

21.6.1 Fatty acids and dietary cholesterol

Myristic and palmitic acids, derived from dairy products and meat, comprise a substantial proportion of total intake of saturated fatty acids in countries with high fat intakes and high CHD rates. They have a more marked LDL-raising effect than other saturated fatty acids. There is impressive evidence, both from prospective epidemiological studies and intervention trials, that substituting ω-6 polyunsaturated fatty acids (chiefly linoleic acid) for a proportion of the saturated fatty acids results not only in a predictable reduction in LDL cholesterol but also in a reduction in risk of cardiovascular events and death. Thus the evidence for the promoting effect of these saturated fatty acids and protective effects of linoleic acid is regarded as convincing. However, excessive intakes of ω-6 – PUFA (>10% total energy) may reduce HDL levels and promote oxidation of LDL. Thus very high intakes should be avoided.

Stearic acid does not appear to adversely effect lipoproteins, but the relationship with other risk factors remains to be clarified. Current evidence suggests no important relationship with CHD. Lauric acid does elevate LDL but is associated with an almost equivalent increase in HDL, which may mitigate at least to some extent any lipoprotein-mediated adverse effects. There is also no corroborative epidemiological evidence of increased CHD risk, hence its classification as a possibly related factor. trans-Unsaturated fatty acids, mostly found in deep-fried fast foods, baked goods, and some fat spreads, are associated with an even more atherogenic plasma lipid profile (increased LDL and lipoprotein(a) and decreased HDL) than saturated fatty acids. Furthermore, several large cohort studies have reported a linear association between their intake and subsequent CHD risk.

ω-3 Polyunsaturated oils (EPA and DHA from fish oils) have potentially powerful beneficial effects on several cardiovascular risk factors (notably, they are antiplatelet and anti-inflammatory) and physiology (endothelial function, arterial compliance, vascular reactivity, cardiac electrophysiology), and randomized trials suggest clinical benefit. Although these fatty acids can lower triglycerides, the benefit is believed to be mediated principally through pathways other than lipoproteins. While the evidence relating to the protective effects of these polyunsaturated fatty acids is regarded as convincing, the potentially protective effects of oleic acid, derived from olive oil, canola, and nuts and plant sources of ω-3 fatty acids (α-linolenic acid, which is high in flaxseed, canola, and soybean oils) are considered to be probable. The beneficial effect of oleic acid on LDL is less marked, and while there is epidemiological evidence for a protective role, oleic acid has not been used as a sole replacement for saturated fat in any randomized controlled trial. α-Linolenic acid (see Section 21.5) from plant foods has been found to be inversely related to CHD in prospective studies, but in the Lyons Heart trial, in which intake was increased, it was only one of the several dietary variables that were modified.

Cholesterol in the blood is derived from endogenous synthesis and dietary intake, principally from dairy fat and meat, which are also important sources of saturated fatty acids, and eggs, which are not. Dietary cholesterol raises plasma LDL and plasma cholesterol, especially when consumed in substantial amounts and when intake of saturated fatty acids is also high. There is some, though not entirely consistent, evidence from observational studies that increasing intakes are associated with increasing CHD risk. However, no clinical trial has examined the effect of reducing dietary cholesterol without also substantially reducing saturated fatty acids. From a practical point of view, restriction of saturated fatty acids will be associated with a reduction in the dietary cholesterol except in individuals with an unusually high intake of egg yolk. Plant sterols and stanols, when incorporated into functional foods, notably margarines and spreads, are associated with appreciable reductions in LDL and cholesterol, by inhibiting cholesterol absorption. Products are widely available but long-term effects have not been examined. It is perhaps surprising that this category was included in the 'probable' list.

21.6.2 Sodium and potassium

Sodium and potassium are considered to be, respectively, convincingly promotive and protective against cardiovascular disease because of their effects on blood pressure (see Section 21.4.4). Although potassium supplements have been shown to be associated with reductions in blood pressure, fruit and vegetables, which are sources of potassium, rather than supplements, are recommended.

21.6.3 Nonstarch polysaccharides and wholegrain cereals

Dietary fibre is a heterogeneous mixture of nonstarch polysaccharides that are not digested and absorbed in the small intestine. Water-soluble fibres (notably pectins, gums, mucilages, and some hemicelluloses) reduce total and LDL cholesterol, and several large cohort studies have reported that high intakes of dietary fibre, as well as diets high in wholegrain cereals, protect against CHD. Thus, although the mechanisms are not clear, dietary fibres are regarded as probably protective factors against CHD.

21.6.4 Antioxidant nutrients and flavonoids

Experimental evidence has clearly demonstrated the potential for antioxidant nutrients (e.g. vitamin E, vitamin C, β-carotene) to reduce the oxidizability of LDL *in vitro*, and prospective studies have shown a decreasing risk of CHD with increasing intakes of these nutrients and flavonoids, which occur in a variety of foods of vegetable origin such as onions, berries, apples, and tea. However, several large, clinical

trials in which vitamins E and C and β-carotene have been given as supplements have shown no consistent benefit. Indeed, vitamin E supplementation has been studied in a sufficient number of studies for meta-analyses to confirm absence of benefit in terms of reducing cardiovascular risk (Table 21.5).

21.6.5 B vitamins

Increasing homocysteine levels appear to increase CHD risk in case–control and cohort studies. Dietary folate and folic acid as a supplement or fortificant result in lowering of homocysteine by facilitating the methylation of homocysteine to methionine (see Chapter 13) and vitamins B_6 and B_{12} may further reduce homocysteine. Although the first trial of homocysteine lowering by supplemental B vitamins suggested clinical cardiovascular benefit, the results have not been confirmed in subsequent randomized controlled trials. The reasons may be the same as those suggested for failing to show benefit of antioxidant nutrients. Had the results of all these trials been available at the time of the WHO deliberations, folate may not have been listed in the 'probable' category.

21.6.6 Food items and food groups

Fruit and vegetables Consumption of fruit and vegetables has long been believed to promote good health, but it is only relatively recently that ecological and prospective studies have reported their potential to reduce both CHD and stroke. The series of DASH trials has shown convincing benefits in terms of reducing blood pressure levels, especially when fruits and vegetables are consumed together with relatively high intakes of low-fat dairy products and a reduced intake of sodium. Additional benefit in terms of cardiovascular risk reduction may accrue as a result of the high intake of antioxidant nutrients and flavonoids in fruits, berries and vegetables, some of which may also be high in dietary fibre.

Fish Many prospective studies have shown a reduced risk of CHD in association with fish consumption, especially fatty fish, with one recent systematic review suggesting that high-risk populations might halve CHD deaths if fish intake was increased to 40–60 g/day. All-cause mortality may also be reduced by an increase in fish consumption. The DART and GISSI-Prevenzione trials support the clinical benefits of regular consumption of fish and fish oils (C20:5, C22:6), especially in high-risk individuals with established cardiovascular disease.

Nuts Several large epidemiological studies have reported decreased CHD risk in association with frequent consumption of nuts. The studies have generally considered nuts as a group. Nuts are high in unsaturated fats, and regular consumption results in a favourable alteration in the fatty acid profile of plasma lipids, as well as some reduction in atherogenic lipoproteins. It is clearly impossible to conduct a long-term clinical trial in which increased intake of nuts is the sole dietary modification. Nevertheless, the evidence is deemed to be sufficient to regard nuts as probably protective against CHD. Any recommendations to include nuts in the diet must be tempered with a reminder of their relatively high energy content to ensure that an increase in intake does not result in energy imbalance.

Soy Soy protein has a favourable effect on several cardiovascular risk factors. An overview of 38 clinical studies suggests that a consumption of 47 g of soy protein daily leads to a 9% decline in total cholesterol and a 13% fall in LDL cholesterol. Soy isoflavones have been shown to lower blood pressure, and there is some evidence of beneficial effects on vascular and endothelial function, platelet aggregation, smooth muscle cell proliferation, and LDL oxidation. Soy protein has been shown to inhibit atherosclerosis in animals, but human data are regarded as insufficient to classify the potential benefits as being greater than 'possible'.

Alcohol Ecological, case–control, and cohort studies all suggest a protective effect of low-to-moderate alcohol consumption. The effect is apparent for all alcoholic drinks and has been attributed to the HDL-raising effect of alcohol, or perhaps to the antioxidant content of some alcoholic beverages. It is noteworthy that the benefits in absolute terms apply only to middle-aged and older individuals. Other cardiovascular and health risks associated with alcohol, especially when consumed in excess, argue strongly against a general recommendation for its use.

Coffee Boiled unfiltered coffee raises total and LDL cholesterol because of the cafestol content of coffee beans. Such unfiltered coffee is still widely consumed in Greece, the Middle East, and Turkey. A shift from coffee prepared in this way to filtered coffee is reported to have contributed appreciably to the decline in plasma cholesterol in Finland.

21.6.7 Dietary patterns

Early dietary advice aimed at reducing cardiovascular risk centred principally around a reduction in saturated and an increase in polyunsaturated fatty acids. More recently, there has been interest in certain dietary patterns that are regarded as protective against CHD. The traditional Mediterranean diets of Italy, Greece, and Spain have been singled out as being of particular benefit, perhaps because populations consuming the traditional diets of countries surrounding the Mediterranean Sea had remarkably low rates of CHD. The fact that, from a culinary point of view, such dietary patterns are regarded as especially attractive may also have contributed.

Vegetarian diets have also been promoted for their apparent cardioprotective effect. Vegetarians are indeed at lower risk of CHD than meat eaters, but it has not been established which attributes of the vegetarian diet might be protective, since there are many aspects other than the avoidance of meat that characterize these diets. One study suggests that the lower rates might be due to the relatively low intake of saturated fatty acids, rather than meat avoidance.

The substantial body of epidemiological, experimental, and clinical trial data provide strong evidence that while Mediterranean and vegetarian diets may indeed be associated with reduced cardiovascular risk, there are other equally cardio-protective dietary patterns. The attributes of cardi-oprotective diets listed in Table 21.6 are seen in many traditional diets (e.g. most Asian diets), and indeed the so-called typical Western diet can be modified to follow these dietary principles. It is important to note that adopting individual attrib-utes of potentially appropriate cardioprotective diets may not confer benefit. For example, con-suming substantial quantities of olive oil, a well-recognized feature of Mediterranen diets, in the context of an otherwise inappropriate diet may confer little or no advantage. Failure to ensure appropriate energy balance may negate the bene-fits of adhering to many of the other attributes listed in Table 21.6 because obesity-mediated car-diovascular risk (see Chapter 17) may outweigh favourable trends in other risk factors. There are other caveats too. The so-called 'prudent diet', in which carbohydrate is recommended to replace saturated fatty acids, needs to be implemented with caution. It is essential that fibre-rich who-legrains, vegetables, and fruits are the major car-bohydrate sources, rather than sugars and starches. High intakes of sugars and starches may lead to an increase in triglycerides and reduction in HDL. Modest increases in *cis*-unsaturated fatty acids and protein may be appropriate nutrients to par-tially substitute for saturated fatty acids for those not willing to consume large quantities of fibre-rich wholegrains, vegetables, and fruit, carbohy-drate sources which are not associated with

Table 21.6 Attributes of cardioprotective dietary patterns

- Low intakes of saturated fatty acids
- High intakes of raw or appropriately prepared fruits and vegetables
- Wholegrains and lightly processed cereal foods are preferred
- Fat intakes are predominantly derived from unmodified vegetable oils[a]
- Fish, nuts, seeds, and vegetable protein sources are important dietary components
- Meat, when consumed, is lean and eaten in small quantities
- Energy balance reduces rates of obesity

[a]Coconut oil and palm oil are not encouraged because they tend to elevate cholesterol and LDL.

unfavourable consequences in terms of triglycer-ide and HDL.

Unfortunately, some populations that previously consumed cardioprotective diets and had low rates of CHD have introduced foods not traditionally con-sumed. For instance, some modern Mediterranean or Asian diets may be high in saturated fatty acids and thus, at least to some extent, have lost their health benefits.

21.7 Nutritional strategies for high-risk populations

It is essential in countries with high CHD rates to have in place a nutritional strategy that is aimed at the entire population. Individuals with extreme lev-els of risk factors or with several different risk fac-tors are at the highest risk of CHD and will benefit most, as individuals, from dietary modification. However, the majority of cases of CHD will occur in people at moderate risk, i.e. those with one or two risk factors that may be modestly elevated. This is

simply because there are far more such individuals in the population than people at very high risk. Thus, in order to reduce (or in those countries where rates are already coming down to further reduce) the epidemic proportions of CHD, popula-tion change is essential. The disadvantage of the 'population approach' is that many individuals are being asked to make changes that are likely to pro-duce a relatively small reduction in their personal

Table 21.7 Ranges of population nutrient intake goals as recommended by WHO and FAO for adults

	AMDR	U-AMDR	L-AMDR
Total fat	20–35%	35%	15%
Saturated fatty acids (SFA)		10%	
Total polyunsaturated fatty acids (PUFA)	6–11%	11%	6%
n-6 PUFA	2.5–9%		Adequate intake: 2.5–3.5%
n-3 PUFA	0.5–2%		
cis-Monounsaturated fatty acids	By difference[a]		
trans-Fatty acids (TFA)		< 1%	
Dietary cholesterol	<300 mg/day		
Total carbohydrate	50–75%		
Free sugars[b]	<10%		
Dietary fibre (NSP)	From foods		
Protein	10–15%		
Sodium chloride	<5 g/day		
Fruit and vegetables	>400 g/day	Encouraged	

Goals are expressed as percentage of total energy, unless otherwise stated.

AMDR, acceptable macronutrient distribution ranges for adults; L, lower; PUFA; polyunsaturated fatty acids; SFA, saturated fatty acids; U, upper.

[a]Total fat = SFA + PFA + TFA.

[b]All monosaccharides and disaccharides added to foods by manufacturer, cook, or consumer, plus sugars naturally present in honey, syrups, and fruit juices.

These targets may be readily translated into food-based dietary guidelines appropriate to food preferences of different population groups.

Source: WHO/FAO (2003) Diet, nutrition and the prevention of chronic diseases. WHO Technical Report Series 916. Geneva, World Health Organization,WHO/FAO (2003) updated following WHO/FAO (2007) Joint FAO/WHO Scientific Update on Carbohydrates in Human Nutrition. EJCN, 61 (Suppl 1) Joint FAOWHO Scientific Update on Carbohydrates in Human Nutrition (2007) and WHO/FAO (2009) Fats and fatty acids in human nutrition. Proceedings of the Joint FAO/WHO Expert Consultation. November 10–14, 2008. Geneva, Switzerland. Ann Nutr Metab, **55**, 5–300.

CHD risk (the 'prevention paradox') and those who are at high risk will still need to be individually identified because they are likely to require more radical and individually designed lifestyle changes and perhaps medication.

Most high-risk countries have in place nutrient and food targets aimed at reducing CHD rates, and more global targets have been set by the WHO. Table 21.7 summarizes the targets suggested by WHO/FAO for adults.

21.8 Dietary advice for high-risk individuals

High-risk individuals are those who have markedly elevated levels of a single risk factor (e.g. those with familial hyperlipidaemia), those with multiple risk factors (Table 21.2), or those who have already developed clinical CHD. They may be identified because of a personal or family history of CHD or in screening programmes. It is clearly important in such individuals to attempt to achieve the lowest possible degree of risk with regard to all identifiable risk factors. From a dietary point of view, the principles are similar to those recommended for the general population, but further changes from the current Western diet are often required. Emphasis on dietary advice specific to particular risk factors is needed (Box 21.1). For those who are overweight or obese, weight loss should be a primary consideration (see Chapter 17). For most high-risk individuals, intakes of saturated plus *trans*-fatty acids 7–10% total energy will help to achieve the lowest possible level of LDL. Regular intakes of soluble-fibre-rich foods and the use of margarines and spreads to which plant sterols or stanols have been added also facilitate LDL reduction. For those with high triglyceride and low HDL levels, rapidly digested (high glycaemic index) carbohydrate intake should be low and carbohydrate should be derived principally from intact fruits, vegetables, and wholegrain cereals.

Indeed, it may be helpful for such individuals to have a lower than average intake of total carbohydrate provided that any relative increase in fat intake derives from mono- and polyunsaturated fatty acids with *cis* configuration and that energy balance is maintained. The presence of hypertension necessitates emphasis on salt restriction and increased intake of fruit, vegetables, and low-fat dairy products. Individually tailored advice from a dietitian and regular monitoring of dietary intake and risk factor levels are usually necessary.

The fact that clinical trials involving cholesterol lowering by means of statin drugs results in clinical benefit in people aged over 70 suggests that older people should also be given dietary advice. The absolute risk of cardiovascular disease increases steadily with age, although the relative risk associated with individual risk factors might decrease. No doubt there is an age beyond which there are minimal advantages to dietary change, but those who might be expected to otherwise have a reasonable life expectancy should be given advice similar to that given to younger people. When giving lipid-lowering advice to older people, it is necessary to ensure an adequate intake of essential nutrients, because they usually have a reduced intake of total energy.

The widespread use of several cardioprotective drugs shown in randomized controlled trials to be of benefit to people at high risk of cardiovascular disease in no way reduces the need to comply with dietary advice. Statins are principally prescribed to reduce total and LDL cholesterol, β-blockers, and angiotensin-converting enzyme inhibitors to lower blood pressure, and aspirin and other antiplatelet drugs to reduce the risk of thrombosis. While these drugs may have some benefits beyond favourably altering the risk factors for which they have been prescribed, a cardioprotective diet influences a wide range of risk determinants. In addition, dietary compliance may enhance the effect of the drug. For example, appreciable reduction of saturated fatty acids will result in lipid lowering beyond that which can routinely be achieved by statins alone, and following the DASH diet will enhance the blood pressure-lowering effect of hypotensive agents. The case studies presented in Box 21.3 give examples of the approach to two patients identified in a screening programme.

21.9 Gene–nutrient interactions

It has long been appreciated that not everyone exposed to a risk factor for CHD will develop the disease and that exposure to foods or nutrients known to influence risk factors will produce a range of

BOX 21.1 Dietary advice for individuals at high risk of coronary heart disease

Increase or include	Changing the dietary pattern	Serving sizes
Cis-unsaturated fats	Use small amounts of soft or plant sterol margarine and oils* in place of butter and hard fats	1–3 tsp
	Include fresh nuts and seeds; avocado; hummus	2 tbsp nuts or seeds (30 g), avocado, hummus
Lean protein sources	Choose low-fat dairy products in place of high-fat dairy products	1 glass milk, 1 small container yoghurt, 2 cm cube cheese
	Use lean meat and poultry—remove any meat fat and poultry skin	2 slices lean meat (100 g cooked) 1 small chicken breast
	Egg plainly cooked—not in fat	Egg (1) 3–4 per week
Fish	Eat fish (not fried), especially oily varieties—if not eating any oily fish then include canola oil, linseeds, walnuts, and wheat germ	2 small fillets of fish (150–200 g cooked)
Fibre and slowly absorbed carbohydrate	Include oats, legumes, and soy products	⅔ cup cooked beans, chickpeas, lentils
Wholegrain products	Choose wholegrain bread, cereal, rice, pasta starchy vegetables with skins	1 slice bread, ½ cup pasta, ⅓ cup rice, cup cereal, 1 small potato, sweet potato, ½ cup parsnip, yams, corn, or equivalent
Fruit and vegetables	Eat plenty of coloured non starchy vegetables	½–1 cup cooked vegetables, 1 cup raw salad, 1 medium raw fruit, ½–1 cup berries (grapes ½ cup), cooked or canned in water or juice, ½ banana
	Eat fruit frequently—a variety of colours	
Nutrient dense foods rich in protective micronutrients but low in energy	Drink water in place of sweetened beverages/alcohol	**Aim for per day** 2–3 servings fruit
Decrease or exclude	**Avoid/reduce intake of:**	3–4+ servings coloured vegetables
Saturated and *trans*-unsaturated fat	High-fat meat products and takeaways; coconut fat, palm oil, partially hydrogenated fat, deep-fried food, butter	2–3 servings low-fat dairy products
Dietary cholesterol		6+ servings cereals mostly wholegrain

Highly refined carbohydrate	High-fat cakes, pastries, desserts, biscuits, sweets, cream, sweet sauces, full-fat ice cream	3–4 servings oils, margarines/table spreads
Excess energy	High-fat high-salt crackers, snacks, sauces, cheeses, sour cream, cream cheese	6–8 cups fluid—water, tea, coffee, sugar-free drinks
Dietary sodium/salt	Avoid high-sodium pre-prepared products, if using salt, then small amounts of iodized salt	If drinking alcohol, then no more than 2 standard drinks for men, 1 for women
Sugary drinks, alcohol	High-sugar drinks, alcoholic drinks (ready mixed), alcohol (beer, wines, spirits)	
Nutrient aims	**Cooking methods**	1–2 servings or less lean meat or poultry
Total fat 25–33% T En	Use low-fat cooking methods	**Aim for per week**
SFA + TFA 7–10% T En	Baking, steaming, boiling, microwaving, grilling	1–2 servings fish, 1 oily
Cis MUFA 10–20%	Cooking in a casserole/crock pot	2–3 servings or more legumes
PUFA (plant and marine ω-3) 5–9% T En	Cooking in a wok without fat	3–5+ (30 g) servings unsalted raw nuts—regular use of seeds, avocado
Dietary cholesterol <200–300 mg/day	If using oil, use small quantities of a variety of named oils, e.g. olive, sunflower, rice bran	
Protein 12–25% T En		
Carbohydrate 40–60% (Fibre 30 g + /day, ½ soluble)		

* oils (grapeseed, safflower, soy, sunflower, canola, olive, peanut, rice bran)

BOX 21.2 Predictive equations for estimating changes in plasma cholesterol and lipoprotein concentrations in response to changes in dietary fatty acids and cholesterol. More sophisticated equations were developed when the effects of different saturated and unsaturated fatty acids were identified. TC and LDL-C given in mg/dL. For mmol/L, multiply by 0.02586.

Authors	Equations
Keys *et al.* (1965)	$\Delta TC = 1.35\,(2\Delta S - \Delta P) + 1.52\Delta Z$
Mensink and Katan (1992)	$\Delta TC = 1.51\Delta S - 0.12\Delta M - 0.60\Delta P$
	$\Delta LDL\text{-}C = 1.28\Delta S - 0.24\Delta M - 0.55\Delta P$
Yu *et al.* (1995)	$\Delta TC = 2.02\,(\Delta C12{:}0 + \Delta 14{:}0 + \Delta 16{:}0) - 0.03$
	$(\Delta 18{:}0) - 0.48\Delta MUFA - 0.96\Delta PUFA$
	$\Delta LDL\text{-}C = 1.46\,(\Delta 12{:}0 + \Delta 14{:}0 + \Delta 16{:}0) + 0.07$
	$(\Delta 18{:}0) - 0.69\Delta MUFA - 0.96\Delta PUFA$

Abbreviations:

Δ, change; LDL-C, LDL cholesterol; M/MUFA, percentage of monounsaturated fatty acids; P/PUFA, percentage of polyunsaturated fatty acids; S, percentage of saturated fatty acids; TC, total cholesterol; all as percentage of total energy intake.

C12:0, C14:0, C16:0, percentage saturated fatty acids with 12, 14, or 16 carbon atoms.

Z, square root of daily dietary cholesterol.

Source: Kris-Etherton, Y., Yu-Poth, S., Sabaté, J., *et al.* (1999) Nuts and their bioactive constituents: Effects on serum lipids and other factors that affect disease risk. *Am J Clin Nutr*, **70**, 5045–115.

responses within a group of individuals all consuming the same diet. For example, while modifying dietary fatty acid composition may alter total and LDL cholesterol to an extent that may, in a population or group of individuals, be predicted by a formula (Box 21.2), some individuals may show little or no change, whereas others will have striking changes in their levels when the nature of dietary fat changes (Fig. 21.9). In the clinical context, failure to respond to dietary modification has often been attributed to failure to comply with dietary advice. While non-compliance is indeed associated with absence of

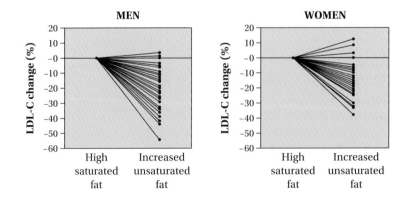

Fig. 21.9 Individual changes in low-density lipoprotein cholesterol (LDL-C) when *cis*-unsaturated fatty acids replace some of the saturated fatty acids in the diet.

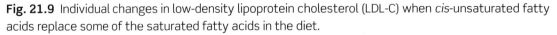

Source: Schaefer, E.J. (2002) Lipoproteins, nutrition, and heart disease. *Am J Clin Nutr*, **75**, 191–212.

response or reduced response, variation has been confirmed in carefully controlled dietary experiments in which all participants were fed identical diets. Genetic factors undoubtedly account for this variability, and several genetic polymorphisms that predict plasma lipid responses to change in dietary fat have now been identified. For example, individuals carrying the *APO E4* allele of the *APO E* gene will show a more marked reduction in total and LDL cholesterol than those who do not carry it, when changed to a diet that is reduced in both fat and cholesterol. A common genetic polymorphism in the promoter region of the *APO AI* gene determines the extent to which HDL responds to substantial increases in polyunsaturated fatty acids.

Such observations have led to speculation that this study of 'nutrigenetics' will soon lead to the development of 'designer diets', which will enable individualized dietary advice to be based on genetic characteristics. However, while this type of nutrigenetic research will no doubt continue to flourish, such expectations are premature for several reasons: polygenic, rather than monogenic, factors are almost certainly responsible for most of the heterogeneity in risk factor response to diet; no studies carried out thus far have involved sufficient participants to study the interaction of many genes; most research to date has centred on the variability in plasma lipid and lipoprotein response to changes in nature of dietary fat, and many other risk factors and nutrients are involved; and finally—and perhaps of greatest importance—there is convincing evidence that compliance with cardioprotective dietary patterns can profoundly reduce cardiovascular risk in high-risk populations and the majority of individuals who have raised risk factor levels.

Nutrigenomic research explores how nutrients influence gene expression, rather than the interindividual differences in relation to the effects of nutrients. Of particular relevance to cardiovascular disease has been the research that has shown the profound effect of ω-3 fatty acids on the activation of nuclear receptors, which are associated with inflammation and lipid metabolism, thus helping to explain their cardioprotective effect.

Cerebrovascular disease

Cerebrovascular disease presents clinically as a stroke, which, like the clinical manifestations of CHD, also has a major impact on public health because of its high frequency in most affluent and developing countries. There are several different types of stroke.

One cause of stroke is a bleed from one of the cerebral arteries (haemorrhagic stroke); it may be associated with a congenital abnormality (aneurysm) and/or raised levels of blood pressure. Thus, nutritional determinants of hypertension are contributory causal factors. Ischaemic strokes are more common and result from thrombosis and atheroma, the process being similar to that which results in myocardial infarction.

The clinical features of stroke (typically loss or slurring of speech and weakness of one side of the body) result from the loss of blood supply to a section of the brain. Although the nutritional determinants have been far less studied than is the case for CHD, the risk factors for the two sets of conditions are similar, and therefore nutritional factors that predispose to CHD should also apply. However, in the relatively limited number of studies of stroke that have been carried out, some food groups emerge as being particularly relevant. Most striking is the protective effect of fruit and vegetables, as demonstrated in six of the seven large prospective studies that examined the relationship. Although it appears most categories of fruit and vegetables may be protective, the effect is particularly striking for cruciferous vegetables, green leafy vegetables and citrus fruits. Blood pressure is also a particularly important risk factor for ischaemic stroke, so that, once again, all the nutritional determinants of hypertension can be regarded as especially relevant.

Of the remaining nutrients and food groups that have been identified as causal or protective in terms of CHD, ω-3 fatty acids, regular fish consumption, and intake of wholegrains have been shown to be protective against ischaemic stroke.

Thus, although there have been no intervention studies specifically to examine the effect on clinical outcome, implementing a cardioprotective dietary pattern can be expected to reduce the risk of both haemorrhagic and ischaemic stroke (see Box 21.3).

BOX 21.3 Case studies

Screening for cardiovascular risk factors and diabetes is recommended for men and women from middle age (younger in high-risk ethnic groups or those with a family history of premature CVD or diabetes) in many countries. Risk equations which are based on age, sex, smoking habits, presence or absence of diabetes, and measurements of blood pressure and total and HDL cholesterol are used to generate risk estimates during the subsequent 5–10 years. Lifestyle advice (dietary modification and usually increased physical activity) is the cornerstone of management, though drug treatment may also be required. The intensity of treatment is based upon degree of risk, a 10–15% chance of a cardiovascular event within the next 5 years generally indicating the need for intensive dietary management and if indicated, drug treatment. The equations do not take family history, obesity, ethnicity, and some of the more recently indentified risk factors into account, but have been shown to be generally robust in several different populations. Such information may be used qualitatively to reinforce advice regarding treatment.

Case 1

Mr AL, aged 53 years, who considered himself to be generally healthy having had no contact with this doctor throughout his adult life volunteered for screening. The questionnaire he was asked to complete revealed a strong family history of premature cardiovascular disease (his father and two uncles had had coronary events in their late 40s or early 50s). AL was not a smoker, his BMI was 28.3 kg/m² and his blood pressure was elevated when measured on several occasions, between 160 and 170 mmHg systolic and 100 and 110 diastolic. His fasting blood glucose levels were normal (4.8 and 5.2 mmol/L) but fasting

lipid levels were not (total cholesterol 8.9 mmol/L, LDL cholesterol 6.4 mmol/L, HDL cholesterol 0.7 mmol/L, and triglyceride 4.9 mmol/L). His risk of a cardiovascular event during the next 5 years was estimated to be 15–20%, but this does not take into account his worrying family history which, together with his lipid levels, suggest that he may have familial combined hyperlipidaemia and that his actual risk may be appreciably greater than indicated by the risk calculator which does not take family history into account. Intensive intervention, including referral to a specialist dietitian, was indicated. Table 21.8a provides an indication of a typical day's diet and the calculated intake of macronutrients. Specific dietary advice (Box 21.1) was offered using a standard behavioural approach (see Chapter 38). Reduction of total energy intake by reducing portion sizes, total and saturated fat, sugars, and alcohol are key aspects of management. Some substitution with ω-3 and ω-6 polyunsaturated fats and cis-monounsaturated fats is appropriate. Ongoing encouragement (see Chapter 17) was considered to be a pivotal component of treatment.

After 6 months, Mr AL had lost 10 kg in weight, his BMI was 24.9 kg/m², blood pressure was 155 systolic, 90 diastolic, and lipid levels had appreciably improved (total cholesterol 7.0 mmol/L, LDL cholesterol 4.7 mmol/L, HDL cholesterol 1.2 mmol/L and triglyceride 3.3 mmol/L. Although this was considered to be an impressive improvement in terms of cardiovascular risk, he was nevertheless prescribed a statin drug in the expectation of even further risk reduction. Simvastatin 20 mg enabled him to reach target LDL cholesterol of 2 mmol/L and Cilazapril 2.5 mg to target levels of blood pressure. However, it should be noted that dietary

Table 21.8a Mr AL's typical day's diet

Food	Number of servings
Cereal—sweetened	1 large
Milk—standard	3½ (800 mL)
Dairy products—not fat-reduced	4 large
Fruit	2 servings (1 raw)
Bread—rolls or bagels	3 large
Baked products—cakes, buns, or muffins	2 large
Butter—as spread	8 tsp (40 g)
Vegetables	2 average
Salad (with olives and sundried tomatoes)	1 small
Rice, pasta, or potatoes	1 large
Coffee—all freshly brewed	4 cups (800 mL)
Sugar—in coffee	12 tsp (60 g)
Meat or chicken	1 serving (200 g)
Smoked salmon or tuna	1 small (30 g)
Wine	2 units (200 mL)
Snack foods—salty	2 average
Snacks—sweet	2 small
Analysis	
Energy	18.5MJ/4500 kcal
Protein	11% TEn
Total fat	44% TEn
SFA	20% TEn
MUFA	14% Ten
PUFA	5% TEn
Carbohydrate	37% TEn
Cholesterol	500 mg/day
Total dietary fibre	30 g/day

modification had achieved risk reduction by influencing several risk factors. Furthermore, diet modification enabled targets to be achieved with lower drug doses than might otherwise have been the case.

Case 2

Mr JB, aged 45 years, also participated in a screening programme. He too had had little previous contact with health professionals. He had no family history of early cardiovascular disease, a BMI of 23 kg/m², a normal blood pressure (118 mmHg systolic and 84 diastolic) and the following lipid profile: total cholesterol 6.8 mmol/L, LDL cholesterol 4.7 mmol/L, HDL 1.2 mmol/L, triglyceride 0.8 mmol/L. His risk of a cardiovascular event within the next 5 years was 2.5–5%. However, it was pointed out to him that although his risk at present was not particularly high, in 10 years' time, if left untreated, risk would be 10–15% or higher as cholesterol levels tend to rise with age. He was diagnosed as having polygenic hypercholesterolaemia and was given general dietary advice along the lines of that described in the list below and encouraged to purchase an appropriate recipe book.

General dietary advice for Mr JB

1 Choose a wide variety of foods, for 3 meals/day.

2 Always choose lean meat, remove visible fat, and consider two or more fish meals each week.

3 Include fruits and/or coloured vegetables at most meals and aim for at least 6 servings daily.

4 Include beans and legumes at least twice a week.

5 Choose wholegrain breads and cereals.

6 Use small amounts of unsaturated oils, margarine, plain unsalted nuts, and seeds

7 Use lower fat preparation and cooking methods with little or no dairy fat, meat fat, or deep-fried foods. Limit sugar and salt.

8 Use low-fat milk and milk products, in 2–3 servings daily.

Table 21.8b Dietary changes achieved by Mr JB

Substituting *cis*-unsaturated for saturated fats	Using soft table spread instead of butter Olive or sunflower oil instead of hard cooking fats Eating 30 g raw unsalted nuts or seeds 5–7 day/week
Substituting lower-fat for full-fat dairy products	Reduced-fat milk Lower-fat hard cheeses such as Edam instead of medium-fat cheese Cottage cheese mixed with a little grated tasty cheese Natural or reduced-fat unsweetened yoghurt instead of cream
Using higher-grain bread and unrefined cereals	Wholegrain or heavier bread for white or soft grain bread Wholegrain oat cereal, brown rice, wholemeal pasta
Increasing fruit and vegetable intake	Larger servings cooked vegetables, all colours, at dinner Salad with lunch Raw fruit 2–3/day
Using lower-fat protein foods	Removing visible fat from meat, reducing serving size Choosing lean poultry Including fish 1–2 servings/week
Changing recipes	Incorporating wholegrain cereals in recipes Including beans and legumes in recipes Using *cis*-unsaturated fats and oils and lower-fat dairy products Reduced sugar

9 Drink plenty of fluids daily, especially water, limit sugar sweetened drinks and alcohol.

10 If choosing ready-prepared foods, then low in fat, salt and sugar.

11 Mostly avoid or limit butter, deep-fried and fatty foods, and sweet, fatty, bakery products.

With the support of his wife, who did most of the cooking, Mr JB made some quite substantial dietary changes (Table 21.8b) and after 6 months, his lipid levels had markedly improved (total cholesterol 5.0 mmol/L, LDL cholesterol 3.3 mmol/L, HDL cholesterol 1.5 mmol/L, triglyceride 0.7 mmol/L).

The estimated 5-year risk of a cardiovascular event had reduced to <2.5%. Although LDL cholesterol had not quite reached the target <2 mmol/L, drug treatment was not considered necessary in the context of primary prevention in a relatively low-risk individual. However long-term encouragement and follow-up is an important component of treatment.

Further Reading

1. **Ascherio, A., Rimm, E.B., Giovannucci, E.L., *et al.** (1996) Dietary fat and risk of coronary heart disease in men: Cohort follow-up study in the USA. *BMJ*, **313**, 84–90.
2. **Beaglehole, R.** (1999) International trends in coronary heart disease mortality and incidence rates. *J Cardiovasc Risk*, **6**, 63–8.
3. **Burr, M.L., Gilbert, J.F., Holliday, R.M., *et al.** (1989) Effects of changes in fat, fish and fibre intakes on death and myocardial reinfarction: Diet and Reinfarction Trial (DART). *Lancet*, **ii**, 757–61.

4. **Czernichow, S., Thomas, D., and Bruckert, E.** (2010) n-6 Fatty acids and cardiovascular health: A review of the evidence for dietary intake recommendations. *BJN,* **104,** 788–96.

5. **Dayton, S., Pearce, M.L., Hashimoto, S.,** *et al.* (1969) A controlled trial of a diet high in unsaturated fat in preventing complications of atherosclerosis. *Circulation,* **39/40** (Suppl. II), 1–63.

6. **de Lorgeril, M., Renaud, S., Mamelle, N.,** *et al.* (1994) Mediterranean α-linolenic acid-rich diet in secondary prevention of coronary heart disease. *Lancet,* **343,** 1454–9.

7. **Elliott, P., Stamler, J., Nichols, R.,** *et al.* (1996) Intersalt revisited: Further analysis of 24 hour-sodium excretion and blood pressure within and across populations. *BMJ,* **312,** 1249–53.

8. **GISSI-Prevenzione** (1999) Dietary supplementation with n-3 polyunsaturated fatty acids and vitamin E after myocardial infarction: Results of the GISSI-Prevenzione trial. Gruppo Italiano per lo Studio della Sopravvivenza nell'Infarto miocardico. *Lancet,* **354,** 447–55.

9. **Hertog, M.L., Feskens, E.J.M., Hollman, P.C.H., Katan, M.B., and Kromhout, D.** (1993) Dietary antioxidant flavonoids and risk of coronary heart disease. *Lancet,* **342,** 1007–17.

10. **Hjermann, I., Byer, K., Holme, I.,** *et al.* (1981) Effect of diet and smoking intervention on the incidence of coronary heart disease. *Lancet,* **ii,** 1303–10.

11. **Keys, A.** (1980). *Seven countries: A multivarate analysis of death and coronary heart disease.* Massachusetts, Harvard University Press.

12. **Keys, A., Anderson, J.T., and Grande, F.** (1965) Serum cholesterol response to changes in the diet. IV Particular saturated fatty acids in the diet. *Metabolism,* **14,** 776–87.

13. **Keys, A., Menotti, A., Karvonen, M.J.,** *et al.* (1986) The diet and 15-year death rate in the Seven Countries Study. *Am J Epidemiol,* **124,** 903–15.

14. **Kris-Etherton, Y., Yu-Poth, S., Sabaté, J.,** *et al.* (1999) Nuts and their bioactive constituents: Effects on serum lipids and other factors that affect disease risk. *Am J Clin Nutr,* **70,** 5045–115.

15. **Knekt, P., Ritz, J., Pereira, M.A.,** *et al.* (2004) Antioxidant vitamins and coronary heart disease: A pooled analysis of cohorts. *Am J Clin Nutr,* **80,** 1508–20.

16. **Law, M.R., Frost, C.D., and Wald, N.J.** (1991) By how much does dietary salt reduction lower blood pressure? Analysis of data from trials of salt reduction. *BMJ,* **302,** 819–24.

17. **Liu, S., Manson, J.E., Stampfer, M.J.,** *et al.* (2000) Wholegrain consumption and risk of ischemic stroke in women: A prospective study. *J Am Med Ass,* **284,** 1534–40.

18. **Mann, J.I., Appleby, P.N., Key, T.J., and Thorogood, M.** (1997) Dietary determinants of ischaemic heart disease in health conscious individuals. *Heart,* **78,** 450–5.

19. **Margetts, B.M., Beilin, L.J., Vandongen, R., and Armstrong, B.K.** (1986) Vegetarian diet in mild hypertension: A randomized controlled trial. *BMJ,* **293,** 1468–71.

20. **Martin, M.J., Hulley, S.B., Browner, W.S.,** *et al.* (1968) Serum cholesterol, blood pressure, and mortality: Implications from a cohort of 361,662 men. *Lancet,* **2,** 933–6.

21. **Mellen, P.B., Walsh, T.F., and Herrington, D.M.** (2008) Wholegrain intake and cardiovascular disease: A meta-analysis. *Nutr Med Cardiovasc Dis* **18,** 283–90.

22. **Mensink, R.P. and Katan, M.B.** (1992) Effect of dietary fatty acids on serum lipids and lipoproteins. A meta-analysis of 27 trials. *Arterioscler Thromb,* **12,** 911–19.

23. **Mensink, R.P., Zoch, P.L., Kester, A.D., and Katan, M.B.** (2003) Effects of dietary fatty acids and carbohydrates on the ratio of serum total to HDL cholesterol and on serum lipids and apoliproteins: A meta-analysis of 60 controlled trials. *Am J Clin Nutr,* **77,** 1146–55.

24. **Ordovas, J.M.** (2004) The quest for cardiovascular health in the genomic era: Nutrigenetics and plasma lipoproteins. *Proc Nutr Soc,* **63,** 145–52.

25. **Rimm, E.B., Ascherio, A., Giovannucci, E.,** *et al.* (1996) Vegetable, fruit, and cereal fiber intake and risk of coronary heart disease among men. *JAMA,* **275,** 447–51.

26. **Robinson, S.M. and Barker, D.J.** (2002) Coronary heart disease: A disorder of growth. *Proc Nutr Soc,* **61,** 537–42.

27. **Sacks, F.M., Svetkey, L.P., Vollmer, W.M., *et al*.** (2001) Effects on blood pressure of reduced dietary sodium and the Dietary Approaches to Stop Hypertension (DASH) Diet. *N Eng J Med*, **344**, 3–10.

28. **Schaefer, E.J**. (2002) Lipoproteins, nutrition, and heart disease. *Am J Clin Nutr*, **75**, 191–212.

29. **Scientific Advisory Committee on Nutrition** (2003) *Salt and health*. The Stationery Office, London.

30. **Stampfer, M.J. and Rimm, E.B.** (1995) Epidemiological evidence for vitamin E in prevention of cardiovascular disease. *Am J Clin Nutr*, **62**, 1365S–9S.

31. **Strassullo, P., Scalfi, L., Branca, F., *et al*.** (2004) Nutrition prevention of ischaemic stroke: Present knowledge, limitations and future perspectives. *Nutr Metab Cardiovasc Dis*, **14**, 97–114.

32. **The Heart Outcomes Prevention Evaluation Study Investigators (HOPE)** (2000) Vitamin E supplementation and cardiovascular events in high-risk patients. *N Engl J Med*, **342**, 154–60.

33. **Truswell, A.S.** (2010) *Cholesterol and Beyond. The research on diet and coronary heart disease 1900–2000*. Dordrecht, Heidelberg, London, New York, Springer.

34. **Ulbricht, T.L.V., and Southgate, D.A.T.** (1991) Coronary heart disease: Seven dietary factors. *Lancet*, **338**, 985–92.

35. **WHO** (2002) *Death and DALY estimates*. Geneva, World Health Organization. http://www.who.int/healthinfo/en/.

36. **WHO/FAO** (2003) *Diet, nutrition and the prevention of chronic diseases*. WHO Technical Report Series 916. Geneva, World Health Organization.

37. **WHO/FAO** (2007) Joint FAO/WHO Scientific Update on Carbohydrates in Human Nutrition. *EJCN*, **61** (Suppl. 1).

38. **WHO/FAO** (2009) Fats and fatty acids in human nutrition. Proceedings of the Joint FAO/WHO Expert Consultation. November 10–14, 2008. Geneva, Switzerland. *Ann Nutr Metab*, **55**, 5–300.

39. **Yu, S., Derr, J., Etherton, T. D., et al.** (1995) Plasma cholesterol-predictive equations demonstrate that stearic acid is neutral and monounsaturated fatty acids are hypocholes terolemic. *Am J Clin Nutr*, **61**, 1129–39.

Useful Websites

To see topical and scientifically robust updates on nutrition associated with this textbook and web links to many of the journals in the Further Reading sections, please see the dedicated Online Resource Centre at **http://www.oxfordtextbooks.co.uk/orc/mann4e/**

Nutrition and cancer

22

Martin Wiseman

22.1 General epidemiology of cancer

Worldwide, some 13% of deaths are caused by cancer, but there is marked variation. For instance, cancers account for 5% of deaths in Africa, but about one-quarter of deaths in industrialized nations. In England in 2008, 30% of deaths in males and 25% in females were due to cancers, second only to cardiovascular diseases.

For the most common cancers, age is a major determinant of risk. Adult cancers tend to be rare below the age of 40, with a marked increase after 65 years (Fig. 22.1). Therefore, as life expectancy increases in many regions of the globe, cancers can be expected to become more common, with attendant social and economic costs. Current approaches to controlling cancer focus on screening to detect cancers at an early stage and on the surgical, chemotherapeutic, and radiotherapeutic management of existing clinical disease. However, screening is an appropriate option for only some cancers, due to inadequacies in screening methods or lack of evidence of efficacy, or of safety of interventions. Equally, treatments can be remarkably successful for some cancers (such as testicular cancer), but for many, and the most frequent, cancers (lung, breast, colon, cervix, stomach) they are often only incompletely effective, especially if the disease is advanced at diagnosis. In addition, screening for and management of existing cancers are expensive options, not always available to lower-income nations.

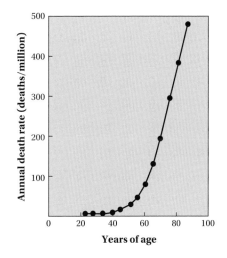

Fig. 22.1 Rates of colon cancer rise steeply with age compatible with multistep, time-dependent tumour progression.

Consequently, it will become increasingly important to identify means of primary prevention as a major thrust in controlling the burden of cancer worldwide. Rational approaches to primary prevention rely on a sound understanding of cause of disease, and understanding the causes of cancers is therefore an essential prerequisite.

Table 22.1 shows the most common cancers (excluding skin) in higher-income compared with lower-income countries. The incidence of specific cancers varies markedly between different geographical regions. For instance, age-standardized rates for nasopharyngeal cancer are around 100 times higher in regions of China than in Western industrialized nations, for colon cancer 20 times higher in the USA than in India, and for breast cancer they are seven times higher in the USA than in non-Jews in Israel (WCRF, 1997). Furthermore, these geographical variations are not static. For example, in Japan, colorectal cancer was extremely rare in the 1960s, but by 1985, rates had risen to become comparable with those in Western industrialized nations (Fig. 22 .2).

Worldwide, stomach cancer rates have fallen steeply over the past half-century. In addition, cancer rates may change when populations migrate. The low rates of breast and colon cancer, and high rates of stomach cancer, that were typical of the

Table 22.1 Common sites of cancer (listed in rank order) in developed countries and developing countries

Developed countries	Developing countries
Lung	Cervix
Large bowel	Stomach
Breast	Mouth
Stomach	Oesophagus
Prostate	Breast
Bladder	Lung

Skin cancers are not included because of difficulties involved in estimating incidence. The most serious of these, malignant melanoma, is more common in some countries, especially where fair-skinned people have a high exposure to sunlight (e.g. Australia, New Zealand, and South Africa).

Miyagi region of Japan were transformed amongst migrants from this population to Hawaii to resemble the local rates, with high incidence of colon and breast cancer and lower rates of stomach cancer, within one or two generations (Fig. 22.3).

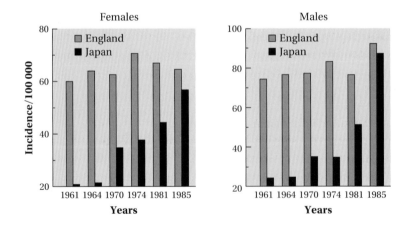

Fig. 22.2 Colorectal cancer incidence in women and men aged 55–60 in Miyagi, Japan and Birmingham, England.

Source: Parkin, D.M., Muir, C.S., Whelan, S.L., *et al.* (1992) *Cancer incidence in five continents.* Vol. I–VI. IARC, Lyon.

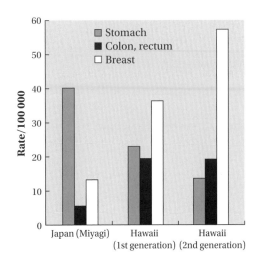

Fig. 22.3 Incidence of stomach, colon/rectum, and breast cancers in Japanese women by generation in Japan and Hawaii, 1968–1977.

The marked plasticity of these variations is amongst the strongest evidence for a major environmental determination for the patterns and rates of the common adult cancers, though childhood cancers do not appear to show the same effect. Twin studies also suggest that inherited genetic factors in general contribute only a small proportion to cancer risk, in the absence of uncommon germline mutations in specific genes, such as *BRCA1* and *BRCA2* for breast cancer. For instance, the identical twin of a male with bowel cancer has a 9% probability of developing the same cancer. Several studies over the past two decades have implicated food and nutrition as key environmental determinants of cancer risk. The authoritative review by the World Cancer Research Fund (2009) estimated that in the UK 39% and in the USA 34% of the most common cancers, and at least 26% and 24% of all cancers, could be attributed to poor diet and nutrition (including excess adiposity) and physical inactivity.

22.2 Biology of cancer

Cancer is a disease characterized by the development of a population of cells that have escaped normal regulation of growth, replication, and differentiation, and which invades surrounding or distant tissues. The maintenance of cellular and tissue integrity over a lifetime relies upon a tightly regulated series of processes, from cell division and DNA replication, through growth and differentiation, to programmed cell death (apoptosis). Cancer develops when a clone of abnormal cells acquires the ability to escape that regulation. At root, cancer results from abnormal cellular function and these abnormalities are the result of mutations—alterations in the nucleotide structure of DNA—most commonly acquired during life (somatic mutations). Nevertheless, in a few rare but important cases, such as familial polyposis coli, the abnormalities may be inherited (germline mutations).

The normal cell cycle incorporates several critical points that determine the future for that cell—whether to replicate, to terminally differentiate, or to undergo apoptosis. The cellular environment, including its nutrient environment, is an important determinant of the progress of the cell cycle. Cell division and DNA replication offer opportunities for errors to occur, resulting in mutation. Increasing elucidation of the regulation of cell division has enhanced understanding of those characteristics of cells that determine their behaviour, in particular whether or not they develop into an invasive tumour. An average human adult contains some 10^{10} cells, and over a lifetime will produce around 10^{16} cells, so perhaps the most remarkable phenomenon is the fact that abnormalities of these processes are not more common.

A developing body of evidence has led to an increasingly sophisticated understanding of the nature of the cellular characteristics that lead to cancer, and of the processes that influence them. Cancer cells display specific characteristics that confer particular capabilities, which are not present in normal cells; taken together these account for their abnormal behaviour. These abnormal capabilities influence aspects of cell growth, replication, and differentiation, as well as the way cells interact with their neighbouring cells and the extracellular environment.

Six of these phenotypic characteristics have been termed the 'hallmarks of cancer' and they are the basis for the abnormal behaviour of cells that leads to cancer. The six capabilities that characterize cancer cells but not normal cells are shown in Fig. 21.4.

Cells usually respond both to stimulatory and to inhibitory external growth signals, but cancer cells develop autonomy in growth that escapes the normal control mechanisms. Normal cells after a number of divisions usually undergo programmed cell death (apoptosis), a process that appears to protect the structural and functional integrity of cells and tissues, but cancer cells do not display this. On the contrary, the usual process whereby cells fail to divide further following a certain number of cell divisions is also disrupted, and abnormalities in the function of tel-

omeres (at the ends of DNA strands) appear to allow clones of cells to develop immortality through continuing division. Finally, the relations of cells with their external environment are altered. While normal cells closely constrain vascular development in growing tissues through secretion of chemoactive substances, cancer cells continue to promote unconstrained angiogenesis, thus allowing the development of a tumour mass. The several processes that ensure the controlled interaction between neighbouring cells is also lost, allowing a clone of cells with a selective growth advantage to exploit that by invading neighbouring tissues and eventually spreading to distant sites. Alone, each abnormality will not be sufficient to cause cancer, but together these characteristics are required for cells to behave as cancers. Each

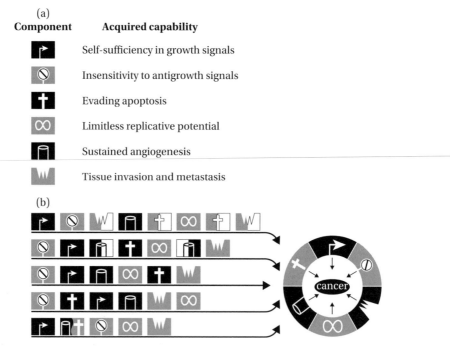

Fig. 22.4 The six capabilities needed for a cell to become cancerous can be acquired through different patterns of mutation. Five different possible pathways that all culminate in acquisition of these six characteristics by a cell are shown schematically. Each phenotypic capability may follow a single mutation, but may also result from two separate mutations. In contrast, a single mutation may cause (or contribute to) one (or more than one) phenotypic abnormality. For instance, in the eight-step pathway, two mutations are required each for tissue invasion and metastasis, and for evading apoptosis, whereas the other pathways require only one. In the five-step pathway, evading apoptosis and sustained angiogenesis both arise from one mutation.

represents a phenotypic abnormality that results from genetic mutation due to DNA damage, which has been acquired during the life of the cell or passed on from a parent cell. Each capability represents a complex set of functions, and may result from one mutation, or from a combination of mutations. Equally, a single mutation might contribute to more than one abnormal capability (Fig. 22.4). A cell has to accumulate all of these characteristics in order to generate the clone of cells that becomes a clinical cancer in a process of serial accumulation of DNA mutation leading to phenotypic abnormalities, in no special chronological sequence. This is a development from the previous model, which suggested three distinct chronological elements of initiation, promotion, and progression, based on studies of experimentally induced cancer using carcinogenic agents. It is estimated that the accumulation of sufficient genetic damage leading to clinically apparent tumours typically occurs over a period of one or two decades. This multistep time-dependent model is supported by the nonlinear, exponential increase in cancer with age (Fig. 22.1).

Table 22.2 lists the main known causes of cancers. These may exert their effects directly, for instance by causing DNA damage and mutation (e.g. ionizing radiation) or indirectly by promoting cell replication. The process of cell division and replication is itself a critically vulnerable time for DNA to accumulate and pass on errors to subsequent generations of cells. Factors that promote cell division therefore expose more cells to any environmental causes of cancer, whether nutritional or otherwise, and so increase the likelihood of mutation. Common factors that promote cell division include inflammation, especially chronic inflammation, and exposure to growth factors such as insulin-like growth factors (IGFs) or sex hormones, which promote growth in specifically sensitive tissues. Nutrition may further influence the intracellular environment directly, for instance by altering the concentration of specific nutrients involved in the regulation of the cell cycle. It may also contribute indirectly by influencing these general processes of inflammation or growth factors.

Nutritional factors that influence the intracellular environment directly or indirectly therefore have

Table 22.2 Factors increasing cancer risk

Environmental
Carcinogenic chemicals
Occupational
Food contamination
Smoking
Pollution
Infectious agents
Viruses (e.g. human papilloma virus, Epstein–Barr virus)
Bacteria (e.g. *Helicobacter pylori*)
Fungi (e.g. *Aspergillus* spp. producing mycotoxin)
Ionizing radiation
Exogenous hormones, e.g. growth factors
Intrinsic
Inherited germline mutations
Endogenous hormones, e.g. growth factors
Inflammation

potential to affect various aspects of the cell cycle, including abnormalities in DNA replication, and so also the likelihood of mutation. However, phenotypic expression depends on more than simply the genetic code based on the nucleotide sequence in DNA, which is altered by mutation. So-called epigenetic effects (those that result in altered gene expression without a change in the nucleotide sequence of DNA) may also have a profound impact on cellular phenotype. Alterations in histone (the protein core around which DNA helices are wound) can influence the overall stability of the genome, and DNA methylation can influence the expression of particular genes.

Therefore, nutritional factors that influence cell-cycle processes have potential for affecting the likelihood that a cell may eventually become cancerous, though the complexities of the processes make it likely that any impact will be the result of the interplay among many different influences.

22.3 Cause and prevention

A *cause* of any disease is any usual exposure that, if removed, reduces the likelihood of the disease developing, or its severity. Most conditions do not have a single cause, but are the result of an interaction among many causal factors. A factor that alone can result in a disease is a called a *sufficient* cause; if more than one factor is required, these are termed *contributory* causes; if a disease cannot occur in the absence of a factor, it is termed a *necessary* cause. Cancer is a condition that generally has several contributory causes. A key focus of research is to identify those factors or combinations of factors that are either necessary or sufficient for the development of cancer.

Controlled trials offer a robust way of testing causation directly by altering exposure in an experimental setting, so that, in well-designed studies, the outcomes can be attributed with confidence to the intervention applied. However, because there are many likely nutritional exposures of interest, and they are likely to interact, both amongst themselves and with other non-nutritional factors, conducting trials that are both well designed and encompass an appropriate range of exposures is usually impractical. Furthermore, trials are unlikely to take place over more than a small part of the many years during which the process of cancer development occurs. Consequently, well-designed trials exploring the causes of cancer tend to use high-risk individuals because they are more likely to progress to measurable outcomes, and to do so in a shorter time, than subjects drawn from the general population. Also, the exposures employed as interventions tend to be single nutrients given as supplements, often at unusually high doses, although some true diet intervention trials have been conducted. Finally, it is difficult either to conduct trials of diet in a truly blinded fashion, or to achieve sufficient sustained dietary change to differentiate between intervention and control groups. This means that, while positive results from such trials can be informative, negative results must be interpreted with caution.

Much of the evidence on the relationship between nutrition and cancer comes from observational epidemiology. These studies have the advantage that they can explore the relationship between hard outcomes and typical exposures in representative populations, but the lack of experimental design means that they are subject to confounding. Confounding distorts the apparent association between an exposure and outcome due to the effect of a third factor, which itself is a cause of the outcome but is also associated with the exposure. This means that by itself an association found between any nutritional factor and cancer in observational epidemiological studies cannot be assumed to be a causal one, although there are characteristics of the data that help to judge the likelihood of whether any such association is truly causal (such as the size of the effect or whether there is a dose–response effect). There are broadly two main types of epidemiological studies of individuals: prospective studies (often in cohorts of people followed up for many years), which record exposures such as diet or physical activity prior to diagnosis; and retrospective studies (often case–control), which record past exposure after diagnosis. It has become clear that, at least for diet and physical activity, retrospective assessments even in otherwise well-designed studies are subject to serious recall bias, making interpretation of data from them difficult.

In addition, as well as trials and epidemiology, there is a considerable body of evidence drawn from laboratory experiments, much of it on animals or from *in vitro* work on isolated tissues or cell lines. Although the direct relevance of much of this work to human cancer is remote, some types of experimental evidence are valuable contributors to understanding the mechanisms that might underpin observed associations in humans, particularly the more recent development of genetic manipulation (e.g. knockout models).

Consequently, in relation to causation of cancer, no single type of study can be regarded as paramount, and interpretation needs to embrace a consideration of several different sources of evidence.

The term 'prevention' is often taken to mean complete avoidance of an outcome. However, it can equally be applied to delay in its appearance (so deferring any adverse outcome, possibly beyond the natural lifespan) or to reduce risk in an individual, which translates to reduction in incidence in a population. In the latter case, an intervention that lowered incidence of an event from 50% to 25% will truly have prevented half the events, although it may never be possible to identify those particular individuals who would otherwise have been affected in the absence of the intervention. In the case of cancer, which has several contributory causes and probably no single necessary cause, interventions on some of them would not be expected to completely prevent cancer, but to reduce the likelihood of its occurrence or defer its appearance—this is also prevention.

22.4 Causes of cancer

There are several established classes of factors that are known to increase risk of developing cancer, due to increasing the likelihood of acquiring mutations in DNA that contribute to the cellular dysregulation characteristic of cancer (Table 22.2). Some factors may directly damage DNA as certain viruses or carcinogenic chemicals do, and others may promote replication and so increase the opportunity for other factors to operate, such as growth factors or inflammation (see Section 22.2).

Nutritional factors may operate either directly through one or more of these mechanisms or may interact with them, either reducing or enhancing their effects.

22.5 Nutrition and cancer

There is some evidence for a link between nutrition and most adult cancers. In addition, nutritional factors may show effects at more than one cancer site. These links were comprehensively reviewed by an expert panel based on a series of systematic reviews commissioned by the World Cancer Research Fund (2007). This report drew conclusions on the likely causality of associations between the principal adult cancers and foods, food components, physical activity, and obesity. They are set out together with known other causes in Table 22.3.

Because most evidence derives from observational epidemiology and from laboratory data on mechanisms, with only a few clinical trials, which are often difficult to interpret, the confidence of the conclusions on causal nutritional factors varies. In general, the confidence is greater for foods or food groups than for individual food components, because of the difficulty of excluding confounding by other food components. Similarly, direct anthropometric measures provide more reliable information than questionnaire-derived data. The number of nutritional factors listed in Table 22.3 is lower than appears in some other reviews because only those factors judged to be convincingly or probably causal factors have been highlighted. There is a plethora of food components for which a body of evidence exists, but which is inconclusive or limited either by the amount, nature, or quality of evidence. Increasingly, evidence is accruing of the influence of genetic and epigenetic variation on how nutritional factors affect the risk of various cancers. Such factors will be helpful in addressing some of these limitations, but methodological issues in the developing area mean that new data need careful interpretation (see Chapter 2).

Box 22.1 illustrates and explains the results of a meta-analysis of the observational studies that have examined the relationship between waist circumference and postmenopausal breast cancer.

Table 22.3 Associations between nutritional factors and common cancer sites. Other known causes of the cancers are also listed

Cancer site	Known causes	Nutritional factors decreasing risk	Nutritional factors increasing risk	Nutritional factors under investigation
Bladder	Tobacco smoking			
Breast (premenopausal)		Lactation ↓↓ Obesity ↓	Alcohol ↑↑ Greater growth in early life ↑	
Breast (postmenopausal)		Lactation ↓↓ Physical activity ↓	Alcohol ↑↑ Greater growth in early life ↑↑ Obesity ↑↑ Central obesity ↑ Adult weight gain ↑	
Cervix	Human papilloma virus			Folate ↓
Colorectum		Physical activity ↓↓ Foods containing nonstarch polysaccharide (dietary fibre) ↓ High-calcium diets ↓ Garlic ↓	Processed and red meat ↑↑ Obesity ↑↑ Greater growth in earlier life ↑↑ Alcohol ↑ (women), ↑↑ (men)	Vitamin D ↓ Fish and poultry ↓
Endometrium		Physical activity ↓	Obesity ↑↑ Central obesity ↑	
Gallbladder	Gallstones		Obesity ↑	
Kidney	Cigarette smoking		Obesity ↑↑	
Liver	Hepatitis and cirrhosis (viral, alcoholic)		Aflatoxin ↑↑ Alcohol ↑	
Lung	Tobacco smoking, radon	Fruits ↓	High-dose β-carotene supplements ↑↑ Arsenic ↑↑	
Mouth, larynx, and pharynx	Tobacco smoking	Fruits and vegetables ↓	Alcohol ↑↑	
Nasopharynx	Epstein–Barr virus		Cantonese-style salted fish ↑	

Table 22.3 *(Continued)*

Cancer site	Known causes	Nutritional factors decreasing risk	Nutritional factors increasing risk	Nutritional factors under investigation
Oesophagus	Tobacco smoking	Fruits and vegetables ↓	Obesity (adenocarcinoma) ↑↑ Alcohol ↑↑ Hot drinks (maté) ↑	
Ovary			Greater growth in early life ↑	
Pancreas	Tobacco smoking	Foods containing folate ↓	Obesity ↑ Central obesity ↑ Greater growth in early life ↑	Physical activity ↓
Prostate		Foods containing selenium ↓	High calcium diets ↑	Vitamin E ↓ Vitamin D ↓
Stomach	*Helicobacter pylori*	Fruit and vegetables ↓	High salt intake ↑	
Skin	Ionizing radiation		Arsenic ↑	
Testis				

↑↑, Convincingly causal nutritional factor increases risk; ↑, probably causal nutritional factor increases risk; ↓↓, Convincingly causal nutritional factor decreases risk; ↓, probably causal nutritional factor decreases risk.

BOX 22.1 The relationship between waist circumference and postmenopausal breast cancer

Visit the web page at http://www.oxfordtextbooks.co.uk/orc/mann4e/ to see a forest plot showing the results of a meta-analysis of observational studies of the relationship between waist circumference and postmenopausal breast cancer.

The columns describe the study identifier, the numbers of cases and controls in those with smaller and larger waists, the weight that the study contributed to the statistical analysis, based on factors such as the size of the study and the numbers of cases, and the relative risk with 95% confidence intervals.

The square boxes represent the relative risk for each study and the size of the box is proportional to the weight. The vertical line is the line of no effect. Where the relative risk is less than 1, that is, lower risk with a smaller waist, the box is to the left of the line, and where greater than 1, to the right. The lines through each box represent the 95% confidence intervals. Under each section is a diamond representing the combined summary estimate with 95% confidence intervals. The text to the left describes the statistical calculation of heterogeneity.

The different sections show results for cohort studies and case–control studies separately, first when adjusted for known confounders, and secondly when not so adjusted. The final section is a sub-group analysis cohort data in studies where it was possible to exclude the use of hormone replacement therapy.

(Continued)

BOX 22.1 The relationship between waist circumference and postmenopausal breast cancer (*Continued*)

This analysis shows a highly statistically significantly lower risk of postmenopausal breast cancer with smaller waist circumference from cohort studies. The risk is 39% lower (relative risk 0.61) in those with a waist circumference below compared with above the cut-off. Case–control studies do not show this effect, possibly due to recall bias or reverse causation. Low heterogeneity and the facts both that adjustment for confounders made little difference to the effect, and that the effect was maintained in those who had not had hormone replacement therapy, suggest that the association is robust.

This approach, together with laboratory data on mechanisms, forms the basis of much of our knowledge regarding the lifestyle-related determinants of cancer.

22.5.1 Foods, beverages, and cancer

Vegetables and fruits This broad category embraces a wide variety of different plant foods that might influence cancer risk. Much of the evidence is derived from case–control studies, but in general prospective cohort data and the few intervention trials have been less impressive. Therefore, interpretation needs to be cautious. Table 22.3 indicates that risk of colorectal, stomach, and lung cancers has been found to be lower amongst people with relatively high intakes of vegetables and fruits than among those consuming small quantities. There are several possible mechanisms that might underlie such associations.

Botanically, there is no clear distinction between the category of fruit (the seed-bearing parts of plants) and vegetables (a dietary description relating to the way foods are included as part of the diet). Many vegetables are, in fact, botanically fruits (e.g. courgettes, aubergines). Although there are compositional similarities within the group, different vegetables and fruits may have very different composition in relation to their micronutrient or nonnutrient composition. Even for a single type of vegetable or fruit, composition may vary several-fold with variety, season, and growing condition.

Components of vegetables and fruits that are relevant to their possible role in influencing cancer risk include the following:

- *Nonstarch polysaccharide/dietary fibre* can be fermented by the colonic flora to produce butyrate, which helps to maintain normal differentiation of colonocytes. It may reduce dietary energy density, which may aid energy balance, and it decreases colonic transit time, which may reduce the contact of colonic epithelium with carcinogens (see below).

- *Vitamins C and E and carotenoids* may act as antioxidants to prevent oxidative and possibly other damage to DNA, lipids, or proteins. Vitamin C may prevent formation of nitrosocompounds, which might be important for stomach cancer.

- *Glucosinolates* are found in brassica vegetables. They are enzymatically transformed by myrosinase released when the plant cells are damaged into *isothiocyanates*. These stimulate hepatic phase 2 enzymes, which conjugate and help excrete carcinogens. The effect of brassica vegetables in lung cancer is greatest in people who do not have an enzyme that eliminates isothiocyanates, making the association more likely to be causal.

- *Flavonoids, including phytoestrogens* from soy and other legumes have several antioxidant and potentially anti-oestrogenic actions.

- *Folate* is essential for normal DNA metabolism and for regulating gene expression.

- *Sulphur compounds* from *Allium* species (onions, garlic, etc.) have been shown in experimental studies to demonstrate anticancer potential, but more robust evidence in humans is lacking.

Meat, fish, poultry, and dairy These animal products are important sources of several nutrients, but higher intakes, typical of higher-income countries, have been linked with certain cancers. Processed and red meats have been linked to increased risk of colorectal cancer, while fish and poultry show an inverse association. Caution needs to be applied in interpretation, as definitions of 'processed meat' vary from country to country.

Dietary components associated with animal products that are relevant to their possible role in cancer include the following:

- *Iron* is abundant in meat and meat products as haem, in which form it is more easily assimilated than in the inorganic form in vegetables. Evidence for the proposal that iron might increase risk of colorectal cancer through its action, in its free form, as a pro-oxidant is not convincing. There is some evidence that cooked meat protein can form heterocyclic amines, which might increase colorectal cancer risk, but this remains speculative. It appears that haem, rather than the iron *per se*, from meat and meat products is susceptible to endogenous nitrosation by bacterial flora in the colon, and these *N*-nitrosocompounds can increase the likelihood of neoplastic change. This effect is not shared by fish or poultry.

- *Calcium* is principally found in milk and dairy products in higher-income Western countries, but in many parts of the world these are not a major part of the diet. There is preliminary evidence from epidemiological studies in Western countries, and from trials of a few years duration on recurrence of adenomas (necessary precursors of cancer, though not all progress), that calcium might reduce risk of colorectal cancer, possibly by forming insoluble soaps and limiting any carcinogenic effect of free fatty acids or bile salts. However, because there is also evidence that such diets may promote aggressive forms of prostate cancer, it is not straightforward to make recommendations.

- *Vitamin D* is mainly found in animal products but is also derived from endogenous formation in the skin. As well as its role in calcium and bone metabolism, vitamin D is an important modulator of cell differentiation and communication. There is increasing epidemiological evidence that people with higher blood concentrations of vitamin D have lower risk of colorectal cancer. It has been proposed that the strong effect of latitude on prostate cancer risk might be mediated by vitamin D status, but this is not supported by epidemiological studies.

- *Total fat* may be derived from both animal and vegetable sources, but the predominant sources of fat in high-income countries are animal products. Ecological studies suggest higher rates of breast cancer with higher fat intakes, but large prospective cohorts predominantly from the USA have been negative. A large study showed that an intervention to reduce fat intake, but which also had other effects (reduced meat, increased fruit and vegetables, weight loss), modestly reduced risk of recurrent breast cancer in postmenopausal women. It is not clear whether any effect is due to the total fat itself or the proportions and amounts of different fatty acids (see below), or to other aspects of diet or lifestyle.

- *Fatty acids* may have specific effects on cancer causation. In animal models, a high intake of linoleic acid (around 12% of energy) seems to promote tumour progression, and this effect may be countered by increasing n-3 fatty acid intake; this has not been confirmed in humans. Specific mechanisms have not been identified.

Starchy staples In most parts of the world, starchy staples are the predominant energy source, but this is less so in high-income countries. The amount and type of starchy food consumed has been proposed as a major factor in determining global cancer patterns.

Factors associated with starchy foods that are relevant to any effect on cancer include:

- *Nonstarch polysaccharide (dietary fibre) and resistant starch*. They have long been implicated as protective factors against colorectal cancer. However, because of difficulties of definition, the precise role that undigestible plant components play is not fully resolved. Nevertheless, there is good epidemiological evidence that higher dietary fibre intakes are associated with lower risk of colorectal cancer. Both nonstarch polysaccharide and resistant starch escape digestion in the small bowel and provide substrate for the colonic flora, which ferment them to release short-chain fatty acids, including butyrate, which helps to maintain the integrity of the colonocyte DNA. In addition, fibre increases stool bulk and decreases transit time, both of which may reduce the opportunity for colonocytes to be in contact with faecal carcinogens. Short-term trials using certain forms of dietary fibre supplements have not shown an effect on adenoma recurrence, but it is not clear whether these experimental results can be extrapolated more generally.

More recently, studies have explored the links between wholegrain cereals and cancer risk, but due to variation in definition, these are difficult to interpret. Any mechanisms underlying observed effects are likely to include the role of dietary fibre, intake of which is intimately associated with whole grains.

Selenium Selenium intake in populations is determined by its concentration in the soil, and where this is high, cereal products are the major source. Rich sources include nuts (especially brazil nuts), shellfish, and meat. Selenium is an important cofactor for several enzymes, including glutathione peroxidase, which is a major antioxidant. A trial found unexpectedly that prostate cancer (not a prior stated outcome) was markedly reduced after selenium supplementation, particularly in men with lower selenium status. Although the epidemiology is moderately consistent, a subsequent well-conducted trial failed to find any effect of selenium supplementation.

Salt The main cause of stomach cancer is agreed to be infection with *H. pylori*. High salt intake appears to interact with this to influence risk. Stomach cancer rates are highest in those parts of the world with the highest salt intakes, e.g. China, Japan. In all countries, there has been a marked decline in stomach cancer rates over the past 50 years, attributed in part to lower salt intakes with increased use of other preservative methods. High salt intake increases risk of atrophic gastritis, which

not only may render the stomach more susceptible to *H. pylori* infection, but also increases the susceptibility of the mucosa to neoplastic change once infection is established.

There is also strong evidence that Cantonese-style so-called salted fish increases risk of nasopharyngeal cancer, especially when consumed in childhood. The term 'salted fish' is misleading as this form of fish, while certainly salty, is only partly preserved and is partly putrefied. The presence of *N*-nitrosocompounds in fish resulting from the putrefaction is thought to account for the effect.

Alcohol Alcohol is classed as a carcinogen by the World Health Organization (WHO) International Agency for Research on Cancer. Higher consumption of alcohol increases risk of cancers of the mouth, larynx, and pharynx, where it acts synergistically with tobacco smoking. It also increases risk of breast cancer, with no apparent threshold for an effect. Heavy alcohol consumption can lead to cirrhosis of the liver, which itself increases risk of liver cancer, irrespective of cause. It is less clear that alcohol *per se* has a specific effect. The main cause of hepatitis and cirrhosis worldwide is hepatitis C, though in high-income countries alcohol remains a major cause.

22.5.2 Energy balance, obesity, physical activity, growth, and cancer

Energy Energy restriction is amongst the most consistent and powerful means of reducing cancer in experimental animals, including primates. So long as nutrient demands are otherwise met, energy-restricted animals have lower age-specific cancer incidence and prolonged life. It is not straightforward to extrapolate these findings to free-living humans, but clearly energy metabolism is implicated in modulating cancer risk in whole-body systems.

Obesity Obesity shows one of the most consistent epidemiological associations with cancer, and increases risk of cancers of the colorectum, breast (in postmenopausal women), endometrium, kidney, oesophagus (adenocarcinoma), and gallbladder. Obesity has several metabolic effects that may account for its effects on cancer risk. Obesity increases insulin resistance and plasma concentrations of insulin, affects binding proteins for IGFs, and also influences the sex hormone axes. It is also an inflammatory state. Many of these physiological effects are reversed by weight loss and data from extremely obese subjects who lost weight after bariatric surgery suggest that the increased cancer risk might also be reversible.

Physical activity The level of physical activity is a major modifiable determinant of energy expenditure, and so of risk of obesity. Increasingly, physical activity is also recognized as an independent modulator of cancer risk. Higher levels of physical activity are associated with lower risk of cancers of the breast, colorectum, pancreas, and lung. Physical activity has several metabolic effects that are relevant to cancer risk. Increasing activity increases insulin sensitivity and reduces insulin levels, increases concentrations of binding proteins for IGFs, and influences the sex hormone axes in both men and women. Higher levels of activity decrease colonic transit time.

Growth Increasingly it is recognized that adult health and susceptibility to disease is influenced not only by genetic background and contemporary environmental exposures (including diet), but also by events occurring from conception onward, which may influence development at critical stages of maturation, resulting in permanent alterations. This so-called programming has been best described in relation to cardiovascular disease, but there is evidence for an effect in cancer, though it has so far not been studied in depth. It has long been known that taller women, and earlier menarche, are associated with higher breast cancer risk. It is now thought that this represents an effect of permanent alteration of the IGF axis, manifest by greater early growth. It is likely that the causal component is lifelong exposure to higher levels of growth factors. The secondary effect of early menarche is to increase lifetime exposure to oestrogens, which may have an independent effect.

22.5.3 Contaminants, cooking and dietary supplements, and cancer

Worldwide, food and drink contamination remains a serious problem. High levels of arsenic in drinking water, for instance in Bangladesh, and aflatoxin contamination of grain, for instance in China and Africa, are the principal known contaminants associated with cancer.

Aflatoxin Aflatoxin is a toxin and known carcinogen resulting from fungal infestation of grain stored in warm, humid conditions typical of subtropical regions of Asia, especially China and Thailand, and in parts of Africa, where its consumption is associated with liver cancer. Recent work that relates its effect on liver cancer risk to genetic differences in the ability to metabolize it adds weight to the likelihood of this association being causal.

Cooking Heat causes chemical reactions in proteins and carbohydrates that might have adverse effects. The high-temperature frying of starchy carbohydrates produces significant quantities of acrylamide, a known carcinogen. In addition, charring of meat as in barbecuing produces polycyclic aromatic hydrocarbons and heterocyclic amines that have been shown to have carcinogenic potential in laboratory animals. However, there is no epidemiological evidence to suggest that the carcinogenic potential of these processes and substances is actually realized in free-living humans.

Dietary supplements For practical reasons, intervention studies of diet and cancer usually use purified supplements of micronutrients rather than attempting to achieve sustained dietary change. This methodology has the advantage of providing robust answers, but the disadvantage of being difficult to extrapolate to the usual free-living situation. In general, with the exception of calcium in relation to colorectal cancer (see above), dietary supplementation has failed to demonstrate consistent effects over the short term on cancer risk. The possible reasons for this include a true lack of effect, a failure to address any more complex interactions, inappropriate dose or form of the nutrient, and timing or duration of the intervention. Consequently, the knowledge gained from negative outcomes of such trials is limited.

22.5.4 Nutrition in the management of cancer

This section is not concerned with interventions over the acute stage but rather in the stable situations before or after therapeutic interventions. The relevant question in the context of nutrition interventions in people with cancer is one of efficacy: does this intervention influence outcome in people who have already had a diagnosis of cancer? Outcome may refer to survival, to rate of recurrence, or progression of a cancer, or to development of a new cancer, or to quality of life. Given that the population is easily defined and that outcomes are likely to occur in a relatively short time, randomized controlled trials are an appropriate tool to offer a 'best' answer, especially as retrospective observational data are particularly likely to suffer from several forms of bias in this clinical setting.

Unfortunately, few trials have been reported, and those are mainly small and with diverse interventions and outcome measures. Thus, it is difficult to be confident about what might be an appropriate, safe, and effective nutrition intervention in people with cancer.

The largest study in this situation (the Women's Intervention Nutrition Study) was aimed at reducing fat intake in postmenopausal women who had completed their treatment for breast cancer. The study showed a small but statistically and clinically meaningful reduction in recurrence of breast cancer, although the intervention resulted in many changes other than in fat consumption, including an increase in fruit and vegetable consumption.

There is some prospective observational evidence that obesity at or prior to diagnosis may lead to lower survival. However, there are several stages between baseline and outcome (times to diagnosis, treatment, and post-treatment) and this makes the information difficult to interpret.

Overall, the evidence is weak but suggests that women with breast cancer might benefit from a conventional, balanced diet rich in vegetables and fruits, low in fat, especially saturated fat, and from increasing physical activity and avoiding obesity and overweight.

Table 22.4 Recommendations for the prevention of cancer through food, nutrition, and physical activity

Body fatness	Be as lean as possible within the normal limit
Physical activity	Be physically active as part of everyday life
Foods and drinks that promote weight gain	Limit consumption of energy-dense foods Avoid sugary drinks
Plant foods	Eat mostly foods of plant origin
Animal foods	Limit intake of red meat and avoid processed meat
Alcoholic drinks	Limit alcoholic drinks
Preservation, processing, preparation	Limit consumption of salt Avoid mouldy cereals (grains) or pulses (legumes)
Dietary supplements	Aim to meet nutritional needs through diet alone
Breastfeeding	Mothers to breastfeed; children to be breastfed

Source: WCRF/AICR (2007) *Food, nutrition, physical activity and the prevention of cancer: A global perspective.* Washington, DC, American Institute for Cancer Research.

There is insufficient evidence to make recommendations in respect of other cancers. It cannot be assumed that the response to particular dietary patterns or specific nutrients in cancer patients, whose nutritional demands may differ from normal, would be similar to healthy people.

22.6 Recommendations

Several authoritative reviews have made recommendations for the prevention of cancer through food, nutrition, and physical activity (COMA, 1998; WCRF, 1997; WHO, 2003). The most recent from WCRF (2007) are set out in Table 22.4. Notably, these recommendations for cancer prevention are consonant with recommendations for other chronic disease, in particular cardiovascular disease. Broadly, the recommendations from WCRF are similar to those in the earlier reports and from other authoritative bodies. The similarity of the conclusions and recommendations from these differently constituted groups adds to the robustness of their interpretations.

22.7 Policy implications

The rising numbers of cases of cancer around the world have focused attention on how best to implement the various recommendations for cancer prevention. Simply providing information is recognized as being inadequate to generate change, and to tend to widen socioeconomic inequalities in health. An expert panel commissioned by WCRF based on systematic reviews of the evidence sought to identify evidence-based policy and other action that showed promise in promoting changes in diet, body fatness, and physical activity to help prevent cancer, while recognizing that such changes would also prevent other chronic diseases including obesity, diabetes, and cardiovascular disease (WCRF, 2009).

The conclusions of the report hinge on the need for action across society, by actors in a wide variety of settings, mostly outside the health domain. Success is characterized by integrated action across these settings, and so requires leadership from government and health professionals, though it is necessary for everybody, whether as an individual or in their employment, to recognize that they share responsibility for improving public health.

The groups of actors that were identified are multinational bodies, industry, government, schools, civil society organizations, media, workplaces and institutions, health and other professionals, and people themselves.

It is important to recognize that there is a substantial and growing evidence base for effective actions by actors in all these settings, which would help achieve the recommendations for prevention of cancer and other diseases.

Conclusions

There is considerable epidemiological, clinical, and laboratory evidence for an impact of nutrition, including physical activity, on risk of developing many adult cancers. For methodological reasons, identifying specific links depends on judgement of several different types of evidence, but conclusions can be drawn. In contrast, there is relatively little evidence for the effect of nutrition on outcome in people with cancer.

Most cancers will have several contributory causes. The inherent methodological complexities, and the as-yet unclear impact of genetic and epigenetic variation, mean that the precise roles of different foods, nutrients, and other food components will be unlikely to be fully elucidated in the near future. Although much remains to be learned, a substantial improvement in public health could already be achieved by applying current knowledge both of the links between food, nutrition, physical activity, and cancer and other diseases, and of effective actions and policies.

Further Reading

1. **Committee on Medical Aspects of Food and Nutrition Policy (COMA)** (1998) *Nutritional aspects of the development of cancer*. London, The Stationery Office.
2. **Doll, R. and Peto, R.** (1981) The causes of cancer: Quantitative estimates of avoidable risks of cancer in the United States today. *J Nat Cancer Inst*, **66**, 1191–308.
3. **Hanahan, D. and Weinberg, R.** (2000) The hallmarks of cancer. *Cell*, **100**, 57–70.
4. **International Agency for Research on Cancer** (2002) *Weight control and physical activity*. Lyon, IARC Press.
5. **International Agency for Research on Cancer** (2003) *Fruit and vegetables*. Lyon, IARC Press.
6. **International Agency for Research on Cancer** (2004) *World Cancer Report*. Lyon, IARC Press.
7. **Key, T., Schatzkin, A., Willett, W., Allen, N., Spencer, E., and Travis, R.** (2004) Diet, nutrition and the prevention of cancer. *Publ Hlth Nutr*, **7**, 187–200.
8. **Parkin, D.M., Muir, C.S., Whelan, S.L., et al.** (1992) *Cancer incidence in five continents*. Vol. I–VI. IARC, Lyon.
9. **World Cancer Research Fund (WRCF)** (1997) *Food, nutrition and the prevention of cancer. A global perspective*. Washington, DC, American Institute for Cancer Research.
10. **World Cancer Research Fund (WRCF)** (2007) *Food, nutrition, physical activity, and the prevention of cancer. A global perspective*. Washington, DC, American Institute for Cancer Research.
11. **World Cancer Research Fund (WRCF)** (2009) *Policy and action for cancer prevention*. Washington, DC, American Institute for Cancer Research.
12. **WHO** (2002) *World Health Report*. Geneva, World Health Organization.
13. **WHO** (2003) *Diet, nutrition and the prevention of chronic diseases*. WHO Technical Report, Series 916, Geneva, World Health Organization.

Useful Websites

To see topical and scientifically robust updates on nutrition associated with this textbook and web links to many of the journals in the Further Reading sections, please see the dedicated Online Resource Centre at **http://www.oxfordtextbooks.co.uk/orc/mann4e/**

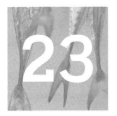

23 Diabetes mellitus and the metabolic syndrome

Jim Mann

Diabetes mellitus

Diabetes mellitus, a condition associated with loss of sugar in the urine, has been diagnosed by physicians for at least three millennia. Until the discovery of insulin in the 1920s, dietary treatment was all that could be offered to people with diabetes. Although dietary advice has altered over the years, reduction and sometimes near elimination of sugars and other carbohydrates formed the cornerstone of management for much of the time until the 1970s, when the merits of a diet low in carbohydrate, and consequently high in fat, were questioned.

The term 'diabetes mellitus' is more appropriately used to describe a group of conditions characterized by raised blood glucose levels (hyperglycaemia) resulting from an absolute or relative deficiency of insulin. In type 1 diabetes (T1DM), previously known as insulin-dependent diabetes, IDDM, there is destruction of the insulin-producing pancreatic islet β-cells usually resulting from an autoimmune process. Insulin treatment, administered by subcutaneous injection, is essential to maintain life. In type 2 diabetes (T2DM), previously non-insulin-dependent diabetes (NIDDM), a key abnormality is resistance to the action of insulin, and in the early stages of the disease, insulin levels may actually be raised as the β-cells of the pancreas produce more insulin in an attempt to overcome the insulin resistance. In many patients with T2DM, the insulin-producing β-cells of the islets in the pancreas may show a degree of failure at some stage during the course of the disease process. Patients with T2DM are initially treated with 'lifestyle modification' therapy. Oral hypoglycaemic (blood glucose-lowering) agents may be added. Insulin may be required later. Impaired glucose tolerance (IGT), impaired fasting glucose (IFG), and gestational diabetes (diabetes developing during pregnancy) may represent the earliest stages of T2DM and are sometimes referred to as prediabetes.

Hyperglycaemia usually leads to glycosuria (glucose in the urine) when the renal threshold for glucose (level up to which glucose is reabsorbed in the renal tubules) is exceeded. Hyperglycaemia and glycosuria result in the classical symptoms of diabetes: polyuria (passing large quantities of urine), polydipsia (thirst), blurring of vision, increased susceptibility to infections, and unintentional weight loss.

23.1 Clinical features of diabetes

T1DM is invariably associated with marked symptoms of hyperglycaemia and often striking unintentional weight loss. If untreated, the absence of insulin leads to severe metabolic disturbances (ketoacidosis), during which the patient may become unconscious and which may be fatal without insulin treatment and correction of fluid and electrolyte imbalance. The diagnosis of T1DM is usually straightforward because blood glucose levels are markedly raised.

In T2DM, symptoms are invariably less severe and ketoacidosis does not occur. IFG, IGT, gestational (pregnancy) diabetes (collectively sometimes known as prediabetes) and about half of all cases of T2DM are without symptoms. Diabetes is diagnosed if random venous plasma glucose is greater than 11.0 mmol/L or the fasting value is greater than 7 (two measurements are required if the person is asymptomatic). A glucose tolerance test (measurement of blood glucose fasting and 2 hours after a 75-g glucose load) may be required to diagnose the prediabetic states and those with borderline blood glucose levels (Table 23.1). The possibility of using haemoglobin A_{1c} (HbA_{1c}) rather than, or in addition to glucose levels as a means of diagnosing diabetes or prediabetes is currently being considered. HbA_{1c} is a measure of glucose levels over a prolonged period of time (the past 6 weeks) to determine the adequacy of diabetes control.

Both types of diabetes may be associated with hypertension and a range of metabolic disturbances, which, together with the hyperglycaemia, help to explain the wide-ranging complications of diabetes that account for much of the ill health and premature death associated with diabetes.

The complications result chiefly from the effects on the arterial and nervous systems. They include diabetic retinopathy, which may lead to blindness, diabetic nephropathy potentially resulting in kidney failure, foot ulceration, which may lead to gangrene, several different neurological conditions, and cardiovascular disease (coronary heart disease and stroke), the most common causes of early death. Interestingly, age-standardized coronary heart disease rates are similar in men and women with diabetes, whereas in the general population, women have appreciably lower rates than men.

Table 23.1 Venous plasma glucose levels for the diagnosis of diabetes, impaired glucose tolerance, and impaired fasting glucose

	Fasting glucose (mmol/L)	2 hours after 75 g glucose (mmol/L)
Diabetes	>7.0	>11.0
Impaired fasting glucose	6.0–7.0	<7.8
Impaired glucose tolerance	<6.0	7.8–11.0
'Normal' glucose tolerance	<6.0	<7.8

23.2 Epidemiology and aetiology of type 2 diabetes

23.2.1 Epidemiology of type 2 diabetes

Worldwide, T2DM is overwhelmingly more common than T1DM. Thus, global statistics relating to 'diabetes' principally reflect frequencies of T2DM. Data relating to trends over time are not particularly reliable because diagnostic criteria have changed, as have diagnostic facilities and rates of screening. These are clearly important determinants of prevalence rates, especially as so many cases are asymptomatic and may not be diagnosed until complications occur. Despite these reservations, there is no longer any doubt about the true worldwide increase in prevalence, resulting both from a tendency towards ageing populations (T2DM has been clearly shown to increase in frequency with age) and increased incidence at all ages. In the developed world in populations principally of European descent, the increase has been steady. However, in some other population groups, there have been dramatic increases in prevalence associated either with migration or with a rapid change from a traditional (non-Western) lifestyle to increased consumption of energy-dense foods, high in fats and sugars, and reduced levels of physical activity. The American Pima Indians, Polynesians and Melanesians in the South Pacific, Australian Aboriginals, and Asian Indian migrants to the UK and other countries are examples of populations in which the process of rapid acculturation has led to diabetes prevalence rates far higher than those observed in European populations. Diabetes is believed to affect 7% of the world's adult population, with 300 million having the condition. India and China have relatively high rates of diabetes and are two of the most populous countries in the world. Thus India is the country with the most people with diabetes, with a current figure of 50.8 million, followed by China with 43.2 million. If the current rates of growth continue unchecked, it has been estimated that by 2030, the total number of people with diabetes worldwide will exceed 435 million. In addition to those with diabetes, there are many with prediabetes. For example, amongst adult Maori, the indigenous people of New Zealand, almost half the adult population have been found to have an abnormality of carbohydrate metabolism. In some of these groups, T2DM, previously regarded as a disease of the middle-aged and elderly, has recently been diagnosed in teenagers and children. Thus, T2DM may be regarded as one of the major epidemic diseases of the twenty-first century. Worldwide prevalence estimates of diabetes are shown in Fig. 23.1.

23.2.2 Aetiology of type 2 diabetes and its complications

From the earliest times until recently, the sugary urine and raised levels of blood glucose have led to the assumption that an excessive intake of sucrose (table sugar) must be an important cause of the condition. While sugar may play a role, it is, on its own, not an important cause. A totally consistent observation in prospective as well as cross-sectional studies is the striking association between risk of T2DM and increasing obesity (Fig. 23.2), particularly when the excess body fat is centrally distributed, i.e. in association with a high waist circumference. It is also clear that there is a strong genetic component to this condition.

The risk of developing T2DM is greatly increased when one or more close family members have the condition, although the precise mode of inheritance has not yet been resolved. It appears therefore that, in predisposed populations or families, genetic and lifestyle factors combine to result in the development of insulin resistance and consequently diabetes. The relative importance of genetic and lifestyle factors is well illustrated by diabetes rates in Pima Indians. Although rates amongst the American Pima Indians are amongst the highest in the world, a genetically similar group living in the mountainous regions of Mexico have relatively low rates. They still follow a traditional way of life unexposed to Western ways and diet and have a high level of physical activity.

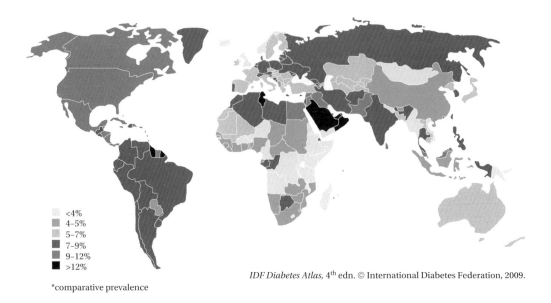

Fig. 23.1 Prevalence (%) estimates of diabetes (20–79 years, 2010).

Source: IDF (2009) *IDF Diabetes Atlas*, 4th edn. Brussels, International Diabetes Federation. http://www.diabetesatlas.org

There have been several attempts to implicate individual foods or nutrients as causal or protective factors in the aetiology of T2DM independent of any association they have with overweight or obesity. It is likely that more than one of the attributes that characterize the Western lifestyle (excessive intakes of energy-dense foods; relatively low intakes of vegetables, fruits, and lightly processed cereal foods with intact cellular structure; inadequate physical activity) contribute to the aetiology. One very large prospective study involving health professionals in the USA has suggested that diets with a high glycaemic load and low cereal fibre content increase the risk of T2DM (Fig. 23.3). The glycaemic load provides an indication of both glycaemic index (GI) (see Chapter 3) and quantity of carbohydrate.

A high intake of saturated fatty acids increases resistance to the action of insulin and is therefore likely to increase the risk of developing T2DM. Intrauterine growth retardation leading to babies born small for dates and prematurity have been suggested as risk factors for the development T2DM in later life. This appears to be especially the case when rapid catch-up growth occurs in infancy and childhood (fetal programming or 'Barker' hypothesis).

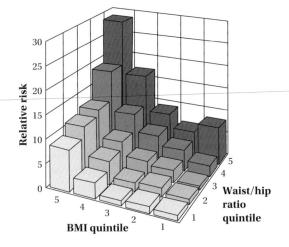

Fig. 23.2 Age-adjusted relative risk of incident diabetes according to quintiles of body mass index (BMI) and waist/hip ratio, Iowa Women's Health Study, 1986 to 1996. Cut points were 22.80, 24.87, 27.06, and 30.21 kg/m² for BMI; 0.762, 0.805, 0.848 and 0.901 for waist/hip ratio.

Source: Folsom, A.R., Kushi, L.H., Anderson, K.E., *et al.* (2000) Associations of general and abdominal obesity with multiple health outcomes in older women: The Iowa Women's Health Study. *Arch Intern Med*, **160**, 2117–28.

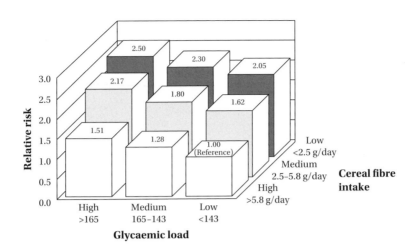

Fig. 23.3 Relative risk of type 2 diabetes mellitus by different levels of cereal fibre intake and glycaemic load. The highest risk is apparent among those who have both a low fibre intake and a diet with a high glycaemic load.

Source: Salmerón, J., Manson, J.E., Stampfer, M.J., *et al.* (1997) Dietary fiber, glycemic load, and risk of non-insulin-dependent diabetes mellitus in women. *JAMA*, **277**, 472–7.

The various lifestyle-related factors considered by the WHO/FAO Expert Consultation on Diet, Nutrition and the Prevention of Chronic Diseases (TR 916) believed to be convincingly or probably related to risk of developing T2DM are shown in Box 23.1. Since the publication of this report, a meta-analysis has suggested a protective effect of green leafy vegetables but not other vegetables and fruits and further evidence has emerged regarding a possible protective role for magnesium. No additional data have emerged regarding the other factors listed in the 'possible' or 'insufficient' columns and obesity continues to be accepted as the principal driver of the diabetes epidemic.

Several complications of diabetes (e.g. retinopathy, nephropathy, and neuropathy) appear to be a result of hyperglycaemia and other metabolic consequences of diabetes and hypertension. Diet plays a role in their prevention and treatment principally by helping to improve blood glucose control and lower blood pressure (see Section 23.5). Cardiovascular disease, which is responsible for the greatest number of deaths and much non-fatal illness in people with T2DM, seems to be even more closely linked to dietary factors. There appear to be some risk factors for coronary heart disease (CHD) which are more important in people with diabetes than in the population at large (Table 23.2). They may help to explain the great excess of CHD in this condition. However, other important determinants of atherogenesis and thrombogenesis seem to be similar in those with and without diabetes. Many are diet-related (see Chapter 21). In countries with low CHD rates in the general population, CHD is also relatively infrequent in people with diabetes. Thus a major focus of dietary recommendations for people with diabetes relates to the need to reduce cardiovascular risk.

23.3 Reducing the risk of type 2 diabetes

While the precise mechanisms by which genes and lifestyle interact to result in T2DM remain elusive, the geographic variation, rapid changes over time, and dietary patterns related to risk suggest that

BOX 23.1 Summary of strength of evidence on lifestyle factors and risk of developing type 2 diabetes

Evidence	Decreased risk	Increased risk
Convincing	Voluntary weight loss in overweight and obese people Physical activity	Overweight and obesity Abdominal obesity Physical inactivity Maternal diabetes[a]
Probable	Non-starch polysaccharides	Saturated fats Intrauterine growth retardation
Possible	ω-3 fatty acids Low glycaemic index foods Exclusive breastfeeding[b]	Total fat intake *trans*-fatty acids
Insufficient	Vitamin E Chromium Magnesium Moderate alcohol	Excess alcohol

[a]Includes gestational diabetes.

[b]As a global public health recommendation, infants should be exclusively breastfed for the first 6 months of life to achieve optimal growth, development, and health.

Source: WHO (2003) *Diet, nutrition and the prevention of chronic diseases.* WHO Technical Report Series 916. Geneva, World Health Organization.

Table 23.2 Risk factors for coronary heart disease (CHD) in people with type 2 diabetes

Risk factors that may be of particular relevance	General CHD risk factors that are also relevant in type 2 diabetes
↑ Triglycerides and very-low-density lipoproteins	↑ Total cholesterol and low density lipoprotein
↑ Small, dense, low-density lipoprotein particles	Hypertension
↓ High-density lipoproteins	Cigarette smoking
↑ Oxidation of low-density lipoprotein	Obesity, especially when centrally distributed
↑ Platelet aggregation	Physical inactivity
↑ Plasminogen activator inhibitor	
↑ Pro-insulin-like molecules	
Microalbuminuria	

↑, increased; ↓, decreased.

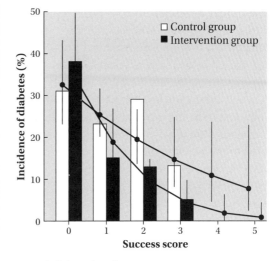

No. with diabetes / Total no.

Intervention group	5/13	10/66	9/69	2/38	0/25	0/24
Control group		15/48	25/107	14/48	2/15	0/11	0/4

Fig. 23.4 Incidence of diabetes during follow-up, according to the success score. At the 1-year visit, each subject received a grade of 0 for each intervention goal that had not been achieved and a grade of 1 for each goal that had been achieved; the success score was computed as the sum of the grades. The association between the success score and the risk of diabetes, with 95% confidence intervals, was estimated by means of logistic-regression analysis of the observed data. The curves show the model-based incidence of diabetes according to the success score as a continuous variable; the curve whose data points align with the open bars represents the model-based incidence for the control group, and the curve whose data points align with the shaded bars represents the model-based incidence for the intervention group.

Source: Tuomilehto, M.D., Lindström, M.S., Eriksson, J.G., *et al.* (2001) Prevention of type 2 diabetes mellitus by changes in lifestyle among subjects with impaired glucose tolerance. *N Engl J Med*, **344**, 1343–50.

lifestyle modification might help to prevent, or at least delay, the onset of T2DM in predisposed individuals. Randomized controlled trials, first reported from Finland, the USA, and China and more recently from other countries, confirm that this is indeed the case. The target interventions (Box 23.2) have generally resulted in an approximately 60% reduction in rates of progression from IGT to T2DM over an approximately 4-year follow-up period. Of particular interest is the fact that in the Finnish study remarkably few of those individuals who complied with most of the five target interventions progressed from IGT to T2DM (Fig. 23.4). Follow-up data suggest that even after withdrawing the intensive intervention provided in the Finnish and US studies, the risk reduction has been maintained for periods of up to 10 years. Similar lifestyle interventions have been shown to increase insulin sensitivity in insulin-resistant individuals prior to the development of IGT or diabetes. These observations suggest

that in groups or populations with high rates of diabetes, it is appropriate to screen high-risk individuals (in particular those with central adiposity, a family history of diabetes, and those with other cardiovascular risk factors) so that preventative measures may be started in those with prediabetes and treatment initiated in those who have already developed the disease. In addition, population-based advice to increase physical activity and to adopt appropriate dietary measures to reduce overweight and obesity will be essential for primary prevention and reducing the epidemic proportions of the disease. The fetal programming hypothesis has led to the reinforcement of the importance of appropriate maternal nutrition as a means of reducing the risk of T2DM, but the strength of evidence regarding the influencing of growth in infancy and childhood by manipulating dietary intake (see Section 23.3) is regarded as insufficient to justify recommendations. The specific recommendations for reducing the risk of T2DM, according to the WHO/FAO Technical Consultation TR916, are shown in Box 23.3.

BOX 23.3 Specific recommendations for reducing the risk of type 2 diabetes

- Prevention/treatment of overweight and obesity, particularly in high-risk groups
- Maintaining an optimum BMI, i.e. at the lower end of the normal range. For the adult population, this means maintaining a mean BMI in the range 21–23 kg/m² and avoiding weight gain (>5 kg) in adult life
- Voluntary weight reduction in overweight or obese individuals with impaired glucose tolerance
- Practising an endurance activity at moderate or greater level of intensity (e.g. brisk walking)

- for 1 hour or more per day on most days per week
- Ensuring that saturated fat intake does not exceed 10% of total energy and for high-risk groups, this should be <7% of total energy
- Achieving adequate intakes of non-starch polysaccharides through regular consumption of wholegrain cereals, legumes, fruits, and vegetables

Source: WHO (2003) *Diet, nutrition and the prevention of chronic diseases.* WHO Technical Report Series 916. Geneva, World Health Organization.

23.4 Epidemiology and aetiology of type 1 diabetes

The frequency of T1DM also shows marked geographic variation. For example, the incidence rates of childhood diabetes (under 15 years) in Europe, ranges from 3.2 cases per 100 000 per year in Macedonia to 40.2 per 100 000 per year in parts of Finland.

In many countries, there have been considerable increases in incidence in recent years. As an example, the increase in incidence in children aged less than 10 in Norway is shown in Fig. 23.5. Although the total number of cases in all countries is appreciably lower than the number of cases of T2DM, the proportional increase has been comparable or greater in many countries. The frequency does not parallel that of T2DM and there is no clear explanation for the

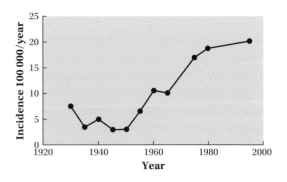

Fig. 23.5 Incidence of diabetes in children under age 10 years in Norway, 1925–1995.

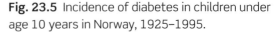

Source: Gale, E. (2002) The rise of childhood type 1 diabetes in the 20th century. *Diabetes,* **51,** 3353–61.

variation from one country to another or the change over time. Genetic factors are important in T1DM, although only about 10% of people with the condition have a clear family history. It is not clear what triggers the autoimmune process that leads to the destruction of the pancreatic islet β-cells. Various nutritional factors have been suggested, but the evidence is far from conclusive. Several epidemiological studies suggest that the early introduction of cow's milk into the diet of infants is associated with an increased risk of developing T1DM later in life, but the extent to which breast milk may be protective or cow's milk detrimental remains to be confirmed. The mechanisms by which infant nutrition might operate as a risk factor are far from clear. It is possible that cow's milk protein might be immunogenic in susceptible individuals. Several immunosuppressive drugs have been suggested as potentially useful means of reducing the risk of T1DM, but these drugs have side effects and none has been demonstrated to be of benefit in randomized controlled trials. Clinical trials involving various infant dietary regimens have also been suggested. Emerging data suggest a possible protective role for vitamin D. As with T2DM, many of the complications of T1DM are associated with unsatisfactory metabolic control, and cardiovascular disease in people with T1DM is associated with risk factors similar to those in the general population. In the aetiology of kidney damage (nephropathy), a high intake of protein, especially animal protein, may be associated, but the evidence is not conclusive.

23.5 Treatments for diabetes

All people with T1DM require insulin replacement treatment. For them, the goals of lifestyle and dietary advice are to minimize short-term fluctuations in blood glucose and especially to reduce the risk of hypoglycaemia by balancing injected insulin with carbohydrate-containing food and physical activity (Box 23.4). Dietary modification also helps to reduce the risk of long-term complications by helping to achieve optimal blood glucose control and satisfactory levels of blood pressure, blood lipids, and other risk factors influenced by diet. Increasingly, 'carbohydrate counting' is being introduced as a means of matching injected insulin with carbohydrate intake and improving glycaemic control in T1DM (see Section 23.5.4). This approach is more flexible than the traditional method of prescribing 'carbohydrate portions', since it permits altering insulin dose on the basis of the quantity of carbohydrate consumed. Carbohydrate portions were formerly prescribed in fixed quantities to match prescribed amounts of injected insulin.

Dietary modification is the cornerstone of treatment for people with T2DM, and many of those who manage to comply with dietary advice will show improvement in the metabolic abnormalities associated with this condition to the extent that oral hypoglycaemic drugs (Box 23.5) and insulin may not be required. Even when drug treatment is required, attention to diet may further improve blood glucose control and modify cardiovascular risk factors in a way that might be expected to reduce risk of CHD and other complications of diabetes.

The principles of dietary advice for people with T1DM and T2DM are similar to those recommended for entire populations at high risk of CHD, and this means that there is no need for people with diabetes to have meals that differ from those of the rest of the family. Evidence-based dietary recommendations for people with diabetes have been issued in most countries; the most widely quoted are those of the American Diabetes Association (ADA) and the Nutrition Study Group of the European Association for the Study of Diabetes (EASD). The two sets of recommendations are broadly comparable and are summarized in Table 23.3. The evidence for the benefit of implementing the recommendations derives principally from trials in which dietary manipulations have been shown to improve glycaemic control or level

BOX 23.4 Balancing injected insulin with carbohydrate-containing food

All those with T1DM require subcutaneous insulin, usually injected by means of an insulin 'pen' two or four times per day. Some people with T2DM also require injected insulin when the pancreatic β-cells are unable to secrete sufficient insulin. Frequently used insulin regimens are: (a) for T2DM, twice daily injections of a mixture of quick-acting (soluble) and longer-acting (isophane) insulins; and (b) for T1DM, soluble insulin, administered shortly before or with the three main meals, and isophane insulin before going to bed. Older forms of soluble insulin need to be injected 15–30 minutes before meals to achieve optimum effects. Recently available insulin analogues are more rapid acting and can be injected immediately before or even after meals, followed by longer-acting insulin before bed time. Carbohydrate-containing food must be consumed at times of peak insulin action to avoid hypoglycaemia (low blood glucose) and slowly released carbohydrate (see Sections 23.5.4 and 23.5.5) at night before going to bed to avoid hypoglycaemia during the night. Insulin dose and type can be adjusted to adapt to preferred quantity and timing of carbohydrate-containing meals and snacks. Some patients with T1DM use insulin pumps, which deliver a continuous supply of small amounts of soluble insulin, boosted at meal times, to reproduce as closely as possible normal insulin secretion.

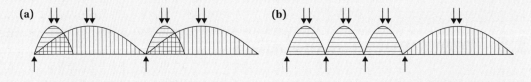

(a) ↑, injection of insulin mixture containing soluble (≡) and isophane (|||) insulins before breakfast and before evening meal.
(b) ↑, injection of soluble (≡) insulin before main meals and isophane (|||) before bed. ↓↓, breakfast, lunch, evening meal, and bed-time snack to provide available carbohydrate at times of peak insulin activity.

BOX 23.5 Oral hypoglyaemic medications. If dietary modification is unable to achieve target blood glucose levels in patients with T2DM, oral hypoglycaemic agents may be prescribed. Several different classes of drugs are available

Drug class	Examples	Comment
Biguanide	Metformin	Reduces gluconeogenesis and glycogenolysis and improves uptake and ultilization of insulin
		Very widely used in overweight patients
Sulphonylureas	Glipizide	Stimulates insulin secretion
	Gliclazide	May be used alone or in conjunction with metformin
Thiazolidinedione	Pioglitazone	Insulin sensitizer
Dipeptidyl Peptidase-4 inhibitor	Sitagliptin Vildagliptin	Increases levels of incretin

of risk factors, which have in turn been shown to influence clinical outcome in people with diabetes.

Dietary recommendations have tended to be less rigid than those in the past and acknowledge that quality of life and needs of the individual must be taken into account when defining nutritional objectives. Healthcare providers are encouraged to achieve a balance between the attempts to achieve optimal control of blood glucose and risk factors and the wellbeing of the patient.

Lifestyle treatments may change with time. The recommendations given here are those of the EASD; they are broadly comparable with those of the ADA. A particularly important feature of these recommendations is the wide range of acceptable macronutrient intakes. While metabolic features guide advice for individuals, this flexibility does enable a considerable degree of personal preference and ensures compatibility with many different dietary patterns. Much publicity has arisen from claims of the 'unique' benefits associated with Mediterranean, high-protein (e.g Zone, CSIRO), high-fibre, low-carbohydrate, and even high-fat (e.g. Atkins) diets for people with diabetes. While the majority of experts would agree that a high-fat diet is undesirable in the long term, the consensus would be that any of these dietary patterns would be acceptable for the majority of people with diabetes, provided they comply with the recommendations for energy and nutrients given below. No single dietary pattern has been shown to be associated with better long-term outcomes than any others.

23.5.1 Energy balance and body weight

The key recommendation for those who are overweight (BMI >25 kg/m²) is that calorie intake should be reduced and energy expenditure increased so that the BMI moves towards the recommended range (18.5–25 kg/m²). Prevention of weight regain is an important aim once weight loss has been achieved. For those who are overweight or obese, reducing energy-dense foods (those high in fats and free sugars) and regular exercise are usually sufficient to achieve weight loss, prescription of precise energy requirements only being necessary for those unable to achieve the desired weight reduction. Even modest weight reduction (a loss of less than 10% body weight) in the overweight or obese improves insulin sensitivity, glycaemic control, body lipids, blood pressure, and other cardiovascular risk factors. Weight loss may reduce or even eliminate the need for hypoglycaemic drug therapy in T2DM and lead to a reduction of insulin dose and improved glycaemic control in T1DM. The reduced life expectancy of overweight people with diabetes is improved in those who lose weight.

Table 23.3 Key aspects of the current recommendations for diabetic diet and lifestyle

Dietary energy and body weight	Achieve and/or maintain BMI of 18.5–25 kg/m²
	Diet and exercise important
Dietary fat	Saturated plus *trans*-unsaturated fatty acids: <10% total energy, <8% if low-density lipoprotein cholesterol raised
	Polyunsaturated fatty acids: 6–10% total energy
	Monounsaturated fatty acids: 10–20% total energy
	Total fat: <35% total energy (if overweight <30%)
	Oily fish, soybean and rapeseed oil, nuts, and green leafy vegetables to provide ω-3 fatty acids
	Cholesterol: <300 g/day

(Continued)

Table 23.3 Key aspects of the current recommendations for diabetic diet and lifestyle *(Continued)*

Carbohydrate	Total carbohydrate: 45–60% total energy, influenced by metabolic characteristics
	Vegetables, fruits, legumes, and cereal-derived foods preferred
Dietary fibre and glycaemic index	Naturally occurring foods rich in dietary fibre are encouraged
	Ideally dietary fibre intake should be more than 40 g/day (or 20 g/1000 kcal/day), half soluble (lesser amounts also beneficial)
	Five servings/day of fibre-rich vegetables and fruit and four or more servings of legumes/week help to provide minimum requirements
	Cereal-based foods should be wholegrain and high in fibre
	Carbohydrate-rich low-glycaemic-index foods are suitable choices, provided other attributes are appropriate
Sucrose and other free sugars	If desired and blood glucose levels are satisfactory, free sugars up to 50 g/day may be incorporated into the diet
	Total free sugars should not exceed 10% total energy (less for those who are overweight)
Protein and renal disease	Total protein intake at lower end of normal range (0.8 g/kg/day) for type 1 patients with established nephropathy
	For all others, protein should provide 10–20% total energy
Vitamins, antioxidant nutrients, minerals, and trace elements	Increase foods rich in tocopherols, carotenoids, vitamin C and flavonoids, trace elements, and other vitamins
	Fruits, vegetables, and wholegrains, rather than supplements, recommended
	Restrict salt to less than 6 g/day (less than 2.3 g sodium)
Alcohol	Up to 10 g for women and 20 g for men per day is acceptable for most people with diabetes who choose to drink alcohol
	Special precautions apply to those on insulin or sulphonylureas, those who are overweight, and those with hypertriglyceridaemia
Special 'diabetic' or foods, functional foods, and supplements	Non-alcoholic beverages sweetened with non-nutritive sweeteners are useful
	Other special foods not encouraged
	No particular merit of fructose and other 'special' nutritive sweeteners over sucrose
Families	Most recommendations suitable for whole family

Source: Derived from the 2004 recommendations of the Nutrition Study Group of the European Association for the Study of Diabetes: Mann, J.I., De Leeuw, I., Hermansen, K., *et al.* (2004) Evidence-based nutritional approaches to the treatment and prevention of diabetes mellitus. *Nutr Metab Cardiovasc Dis*, **14**, 373–94.

23.5.2 Protein

Protein intake in most Western populations ranges between 10 and 20% total energy, corresponding to 0.8–2.0 g/kg body weight. Intakes at the higher end of the range are appropriate for people with diabetes who do not have evidence of diabetic renal disease and where preference is to have lower intakes of carbohydrate. In patients with T1DM and evidence of established nephropathy, protein intakes should be at the lower end of this range (0.8 g/kg body weight/day). Such restriction has been shown to reduce the risk of end-stage renal failure or death when compared in randomized controlled trials with more usual intakes (1.2 g/kg/day). The evidence for appreciably reducing protein intake is less convincing for T2DM patients with established nephropathy or for T1DM or T2DM patients with microalbuminuria (incipient nephropathy). However, in those with no nephropathy or microalbuminuria it is suggested that protein intake not exceed 20% total energy, since there is evidence that beyond this level of intake renal function may deteriorate, especially in the presence of hypertension or poor glycaemic control.

23.5.3 Dietary fat

The striking relationships between saturated and *trans*-unsaturated fatty acids, total and low density lipoprotein cholesterol and CHD justify their combined restriction to less than 10% total energy, or less than 8% if low-density lipoprotein (LDL) is raised (see Chapter 21).

The wide range of acceptable intakes of *cis*-monounsaturated fatty acids (10–20% total energy) reflects their beneficial effect when compared with saturated fatty acids or low-fibre, high-glycaemic index, carbohydrate-containing foods on lipids, lipoproteins, and insulin sensitivity. The range also permits a more flexible approach to the selection of food choices and dietary patterns (see Section 23.5.10) provided total fat intake does not exceed 35% total energy or 30% in the overweight or obese. The reasons for recommending an upper level of intake for total fat include the potential to increase insulin resistance at higher levels and the high energy density associated with high fat intakes. ω-6 polyunsaturated fatty acids facilitate LDL lowering, but intakes greater than 10% total energy are not advised because of a possible increased risk of lipid oxidation or reduction in high-density lipoprotein (HDL) associated with high intakes. The optimal ratio of ω-3 to ω-6 polyunsaturated acids is unknown but ω-3 fatty acids are essential and have a number of potentially beneficial effects in terms of reducing cardiovascular risk. Regular intakes of oily fish, rapeseed (canola) or soybean oil, nuts, and some green leafy vegetables ensure adequate intakes. Modest restriction of cholesterol to less than 300 mg/day (further reduction if LDL is raised) is based on the adverse effects of large quantities on LDL (particularly in the presence of relatively high intakes of saturated fatty acids) and evidence from some prospective studies that substantial intakes are related to increased risk of cardiovascular disease.

23.5.4 Carbohydrate

The recommended range of intakes, 45–60% total energy, is based on the limits for fat and protein and the acceptability in terms of glycaemic control and risk factor status across the wide range. However, the nature of the carbohydrate is important, especially with intakes at the upper end of the range. Vegetables, legumes, intact fruits, and wholegrain cereals are always the preferred carbohydrate sources because of their favourable effect on glycaemic control and their potential for reducing cardiovascular risk. High intakes of starchy or highly processed foods with a high glycaemic index (Table 23.3) may give poor glycaemic control, increased triglycerides, and low levels of HDL. Thus, metabolic characteristics, as well as personal preferences, should determine the level of intake. Those with dyslipidaemia (high triglycerides, low HDL) and poor glycaemic control may be more satisfactorily controlled in terms of their metabolic derangement, on intakes at the lower end of the range. For them it is particularly important that carbohydrate-containing foods should be rich in dietary fibre and have a low glycaemic index.

For those on tablets to lower blood glucose or insulin, timing and dosage of medication should match quantity, nature, and timing of carbohydrate intake. Failure to do so may result in symptoms of hypoglycaemia and reduce the potential to achieve good blood glucose control. Measurement of glucose on a finger prick blood sample by patients at home, using one of the many meters now available, enables them not only to assess blood glucose control, but for those with T1DM, to adjust insulin dose according to carbohydrate content of their meal (carbohydrate counting) and the preprandial blood glucose measurement.

23.5.5 Dietary fibre and glycaemic index

Randomized controlled trials have shown the potential of naturally occurring foods, rich in dietary fibre, especially soluble forms, to improve glycaemic control and lipid profile in patients with T1DM and T2DM, hence the recommendation to encourage such foods and a fibre intake of 40 g or more (or 20 g/1000 kcal) daily. About half the dietary fibre should be soluble. Five or more servings per day of fibre-rich vegetables and fruit and four or more servings of legumes per week help to provide minimum requirements for fibre intake, when most cereal-based foods are wholegrain-fibre-rich. Beneficial effects are also obtained with lower, and for some, more acceptable amounts.

Diets rich in low-glycaemic-index foods have also been shown to produce improved glycaemic control, especially in patients with T2DM (see Chapter 3). Most (but not all) of such foods are high in dietary fibre. Low-glycaemic-index foods are therefore suitable food choices for people with diabetes. However, there are some important limitations to the use of glycaemic index. Foods high in fat and sugars generally have a low glycaemic index, yet they may be energy-dense and include inappropriate fat sources and are therefore poor food choices for people with diabetes. Thus, glycaemic index concept is only meaningful when used to classify predominantly carbohydrate-containing food and when comparing foods within a comparable food group (e.g. breads, fruits, pasta, and rice). The glycaemic index of foods must be interpreted in relation to energy content and content of other macronutrients.

23.5.6 Sucrose and other free sugars

When incorporated in modest amounts (< 50 g/day) into diets of appropriate macronutrient composition and energy content, sucrose appears not to be associated with any measurable untoward clinical or metabolic effect, hence the recommendation that such modest amounts of free sugars might be included in a diabetic dietary prescription. As for the general population, it is advised that total free sugars do not exceed 10% total energy, though more restrictive advice concerning free sugars may be useful for those needing to lose weight, those with poor glycaemic control, and those with dyslipidaemia (high triglycerides, low HDL).

23.5.7 Antioxidant nutrients, vitamins, minerals, and trace elements

Foods naturally rich in dietary antioxidants (tocopherols, carotenoids, vitamin C, flavonoids), trace elements, and other vitamins are encouraged. Daily consumption of a range of vegetables, fruits, and wholegrain breads and cereals should provide adequate intakes of vitamins and antioxidant nutrients and there is currently no evidence that dietary supplements confer benefit. Given the tendency towards high levels of blood pressure in people with diabetes, restriction of salt intake to less then 6 g/day is advised, with further restriction considered appropriate for those with elevated blood pressure levels.

23.5.8 Alcohol

A limited amount of information tends to confirm that people with T2DM, like adults in the general population, who have a moderate intake of alcoholic drinks may have a reduced risk of CHD. On the other hand, alcohol may be a relevant source of energy in those who are overweight and may be associated with raised levels of blood pressure, increased triglycerides, and an increased risk of hypoglycaemia, especially in insulin-treated individuals or those on some oral hypoglycaemic agents. Thus, it is recommended that moderate use of alcohol (up to 10 g/day for women and 20 g/day for men) is acceptable rather than beneficial for those with diabetes who choose to drink alcohol. When alcohol is taken by those on insulin, it is essential that it be taken with carbohydrate-containing food in order to avoid the risk of potentially profound and prolonged hypoglycaemia. Alcohol should be limited by those who are overweight, hypertensive, or hypertryglyceridaemic. Abstention is advised for women who are pregnant and those with a history of alcohol abuse or pancreatitis, appreciable hypertriglyceridaemia, and advanced neuropathy.

23.5.9 Diabetic foods, functional foods, and supplements

Foods advertised as being of particular benefit for people with diabetes ('diabetic' foods) are generally sucrose-free but may nevertheless be high in fructose or other nutritive sweeteners, and sometimes also fat. These have no substantial advantages over sucrose-containing foods for people with diabetes and should not be encouraged. Non-nutritive sweeteners (e.g. aspartame) may be useful, especially in drinks. Many functional foods and supplements are currently also being promoted for diabetes management or for reducing the risk of diabetes or its complications. These include fibre-enriched products and margarines containing plant sterols or stanols and supplements containing various dietary fibres, ω-3 fatty acids, minerals, trace elements, and some herbs. Most of these products have not been tested in long-term clinical trials and are therefore not encouraged at present.

23.5.10 Translating nutritional principles into practice

Most medical practitioners do not have the training or the time to help people with diabetes translate the nutrition principles described here into practice. Dietitians or appropriately trained nutritionists play a key role in translating these general principles into specific advice for individuals. The high intakes of total and saturated fat by people with diabetes in Europe (Fig. 23.6) provide an indication of the extent of dietary change required by many. The wide ranges of acceptable intake for monounsaturated fatty acids and carbohydrates

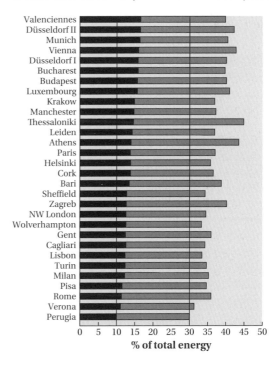

Fig. 23.6 Intake of total (■) and saturated (■) fatty acids as proportion of total dietary intake, calculated from 4-day diet records collected from people with T1DM. Data from European centres participating in the EURODIAB study.

Source: Toeller, M., Klischan, A., Heitkamp, G., et al. (1996) Nutritional intake of 2868 IDDM patients from 30 centres in Europe. EURODIAB IDDM Complications Study Group. *Diabetologia*, **39**, 929–39.

enable the nutrient recommendations to be translated into a variety of dietary patterns. There has been a trend in some countries for conventional, as well as alternative health practitioners to recommend low-carbohydrate (comparable with that recommended in the early and middle years of the twentieth century) or very-low-carbohydrate (Atkins type) diets as the preferred option for the treatment and prevention of diabetes. The justification for such a recommendation stems from the claim that such a diet facilitates weight loss and weight loss maintenance and also that high-carbohydrate diets induce dyslipidaemia and hyperglycaemia. There is no justification for the former claim. Meta-analyses have confirmed that in the medium-to-long term, macronutrient distribution does not determine extent of weight loss. Furthermore, while not recommending high-carbohydrate diets for those with marked metabolic derangements, a relatively adverse metabolic profile is only associated with high carbohydrate intake if sugars and starches, rather than high-fibre vegetables, fruits, and wholegrains, are the predominant sources of carbohydrate calories. The importance of increased physical activity as well as dietary advice for those who are overweight cannot be over-emphasized. Behaviour modification techniques and various special lifestyle programmes can be of considerable value. Ongoing encouragement and reinforcement of lifestyle changes are essential, and one-off advice is rarely adequate.

The case study in Box 23.6 describes the experience of one of our patients and provides a good indication of what can be achieved in practice by closely following dietary advice.

BOX 23.6 Case study

A 63-year-old school principal, Mr AD, with T2DM was referred to our hospital diabetes clinic. He was being treated with tablets (maximum doses of gliclazide, metformin, and pioglitazone (Box 23.5) and was in theory following a 'diabetic diet'. His general practitioner had referred him for conversion to insulin treatment believing that this was the only option for improving diabetes control, considered to be essential and of some urgency, given that he had had a myocardial infarction a year previously and been found to have diabetic retinopathy on a recent routine examination of his eyes. His BMI was 32 kg/m^2 and his HbA$_{1c}$ was 9.6% (81 mmol/ml), indicating poor blood glucose control. At his first visit Mr AD indicated his willingness to start insulin provided he could be taught injection techniques immediately so that he could return to work without delay ('In my job, I don't have any more time to devote to myself'). With some difficulty, he was persuaded to talk briefly to the clinic dietitian. She soon discovered that his 'diabetic diet' involved avoiding added sugars and whenever possible foods known to be high in sugars (e.g. chocolates, sweets, and puddings). However, it appeared that portion sizes were extremely large, that sweet foods had been replaced by energy-dense high-fat foods (e.g. a meat pie, or a battered fried fish almost every day for lunch ('I thought these were good choices as they don't contain sugar') and that fruit and vegetables, other than potatoes, were not a major feature of his dietary pattern. As a result he was persuaded that dietary modification with some regular daily exercise should precede the initiation of insulin treatment. The possibility that insulin treatment might promote further weight gain provided the impetus required for Mr AD to agree to devote some time to think about his lifestyle in relation to his health. The dietary advice was relatively simple: a reduction in portion size, radical reduction in high-fat, energy-dense foods, an increase in fruit and vegetables other than potatoes, and the use of dense wholegrain, low-glycaemic-index bread instead of his usual white bread. Being an intelligent man, having been persuaded to make the changes, he was meticulous regarding implementation. Within days and before his weight had changed, his blood glucose levels were down to single figures throughout the day. After 3 weeks he had lost nearly 5 kg in weight and was experiencing some hypoglycaemic episodes. Over the subsequent months his weight continued to fall and the pioglitazone dose was reduced and then stopped. As HbA$_{1c}$ continued to improve, the gliclazide dose too was reduced and then stopped and by the end of the year after first referral, his BMI was 26 kg/m^2, his HbA$_{1c}$ was 6.8% 50 mmol/L, and metformin was his only hypoglycaemic medication. At the time of writing, some 5 years after the referral, this satisfactory situation continues. In addition to the improvement in glycaemic control, blood pressure and lipid profile have also improved with the dietary modification and weight loss. However, he continues on his statin drug and other cardiac medications prescribed following his myocardial infarction. Mr AD has recently retired, taken over much of the meal preparation from his wife, and faces the next phase of his life course with a much improved prognosis. Interestingly, he no longer misses his earlier dietary pattern and enjoys being adventurous in his newfound culinary skills.

Comment

The responses such as that described here are not uncommon in people with type 2 diabetes who are prepared to make major changes in their diet and physical activity patterns. Indeed we have recently demonstrated in a formal randomized controlled trial (Coppell *et al.*, BMJ, 2010) that even in people whose medical treatment (including, if necessary, insulin) has been optimized according to current guidelines, intensive lifestyle changes can result in significant improvement in diabetes control as measured by HbA$_{1c}$. While almost everyone will benefit from improved diet and exercise habits, whether or not tablet treatment can be reduced or stopped and whether insulin is required will vary from patient to patient, given that type 2 diabetes is a heterogeneous condition. Dosage of tablets may be reduced if blood sugar levels are consistently low or patients experience hypoglycaemia, as happened in the case of Mr AD. Typically, metformin is continued since this drug tends to enhance insulin sensitivity. Many patients with T2DM do require insulin treatment after having had the condition for many years. The β-cells become 'exhausted' after a prolonged period of producing larger than usual amounts of insulin in an attempt to overcome insulin resistance, the underlying abnormality in most people with T2DM. While it is never too late to recommend enhanced lifestyle advice, the most striking results are seen when it is implemented relatively early in the disease process.

23.6 Families and communities

Individual compliance with dietary advice is improved if the general aspects of advice are understood by the family and are of potential benefit to them. In view of the strong genetic component to T2DM, the possibility that lifestyle changes might reduce the risk of developing the condition and that the dietary principles are similar to those that reduce CHD risk, it seems perfectly reasonable to suggest that foods and meals that are suitable for people with diabetes are appropriate for their families. In countries with high rates of T2DM, community programmes are needed but, as with CHD prevention, appropriate food labelling and availability of appropriate foods at reasonable cost are essential components of such initiatives. In both families and communities, avoidance and treatment of overweight and obesity provide the best means of reducing diabetes risk. There is at present insufficient evidence to justify programmes aimed at identifying people at risk of T1DM.

Metabolic syndrome

Resistance to the action of insulin, an important underlying abnormality in T2DM, is also associated with a range of additional clinical and metabolic abnormalities (Box 23.7) that are often seen in

---

BOX 23.7 Clinical and metabolic features other than hyperglycaemia associated with insulin resistance

- Central obesity
- Raised blood pressure
- Dyslipidaemia
  - Increased triglyceride
  - Low HDL
  - Predominance of small, dense LDL particles
  - Increased uric acid and gout
- Increased plasminogen activator inhibitor (PAI-1)
- NASH (non-alcoholic steatohepatitis)
- Endothelial dysfunction
- Increased proinflammatory cytokines
- Increased homocysteine

---

association with T2DM, IGT, or IFG, but may also occur with normal blood glucose levels. Several national and international organizations have suggested sets of diagnostic criteria for what has become known as the metabolic syndrome (Box 23.8). The validity of describing this constellation of abnormalities as a 'syndrome' has been questioned on the grounds that the criteria are clearly arbitrary and its causes ill understood. Nevertheless, its existence does help to define a group of individuals who are at high risk of cardiovascular disease and of developing T2DM if they have not already done so. As many as one-quarter (and in some instances appreciably more) of all adults in many affluent and some developing countries will fit the criteria set by the WHO and the US National Cholesterol Education Programme (NCEP). However, this figure is appreciably greater if the criteria suggested by the International Diabetes Federation are implemented. Lifestyle-related risk factors are identical to those described for T2DM, as are the measures for prevention and treatment.

BOX 23.8 Diagnostic criteria suggested for the metabolic syndrome by different international organizations

WHO (1999)	NCEP, ATP111 (2001)	IDF (2005)
Hyperglycaemia or insulin resistance Plus two or more of:	Three of more of:	Central obesity: Waist (ethnic specific) Europeans ≥94 cm (M), ≥80 cm (F) South Asians/Chinese ≥90 cm (M), ≥80 cm (F)
Obesity: W/H >0.9 (M), 0.85 (F) or BMI >30 kg/m²	Central obesity: Waist >102 cm (M), 88 cm (F)	Plus two of: Fasting glucose ≥5.6 mmol/L
	Fasting glucose ≥ 6.1 mmol/L	
Dyslipidaemia: Triglyceride ≥1.7 mmol/L or	Hypertriglyceridaemia: Triglyceride ≥1.7 mmol/L	Treated dyslipidaemia: or Raised triglyceride ≥1.7 mmol/L
HDL <0.9 mmol/L (M), 1.0 mmol/L (F)	Low HDL <1.0 mmol/L (M), 1.3 mmol/L (F)	Reduced HDL ≥1.03 mmol/L (M), ≥1.29 mmol/L (F)

BOX 23.8 Diagnostic criteria suggested for the metabolic syndrome by different international organizations *(Continued)*

WHO (1999)	NCEP, ATP111 (2001)	IDF (2005)
Hypertension:	Hypertension:	Treated hypertension or:
Blood pressure ≥140/90 mmHg	Blood pressure ≥135/85 mmHg	Raised blood pressure:
	or treatment	>130 systolic or >85 diastolic
Microalbuminuria		

ATP, adult treatment panel; BMI, body mass index; F, female; HDL, high-density lipoprotein; IDF, International Diabetes Federation; M, male; NCEP, National Cholesterol Education Programme; W/H, waist/hip ratio; WHO, World Heath Organization.

Source: WHO (1999) *Definition, diagnosis and classification of diabetes mellitus and its complications.* Report of a WHO consultation. Geneva, Switzerland, World Health Organization; NCEP, ATP 111 (2001) Executive summary of the Third Report of The National Cholesterol Education Program (NCEP) Expert Panel on Detection, Evaluation, And Treatment of High Blood Cholesterol In Adults (Adult Treatment Panel III). *JAMA*, 285, 2486–97; Alberti, K.G., Zimmet, P., and Shaw, J. (2005) The metabolic syndrome—a new worldwide definition. *Lancet*, **366**, 1059–62.

Lifestyle modification is the pivotal component of management, since weight loss associated with increased physical activity and the appropriate dietary measures offers the only means of favourably influencing the broad range of abnormalities associated with the syndrome.

Further Reading

1. **Alberti, K.G.M.M. and Zimmet, P.Z.** (1998) Definition, diagnosis and classification of diabetes mellitus and its complications, part 1: Diagnosis and classification of diabetes mellitus provisional report of a WHO consultation. *Diabet Med*, **15**, 539–53.

2. **Alberti, K.G., Zimmet P., and Shaw J.** (2005). The metabolic syndrome—a new worldwide definition. *Lancet*, **366**,1059–62.

3. **American Diabetes Association (ADA)** (2008) Clinical practice recommendations. *Diabetes Care*, **31** (Suppl. 1), S61–78.

4. **Anderson, E.J., Richardson, M., Castle, G. et al.** (1993). Nutrition interventions for intensive therapy in the Diabetes Control and Complications Trial. The DCCT Research Group. *J Am Diet Assoc* **93**, 768–72.

5. **Coppell, K.J., Kataoka., M, Williams, S.M., et al.** (2010). Nutritional intervention in patients with type 2 diabetes who are hyperglycaemic despite optimised drug treatment—Lifestyle Over and Above Drugs in Diabetes (LOADD) study: Randomised controlled trial. *BMJ*, **341**, c3337.

6. **Folsom, A.R., Kushi, L.H., Anderson, K.E., et al.** (2000) Associations of general and abdominal obesity with multiple health outcomes in older women: The Iowa Women's Health Study. *Arch Intern Med*, **160**, 2117–28.

7. **Gale, E.** (2002) The rise of childhood type 1 diabetes in the 20th century. *Diabetes*, **51**, 3353–61.

8. **Gale, E.A.** (2005) The myth of the metabolic syndrome. *Diabetologia*, **48**, 1679–83.

9. **Gillies, C.L., Abrams, K.R., Lambert, P.C., et al.** (2007) Pharmacological and lifestyle interventions to prevent or delay type 2 diabetes in people with impaired glucose tolerance: Systematic review and meta-analysis. *BMJ*, **334**, 299.

10. **IDF** (2009) *IDF Diabetes Atlas*, 4th edn. Brussels, International Diabetes Federation (IDF). http://www.diabetesatlas.org.

11. **Jarvi, A.E., Karlström, B.E., Grandfeldt, Y.E., et al.** (1999) Improved glycaemic control and lipid profile and normalized fibrinolytic activity in a low-glycaemic index diet in type 2 diabetic patients. *Diabetes Care*, **22**, 10–18.

12. **Knowler, W., Fowler, S., Hamman R, et al.** (2009) 10-year follow-up of diabetes incidence and weight loss in the Diabetes Prevention Program Outcomes Study. *Lancet*, **374**, 1677–86.

13. **Lindström, J., Ilanne-Parikka, P., Peltonen, M., et al.** (2006) Sustained reduction in the incidence of type 2 diabetes by lifestyle intervention: Follow-up of the Finnish Diabetes Prevention Study. *Lancet*, **368**, 1673–9.

14. **Mann, J.** (2000) Stemming the tide of diabetes. *Lancet*, **356**, 1454–5.

15. **Mann, J.I., De Leeuw, I., Hermansen, K., et al.** (2004) Evidence-based nutritional approaches to the treatment and prevention of diabetes mellitus. *Nutr Metab Cardiovasc Dis*, **14**, 373–94.

16. **NCEP, ATP 111** (2001) Executive summary of the Third Report of The National Cholesterol Education Program (NCEP) Expert Panel on Detection, Evaluation, And Treatment of High Blood Cholesterol In Adults (Adult Treatment Panel III). *JAMA*, **285**, 2486–97.

17. **Salmeron, J., Ascherio, A., Rimm, E.B., et al.** (1997) Dietary fibre, glycaemic load and risk of NIDDM in men. *Diabetes Care*, **20**, 545–50.

18. **Salmerón, J., Manson, J.E., Stampfer, M.J., et al.** (1997) Dietary fiber, glycemic load, and risk of non-insulin-dependent diabetes mellitus in women. *JAMA*, **277**, 472–7.

19. **Stumvoll, M., Goldstein, B., and van Haeften, T.** (2005) Type 2 diabetes: Principles of pathogenesis and therapy. *Lancet*, **365**, 1333–46.

20. **Toeller, M., Klischan, A., Heitkamp, G., et al.** (1996) Nutritional intake of 2868 IDDM patients from 30 centres in Europe. EURODIAB IDDM Complications Study Group. *Diabetologia*, **39**, 929–39.

21. **Tuomilehto, M.D., Lindström, M.S., Eriksson, J.G., et al.** (2001) Prevention of type 2 diabetes mellitus by changes in lifestyle among subjects with impaired glucose tolerance. *N Engl J Med*, **344**, 1343–50.

22. **Vessby, B., Uusitupa, M., Hermansen, K., et al.** (2001) Substituting dietary saturated for monounsaturated fat impairs insulin sensitivity in healthy men and women: The KANWU Study. *Diabetologia*, **44**, 312–19.

23. **WHO** (1999) *Definition, diagnosis and classification of diabetes mellitus and its complications*. Report of a WHO consultation. Geneva, Switzerland, World Health Organization.

24. **WHO** (2003) *Diet, nutrition and the prevention of chronic diseases*. WHO Technical Report Series 916. Geneva, World Health Organization.

Useful Websites

 To see topical and scientifically robust updates on nutrition associated with this textbook and web links to many of the journals in the Further Reading sections, please see the dedicated Online Resource Centre at **http://www.oxfordtextbooks.co.uk/orc/mann4e/**

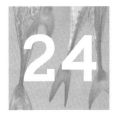

24 The eating disorders: anorexia nervosa, bulimia nervosa, and EDNOS

Hannah Turner and Robert Peveler

For many years the term 'eating disorders' has been taken to include two principal conditions, anorexia nervosa (AN) and bulimia nervosa (BN). However, it is now recognized that a significant proportion of patients seen in routine clinical practice present with a syndrome that falls short of the 'full-blown' AN or BN, which is usually termed 'eating disorder not otherwise specified' (EDNOS). Thus, there is now some debate about the threshold of 'clinical' eating disorders. Although descriptions of AN date back to 1873, BN was not described as a clinical disorder until 1979. The term EDNOS has only been in use since 1980. Eating disorders are a significant cause of physical and psychosocial morbidity, particularly among female adolescents and young adult women.

24.1 Definitions

24.1.1 Anorexia nervosa

The diagnostic criteria for AN (as given in the fourth edition of the *Diagnostic and Statistical Manual of Mental Disorders* (DSM-IV)) are shown in Table 24.1. The first is the maintenance of body weight at least 15% below that expected for age and height (body mass index, BMI <17.5 kg/m^2 in adults). Weight loss is commonly achieved through extreme dietary restriction, although a subgroup of patients will also engage in other weight loss behaviours such as compulsive and driven exercise, self-induced vomiting, and laxative misuse. The second feature is a characteristic set of attitudes and values concerning shape and weight. Patients often experience intense feelings of fatness, as well as extreme fear of loss of control over eating and weight gain. They express a level of dissatisfaction with their body weight and shape that far exceeds that typically seen in the general population, and they tend to judge their self-worth almost solely in terms of their weight, shape, and ability to control their food intake. The third diagnostic feature is amenorrhoea (in postmenarchal females who are not taking an oral contraceptive), and both men and women may report loss of sex drive.

24.1.2 Bulimia nervosa

The DSM-IV diagnostic criteria for BN are also shown in Table 24.1. The first is recurrent episodes of binge eating during which an objectively large amount of food is consumed, with associated loss of perceived control of eating. The second feature is the use of compensatory behaviours designed to prevent weight gain. These include dietary restriction, self-induced vomiting, misuse of laxatives or diuretics, and excessive exercise. The third feature is the same set of attitudes and values seen in AN, with self-worth being determined almost exclusively on the basis of weight, shape, and ability to control food intake. Although

Table 24.1 Diagnostic criteria for anorexia nervosa and bulimia nervosa and EDNOS

Anorexia nervosa
A refusal to maintain body weight at or above a minimally normal weight for age and height (e.g. weight loss leading to a maintenance of body weight less than 85% of that expected, or failure to make expected weight gain during period of growth, leading to body weight less than 85% of that expected)
Intense fear of gaining weight or becoming fat, even though underweight
Disturbance in the way in which one's body weight or shape is experienced, undue influence of body weight or shape on self-evaluation, or denial of the seriousness of the current low body weight
In postmenarchal females, amenorrhoea (i.e. the absence of at least three consecutive cycles)
Bulimia nervosa
Recurrent episodes of binge eating. An episode of binge eating is characterized by: (1) Eating, in a discrete period of time (e.g. within any 2-hour period), an amount of food that is definitely larger than most people would eat during a similar period of time and under similar circumstances; and (2) a sense of lack of control over eating during the episode
Recurrent inappropriate compensatory behaviour in order to prevent weight gain, such as self-induced vomiting; misuse of laxatives, diuretics, enemas, or other medications; fasting or excessive exercise
The binge eating and inappropriate compensatory behaviours both occur, on average, at least twice a week for 3 months
Self-evaluation is unduly influenced by body shape and weight
The disturbance does not occur exclusively during episodes of AN
Examples of EDNOS include:
All the criteria for anorexia nervosa, except that the individual's current weight is in the normal range, or for females, regular menstruation continues
All of the criteria for bulimia nervosa, except that the binge eating and inappropriate compensatory mechanisms occur at a lower frequency than that required for a full diagnosis
Use of inappropriate compensatory behaviours by an individual of normal body weight after eating small amounts of food
Repeatedly chewing and spitting out, but not swallowing, large amounts of food
Binge-eating disorder

most people with BN are within the normal weight range, a proportion will have a history of AN. Where BN occurs in the context of AN, the latter diagnosis takes precedence.

24.1.3 EDNOS

Although recent findings suggest that EDNOS is commonly seen in clinical practice, this group of patients has less often been the focus of research and thus their characteristics remain poorly described. However, a number of subgroups have been suggested (see Table 24.1). For example, a proportion present with all the key features of BN but fail to fulfil the diagnostic criteria relating to frequency of occurrence of behavioural symptoms. Others may present with all the diagnostic features of AN but (in the case of women) may continue to menstruate at a BMI of $17.5 \, \text{kg/m}^2$ or below. It has also been documented that a subgroup with AN are aware that they are underweight and do not experience feelings of fatness.

24.2 Epidemiology

About 1 in 250 females and 1 in 2000 males will experience AN, most often in adolescence and young adulthood. About five times that number will suffer from BN. In community studies, prevalence rates of BN have been estimated at between 0.5% and 1.0% in young women. AN is less common, with prevalence estimated at 0.3% in young women. The prevalence of EDNOS remains unclear, although reports suggest that it is the most common presentation seen in clinical practice.

24.3 Anorexia nervosa

24.3.1 Development of the disorder

The onset of AN is usually in adolescence, although cases of prepubertal and adult onset have been reported. The disorder typically starts with an episode of dieting, although the path into this behaviour can vary. For some, natural bodily changes that accompany puberty, or a negative weight-related or shape-related comment from another person, may lead to a conscious decision to diet. For others, an episode of physical illness with associated weight loss, such as glandular fever, may lead to more intentional dietary restriction. Commonly occurring in the context of low self-worth, positive feedback in the form of attention from others initially serves to reinforce dieting behaviour and further weight loss. Patients with AN often report a sense of euphoria at being in control of their weight. For others, it brings feelings of success and a fleeting sense of superiority at achieving something few in the general population can accomplish. An example of a food diary for a patient with anorexia nervosa is given in Fig. 24.1.

24.3.2 Clinical features

As dieting intensifies, so weight falls, and the physiological and psychological effects of starvation develop. Behaviours around food become increasingly rigid and deceptive, and the range of acceptable foods slowly diminishes. Foods that are viewed as fattening are typically avoided and vegetarianism is common. The average energy intake is in the region of 600–900 kcal/day, with the proportion of energy derived from fat being particularly low. Mineral intake is also low, although mineral deficiencies are rare. It is possible that zinc deficiency

Food Diary

Time	Food and drink consumed	Place	*	V/L	Comments
7 am	Black tea 2 crackers	Kitchen			Feel OK
12 pm	Salad of lettuce, cucumber and tomato 3 crab sticks 1 cracker Black coffee	Lounge			Worried that I've eaten too much
2 pm	Apple Glass of water	Kitchen			
6 pm	Steamed vegetables 1/2 piece of chicken	Lounge			Feel full + bloated Worried that my weight will go up tomorrow

* = binge, V = vomiting, L = laxatives

Fig. 24.1 Example food diary for a patient with anorexia nervosa.

may contribute to the maintenance of the disorder through an effect on appetite and taste. However, true 'anorexia' is rare in so far as most patients report feeling persistently hungry. A proportion will feel driven to engage in excessive exercise, leading to further weight loss. Some will also engage in other forms of weight-control behaviour, such as self-induced vomiting or laxative misuse. A minority of patients will intermittently lose control over their eating and binge, although the amounts consumed tend not to be large.

Reduction in food intake is accompanied by a number of cognitive changes. Many will view either their body, or particular parts, as being bigger than their true size, and this is typically accompanied by an intense dislike or loathing of the body or body part. Cognitive rumination about weight and shape becomes all-consuming and an increasing amount of time is given to thinking about food. Over time, general functioning becomes increasingly impaired, interest in other areas of life diminishes, and day-to-day routines become characterized by social withdrawal and isolation. Depression, irritability, and anxiety are common, as are obsessional features. Typically, all features get worse with further weight loss.

Chronic presentations may also be accompanied by thoughts of hopelessness and suicide.

Physical health AN is associated with a range of physical abnormalities, most of which are now believed to be secondary to disturbed patterns of eating and low weight. Although patients often present with few physical complaints, further enquiry often reveals heightened sensitivity to cold and a variety of gastrointestinal symptoms including constipation, fullness after eating, bloatedness, and vague abdominal pains. Other symptoms include restlessness, lack of energy, low sexual appetite, early morning wakening, and dizziness on standing. In postmenarchal females who are not taking an oral contraceptive, amenorrhoea is often present, with infertility posing a concern for many women. On examination, patients are typically emaciated and underweight. Those with a prepubertal onset may be short in stature and show failure of breast development. Often there is fine downy hair (lanugo) on the back, arms and side of the face. The skin tends to be dry and the hands and feet cold. Blood pressure and pulse are low and there may be dependent oedema. The findings on investigation are shown in Table 24.2.

Table 24.2 Anorexia nervosa and bulimia nervosa: common abnormalities on investigation

ANOREXIA NERVOSA
Endocrine
Low levels of female sex hormones (luteinizing hormone, follicle stimulating hormone, and oestradiol)
Low triiodothyronine (T3) level but normal levels of thryoxine (T4) and thyroid-stimulating hormone
Raised growth hormone and cortisol levels
Cardiovascular
Low blood pressure (especially postural)
Bradycardia
Other arrhythmias
Haematological
Slightly lowered white cell count
Anaemia (normocytic normochromic)
Low erthyrocyte sedimentation rate
Other metabolic abnormalities
Raised blood cholesterol
Increased serum carotene
Low blood sugar
Dehydration
Electrolyte disturbance (in those who vomit frequently or misuse large quantities of laxatives or diuretics), especially hypokalaemia
Other findings
Skeletal abnormalities (raised rate of osteopenia with risk of fractures)
Delayed gastric emptying and prolonged gastrointestinal transit time
Hypertrophy of salivary glands (especially parotids)
Enlarged cerebral ventricles and external cerebrovascular fluid spaces ('pseudoatrophy')
BULIMIA NERVOSA
Endocrine
Electrolyte disturbance, especially hypokalaemia, in those who vomit frequently or misuse large quantities of laxatives or diuretics
Gastrointestinal
Prolonged digestion
Oesophageal damage and/or irritation of the oesophagus and/or pharynx due to contact with gastric acids
Perforation of upper digestive tract, oesophagus, or stomach
Abdominal pain and distention
Hypertrophy of salivary glands

(*Continued*)

Table 24.2 Anorexia nervosa and bulimia nervosa: common abnormalities on investigation (*Continued*)

Cardiac
Cardiac arrhythmias
Other
Dental erosion—gastric acids may cause deterioration of tooth enamel (perimolysis)
Hand callouses
Blood in vomit
Sore throat
Fatigue
Nausea
Weight gain

24.3.3 Aetiology

Predisposing factors AN is a complex illness that develops over time, often as a result of multiple influences. Dieting appears to be a general risk factor, although only a small percentage of those who diet go on to develop a clinical eating disorder. This suggests the importance of other aetiological factors. Other risk factors identified in the literature include a history of obesity, and premorbid characteristics such as long-standing low self-esteem and perfectionism. Patients with AN are often high achievers who have an intense need to be accepted by others. Family relationships are often disturbed, although it remains unclear as to whether this is a cause or consequence of the eating disorder, or both. A history of eating disorders and depression are also commonly seen within patients' families, and genetic studies have shown a significant linkage on chromosome 1 for restricting AN.

Maintaining factors As weight loss continues, so the physical and psychological sequelae of starvation become more prominent, some of which perpetuate the disorder. For example, delayed gastric emptying results in fullness even after eating small amounts of food, a situation that can fuel concern about uncontrollable weight gain. Weight loss may initially be accompanied by positive feedback from others, but over the course of time, social withdrawal can lead to isolation from peers. Controlling food intake can lead to a powerful sense of self-control and often serves to enhance self-esteem. Those with AN can also hold a powerful position with the family.

24.3.4 Assessment

A large proportion of people with AN are ambivalent about seeking treatment and many will have been persuaded to seek help by concerned relatives or friends. Thus, assessment forms a crucial part of the treatment process. Assessment should cover psychological, social, and physical needs, as well as assessment of risk to self and others. Where possible, the diagnosis should be made using a standardized diagnostic instrument, such as the Structured Clinical Interview for DSM-IV (SCID-I). No physical tests are required to make the diagnosis, and unless there are positive reasons to suspect the presence of another physical condition, no tests are required to exclude other medical disorders, when it is apparent that weight loss is self-induced.

A proportion of patients will present in a general medical setting and will report physical symptoms such as gastrointestinal symptoms, amenorrhoea, or infertility. However, once it is been established that weight loss has been self-induced, a diagnosis of AN can be explored. All patients with AN should have a thorough physical examination. Those who vomit frequently or misuse significant quantities of laxatives or diuretics should have their electrolytes checked. Given the increased risk of osteoporosis, it can be useful to conduct a dual energy X-ray absorptiometry (DEXA) scan to assess bone density in patients who have been underweight for an extended period of time. It may also be helpful to conduct a pelvic ultrasound to assess ovarian and uterine maturity in those with persisting amenorrhoea.

24.3.5 Management

There are three aspects to the management of AN. The first is to help patients to recognize that they have an illness. Acceptance and motivation to change are crucial given the recalcitrant nature of the illness. The second goal is the normalization of eating habits and weight restoration. Due to the risk of refeeding syndrome, calorie intake should be increased gradually and it may be necessary to monitor phosphate levels during this initial phase. Weight gain may be achieved through outpatient, day-patient, or inpatient treatment, and is typically facilitated through providing a combination of nutritional advice and psychological support. Drugs have almost no role, although dietary supplements can be of value in assisting weight restoration. The third aspect involves addressing patients' overevaluation of weight and shape, their extreme control over eating patterns and underlying psychosocial functioning. These aspects of treatment are typically addressed in specialized treatments such as family therapy, cognitive behaviour therapy, or cognitive analytic therapy.

24.3.6 Course and outcome

Response to treatment varies widely. For those who are willing and able to change, the illness duration can be relatively short. However, for others it can become a chronic problem commonly characterized by a resistance to change, despite a wish to recover. Although there are few consistent predictors of outcome, a long history and late onset have both been associated with a poor prognosis. Low weight and a history of premorbid psychosocial problems also tend to be associated with a poor outcome.

Long-term follow-up studies indicate that at 6-year follow-up, 55% had no eating disorder, 27% continued with AN, 10% had BN, 2% were classified with EDNOS, and 6% were deceased. AN is associated with increased mortality, the standardized mortality ratio over the first 10 years after presentation showing a 10-fold increased risk. Most deaths are either a direct result of medical complications or due to suicide. The mortality rate appears to be the highest for those presenting with lower weight during their illness and for those presenting between 20 and 29 years of age.

24.4 Bulimia nervosa

24.4.1 Clinical features

As in AN, those with BN tend to judge their self-worth almost exclusively on the basis of their weight and shape and their ability to control their food intake. They also use extreme forms of weight control, such as fasting and self-induced vomiting. However, people with BN tend to lie within the normal weight range, and they regularly engage in episodes of 'binge eating'. Binges will vary in size; they typically involve the consumption of 2000 kcal or more and tend to consist of foods the person is attempting to avoid. Patients typically become stuck in a vicious cycle of dietary restriction, bingeing, and purging, and are plagued by a constant fear of weight gain. This cycle invariably has a detrimental impact on other areas of functioning, such as work and social relationships, and it can have significant financial implications, leading some to steal money or food from others. People with BN tend to 'value' their symptoms less compared with those with AN and often binge and purge in secret.

Evidence suggests that a significant proportion of people with BN have difficulty regulating their emotions, and for many bingeing may serve as a form of emotional regulation: a means of reducing the intensity of emotions when they become intolerable. Many also have impulse control problems and a history of interpersonal difficulties. A subgroup will also present with comorbid depression and/or borderline personality disorder, and many of these will engage in a range of self-destructive behaviours such as cutting, overdosing, and substance misuse, with the dominant behaviour changing over time.

Physical health Physical complications most commonly associated with BN include irregular or absent menstruation, weakness and lethargy, vague abdominal pains, and toothache. On examination, appearance is usually unremarkable. Parotid gland enlargement may be present and there may be significant erosion of the dental enamel, particularly on the lingual surface of the upper front teeth. The most important abnormality on investigation is the electrolyte disturbance that is encountered in those who vomit frequently and in those who take large quantities of laxatives or diuretics. Clinically serious electrolyte disturbance may require treatment with potassium supplements until the eating disorder has been resolved. An example of a food diary for a patient with bulimia nervosa is given in Fig. 24.2.

24.4.2 Aetiology

Although many patients with BN will report a history of AN, a number of factors have been identified that preferentially increase the risk of BN. These include childhood and parental obesity, early menarche, and parental alcoholism. A history of trauma, including childhood sexual abuse (CSA) has also been associated with BN. However, while the rate of CSA in patients with BN is higher than

that amongst matched subjects in the general population, it is not higher than that found amongst young women with other psychiatric disorders. This suggests it may serve as a general risk factor for psychiatric disorder, rather than for BN *per se*.

24.4.3 Assessment

Many patients with BN feel too guilty and ashamed of their illness to ask for help, and often live with their disorder for years before seeking treatment. As with AN, they may present complaining of physical symptoms such as gastrointestinal or gynaecological symptoms. The lack of clear markers can make diagnosis difficult and highlights the importance of conducting a thorough assessment.

Those with BN typically present with a loss of control over their eating that is characterized by frequent episodes of binge eating and compensatory behaviours. Assessment and diagnosis is often relatively straightforward, although chaotic eating patterns can sometimes make it difficult to establish the presence of discrete episodes of binge eating. As with AN, no physical tests are needed to establish the diagnosis. However, the electrolytes should be checked of all those who vomit frequently or misuse large quantities of laxatives or diuretics.

24.4.4 Management

Most patients with BN can be treated on an outpatient basis. Cognitive behavioural therapy (CBT) represents the most extensively researched and validated psychological therapy for BN. CBT is a time-limited intervention that focuses on modifying disturbed eating habits and addressing the overvaluation of shape and weight. An alternative treatment is interpersonal psychotherapy (IPT), an intervention that targets interpersonal problems rather than eating patterns *per se*. Both treatments can be administered on an outpatient basis. A subset of patients will respond well to less intensive behavioural interventions, such as guided self-help programmes, although this is unlikely to be sufficient for the majority. Antidepressant drugs have

Food Diary

Time	Food and drink consumed	Place	*	V/L	Comments
9 am	Black coffee	Kitchen			Feel OK — today is going to be a good day
1 pm	Ham and Salad sandwich	Office desk			So far so good
6 pm	2 cheese rolls	Kitchen			Ate whilst preparing dinner—wish I hadn't but know I'll bring it up later
6:30 pm	Lasagne and garlic bread	Kitchen	*	V	Shouldn't have had seconds
7 pm	Bowl of cereal 2 bowls of ice-cream Chocolate bar 2 slices of toast Bottle of coke (small)	Lounge " " " "	*	V	Feel horrible — can't believe I lost control after being so good at work

* = binge, V = vomiting, L = laxatives

Fig. 24.2 Example food diary for a patient with bulimia nervosa.

been shown to have an antibulimic effect, leading to a rapid decline in the frequency of binge eating and purging and an improvement in mood. However, the effect is not as great as that obtained with CBT and evidence suggests that improvements are not maintained.

24.4.5 Course and outcome

Relatively little is known about the long-term course and outcome of BN. Outcome studies conducted to date suggest that at best only 50% of those who receive CBT are likely to be free from their symptoms at follow-up, 20% can expect to continue with a full diagnosis, while the remaining 30% will experience episodes of relapse or will continue with a subclinical form. Evidence has also shown IPT to be equally as effective as CBT at 18-month follow-up.

24.4.6 Binge-eating disorder

Binge-eating disorder is the most well-recognized subgroup within EDNOS. These patients present with all the characteristic features of BN but do not engage in compensatory behaviours. Other key characteristics include eating much more rapidly than normal, eating until feeling uncomfortably full, eating large amounts of food when not feeling physically hungry, and feeling disgusted with oneself or very guilty after overeating. Binge-eating disorder is commonly associated with obesity and it affects between 5% and 10% of obese patients seeking weight-loss treatment. Modified versions of the standard treatments for BN have been developed for use with those presenting with binge-eating disorder, and it is recommended that these interventions are used where appropriate. Studies examining the natural course of binge-eating disorder suggest recovery rates of up to 85% at 5 years.

24.5 Eating disorders and comorbidity

A number of other high-risk groups have also been identified. These include those presenting with an

eating disorder and type 1 diabetes mellitus (T1DM), and athletes with eating disorders. In relation to the former, it has been suggested that full and subclinical eating disorders may be more common among those with T1DM compared with aged-matched peers. Patients with T1DM may adopt the underuse or omission of insulin as a means of weight control, and it has been shown that even relatively short periods of impaired metabolic control can lead to increased risk of the physical complications associated with diabetes, such as retinopathy, nephropathy, or neuropathy, as well as increased mortality. There is little primary research concerning the treatment of diabetic patients with an eating disorder and advice is therefore based on guidelines provided for the treatment of nondiabetic patients. However, the coexistence of diabetes with an eating disorder invariably complicates psychological interventions, and thus the clinical management of this group remains a challenge.

Female athletes have also been identified as a group at increased risk of developing disturbed eating and associated problems. Pressure to conform to a sport-specific 'ideal' in disciplines such as distance running, gymnastics, and figure skating may lead a proportion to diet in order to improve performance. In order to capture the risks associated with eating disorders in athletes, terms such as 'anorexia athletica' and the 'female athlete triad' have been developed, the latter referring to the following three conditions: disordered eating, amenorrhoea, and osteoporosis. Identifying disordered eating among athletes must include the identification and assessment of a wide range of weight-control behaviours.

Summary

Although traditionally equated with AN and BN, it is now recognized that a significant proportion of the eating-disorder population present with EDNOS. Eating disorders are associated with significant psychological and physical complications. While many of these features will remit with weight restoration and/or cessation of weight-control behaviours, those presenting with a chronic course may experience long-term complications such as osteoporosis and infertility. The co-occurrence of subclinical disordered eating and conditions such as T1DM is also associated with significant physical morbidity and mortality. Patients with eating disorders present in a range of clinical settings and thus careful assessment is crucial for accurate identification and diagnosis. Comprehensive treatment requires the management of both physical and psychological aspects of the illness. While a proportion of patients will recover, a minority will present with an unremitting pattern of symptoms that may require longer-term management.

Further Reading

1. **American Dietetic Association** (2006) Position of the American Dietetic Association: Nutrition intervention in the treatment of anorexia nervosa, bulimia nervosa, and other eating disorders. *J Amer Diet Assoc*, **106**, 2073–82.

2. **Birmingham, C.L. and Beumont, P.J.V.** (2004) *Medical management of eating disorders: A practical handbook for healthcare professionals.* Cambridge, Cambridge University Press.

3. **Fairburn, C.G.** (2008) *Cognitive behavioural therapy and eating disorders.* Guilford Publications.

4. **Fairburn, C.G. and Brownell, K.D.** (2002) *Eating disorders and obesity: A comprehensive handbook.* 2nd edition. New York, Guilford Press.

5. **National Collaborating Centre for Mental Health** (2004) *Core interventions in the treatment and management of anorexia nervosa, bulimia nervosa and related eating disorders.* London, British Psychological Society.

6. **Treasure, J., Schmidt, U., and van Furth, E.** (2003) *Handbook of eating disorders.* 2nd edn. London, Wiley.

7. **Treasure, J., Clandino, A.M., and Zucker, N.** (2010) Eating disorders. *Lancet*, **375**, 583–93.

8. **Turner, H., Bryant-Waugh, R., and Peveler, R.** (2010) The clinical features of EDNOS: Relationship to mood, health status and general functioning. *Eat Behav*, **11**, 127–30.

Useful Websites

 To see topical and scientifically robust updates on nutrition associated with this textbook and web links to many of the journals in the Further Reading sections, please see the dedicated Online Resource Centre at **http://www.oxfordtextbooks.co.uk/orc/mann4e/**

Part 4

Foods

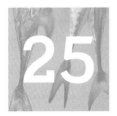

Food groups

Trish Griffiths, Bernard Venn, Margaret Allman-Farinelli, Stewart Truswell, Meika Foster, Anita S. Lawrence, Samir Samman, Kim Bell-Anderson, and Laurence Eyres

25.1 Breads and cereals
Trish Griffiths

Cereals, the 'seeds of civilization,' have constituted much of the food eaten by humans for thousands of years. It was not until the nomadic hunter-gatherers learned to farm crops that permanent settlements arose. Cultivation of wheat can be traced back to about 7000 BC in the Euphrates valley, while cultivation of rice dates back to around 3000 BC in China and shortly after in India. Maize (corn) was first cultivated about 5000 BC in Mexico. Food patterns were, and still are, most often built around a cereal. Wheat and barley were the staple foods of ancient Egypt, Greece, and Rome; rice in India and Southern China; maize the staple of the early Americans; oats and rye staples in the colder regions of Europe, and millets (including sorghum) were important in Africa and parts of Asia. Early breads were made from crude flours produced by pounding grains with a stone. Water was then added and the dough baked to a flat bread. Leavened bread dates back to Egypt in about 2000 BC.

Wheat, rice, and maize are currently the predominant cereals in both the land devoted to them and their consumption. Wheat covers more of the earth's surface than any other crop, largely having replaced rye, barley, and oats in Northern Europe, and increasingly replacing sorghum and millet in Africa. About 50% of the food protein available on the globe is derived from cereals, with consumption greatest in the developing countries (providing two-thirds of energy and protein). With increasing income, cereal consumption tends to decrease, while the intake of animal products and refined carbohydrates increases.

Broadly speaking, the nutritional value of different cereal grains is essentially similar, with some variation due to genetic factors and environmental conditions such as soil type and temperature (Table 25.1). Cereals are an important source of energy, providing between 1400 and 1600 kJ per 100 g of whole cereal. Cereals provide starch and dietary fibre (soluble and insoluble), which together comprise 70–77% of the grain. Grains are usually processed and cooked so that the starch is digestible. Protein accounts for 6–15% of the grain and the limiting amino acid is lysine, with maize additionally low in tryptophan. Gluten is the major protein in wheat and rye and oryzenin the major protein in rice. All cereals are low in fat, oats have more; most of the fat is polyunsaturated. Whole grains are a good source of thiamin, their germ is rich in vitamin E, and they contain significant amounts of minerals, especially potassium, phosphorus, magnesium,

iron, and zinc plus selenium, copper, and manganese. The net contribution of cereals to mineral intake may be less than anticipated because phytate in the outer bran layers binds some minerals and inhibits their absorption. Bioavailability of minerals is better from refined products but because the mineral content is less, overall more minerals will be provided by whole grains. During fermentation, as in bread making, the enzyme phytase is produced, which breaks down phytate.

Wholegrain cereals are rich in fibre and 'bioactive' components, including antioxidants (especially phenolics), phyto-oestrogens (lignans), phytosterols, vitamins, minerals, and trace elements. Epidemiological studies suggest consumption of whole grains is associated with reduced risk of chronic diseases and this is thought to be due to their content of bioactives.

25.1.1 Processing of cereal grains for human consumption

Wheat requires some processing to increase its digestibility. This is achieved by milling, which involves a series of grinding and sifting steps to

Table 25.1 Nutrient content of grains

	Nutrients per 100 g (raw grains)				
	Wheat[a]	Brown rice[b]	Maize[b]	Millet[b]	Oats[b]
Water (g)	11.0	12.0	13.8	11.8	8.3
Protein (g)	12.6	7.5	9.0	10.0	15.0
Fat (g)	2.7	1.9	3.9	2.9	7.0
Carbohydrate (g)	72.4	77.4	72.2	72.9	69
Thiamin (mg)	0.5	0.34	0.37	0.73	0.6
Niacin (mg)	6.1	4.7	2.2	2.3	1.0
Calcium (mg)	35.0	32.0	22.0	20.0	53.0
Iron (mg)	3.7	1.6	2.1	6.8	4.5

Source: [a]Bread Research Institute of Australia; [b]Lorenz, K.J., and Kulp, K. (eds) (1991) *Handbook of cereal science and technology*. New York, Marcel Dekker.

produce flour. The nutritional value of flour varies with the extraction rate (the number of parts by weight of flour produced after milling 100 parts of grain). Starch and protein are in the endosperm, so are reduced little by this processing. Typically, fibre, vitamins, and minerals are concentrated in the outer bran and aleurone layers of grains and the extent to which these layers are removed during milling determines the nutrient content of flour. White flour has a lower micronutrient content than wholemeal, but white flour products such as bread still make a significant contribution to the diet. In many industrial countries, cereal products are fortified with added vitamins or minerals (e.g. thiamin, niacin, calcium, iron). The protein content and 'hardness' of wheat determines how it is used. Hard, high-protein wheat is most suitable for bread; soft, low-protein wheats are most suitable for biscuits, and extra-hard durum wheat is used almost exclusively to make pasta. In addition to flour, milling produces bran, germ, and semolina. Bread, one of the most widely eaten foods in the world, is the major product made from wheat flour. White, wholemeal, and mixed grain breads are popular in Western countries; flatbreads are common in the Middle East and steamed breads in China.

Rice is the staple food of over half the world's population. After harvesting, paddy rice is cleaned and de-hulled but the bran layer is retained to produce brown rice. Alternatively, the brown rice can be further milled and polished to give white rice. Brown rice has a higher protein, mineral, and vitamin content than milled rice but also has a higher content of phytate and fibre. The practice of extensive abrasive polishing of rice is of concern in many Asian nations, where the majority of food eaten is rice and loss of nutrients like protein, thiamin, and iron becomes critical. The practice of parboiling rice before milling is encouraged as this results in an inward migration of water-soluble vitamins (including thiamin) to the endosperm. The process of rice enrichment may also improve nutrient intake. This involves mixing the ordinary white rice in a fixed proportion with rice that has been treated with a vitamin mixture and often iron. Lastly, 'Golden rice' is a new strain of rice genetically modified to produce β-carotene in the grain (which the body turns into vitamin A). It was developed in an attempt to reduce vitamin A deficiency and childhood blindness in developing countries. It remains controversial because of its genetically modified status. In developed countries, people have been enticed to eat more rice by a range of novel products such as rice cakes, rice bran, rice noodles, and rice crackers.

Maize (American corn) may be either dry milled (the protein and starch fractions are not separated) or wet milled (the protein and starch are separated). Dry milling produces grits, meals, flour, and hominy feed, while wet milling yields starch, dextrose, corn syrup solids, and glucose. Immature maize is often eaten fresh as a vegetable, i.e. sweet corn. Maize kernels can also be frozen or canned. Maize is used in the production of corn meals, corn flour, corn chips, tacos, and tortillas and consumption of these foods is no longer confined to Mexico. In African countries, maize is widely consumed as a porridge, either a stiff porridge (ugali) or thin gruel (uji), which can also be used as the basis for alcoholic or non-alcoholic beverages. Maize is also processed to make flaked breakfast cereals (corn flakes). While maize contains little niacin or its amino acid precursor, tryptophan, the traditional Central American cooking method (using a lime cooking step) for tortillas increases the availability of niacin and apparently prevents widespread pellagra in populations relying on maize tortillas as a staple food.

Oats are processed by steaming or kiln-drying before de-hulling. The resultant 'groats' can be cut to produce a coarse meal, which is steamed, then rolled to make oat flakes, or granulated to produce a fine oatmeal. Oats are generally eaten as a breakfast cereal (porridge or muesli). Consumption of oat bran became popular because of the cholesterol-lowering properties of its soluble fibre. However, the amounts usually consumed often have only a minor effect.

Barley is used in the form of pearled grains for soups, flour for flatbreads and ground grain for porridge. Barley flour is generally milled by conventional roller milling as used for wheat. Malted barley is important in the brewing (for making beer and some whiskies) and baking industries and is also used in making vinegar and for flavouring breakfast cereals.

Rye is milled in a similar fashion to wheat. Cracked rye is used for porridge and other breakfast cereals and rye flour can be baked into bread, pumpernickel, and crispbreads.

Millet is a name given to a group of cereals that includes sorghum. These are consumed in Africa, parts of India, Pakistan, and China. The grains are pounded into flour and mixed with water to make porridge. In Ethiopia, finely ground millet grains are left to ferment slightly before being baked into flatbreads called injera.

While it has been common practice to highly refine cereals such as wheat and rice, there appear to be significant benefits from eating more wholegrain foods. In addition to their higher nutrient content, consumption of wholegrains is associated with protection from coronary heart disease, ischaemic stroke, and type 2 diabetes, and with bowel health. These foods have more slowly digested carbohydrate, which is useful in the control of blood glucose in people with diabetes (lower glycaemic index).

Further Reading

1. **Juliano, B.** (1993) *Rice in human nutrition. Food and Nutrition Series No. 26.* Rome, IRRI and FAO.
2. **Lorenz, K.J. and Kulp, K.** (eds) (1991) *Handbook of cereal science and technology.* New York, Marcel Dekker.
3. **Montonen, J., Knekt, P., Jarvinen, R., Aromaa, A., and Reunanen, A.** (2003) Whole grain and fibre intake and the incidence of type 2 diabetes. *Am J Clin Nutr,* **77**, 622–29.
4. **Slavin, J.** (2003) Why whole grains are protective: Biological mechanisms. *Proc Nutrition Society (UK),* **62**, 129–34.
5. **Tang G, Qin J, Dolnikowski GG, Russell RM., and Grusak MA** (2009) Golden rice is an effective source of vitamin A. *Am J. Clin Nutr,* **89**: 1776–83.
6. **Truswell, A.S.** (2002) Cereal grains and coronary heart disease (review). *Eur J Clin Nutr,* **56**, 1–14.

25.2 Legumes

Bernard Venn

Legumes are the edible seed from the Leguminosae family (Fabaceae) and include dried peas, beans, soya beans, lentils, and dhal. Peanuts are also legumes. Cultivated since the earliest civilizations, legumes were often considered an inferior food eaten by peasants, described as being 'poor man's meat'. Leguminous plants grow in a wide range of climates and are often used in crop rotations or intercropping as way of introducing nitrogen into the soil as a sustainable alternative to adding nitrogenous fertilizers. Legumes never assumed the importance of a staple food as did the cereal crops, yet, they play an important synergistic role with cereals both in meeting nutritional requirements and fertilizing the soil.

The cereal-and-bean combination is a feature of many cuisines. Mexicans eat kidney beans and tortillas, Indians top their rice with dhal, the Chinese enjoy soy products with rice, those in the Middle East combine lentils with rice, while the English put baked beans on toast. The ratio of quantities of cereal and beans consumed is similar among cuisines, with cereals providing the main source of energy and legumes used as accompaniments.

Of all the foods, legumes most adequately meet the recommended dietary guidelines for healthful eating. They are high in carbohydrate and dietary fibre, mostly low in fat, and supply adequate protein while being a good source of minerals and vitamins, although lacking in vitamin B_{12}. Cooked legumes contain about 6–9% protein, about twice as much protein as in cereal foods. The exceptions are soybeans and peanuts, which contain 14% and 24% respectively, when cooked. The limiting amino acids of legumes are the sulphur-containing methionine and cysteine but, being rich in lysine, legume proteins are well complemented by cereals. Reports suggest that the amount of indispensable amino acids in soy protein products is sufficient to meet protein requirements for normal human growth and development. Soy protein has been shown to have a beneficial role in the control of blood lipids.

Legumes provide around 10–13 g carbohydrate that is the slowly digested type, and 6–9 g of fibre per 100 g of cooked beans. Some of the fibre is soluble fibre, which might lower blood cholesterol. Legumes also contain oligosaccharides, which escape digestion in the gut to be fermented by bacteria in the large bowel. This is responsible for the abdominal discomfort and flatulence often experienced and is perhaps the factor limiting consumption. However, these compounds may have beneficial effects for gastrointestinal health. Legumes are low in fat (~2.5%) but soybeans and peanuts contain 8% and 47% fat, respectively. This fat is mostly monounsaturated or polyunsaturated. Soybeans contain the ω-3 fatty acid linolenic acid.

Legumes supply vitamins and minerals including thiamin, niacin, iron, zinc, calcium, and magnesium (Table 25.2). Legumes have several food qualities that are associated with the prevention of chronic diseases. In particular, high fibre, high satiety, and low energy density are qualities compatible with recommendations aimed at countering obesity and its consequential health risks. Soybeans contain phyto-oestrogens isoflavones, and lignans. It is reported that phyto-oestrogens may be a useful treatment for menopausal symptoms, including maintenance of bone density. There are, however, several substances in uncooked legumes that inhibit their nutritional quality. Most of these toxic substances are destroyed or inactivated by normal cooking or processing.

Trypsin inhibitors may reduce the effectiveness of the digestive process; haemagglutinins appear to reduce the efficiency of absorption of digestive products; phytate binds metals, like zinc and iron, decreasing their absorption; goitrogens interrupt the absorption of iodine. Apart from antinutrient toxins, other substances in beans can cause specific diseases. *Lathyrus sativus* is drought-resistant but can precipitate lathyrism (a neurological disorder that occurs in India) when consumed in large amounts. Broad beans may result in favism, a haemolytic anaemia, in individuals of Mediterranean descent who are genetically susceptible to this disease. Some legumes contain toxic cyanide and alkaloids. Peanuts are common food allergens and can cause anaphylaxis (see Chapter 34). Peanuts are susceptible to *Aspergillus* mould, which produces aflatoxin, a potent liver carcinogen. Careful storage and monitoring are essential to avoid this contamination. Bacteria capable of causing food poisoning may be present on bean sprouts, even in developed countries. For this reason, the US Food and Drug Administration advise that children, the elderly, and people with a compromised immune system should not eat raw or lightly cooked sprouts.

25.2.1 Products from the basic food

Uncooked dried legumes are virtually indigestible, tasteless, and too hard to eat anyway. Processing is essential to make beans edible and improve the nutritional quality and digestibility of the bean. Pre-soaking and rinsing with cold water is recommended to remove anti-nutrients and to minimize gastrointestinal discomfort and flatulence that may occur in some people. Cooking and processing inactivates most antinutrients and toxins. Germination and fermentation improve the nutritional quality of the bean, resulting in increases in vitamin C, niacin, riboflavin and thiamin, and vitamin E content.

Table 25.2 Nutrient content of legumes

Nutrient	Nutrients per 100 g cooked beans
Protein (g)	6.2 (cannelini) to 24.7 (peanuts)
Fat (g)	0.4 (lentils) to 7.7 (soybeans)
Carbohydrate (g)	1.4 (soybeans) to 12.6 (haricot beans)
Dietary fibre (g)	3.7 (lentils) to 8.8 (haricot beans)
Thiamin (mg)	0.06 (lima beans) to 0.79 (peanuts)
Riboflavin (mg)	Trace (kidney beans) to 0.07 (soybeans)
Niacin equivalents (mg)	1.6 (lima beans) to 19.8 (peanuts)
Calcium (mg)	13.0 (split peas) to 76.0 (soybeans)
Iron (mg)	1.1 (split peas) to 2.2 (soybeans)
Zinc (mg)	0.6 (split peas) to 1.6 (soybeans)

Source: NUTTAB 2010 online searchable database.

In India and some parts of Africa, raw legumes are milled to remove fibrous seed coats. Cotyledons are split along natural cleavage lines to form two split peas or dhal. The peas or beans are then boiled, roasted, fermented, germinated, or ground into flour or paste. In Western countries and South America and much of Africa, the seeds are soaked and cooked for long periods of time to inactivate toxic substances and improve digestibility. The beans are either eaten whole, puréed and fried, or made into cakes. In Asia, immature beans are eaten whole in salads, vegetable dishes, or soups; mature soybeans are not usually eaten as whole beans but rather processed into curd, cheese, sauces or pastes, or sprouted as a vegetable.

Today, peanuts and soybeans account for most of the legume products. Soybeans are made into a range of products, including soy proteins and concentrates or isolates, extrusion-textured products, soy flour, soy milk, and tofu. Many soy products are used in manufactured food products, including bread and baked goods, processed meat products, soy ice-cream, sauces and low-fat spreads. Peanuts are made into butters and used in confectionary and baked goods.

Further Reading

1. **Darmadi-Blackberry, I., Wahlqvist, M.L., Kouris-Blazos, A.,** *et al.* (2004) Legumes: The most important dietary predictor of survival in older people of different ethnicities. *Asia Pacific J Clin Nutr,* **13**, 217–20.
2. **FAO** (1989) Utilization of tropical foods: Tropical beans. Food and Nutrition Paper 47/4. Rome, Food and Agricultural Organization.
3. **McGee, H.** (2004) Legumes: Beans and peas. In: McGee, H. *On food and cooking. The science and lore of the kitchen*. 2nd edition. New York, Scribner, pp. 483–501.
4. **Messina, M.** (ed.) (2000) Proceedings of the third international symposium on the role of soy in preventing and treating chronic disease. *J Nutr*, **130**, 653S–711S.

25.3 Nuts and seeds
Margaret Allman-Farinelli

Nuts and seeds have been valued for their oils as much as for a food in itself and were an important source of nutrients and energy since the earliest civilizations. Traditional cuisines have utilized the locally grown nuts and seeds for both savoury and sweet dishes. In recent years, there has been much interest in the nutritional properties of nuts that promote health. Today, nuts and seeds are processed for their oil, ground into pastes, used as ingredients in baked goods, eaten raw, or roasted as snack foods.

Common types of nuts include almonds, walnuts, pecans, cashews, brazil nuts, macadamias, hazelnuts, pine nuts, and pistachios. Sunflower, sesame, and pumpkin seeds are the most common seeds eaten as foods. Caraway and poppy seeds are used as seasonings.

Nuts and seeds have similar nutritional qualities; their low water content and high content of energy, protein, vitamins and minerals makes them nutritious foods (Table 25.3). The energy content of nuts is mostly due to their high fat content. The fat in nuts varies in both quantity and type. Chestnuts are low in fat, but other nuts contain from 45% to 75% fat. The majority of nuts contain unsaturated fatty acids, either monounsaturated (e.g. macadamia) or polyunsaturated. Walnuts are rich in ω-6 polyunsaturated fatty acids but also a good source of ω-3 linolenic acid. The protein content of nuts ranges from 2% to 25%; lysine is the limiting amino acid. They are good sources of dietary fibre, B vitamins (thiamin, riboflavin, and niacin), vitamin E, and iron, zinc, magnesium, potassium, and calcium. Nuts and seeds contain no vitamin C.

Several epidemiological studies indicate that people eating nuts four or five times per week may have a lower risk of coronary heart disease. The constituents likely to confer these benefits are the amino acid arginine, vitamin E, and/or unsaturated fat. There is a danger here of confounding. Nuts make up only a small percentage of the total diet. Studies have also indicated that people regularly consuming nuts have either the same or a lower body weight than those not eating nuts. Thus, nuts are a useful addition to the diet for most people. However, an estimated 1% of people are allergic to tree nuts or peanuts.

Table 25.3 Nutrient content of raw nuts and seeds

Nutrient	Nutrients per 100 g
Protein (g)	2.0 (chestnuts) to 24.4 (pumpkin seeds)
Fat (g)	2.7 (chestnuts) to 77.6 (macadamias)
Carbohydrate (g)	3.1 (brazil nuts) to 36.6 (chestnuts)
Dietary fibre[a] (g)	1.9 (pine nuts) to 7.9 (sesame seeds)
Thiamin (mg)	0.18 (roasted peanuts) to 0.93 (sesame seeds)
Riboflavin (mg)	0.06 (macadamias) to 0.75 (almonds)
Niacin equivalents (mg)	0.9 (chestnuts) to 9.1 (sunflower seeds)
Calcium (mg)	11.0 (pine nuts) to 670.0 (sesame seeds)
Iron (mg)	1.6 (macadamias) to 10.4 (sesame seeds)
Zinc (mg)	0.5 (chestnuts) to 6.6 (soybeans)

[a]Englyst method (see Section 29.2.4).
Source: Holland, B., Unwin, I.D., and Buss, D.H. (1992) *Fruit and nuts*. First supplement to: *McCance and Widdowson's: The composition of foods*, 5th edition. London, Royal Society of Chemistry, MAFF.

Further Reading

1. **Albert, V.M., Gaziano, J.M., Willett, W.C., and Manson, J.E.** (2002) Nut consumption and decreased risk of sudden death in the Physician's Health Study. *Arch Int Med*, **162**, 1382–87.
2. **Holland, B., Unwin, I.D., and Buss, D.H.** (1992) *Fruit and nuts.* First supplement to: *McCance and Widdowson's: The composition of foods.* 5th edition. London, Royal Society of Chemistry, MAFF.
3. **Hu, F.B., Stampfer, M.J., Manson, J.E., et al.** (1998) Frequent nut consumption and risk of coronary heart disease in women: Prospective cohort study. *BMJ*, **317**, 1341–5.
4. **Sabate, J.** (1999) Nut consumption, vegetarian diets, ischaemic heart disease risk, and all cause mortality: Evidence from epidemiologic studies. *Am J Clin Nutr*, **70** (Suppl. 3), 500S–3S.
5. **Sicherer, S.H., Munoz-Furlong, A., and Sampson, H.A.** (2003) Prevalence of peanut and tree nut allergy in the USA determined by means of a random-digit dial telephone survey: A 5-year follow-up study. *J Allergy Clin Immunol*, **112**, 1203–7.
6. **Spaccarotella K.J., Kris-Etherton P.M., Stone W.L., et al.** (2008) The effect of walnut intake on factors related to prostate and vascular health in older men. *Nutrition Journal*, **7**, 13.

25.4 Fruit

Stewart Truswell

In its strict botanical sense, a 'fruit' is the fleshy or dry ripened ovary of a plant enclosing the seed and so includes corn grains, bean pods, tomatoes, olives, cucumbers, and almonds and pecans (in their shells). We usually restrict the term 'fruit' to mean the ripened ovaries that are sweet and either succulent or pulpy and usually eaten as an appetizer or a dessert. Fresh fruits were formerly only available seasonally, but with technology and imports, many are available most of the year. Most of us eat more species in the fruit food group than in any other food group, for example, 30 or more species: some daily (e.g. apples, oranges, bananas) and others rarely (e.g. golden berries, elderberries, mulberries, loganberries, passion fruit).

Our ancestors originally ate fruits for their sweetness. They learned that those fruits that were not bitter were unlikely to be toxic. The sugar that makes them sweet provides energy and may be fructose, glucose, and/or sucrose and others (such as sorbitol). Fruits generally provide useful amounts of potassium, vitamin C, carotenoids, and folate (Table 25.4). Avocados are unusual because they have a high content of fat (mostly monounsaturated) and contain a 7-carbon sugar.

Fruits are preserved in jams by boiling with sugar; the pectin (soluble dietary fibre) they contain makes a gel. Some fruits are dried: especially grapes, plums, dates, bananas, and apricots (dried fruits have lost the vitamin C).

Quite large amounts of some fruits, especially citrus and apples, are consumed in the form of fruit juices, which contain most of the nutrients but less of the fibre, and give less satiety.

Grapes are high in sugar (glucose), which makes crushed grapes a good substrate for fermentation into wine; apples are fermented to make cider.

Most fruits taste somewhat sour, because they contain organic acids such as citric, malic, tartaric, ascorbic, and in some cases, benzoic or sorbic acids. Only citric and malic acids provide small amounts of energy in the mammalian body. Because of the sourness, sugar is added to some fruits to make them palatable.

Fruits contain other substances, not classical nutrients, which can be biologically active, for example flavonoids, salicylates, and limonoids. Tiny amounts of many different natural esters, aldehydes, and ketones contribute the distinctive volatile flavours of fruits (e.g. in an apple, 103 flavour compounds have been identified).

Table 25.4 Nutrients of interest in fruits per 100g raw edible portion

Nutrient	Lowest concentration	Typical fruit (orange)	Highest concentration
Protein (g)	0.3 (apples)	1.1	2.6 (passion fruit)
Fat (g)	0.1 (most)	0.1	19.5 (avocado)
Sugars (g)	trace (olive)	8.5	20.9 (bananas)
Dietary fibre (g)	0.1 (watermelon)	1.7	3.7 (guava)
β-Carotene (mg)	7.0 (lemon)	47	700 (mangoes)
Vitamin C (mg)	3.0 (grapes)	54	230 (guava)
Folate (mg)	trace (nectarines)	31	34 (blackberries)
Potassium (mg)	88.0 (watermelon)	150	400 (banana)
Sodium (mg)	1 (peaches)	5	32 (honeydew melon)

Source: Food Standards Agency (2002) *McCance and Widdowson's: The composition of foods*, 6th summary edition. Cambridge, Royal Society of Chemistry.

People have taken these other substances for granted. It was a surprise when Canadian pharmacologists discovered that grapefruit juice increases the blood concentrations of a number of commonly used potent drugs, for example, most statins and felodipine, by downregulation of cytochrome P450 3A4, which is involved in their first-pass metabolism. The active substance in grapefruit is probably 6′,7′-dihydrobergamottin, a furanocoumarin.

People cannot live for long on fruits alone unless they include nuts. Fruits are inadequate in protein, sodium, calcium, iron, and zinc. Nutritionists, however, look very favourably on fruit as part of a mixed diet and urge people to eat plenty of fruits each day. This is because they are low in energy, fat, and sodium and make valuable contributions to the intakes of vitamin C, carotenoids, folate, and dietary fibre. Numerous epidemiological studies have shown that people who eat above-average amounts of fruit and vegetables (intakes of these two food groups are usually recorded together) have below-average rates of heart disease, stroke, and probably cancer. This may be partly because more fruit is eaten in privileged sections of society, and partly because of the good things in fruits, such as antioxidant nutrients (vitamin C and carotenoids) or other substances yet to be fully elucidated.

There is little to be said about fruits on the negative side, except that in the orchard they are often sprayed with pesticide. These pesticides should have decomposed before sale but it is safer to wash fruits before eating. The seeds or stones of some fruits contain cyanogenic glycosides, which are potentially toxic.

Further Reading

1. **Bailey, D.G., Malcolm, J., Arnold, O., and Spence, J.D.** (1998) Grapefruit juice—drug interactions. *Br J Clin Pharmacol*, **46**, 101–10.

2. **Food Standards Agency** (2002) *McCance and Widdowson's: The composition of foods*, 6th summary edition. Cambridge, Royal Society of Chemistry.

3. **Paine MF, Widmer WW, Hart HL, et al.,** (2006) A furanocoumarin—free grapefruit juice establishes furanocoumarins as the mediators of the grapefruit juice—felodipine interaction. *Am J Clin Nutr*, **83**, 1097–105.

4. **Steffen, L.M.** (2006) Eat your fruit and vegetables. *Lancet*, **267**, 278–9.

5. **Strandhagen, E., Hansson, P.O., Boseaus, I., Isaksson, B., and Eriksson, J.H.** (2000) High fruit intake may reduce mortality among middle aged and elderly men. The study of men born in 1913. *Eur J Clin Nutr*, **54**, 337–41.

25.5 Vegetables
Meika Foster

Vegetables comprise any plant part, other than fruit and seeds, that is used as food. They include roots and tubers such as potatoes, taro, turnips, parsnips, carrots, cassava, and yams; bulbs such as onions; stems like celery; leaves such as lettuce, cabbage, and parsley; and flowers such as broccoli and cauliflower. Some fungi (e.g. mushrooms) are also consumed as vegetables. Zucchini, squash, and tomatoes, although strictly fruits, are usually treated as vegetables by the consumer. Peas and beans are legumes but when immature and green are treated as vegetables. The nutritional composition and the usage pattern of the roots and tubers is somewhat different to that of the stems, leaves, and flowers.

Potatoes have their origins in the New World, being staples of the Incas; other tubers such as yams and taro have been staple foods in the Pacific Islands for many years. Leafy vegetables were grown in monastery gardens during the Middle Ages. Today, most nations have cereal staples like rice or wheat but some countries have vegetable staples. Cassava is a staple energy source for about 200 million people in tropical countries. Potatoes, whether boiled or baked, or as chips, remain a much-consumed commodity in developed nations. While leafy vegetables are commonly eaten in developed countries, they are less popular in developing nations. It is estimated that in India there were 40 species of leaves grown 70 years ago, but that number has now diminished.

Potatoes supply moderate amounts of protein in many people's diets. The biological value is good, with the limiting amino acid being methionine. Stem, bulb, leaf, and flower vegetables usually provide smaller amounts of protein to the diet, although their content may be similar. All vegetables contain negligible fat. Starch predominates in tubers, mainly amylopectin; the other vegetables contain sugars. Vegetables are a good source of dietary fibre. The fibre includes the soluble-type (e.g. pectin) but also insoluble fibre, like cellulose.

Green leafy vegetables have a very high water content and are exceptionally low in energy while relatively high in micronutrients (Darmon *et al.*, 2005), so in a weight-conscious community they are a good food choice. Some vegetables are rich in micronutrients: potatoes are a major source of vitamin C (because of the amount consumed), carrots are exceptionally high in β-carotene, and spinach is rich in folic acid. Dark-green leafy vegetables like spinach are a good source of lutein, and orange capsicums are a good source of zeaxanthin. These two carotenoids function in the macula lutea in the centre of the retina. Broccoli is relatively rich in calcium and spinach in iron, although neither is necessarily consumed in sufficient quantities to make a large contribution to the mineral intake. The other factor to consider is the bioavailability. Studies have shown that β-carotene from vegetables is more poorly absorbed than the pharmaceutical preparation. This is unfortunate because leaves are rich in β-carotene, and blindness from vitamin A deficiency remains a major public health risk in many developing countries. It is well established that the absorption of non-haem iron from vegetables is not as good as the haem form

Table 25.5 Nutrient content of typical leafy vegetables and roots and tubers

Nutrient	Nutrients per 100 g edible portion (Leafy vegetables)			Nutrients per 100 g edible portion (Roots and tubers)		
	Cabbage, chinese	Lettuce, iceberg	Spinach	Carrots	Cassava	Potato
Energy (kJ)	48	58	97	173	667	321
Protein (g)	1.56	0.9	2.86	0.93	1.36	2.02
Fat (g)	0.16	0.14	0.39	0.24	0.28	0.09
Carbohydrate (g)	1.78	2.97	3.63	9.58	38.06	17.47
Fibre (g)	1.0	1.2	2.2	2.8	1.8	2.2
Vitamin C (mg)	26	2.8	28.1	5.9	20.6	19.7
β-Carotene (μg)	2549	299	5626	8285	8	1
Folate (μg)	41	29	194	19	27	16
Calcium (mg)	93	18	99	33	16	12
Iron (mg)	1.04	0.41	2.71	0.30	0.27	0.78
Potassium (mg)	252	141	558	320	271	421
Zinc (mg)	0.17	0.15	0.53	0.24	0.34	0.29

Source: US Department of Agriculture, Agricultural Research Service (2009) USDA National Nutrient Database for Standard Reference, Release 22.

found in meat, but the presence of vitamin C will enhance non-haem iron absorption.

Cooking reduces the vitamin C and folate content of vegetables, often by a considerable amount. Vegetables should be cooked, therefore, for the shortest possible time in a small amount of water.

Apart from the well-recognized nutrients, vegetables contain a variety of substances that may be beneficial for health (Table 25.5). Epidemiological studies indicate that vegetable consumption is associated with a lower prevalence of certain types of cancer like bowel (van Duijuhoven *et al.*, 2009), lung, and stomach. Initially this was attributed to their high content of antioxidant vitamins (β-carotene) but randomized controlled trials with β-carotene were disappointing, and other constituents may be more important. Flavonoids like quercetin and kaempferol, found in onions and broccoli, and glucosinolates,

found in cruciferous vegetables like broccoli and brussels sprouts, may protect against cancer. The flavonoids may also be cardioprotective because they function as antioxidants and may decrease platelet aggregation. In the Nurses Health Study and the Health Professionals Follow-Up (combined cohort of 109 635 subjects) higher vegetable consumption was associated with lower risk of cardiovascular disease (Hung *et al.*, 2004).

While eating vegetables is desirable, there are a few potential toxic effects. Potatoes, especially green ones, contain solanine, a neurotoxin, and this is harmful if excessive amounts are eaten. Sweet potatoes if infected with a certain fungus may contain furanoterpenes that cause lung disorders. Cassava contains cyanogenic glycosides, which liberate cyanide, but this is largely removed by peeling and cooking.

Vegetables are an enjoyable, nutritious food commodity. A number of major epidemiological studies have led to the advice to consume five servings of vegetables and fruit per day. It seems to be generally agreed that the five servings can include one fruit juice, can include frozen and canned fruit or vegetables, and one serving of dried fruit, but presumably not potato chips.

Whether the planet can provide all this fruit and vegetable for all people is another challenge that will need to be addressed. An ongoing debate is the extent to which organic agricultural practices can enhance biodiversity, biological cycles, and soil activity to achieve food production systems that are socially, ecologically, and economically sustainable.

Further Reading

1. **Darmon, N., Darmon, M., Maillot, M., and Drewnowski, A.** (2005) A nutrient density standard for vegetables and fruits: Nutrients per calorie and nutrients per unit cost. *J Am Diet Assoc*, **105**, 1881–7.
2. **Hung, H.C., Joshipura, K.J., Hu, F.B., *et al*.** (2004) Fruit and vegetable intake and risk of major chronic disease. *J Natl Cancer Inst*, **96**, 1577–84.
3. **Tohill, B.C., Seymour, J., Serdula, M., Kettel-Khan, L., and Rolls, B.J.** (2004) What epidemiologic studies tell us about the relationship between fruit and vegetable consumption and body weight. *Nutr Rev*, **62**, 365–74.
4. **US Department of Agriculture, Agricultural Research Service** (2009) USDA National Nutrient Database for Standard Reference, Release 22. http://www.ars.usda.gov/ba/bhnrc/ndl
5. **van Duijuhoven, F.J.B., Bueno-De-Mesquita, H.B., Ferrari, P., *et al*.** (2009) Fruit, vegetables and colorectal cancer risk: The European Prospective Investigation into Cancer and Nutrition. *Am J Clin Nutr*, **89**, 1441–52.
6. **Williams, C.** (1995) Healthy eating: Clarifying advice about fruit and vegetables. *BMJ*, **310**, 1453–5.

25.6 Milk and milk products
Anita S. Lawrence

All mammals produce milk and man consumes a variety of milks from cows, sheep, goats, horses, reindeer, yaks, water buffalos, and camels. Use of animals' milk as a food source presumably coincided with the domestication of animals around 10 000 years ago. Sheep and goats were domesticated first, probably about 8000–9000 BC. Cave paintings show that cows were domesticated by 4000 BC, and traces of cheeses have been found in Egyptian tombs dating back to 2000 BC. Hippocrates recommended milk as a health food and medicine about 400 BC.

Milk is the only food for the first few months of human life. Although human milk has several advantages for babies over cows' milk, it is clear that milk contains all the nutrients that a new growing mammal needs. After weaning, adult milk consumption varies in different parts of the world. In some regions adults consume milk regularly, in other regions they do not habitually consume it. In Western countries, a milk group of foods (milk and products) is one of the food groups recommended for health in nutrition education (see Chapter 37).

25.6.1 Composition

Milk is a good source of high-quality protein. It contains useful amounts of all of the indispensable amino acids. Milk protein is able to complement lysine-deficient protein foods such as wheat and maize. A small proportion of individuals are allergic to milk protein. Prevalence is highest in the first year of life, occurring in approximately 2% of infants. Of these, the great majority (approximately 90% of affected children) grow out of their milk allergy by 3 years of age.

Note: As the main type of milk consumed internationally is cows' milk, for the rest of this chapter the term 'milk' is used to denote cows' milk, unless it is preceded by the name of another animal.

Carbohydrate is present in cow's milk in the form of the disaccharide, lactose. Lactose is normally digested in the small intestine by the enzyme lactase. However, many individuals, particularly those originating from South-East Asia, the Middle East, and parts of Africa, produce reduced levels of lactase after early childhood and some lactose passes to their colon undigested. Its fermentation can cause discomfort and diarrhoea.

Contrary to popular belief, individuals with lactose non-persistence can usually consume two cups of milk each day without any unpleasant symptoms, if they drink them with food at separate meal times. Also, lactose tolerance is improved by regular milk consumption.

The geographic distribution of lactose persistence into adulthood is genetically determined and matches the traditional distribution of dairy farming. Gene analysis indicates that selection occurred relatively recently in the last 5000–10 000 years.

In human milk, lactose is not the only sugar. There are also *oligosaccharides*, with three to ten residues made up of five monosaccharides: galactose, glucose, fucose, N-acetylglucosamine, and sialic acid. Cows' milk and usual infant formulas contain only trace amounts. These oligosaccharides are not absorbed in the small intestine; they pass on to the baby's large intestine, where they promote the growth of (beneficial) bifidobacteria and can reduce access to the body of pathogenic bacteria and their toxins.

Whole, reduced-fat, and skimmed milk typically contain 3.8%, 1.4%, and less than 0.1% fat, respectively (Table 25.6). Milk fat is a very complex natural fat, its triacylglycerols being synthesized from some 400 different fatty acids. About one-quarter are monounsaturated and about two-thirds are saturated. Milk fat includes components thought to be beneficial for health, including fat-soluble vitamins, rumenic acid (*cis*-9, *trans*-11 conjugated linoleic acid), vaccenic acid, sphingolipids, and butyric acid.

Table 25.6 Nutritional composition of cows' milk and milk products per typical portion

	Whole milk (250 mL)	Reduced-fat milk (250 mL)	Skimmed milk (250 mL)	Cheddar cheese (40 g)	Reduced-fat strawberry yoghurt (200 g)
Energy (kJ)	678	510	360	672	696
Protein (g)	8.3	9.8	9.0	10.1	9.8
Fat (g)	9.5	3.5	0.3	13.5	1.8
Carbohydrate (g)	11.8	13.3	12.5	0.0	29.0
Vitamin A (µg) (RE)	120.8	36.3	0	158.6	16.0
Riboflavin (mg)	0.5	0.5	0.5	0.2	0.6
Calcium (mg)	285	343	308	312	320

RE, retinol equivalent.
Source: Australian Dairy Corporation (1999).

Milk provides significant amounts of a range of vitamins, particularly vitamin B_{12}, riboflavin, folate, and, if whole milk, vitamin A. It also contains traces of vitamin D, more if fortified, as in North America.

Milk and its products are generally the richest source of calcium in Western diets as they have a high calcium content per serving and the calcium is highly bioavailable. Few other foods provide the body with as much calcium per serving as dairy foods. Milk also supplies a wide range of other minerals, including phosphorus, magnesium, potassium, zinc, selenium, sodium, and iodine but it is low in iron. As milk contains about 90% water, it is a useful vehicle for rehydration.

Goats' milk provides comparable nutrients to whole cows' milk but is a poor source of folate and riboflavin. Sheep's milk, on the other hand, contains more protein, fat, and vitamins and minerals than cows' milk; it is more nutrient energy-dense.

25.6.2 Processing

Milk is pasteurized to destroy disease-causing bacteria: heating to 72°C for 15 seconds and then cooling immediately is a commonly used method. Milk is available in different forms. In some countries, milk is drunk in a cultured form, e.g. as kefir or as cultured butter milk. Skimmed milks have (almost) all the fat taken out and so do not naturally contain the fat-soluble vitamins A (or D). Spray-dried powdered milk has its moisture removed. It is the basis of infant formulas after adjustments are made to 'humanize' it. Milk powder (which should be fortified with vitamin A) is a major commodity for feeding young children, imported by countries where there is insufficient local dairy supply.

A 200 g portion of reduced-fat *yoghurt* provides a similar range of nutrients to a 250 mL glass of reduced-fat milk, but less lactose. (There is more carbohydrate if sugar is used to sweeten the yoghurt.) In addition to the starter cultures, some types of yoghurt contain probiotic organisms, which can survive the passage through the gastrointestine and have been shown to benefit gastrointestinal health.

Cheese is made using some or all of the following processes: standardization and pasteurization of the milk, addition of rennet (chymosin) and starter cultures, coagulation of the milk, cutting and stirring of the curd, heating, salting, hooping, pressing, maturing, and wrapping. The added salt provides flavour, helps to inhibit the growth of spoilage microorganisms, regulates the structure, and assists in the ripening process of the cheese.

Cheese is a concentrated source of many of the nutrients found in milk, but is much lower in lactose. A 40 g portion of cheese (e.g. Cheddar) provides about the same amounts of energy and calcium as a 250 mL glass of whole milk but more fat and protein, vitamin A, and vitamin K_2. The sodium content varies widely according to the type of cheese; for example, cottage cheese and Cheddar cheese contain about 200 mg and 650 mg per 100 g, respectively. There are probably about 1000 different varieties of cheese but most are not mass produced and from the viewpoint of their nutritional composition they can be grouped. Twenty-five different types are shown in the British food tables.

Left to settle, the fat naturally present in milk rises to the top of the milk. *Cream* consists of about equal proportions of water and dairy fat. If cream is shaken, beaten or churned, it turns into butter and buttermilk. Butter consists of about 80% dairy fat.

25.6.3 Health aspects

A number of randomized controlled studies have demonstrated that increased consumption of milk or other calcium-rich dairy foods increases bone mass at one or more skeletal sites during growth and helps to reduce age-related bone loss in adulthood.

The 2005 Dietary Guidelines for Americans state 'Adults and children should not avoid milk and milk products because of concerns that these foods lead to weight gain'.

Milk fat, butter, and cream containing mostly saturated fatty acids (10% of the fat is myristic) tend to raise plasma low-density-lipoprotein cholesterol and total cholesterol. Yet in 10 cohort epidemiological studies, milk drinking has not been associated with increased cardiovascular disease. Comparing cheese with butter (at the same dairy fat intake) in three separate sets of human experiments, the cheese raised plasma LDL cholesterol less than butter.

Collectively, the data from prospective cohort studies indicate that milk intake is associated with a reduced risk of colorectal cancer.

Milk is noncariogenic (it neither promotes nor reduces the prevalence or incidence of dental caries), and cheese has cariostatic properties (it can help to reduce the risk of dental caries).

Further Reading

1. **Australian Dairy Corporation** (1999).
2. **Bersaglieri, T., Sabeti, P.C., Patterson, N.,** *et al*. (2004) Genetic signatures of strong recent positive selection at the lactase gene. *Am J Hum Genet*, **74**, 1111–20.
3. **Elwood, P.C., Pickering, J.E., Hughes, J., Fehily, A.M., and Ness, A.R.** (2004) Milk drinking, ischaemic heart disease and ischaemic stroke II. Evidence from cohort studies. *Eur J Clin Nutr*, **58**, 718–24.
4. **Miller, G.D., Jarvis, J.D., and McBean, L.D.** (eds) (1999) *Handbook of dairy foods and nutrition*. Florida, CRC Press.
5. **Nestel, P.J., Chronopoulos, A., and Cehun, M.** (2005) Dairy fat in cheese raises LDL-cholesterol less than in butter in mildly hypercholesterolaemic subjects. *Eur J Clin Nutr*, **59**, 1059–63.

25.7 Meat and poultry
Margaret Allman-Farinelli

There is evidence of primitive man hunting for animals from around 500 000 BC but it was not until the end of the last Ice Age (10 000–12 000 years ago) that humans began to domesticate animals along with the development of agriculture. The term 'meat' encompasses not only the muscle tissues but also organs like liver, kidneys, and pancreas (termed offal). The major animals nowadays reared for human consumption are pigs, cattle, sheep, and birds like chicken and turkey. More unusual meats that are consumed include seals by the Eskimos, kangaroos in Australia, deer in Europe (venison), antelopes in Africa, and guinea-pigs in South America.

Muscle meat is generally a good source of protein and minerals, while offal meats offer a rich source of vitamins. Muscle is rich in indispensable amino acids, particularly sulphur amino acids. The greater the proportion of muscle to connective tissue, the greater the digestibility of the protein and its biological value. The mineral content is high, with potassium and phosphorus accounting for the largest proportion. Meat is a major source of readily available iron and zinc, and a good source of magnesium. Liver and kidney are richer in iron and zinc than muscle, and pig liver contains more than that from sheep or beef. The bioavailability of minerals from meat is superior to that from cereal and other plant foods. Meat provides a valuable source of thiamin, niacin, and riboflavin, with pork higher in thiamin than the other meats. Organ meats contain more vitamins A and B_{12}, especially liver because this is where these vitamins are stored (Table 25.7). Liver is so rich in vitamin A that it is no longer advised for pregnant women because too much vitamin A is teratogenic.

In a number of Western countries, there has been a decline in the consumption of meat, especially red meat. One of the reasons is the perceived threat

Table 25.7 Nutrient content of meats

Nutrient	Nutrients per 100 g cooked meats			
	Beef (grilled steak)	Lamb (grilled chop)	Pork (grilled chop)	Chicken (roast, no skin)
Protein (g)	28.6	27.8	32.3	24.8
Fat (g)	6.0	12.3	10.7	5.4
Saturated fatty acids	2.5	5.9	3.8	1.6
Monounsaturated fatty acids	2.8	4.6	4.1	2.5
Polyunsaturated fatty acids	0.2	0.6	1.5	1.0
Carbohydrate (g)	0.0	0.0	0.0	0.0
Vitamin B$_{12}$ (µg)	2	2	2	trace
Iron (mg)	3.5	2.1	1.2	0.8
Zinc (mg)	5.3	4.1	3.5	1.5

Source: Holland, B., Welch., A.A., Unwin, I.D., Buss, D.H., Paul, A.A., and Southgate, D.A.T. (1991) *McCance and Widdowson's: The composition of foods*, 5th edition. London, Royal Society of Chemistry, MAFF.

to good health. In the past, meats had a higher fat content. The fat was largely saturated and it is well known that saturated fat will raise plasma cholesterol. However, there is some question as to whether one of the major fatty acid constituents of meat, stearic acid, will raise cholesterol. Animal producers have made large efforts over the past couple of decades to breed leaner animals and butchers have been altering the type of cuts and trimming meats. This means that the fat content of lean meat is less than many consumers perceive. Meat also contains unsaturated fat, including the very-long-chain ω-6 fatty acid arachidonic acid, which is a predominant fatty acid in cell membranes. Humans can produce this from linoleic acid in vegetable oils, but an intake of preformed arachidonic acid may be important in pregnant and lactating women and the infant for optimal development of the infant brain and retina.

Meat is made into a range of products by curing (e.g. ham and bacon) and by the addition of cereals (e.g. sausages). There is some concern about the nitrate used to cure meat because the nitrites formed have been linked with nitrosamine and cancer in animals. However, the amount permitted to be used has been lowered to the minimum that prevents bacterial growth and we actually obtain more nitrites via conversion of nitrates from plant foods (which obtain it from the soil).

Nutritionists who have researched Paleolithic diets—which all humans lived on before the agricultural revolution—conclude that meats and offal on average provided a higher proportion of total dietary energy and nutrients for our ancestors than they do today, i.e. *Homo sapiens* evolved on a relatively high-meat diet.

Meat provides satiety and it appears to be useful in a low-calorie diet for weight reduction, for example, as part of the 'CSIRO total wellbeing diet'.

Meat has a short shelf-life and must be kept at low temperatures and be cooked adequately to prevent microbial growth. The mode of cooking may be important. Frying or grilling on a hot plate may lead to the development of heterocyclic amines shown to be mutagenic. However, it cannot necessarily be extrapolated that these cause cancer in humans. The relationship between red meat consumption and the development of colorectal cancer remains debatable. In the cohort epidemiological studies, any association of red meat with colorectal cancer is small, but processed meats seem to increase the relative risk.

A major concern for meat eaters was the development of 'mad cow disease' (bovine spongiform encephalopathy), which occurred first in British beef. The link between eating affected meat and neurological disease in man (Creutzfeldt–Jakob disease) has been difficult to understand but as a precaution millions of cattle were destroyed (see Chapter 27).

Chicken and turkey meats are consumed in growing amounts in countries like the USA and Australasia. Chicken is cheaper and people may select 'white' meat over red meat because they believe it to be healthier. More exotic birds consumed include pigeon, pheasant, and partridge. It is not only the muscle that is consumed but also parts like the feet (in China), the liver (goose paté), and even the head. Poultry is a good source of protein, with the fat content dependent on the individual bird; for example, turkey is leaner than chicken, which is leaner than goose or duck. Much of the fat is located just under the skin and can be removed easily. Like red meat, poultry is a good source of protein and minerals, including iron and zinc.

Further Reading

1. **Cordain, L., Brand Miller, J., Boyd Eaton, S., Mann, N., Holt, S.H.A., and Speth, J.D.** (2000) Plant-animal subsistence ratios and macronutrient energy estimations in world wide hunter-gatherer diets. *Am J Clin Nutr*, **71**, 682–92.

2. **Holland, B., Welch., A.A., Unwin, I.D., Buss, D.H., Paul, A.A., and Southgate, D.A.T.** (1991) *McCance and Widdowson's: The composition of foods*, 5th edition. London, Royal Society of Chemistry, MAFF.

3. **Lawrie, R.** (ed.) (1998) *Lawrie's meat science*, 6th edition. Cambridge, Woodhead Publishing.

4. **Norat, T., Bingham, S., Ferrari, P., *et al*.** (2005) Meat, fish and colorectal cancer risk: The European prospective investigation into cancer and nutrition. *J Natl Cancer Inst*, **97**, 906–16.

5. **Truswell, A.S.** (2009) Problems with red meat in WCRF—2. *Am J Clin Nutr*, **89**, 1274–5.

25.8 Fish and seafood

Samir Samman

Man has searched rivers, lakes, and the seas for food since the earliest times. Today most fish are still caught in the oceans, rivers, and lakes but some are produced under intensive farm conditions. Usually, the main edible parts are the flesh but other components, such as roe, are eaten also. Fish, like meat, contains protein of high biological value. The recent nutritional interest in fish, however, is the fat content, which ranges from 0.5% to 15%. It varies according to season and environmental factors such as water temperature. Fish oils contain long-chain ω-3 polyunsaturated fatty acids, mainly eicosapentaenoic acid (EPA) and docosahexaenoic acid (DHA). Oily fish, such as Atlantic salmon, can provide more than 1 g long chain ω-3 polyunsaturated fat per 100 g of fish. In canned fish, more of the fat may be contributed by the oil used in packaging or cooking than by the fish itself. Because of the highly polyunsaturated fats, fish decomposes rapidly.

There is very little carbohydrate in fish and moderate amounts of cholesterol (more in fish roe). It is not usually a good source of fat-soluble vitamins, such as vitamin E, but fish liver and whole-body fish like sardines provide vitamin D. Fish is, however, a source of vitamin B_6, B_{12}, riboflavin, folate, and most inorganic nutrients, notably iodine, selenium, and

Table 25.8 Nutrient content of fish

Nutrient	Nutrients per 100 g raw edible portion
Protein (g)	11.2 (steamed plaice) to 23.8 (steamed halibut)
Fat (g)	0.6 (steamed haddock) to 13.0 (grilled herring)
Calcium (mg)	22.0 (baked cod) to 550 (sardines in oil, drained)
Iron (mg)	0.4 (baked cod) to 4.6 (sardines in tomato sauce)
Zinc (mg)	0.5 (baked cod) to 3.5 (anchovies)

Source: Holland, B., Welch., A.A., Unwin, I.D., Buss, D.H., Paul, A.A., and Southgate, D.A.T. (1991) *McCance and Widdowson's: The composition of foods*, 5th edition. London, Royal Society of Chemistry, MAFF.

fluoride. Calcium, although not found in high amounts in fish flesh, can be eaten as part of the edible soft bones (as in sardines; see Table 25.8). Sodium content is usually low, but as with fat it can be introduced as part of the processing (e.g. fish canned in brine).

Fish obtained from cold, clear, deep water are generally more flavoursome than those obtained from warm, muddy, shallow water. Sauces and garnishes are often used to enhance the flavour of fish, the cooking methods determined by the fish's fat content. Fatty fish, like salmon or mullet, is usually grilled or baked, whereas lean fish (e.g. whiting or cod) is fried. Undercooked fish can present some problems such as tapeworms, which deplete vitamin B_{12}, and thiaminase, which destroys thiamin.

Other potential hazards associated with the consumption of fish are: tetradoxin poisoning (which is mainly associated with puffer fish), poisoning by dinoflagellates (*Ciguatera*), and bacterial spoilage, particularly in tuna and toxic metal contamination (e.g. mercury). The major food authorities advise that pregnant women, women planning pregnancy, and young children should limit their intake of large fish species at the top of the food chain or those that live a long time, as these may accumulate higher levels of mercury.

The health benefits of fish consumption are considerable. Long-term fish consumption may reduce death from heart disease. Fatty fish appears to be the most protective and benefits are most obvious in high-risk populations. These effects may be attributable to the ω-3 fatty acids in the fatty-fish flesh, which can reduce the risk of dangerous arrhythmia and also reduce thrombotic tendency by an array of mechanisms. The consumption of two (oily) fish-containing meals per week is associated with a reduced risk of sudden death from coronary heart disease. Methods used to prepare fish should minimize the addition of saturated fat and salt. With the growth of the world population and increased size of fishing boats and nets, fish species in some seas have meanwhile been depleted of wild fish (Food and Agriculture Organization of the United Nations, Fisheries Department, 2004).

Shellfish (King *et al.*, 1990) are nowadays a luxury food for most people. They have similar nutritional characteristics to fish. Only part of the sterols they contain is cholesterol, some is phytosterols. Oysters are rich in zinc. Some coastal societies, notably the Japanese, enjoy seaweeds and green, brown, and red algae ('vegetables from the sea'), often cultivated. They have a high iodine content.

Further Reading

1. **Food and Agriculture Organization of the United Nations, Fisheries Department** (2004) *The state of worlds fisheries and aquaculture.* FAO, Rome.
2. **Holland, B., Welch., A.A., Unwin, I.D., Buss, D.H., Paul, A.A., and Southgate, D.A.T.** (1991) *McCance and Widdowson's: The composition of foods*, 5th edition. London, Royal Society of Chemistry, MAFF.

3. **King, I., Childs, M.T., Dorsett, C., Ostrander, J.G., and Monsen, E.R.** (1990) Shellfish: Proximate composition, minerals, fatty acids and sterols. *J Am Diet Assoc*, **90**,677–85.

4. **Lee, J.H., O'Keefe, J.H., Lavie, C.J., and Harris, W.S.** (2009) Omega-3 fatty acids: Cardiovascular benefits, sources and sustainability. *Nat Rev Cardiol* **6**: 753–8.

5. **Markmann, P. and Gronbaek, M.** (1999) Fish consumption and coronary heart disease mortality. A systematic review of prospective cohort studies. *Eur J Clin Nutr*, **53**, 585–90.

6. **Ruiter, A.** (ed.) (1995) *Fish and fishery products. Composition, nutritive properties and stability.* Wallingford UK, CAB International.

25.9 Eggs

Kim Bell-Anderson

For Harold McGee, 'the egg is one of the kitchen's marvels and one of nature's. … The cook can use eggs to generate such a variety of structures.' The egg is a convenient nutritional package, providing high-biological-value protein, rich in essential amino acids, and is an excellent source of micronutrients (Table 25.9). Eggs have often been thought to raise plasma cholesterol levels; however, recent cohort studies suggest that consumption of up to one egg per day has little effect on serum cholesterol and only increases the risk of cardiovascular disease marginally in the normal, healthy population. It is still not clear if the risk is greater in individuals with hyperlipidaemia and/or type 2 diabetes.

An egg is an ideal source of nutrition for pregnant women as it supplies extra kilojoules, protein, and important micronutrients such as iron, zinc, folate, and vitamin B_{12}. Children benefit from eggs as a good source of riboflavin and zinc (often both are low in children's diets) and vitamin A, which is essential for growth and eye health. An egg makes a good centre of a meal for someone eating at home on their own.

Table 25.9 Nutrient content and % recommended dietary intake (RDI) in one egg

Nutrient	Per egg	% RDI	Nutrient	Per egg	% RDI
Energy (kJ)	267.0	3.0	Calcium (mg)	30.0	3.7
Protein (g)	5.8	11.5	Iron (mg)	0.7	
Fat (g)	4.5	6.5	Selenium (µg)	14.0	20.0
Saturated (g)	1.4	6.0	Riboflavin (mg)	0.2	10.0
Monounsaturated (g)	1.9		Niacin equ (mg)	1.6	16.0
Polyunsaturated (g)	0.45		Vitamin B_{12} (µg)	0.5	25.0
ω-3 (g)	0.05	2.0*	Folate (µg)	22.0	11.0
Cholesterol (mg)	168.0		Vitamin A (µg)	72.0	10.0
Carbohydrate (g)	0.15		Lutein + zeaxanthin (µg)	131.0	

Values are for one raw egg (large, shell excluded) 45 g.

*= % adequate intake recommendation.

Source: Natoli, S. (2004) *Nutritional and health benefits of eggs*, 2nd edition. Sydney, Australian Egg Corporation Ltd.

Egg allergy is more common in children under 2 years, with tolerance usually developing between the ages of 2 and 4 years. The egg white, which is mainly protein, is the main source of allergens.

Eggs are a bioavailable source of the antioxidants lutein and zeaxanthin, which may help to prevent macular degeneration. Antioxidant (lutein)-enhanced eggs are available in some countries. Other 'designer' eggs may be enriched with vitamin C, selenium, or ω-3 fatty acids. These changes are achieved by changing the hens' rations.

Further Reading

1. **Hu, F.B., Stampfer, M.J., Rimm, E.B., et al**. (1999) A prospective study of egg consumption and risk of cardiovascular disease in men and women. *J Am Med Assoc*, **281**, 1387–94.

2. **McGee, H.** (2004) On food and cooking. *The science and lore of the kitchen*. New York, Scribner.

3. **Natoli, S.** (2004) *Nutritional and health benefits of eggs*, 2nd edition. Sydney, Australian Egg Corporation Ltd.

25.10 Fats and oils

Laurence Eyres

The type and amount of fats consumed today is very different from the days of the hunter-gatherer when lean animals were eaten and fat came from fish, seeds, and nuts. It is necessary for the diet to provide the essential fatty acids, but in most developed countries obtaining sufficient amounts of fat is rarely a problem. Overconsumption of fats and oils, particularly *trans*- and saturated fat, is of far greater concern. The main sources of dietary fat are meats, dairy products, and vegetable oils and spreads and their associated products, particularly baked goods and snack and confectionery products. In the second half of the twentieth century, the vegetable oil industry came to rely increasingly on hydrogenation to produce stable and functional solid vegetable-derived fats used in frying, baking, and table spreads. During the past 30 years, the type of fat consumed has changed from predominantly animal sources like butter, tallow, and lard towards these vegetable-derived fats and oils. In the past 20 years the knowledge that *trans*- and saturated fat are associated with raising blood cholesterol and risk of coronary heart disease has resulted in the emphasis on consumption of more unsaturated fats and the search for functionality without hydrogenation. This has been a serious challenge for the food industry. Consumer demand has seen the development and production of new oils and spreads, as little hard margarine (80% fat) is consumed today. However, the diet remains high in saturated fats because lifestyle changes have resulted in greater use of pre-prepared foods inside the home and particularly fast food consumed outside the home that are manufactured with saturated fats and oils. Baked products (unlabelled) are also high in saturated fats.

The bulk of edible fats and oils are made up of triglycerides (i.e. three fatty acids on a glycerol backbone). The predominant fatty acid present in the oil or fat will determine whether it is classified as a saturated, monounsaturated, or polyunsaturated fat (Table 25.10). The proportions of saturated and unsaturated fatty acids in the structure also determines the physical characteristics such as melting point and solid fat content at a particular temperature. By convention, if a triglyceride is solid at room temperature, it is termed a fat and if liquid then it is oil. Then, canola oil, which has oleic acid as its major fatty acid, is called a monounsaturate, sunflower, soybean, and safflower oils with linoleic acid as the predominant fatty acid are polyunsaturates, and

Table 25.10 Fatty acid composition of common fats and oils (by gas chromatography)

Fat/oil	Saturates (%)	Monounsaturates (%)	Polyunsaturates (%)
Butter fat	64	33[a]	3
Canola	7	63	30
Coconut	91	7	2
Cottonseed	26	22	51
Olive	14	76	10
Palm	51	39	10
Peanut	19	45	36
Safflower	9	14	77
Soybean oil	15	23	62
Sunflower (high oleic)	10	85	5
Sunflower	11	23	66
Tallow	50	47[a]	3

[a]Tallow and butter fat contain about 5% *trans*-fatty acids and appear as monounsaturates in this table. These *trans*-acids are produced by ruminant animals by bio-hydrogenation and are different isomers to those produced by chemical hydrogenation of unsaturated vegetable oils. It is still not certain whether these naturally occurring *trans*-isomers are as atherogenic as those produced chemically.

butter (milk fat) is a saturate. Fats and oils also contribute fat-soluble vitamins to the diet, especially vitamin E and vitamin D in spreads, dairy blends, and margarines. Table 25.11 lists the minor constituents of fats and oils.

25.10.1 Daily intake of fat and fatty acid make-up

There is general agreement that fats and oils should constitute less, between 20% and 30% of the total energy intake (E%). The make-up of this dietary fat intake (65–90 g per day) has been debated for many years but recent agreements and papers produce the following typical composition that should be desirable:

- Saturated and *trans*-fats as low as possible—preferably below 5%
- Polyunsaturated fatty acids ω-6—4–5% provides an adequate intake

Table 25.11 Minor constituents of fats and oils

Fat/oil	Minor constituents
Monoglycerides and diglycerides	One or two fatty acids esterified to glycerol
Free fatty acids	Not combined with any other molecule
Phospholipids	Also known as phosphatides
Sterols	Phytosterols (in plant oils), cholesterol (in animal fats)
Tocopherols (eight isomers)	Vitamin E (antioxidant) compounds, tocotrienols from palm oil.
Carotenoids	Yellow red colours
Chlorophyll	Green pigment (olive and avocado oils)
Vitamins	Vitamin E and perhaps A and D

- Polyunsaturated fatty acids ω-3 as α-linolenic acid—0.5%
- DHA and EPA—a minimum 500 mg/day
- Monounsaturated fatty acids (*cis*)—the bulk of the dietary fatty acid intake.

This has implications for the production of the main edible oils. Palm oil has come under scrutiny for its high saturated fatty acid content and canola seems to be making ground as a major oil at the expense of soy. Monounsaturated versions of sunflower, soy, and canola oils are becoming commercial realities. Unfortunately, the price of the saturated fats such as tallow and palm tends to be below that of the unsaturated vegetable oils, thus encouraging the majority of the population to have a purchase preference for these fats.

25.10.2 Plant sterols

It has been known for many years that plant sterols such as β-sitosterol reduced serum cholesterol by preventing its absorption. The past decade has seen the launch of several margarines worldwide containing significant amounts of plants sterols (8–15%) which have been shown in nutritional trials to reduce serum cholesterol by between 10 and 15%. Over 1.5 g of plants sterols must be consumed on a daily basis to achieve this reduction. The price of plant sterol margarines is very high and hence only tends to be consumed by those people who have been told by their medical adviser to reduce their serum cholesterol.

25.10.3 Issues with oxidized and rancid fats

Recent research has shown that intakes of highly oxidized oils and heat-abused frying fats may well be detrimental to health.

There is growing concern about the effect of oxidized fatty acids on dietary lipids, particularly oxidized cholesterol. Concerns about rancidity implies that all oils should be sold in oxygen-

and-light-impermeable containers such as glass and tin. Unfortunately this is not the case and unsaturated oils are sold in clear plastic, leading to their oxidative and organoleptical deterioration. Polyunsaturated oils also decompose rapidly at high temperatures so are unsuitable for deep fat frying.

25.10.4 Long chain ω-3 fatty acids

The long chain ω-3 fatty acids have been shown to be significant nutrients for humans. There is ongoing debate about whether these long chain ω-3 fatty acids should be consumed as fish or as refined oils in the form of dietary supplements or as functional food ingredients. The long chain polyunsaturates, DHA and EPA are now routinely added to infant formulae. α-Linolenic acid has been widely advertised to the consumer as ω-3 which it is, but the conversion of this acid in the body to long chain polyunsaturates is minimal.

25.10.5 Antioxidants

Whilst there is growing concern about dietary intakes of synthetic antioxidants such as BHA, BHT, and TBHQ, there is a growing emphasis on the inclusion of the necessary 'antioxidants' in the diet. These natural antioxidants include polyphenols from olive oil, herbs and spices, and oleoresins extracted from peppers. A major antioxidant being used in edible oils is Vitamin E (eight isomers). The major source of natural vitamin E is from palm oil distillates. Squalene (a polyunsaturated hydrocarbon) traditionally produced from shark livers is being produced from palm oil and is a significant minor constituent of olive oil. Squalene is consumed as a dietary supplement in Asia and has supposedly beneficial health properties, although its mode of action has never been established, but it has been proposed as a sacrificial antioxidant in the body.

25.10.6 Sources of the main dietary fats and oils

Animal fats are usually obtained by a process called rendering. This involves heating or steaming to remove the adipose tissue from the animal carcass. These fats are most commonly obtained from pigs (lard) and ruminants (tallow). After rendering they contain residual amounts of free fatty acids, pigments, water, and protein, all of which must be removed by bleaching and deodorizing for a high-quality stable product. Fats and oils derived from animal sources contain cholesterol and are usually high in saturated fat.

Vegetable oils and fats are obtained from a wide variety of plants. They can be obtained from seeds (canola (rapeseed), sunflower, cottonseed, safflower, and palm), legumes (soybean and peanuts), fruits (palm, olive, and avocado), and nuts (almond, hazelnut, and walnut). Vegetable oils are pressed from seeds or nuts and then the unwanted components, such as colour pigments, phosphatides, and free fatty acids, are usually removed. In 2010 the main fat produced in the world was palm oil (42 million tonnes), with soybean the second largest (36 million tonnes), rapeseed the third (20 million tonnes), and sunflower the fourth (11 million tonnes). Olive oil is a minor oil, only amounting to 2.5 million tonnes globally.

Solvent extraction may also be used to remove residual fat from the meal. Further processing or refining is usually required when specific sensory properties or functions are required. This produces clear, high-quality oil that is suitable for use as an ingredient, for frying, salad dressings, mayonnaise, and the production of margarine and shortenings. Most crushing of seeds, nuts, and fruits requires a cooking stage prior to pressing to increase oil yields. Cold-pressed oils have this step omitted and the temperature during pressing is controlled. Cold-pressed oils tend to have stronger flavours and odours, which may be desirable in certain foods. The flagship of cold-pressed oil is extra virgin olive oil, which has been consumed in the human diet for millennia. Close attention is paid to minimizing the loss of vitamin E and natural antioxidants like polyphenols during the extraction process.

There are strict standards for extra virgin olive oil and there is a significant price premium which often leads to adulteration.

Margarine is a water-in-oil emulsion produced from vegetable oils (liquid at ambient temperature) and fat (solid or semi-solid 'hard' fraction). The hard fraction is essential to give solidity to the margarine and is now produced by interesterification. The traditional process used for over 50 years, termed hydrogenation, is used less commonly now as it produces *trans*-fatty acids. By blending interesterified fats with liquid oils in varying proportions, the functional and nutritional properties can be altered. Whilst *trans*-fats have now been removed from spreads, there is an increase in the amount of saturated fat in these products due to the use of mainly interesterified fats based on palm oil. Water, skimmed-milk powder, salt, lecithin, emulsifiers, colours, flavours, and vitamins are added to the blend. Spreads containing approximately 40% less fat are becoming popular (as reduced-energy products). These products have the spreading and organoleptic properties of full-fat products but should not be used for cooking or baking because of their high water content.

Other commodities based around fats and oils include animal and vegetable shortenings (with no water, salt, or milk) used by the baking industry and frying oils (stable to heat and moisture) for domestic, small-scale food outlets, and large-scale food production. Salad dressings and mayonnaises are oil-in-water emulsions. Mayonnaise is about 80% oil, which is 'winterized' to prevent crystal formation upon refrigeration that would break the emulsion. For baking and frying, saturated fats such as palm oil, tallow, and lard are still commonly used because they provide the sensory and functional properties that are required as well as being stable. The way a biscuit melts in the mouth is important, and also more saturated oil avoids the problem of oxidation producing off-flavours. Newer products such as high-oleic sunflower oil, canola and soybean, and blends of vegetable oils are now finding their way into the baking and frying sector of the food industry.

Confectionery fats include cocoa butter and hydrogenated and fractionated coconut and palm kernel oils (90% saturated). These are used in cake frostings and in imitation chocolate coatings. Cocoa butter is 65% saturated fat, a fact ignored by most chocolate lovers.

Further Reading

1. **Destaillats, F., Sébédio, J.-L., Dionisi, F., and Chardigny, J.-M.** (ed.) (2009) *Trans fatty acids in human nutrition*, 2nd edition. Bridgwater, UK, The Oily Press.
2. **FAO/WHO** (1994) *Fats and oils in human nutrition*. Report of a Joint Expert Consultation. Rome, Food and Agricultural Organization.
3. **Frankel, E.N.** (2007) *Antioxidants in food and biology*. Bridgwater, UK. The Oily Press.
4. **Gunstone, F.D.** (ed.) (2004) *The chemistry of oils and fats*. Oxford, Blackwell.
5. **O'Connor, C.J.** (ed.) (2007) *Handbook of Australasian edible oils*. Auckland, Oils and Fats Specialist group of NZIC.

25.11 Herbs and spices
Kim Bell-Anderson

The supply of exotic spices such as cinnamon, mace, and nutmeg to 16th- and 17th-century Europe from Asia did much more than contribute distinct flavours to the creation of new food cultures—it helped to define sea routes across the globe. The quest for spices from Asia and America played a major role in shaping the European exploration of the world.

Spices are defined as parts of dried seed, bark, or root. The definition of herbs used for culinary purposes is the fresh or dried leaves of a plant; in herbal medicine, the term more loosely includes any part of a plant that contributes savoury, aromatic, or medicinal properties.

As well as adding distinctive flavour to food and drink, herbs and spices have traditionally been used for spiritual fulfilment and for their medicinal qualities. Before the development of synthetic drugs in the nineteenth century, herbs (not just those used in the kitchen) were the major ingredient in medicines; even now plant extracts are present in some drugs.

Herbs and spices impart overwhelming flavour and aroma to food due to the fusion of volatile chemicals concentrated within the plants. The major chemical families from which these aroma compounds are derived are the terpenes and the phenolics. Terpenes are extremely volatile and reactive molecules, which often contribute to the first flavour or aroma we detect, and quickly dissipate upon heating. Phenolics contribute a more persistent flavour and are more likely to be found in spices. Some spices are valued not for their aroma but for their pungency, which imparts an irritating sensation that is pleasurable. The chemicals responsible include thiocyanates, found in mustards, ginger, horseradish, and wasabi, and alkylamides, for example capsaicin, found in chilli.

Herbs and spices typically contribute minimally to nutrient intake, although some may be a significant source of calcium and iron (e.g. parsley) if eaten in large enough quantities. They are also rich in phosphorus, manganese, and zinc. Fresh herbs contain substantial amounts of β-carotene and vitamin C, although drying and grinding of herbs will remove them. The health-promoting properties of herbs and spices can be mainly attributed to their active phytochemical content, in particular the phenolics and terpenes. Terpenes have been shown to help reduce the body's production of DNA-damaging molecules. Phenolics are powerful antioxidants, and high antioxidant activity has been reported in oregano, sage, peppermint, thyme, bay leaf, dill, rosemary, turmeric, cloves, allspice, cinnamon, and marjoram (50–100 mmol/100 g). Consumption of 1 g of these herbs and spices could make a relevant contribution (>1 mmol) to the dietary intake of antioxidants.

The American National Cancer Institute has recognized some commonly used herbs as having anticarcinogenic qualities. These include basil, mint, oregano, rosemary, sage, thyme, turmeric, ginger, liquorice root, caraway, coriander, cumin, dill, parsley, and tarragon. Turmeric is highly valued for its active ingredient curcumin, which has been shown to suppress the development of tumours in the stomach, breast, lung, and skin. Curcumin is also known for its anti-inflammatory properties in humans.

Other physiological effects of herbs and spices include hypocholesterolaemia and hypolipidaemia

(fenugreek, garlic), anticoagulant, antiemetic (ginger), and immune-stimulating (liquorice).

There are thousands of active phytochemicals in herbs and spices and there is little information known about the bioavailability and bioactivity of these compounds. Furthermore, the concentrations of these chemicals are subject to seasonal variation, species variety, and agricultural processes. It should also be noted that some herbs and spices may be toxic in high amounts.

Seasoning meals with a generous amount of herbs and spices to enhance flavour and increase the appeal and consumption of nutritious foods is a useful means of promoting health, protecting against chronic disease, and reducing our reliance on salt as a flavour enhancer.

Further Reading

1. **Craig, W.J.** (1999) Health-promoting properties of common herbs. *Am J Clin Nutr*, **70**, 491S–9S.
2. **Greenberg, S. and Ortiz, E.L.** (1983) *The spice of life*. London, Mermaid Books/Channel 4 TV.
3. **McGee, H.** (2004) *McGee on food and cooking*. Great Britain, Hodder and Stoughton.

25.12 Food processing
Stewart Truswell

All the foods we eat are living matter, made of cells that contain enzymes, and many foods, especially those of animal origin, are inhabited by microorganisms. Hence food processing is necessary to prevent food decaying and to keep it safe for consumption. Food processing destroys the growth of microorganisms, including pathogens like *Salmonella* and *Listeria*, and will inactivate autolytic enzymes and some natural toxins (e.g. trypsin inhibitors). The storage life of the food is increased, which means that it can be grown some distance from the point of consumption. This enables us to benefit from economies of scale by growing large quantities of food on the most suitable land. Not all processing involves food preservation; some also improves the appearance and flavour of foods, and convenience. One of the major considerations of modern consumers is

the ease and speed with which a meal can be prepared, and more meals are now consumed away from the home. Food processing is essential to meet these consumer needs.

25.12.1 Methods of food processing

Many methods involve *reduction of water content* so that microorganisms cannot grow and autolytic enzymes are inhibited. One of the earliest methods of food preservation used was *drying*. The ancient Greeks sun-dried grapes to produce raisins, which lasted longer than the fresh fruits because of their low water content. In addition to sun drying and smoking of foods, modern technology includes tunnel drying, spray drying, and freeze drying of food to make milk powders, egg powders, and coffee powders.

Freezing, while not removing the water, changes it into a form that is unavailable for normal enzyme functions, and the low temperature decreases both bacterial growth and enzyme activity. Addition of *salt* (as in salting of fish) or inclusion of *sugar* (as in jams) also prevents bacterial growth because of their osmotic effects.

Heat is used in several ways to prevent food spoilage and microbial growth. Pasteurization of milk by heating to 72°C for 15 seconds destroys pathogenic organisms. Blanching of food (75–95°C for 1–8 minutes) before freezing and canning inactivates autolytic enzymes. Canned and sealed foods are sterilized by the application of heat.

Many fruits and vegetables are foods with particularly short shelf-lives. If people are to meet the recommendations made by various health authorities to increase fruit and vegetable consumption, some processing is essential. Fresh fruits need to be harvested and stored using modern technology to increase year-round availability and distribution around the globe. Bananas are picked before they are ripe and shipped and stored at a *controlled temperature* until they are ripened by exposure to ethylene gas (which is naturally given off during ripening of bananas). Californian oranges may be consumed in New Zealand and New Zealand kiwi fruit in California when local production ceases seasonally.

Other food-processing methods include *milling* and *pressing*. Most cereal products such as wheat, maize, and rice are subjected to varying amounts of crushing with metal rollers and sieving to separate coarse and fine components, which eventually produces the different flours and brans. Pressing is used to crush the juice from fruits like grapes (for wine making) and oranges and to press edible oils from oilseeds like canola and sunflower seeds.

Packaging and refrigeration also assist in preventing spoilage of food. Sealing sterilized foods in cans or vacuum packs prevents microbial growth because oxygen is unavailable. Refrigeration retards the multiplication of microorganisms (although some will still reproduce at 4°C).

Food irradiation is a newer technique that can be applied to foods, the flavour of which would be altered by heating (e.g. spices and strawberries). However, the employment of irradiation is an emotive issue (though food that has been irradiated is *not* radioactive). The practice is restricted by legislation in many countries at present. Food irradiation can also be used to inhibit sprouting of potatoes, delay the ripening of fruits, kill insect pests in fruit, grains or spices, reduce or eliminate food spoilage organisms, and reduce microorganisms on meats and seafoods.

25.12.2 Food additives (Table 25.12)

Chemical *preservatives* may be added to specific foods to prevent bacterial growth. Examples include benzoic acid, propionic acid, sorbic acid, and sodium metabisulphite. *Antioxidants* may be added to slow the oxidation of oils and fats, preventing rancidity. *Fermentation* of products will produce acid or alcohol, both of which inhibit autolytic enzymes and bacterial growth.

Other food processing includes the addition of chemicals to provide a variety of functions. Additives such as *emulsifiers* keep the oil and aqueous phases together in mayonnaises and sauces. *Humectants* prevent food from drying out (e.g. glycerol in cake frostings). *Thickeners* may be added to sauces or jams to improve texture. *Anticaking agents* may be added to ensure that powdered foods do not become lumpy (e.g. flavoured coffee mixes). *Food acids* may be used for flavour or to adjust the pH for preservation reasons.

Some foods have their organoleptic properties enhanced by the addition of *colours* and *flavours*. About half of the colours used are from natural sources (e.g. β-carotene).

Artificial sweeteners are used to replace sugars and reduce the energy content of foods because they provide no calories. They have an intense sweet taste but some have other lesser tastes (e.g. bitter) and a better effect is often achieved by combining

Table 25.12 Some common food additives, the code number used in the European Union and other countries, and one of the foods or drinks to which it is added

Food additive	Code no.	Foods
Preservatives		
Sorbic acid	200	Cheesecake
Benzoic acid	210	Fruit juices
Sodium metabisulphite	223	Wine
Lactic acid	270	White bread
Propionic acid	280	Bread
Fumaric acid	297	Confectionery
Antioxidants		
Ascorbic acid	300	Stock cubes
α-Tocopherols	307	Oils
Propyl gallate	310	Gelatin desserts
Butylated hydroxyanisole	320	Ice cream
Emulsifiers		
Lecithins	322	Chocolate
Mono- and diglycerides of fatty acids	471	Potato crisps
Humectants		
Sorbitol	420	Chewing gum
Glycerol	422	Pastilles
Thickeners		
Alginic acid	400	Ice cream
Guar gum	412	Salad dressings
Xanthan gum	415	Bottled sauces
Pectin	440	Jams
Methyl cellulose	461	Jelly
Anticaking agents		
Magnesium carbonate	504	Icing sugar
Food acids		
Acetic acid	260	Tomato ketchup
Malic acid	296	Canned tomatoes
Citric acid	330	Marmalades
Colours		
Curcumin	100	Curry powder
Erythrosine	127	Glacé cherries

(Continued)

Table 25.12 Some common food additives, the code number used in the European Union and other countries, and one of the foods or drinks to which it is added (*Continued*)

β-Carotene	160a	Margarines
Canthaxanthin	161g	Biscuits
Artificial sweeteners		
Acesulphame K	950	Baked goods
Aspartame	951	Soft drinks
Cyclamate	952	Tea and coffee
Saccharine	954	Tea and coffee

two different sweeteners. Saccharine and cyclamate break down with heat so they cannot be ingredient(s) before a food is cooked. All these sweeteners have been researched and monitored for safety; diabetics can consume relatively large amounts. Aspartame is a dipeptide of phenylalanine and aspartic acid. It should be avoided (it must be on the label) by people with phenylketonuria.

Flavours are usually a 'trade secret' so that the names of individual flavours are not declared on the label. However, in most developed nations, food legislation only permits those that have been shown to be safe. In the USA they are known as GRAS, meaning 'generally regarded as safe'.

Other types of food additive are *vitamins* or *minerals*. Some foods may have their micronutrient content *restored* (e.g. the thiamin removed with the bran during milling of flour is replaced), while other food may be *fortified* (for example, foods are being fortified with folic acid so that women of childbearing age can obtain adequate amounts in the diet). Vitamins may be added to a food that becomes a *replacement* for a food in which the vitamin naturally occurs; such an example is margarine, to which vitamin A and D are added, both occurring in butter.

25.12.3 Safety aspects of food additives

A series of strict tests must be conducted before a food additive is permitted. The Food and Agriculture Organization/World Health Organization (FAO/WHO) have a joint expert committee on food additives (JECFA) and most countries have an expert body that prepares food legislation, for example the US Food and Drug Administration (FDA), the European Scientific Committee for Food, the UK Food Standards Agency, and Foods Standards Australia New Zealand (FSANZ). The acute toxicity of the additive must be tested in both male and female animals in a minimum of three species and distribution of the compound in the body is assayed. Short-term feeding trials are conducted in at least two species of animal (only one can be a rodent) and reproduction is studied over two generations. After this, both mutagenicity and carcinogenicity are tested for in bacteria and tissue culture. Effects of food additives in humans are continually reviewed. It is not sufficiently realized that the most likely toxic substances in our foods are naturally occurring ones rather than food additives. Additives are the most thoroughly monitored and tested of all chemicals in the food supply chain (see also Chapter 27).

25.12.4 Effects of food processing on nutrient content

Some nutrient losses will occur during processing but domestic cooking also results in appreciable losses of vitamins and leaching of minerals. Most

Table 25.13 The effect of freezing and boiling on vitamin C content of selected vegetables

Food	Vitamin C mg/100 g
Brussels sprouts (raw)	115
Brussels sprouts (boiled)	60
Brussels sprouts (frozen, boiled)	69
Peas (boiled)	16
Peas (frozen, boiled)	12

Source: Food Standards Agency (2002) *McCance and Widdowson's: The composition of foods*, 6th summary edition. Cambridge, Royal Society of Chemistry.

and easily quantified, unlike those in domestic kitchens. There are some nutritional benefits of food processing: destruction of trypsin inhibitors in legumes, liberation of bound niacin in cereals, and nutrient enrichment with certain foods. In some cases, the nutrient content may be greater when using a processed food than preparing it from the raw product in a domestic kitchen.

25.12.5 Conclusion

Food processing allows an abundant, year-round pathogen-free food supply. No pregnant woman would debate the importance of pasteurization of milk to remove bacteria that could cause miscarriage. Some nutrient losses are inevitable upon processing but they are not usually large. The overall impact of nutrient loss will be dependent on the composition of the total diet (e.g. milling and polishing of rice would only precipitate thiamin deficiency in those people who eat nothing else). If it were not for processing, the food would be unavailable for consumption throughout the year and the nutrient may be missed altogether.

labile of the vitamins are vitamin C and folate, which are unstable with heat, although low pH will protect vitamin C (Table 25.13). The losses during processing by the food industry are standardized

Further Reading

1. **Coultate, T.P.** (2002) *Food: The chemistry of its components*, 4th edition. York, UK, Royal Society of Chemistry.
2. **FAO/IAEA/WHO** (1999) *High dose irradiation: Wholesomeness of food irradiated with doses above 10 kGy*. Report of a Joint Study Group. WHO Technical Report Series 890. Geneva, World Health Organization.
3. **Food Standards Agency** (2002) *McCance and Widdowson's: The composition of foods*, 6th summary edition. Cambridge, Royal Society of Chemistry.
4. **International Food Information Service** (2005) *Dictionary of food science and technology*. Oxford, Blackwell.

Useful Websites

To see topical and scientifically robust updates on nutrition associated with this textbook and web links to many of the journals in the Further Reading sections, please see the dedicated Online Resource Centre at **http://www.oxfordtextbooks.co.uk/orc/mann4e/**

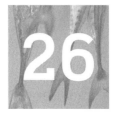

26 Nutrition, the environment, and sustainable diets

Helen Crawley and Tim Lang

This chapter introduces key ways in which the environment shapes human nutrition and, vice versa, how what we eat reflects how we treat and think of the environment. Theoretically, scientifically, and practically, nutrition needs to put the environment at centre stage in the twenty-first century.

Issues such as energy, climate change, biodiversity, water, and soil all shape food systems, the availability of nutrients, and food production. Strong evidence of how the natural world is under stress is encouraging policy makers and food companies to alter their thinking about nature and food's footprint on the planet. Instead of taking the environment for granted, suppliers are beginning to realize the need for longer-term perspectives on how food is produced, distributed, and consumed. The future of food systems is likely to hinge on whether food production and consumption can become more sustainable.

Dietary guidelines have historically been put together to ensure population groups eat a diet which is health-promoting, but these guidelines are likely to have to change as an increasing world population puts pressure on environmental resources. Many countries are now considering what a low-carbon, nutritionally sound diet should look like and nutritionists need to consider their important role in promoting both healthy and sustainable diets.

26.1 Models of the environment–nutrition relationship

Historically, nutrition's core focus has been on the impact of nutrients on human physiology: to clarify what the relationships are and to look at how other factors affect them. The meaning of the 'environment' when we discuss this in relation to nutrition varies. Sometimes it is taken to mean the human body's immediate context, factors such as household, income, age, gender, and family which shape

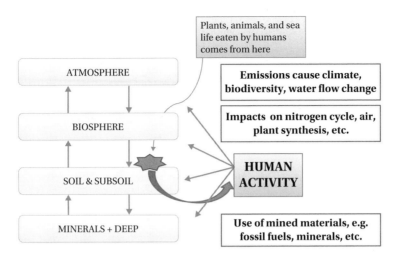

Fig. 26.1 How human activity affects the planetary ecology on which our food capacities depend.

the nutrient–body–health relationship. This meaning of the 'environment' is captured in Dahlgren and Whitehead's rainbow model of determinants of health, in which the individual sits at the centre of an arching set of factors—family, community, government, industry, environment—fanning outwards, but which all shape health. This conceptualization puts the environment at a distance, a factor in nutrition which is mediated through other more immediate filters. But another perspective suggests that how people eat and the means by which the nutrients arrive to the mouth are intimately entwined with the environment. From this perspective, human food is a source coming from a small 'slice' of the earth's crust, affected by the interplay of other forces such as atmosphere, land, sea, and the solar energy which enables plants to photosynthesize and grow (Fig. 26.1). This ecological perspective is increasingly accepted as critical for public health nutrition, not least since the capacity to produce nutrients for humans to ingest is being threatened by the impact of human activity on natural ecology.

Mismanagement of eco-systems can have a direct effect on food production. If soil or any other medium from which food comes is in a poor state, yields and health are directly affected. Human effects include deficiencies of iron, iodine, or vitamin A in the food supply leading to stunting and poor development in humans. In the nineteenth and early twentieth centuries, there was a strong tradition in nutrition science of interest in the role of soil and other environment factors on nutrient uptake. In the mid-to-late twentieth century it seemed momentarily that the earth's productive capacities were limitless, and that the worries about whether production gains could meet population growth were solved. These concerns were first articulated by Thomas Malthus in his 'Essay on the Principle of Population' in 1798. They have been debated ever since. Interest in the relationship between ecology and nutrition have, however, returned in the twenty-first century due to evidence about the potentially devastating impact of climate change, water stress, and biodiversity loss on food production capacity.

26.2 Measuring food's impact on the environment

There are many useful measures for nutritionists to help improve awareness of the mutual dependency of humans, food, and environment. One overall method now commonly used is 'footprinting'. This was a metaphor suggested by Canadian ecologists in the 1990s to generate a composite view of human impacts, like footprints in the sand. The idea has been captured in measures such as those in the Global Footprint reports. These reports merge measures, such as greenhouse gas (GHG) emissions, water use, biodiversity status, land per person available for food production, and CO_2 absorption, and calculate trends. Fig. 26.2 shows how the relationship between resource demand and biocapacity has changed in the US over the past 50 years.

This work has generally concluded that, on current resource use trends, by 2030 two planets will be required to feed, clothe, and maintain existing human lifestyles. Use of productive land and water in 2007 exceeded the Earth's biocapacity—the area actually available to produce renewable resources and absorb CO_2—by 50%. This picture, however, covers a wide disparity between levels of development. If everyone lived like North Americans, five planets would be needed to resource them, if like Europeans, three planets, but if like people on Haiti, only seven-tenths of a planet.

The picture is not all negative. While measures of global biodiversity suggest that there is a serious decline in tropical regions, there are rises in the temperate zones. The message is that improved management and pollution controls can have a positive effect. Nonetheless, the overall figures suggest that human economic activity might now have overstretched the planet's capacity to maintain life.

Various calculations have been made of how different lifestyles and nations consume resources through the food they eat:

- US consumers throw away 25% of all food they purchase, a waste which represents 4% of all US energy use and approximately one-quarter of all water use.

- A pan-European study for the European Commission calculated that food was responsible for one-third of consumers' overall environmental impact. Using life-cycle analysis, it found that meat and dairy products contributed an average of 24% of the environmental impact of the EU 27 member states' consumers, while representing only 6% of consumers' financial spending.

- The Food and Agriculture Organization (FAO) estimates that globally 18% of all GHG emissions are accounted for by the livestock system.

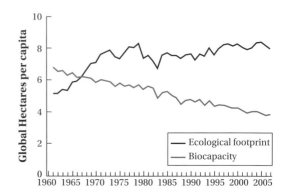

Fig. 26.2 Ecological footprint (resource demand per person) AND biocapacity (resource supply per person) in the USA 1960–2007. Biocapacity varies each year with ecosystem management, agricultural practices (such as fertilizer use and irrigation), ecosystem degradation, and weather.

Source: Global Footprint Network (2010) *Living Planet Report 2010: Biodiversity, biocapactity and development.* Gland, London and Oakland, WWF, Institute of Zoology, Global Footprint Network.

26.3 Key environmental determinants of nutrition

26.3.1 Climate change

Since the late 1800s, the planet's average temperature has increased by 0.4–0.8°C, with further rises predicted by 2100 of 1.4–5.8°C. The majority of this change has occurred over the past five decades. These changes are caused by increasing release of GHG, primarily carbon dioxide and nitrous oxide. Reductions in GHG emissions by 2050 of at least 50% globally and 80% in the developed world are thought to be required to avoid dangerous climate change. Measuring flows of CO_2 in the food supply chain has become one important measure, which food companies are beginning to do for their products. Methane is 24 times more potent as a GHG than CO_2 and, given that animals emit methane when chewing the cud and breaking wind, GHGs tend to be given as CO_2 equivalents (CO_2e). There is not yet an agreed global standard methodology for calculating this, but moves to create one began in the 2000s.

In a developed country like the UK, 18% of total GHGs are due to the food system. Farm animals alone are responsible for 31% of these food GHG emissions and fertilizers for 38% of nitrous oxide (N_2O). Meat and meat products (including meat, poultry, sausages, or similar) are agreed to be the largest contributor, accounting for 4–12% of European's impact on global warming of all consumer products. The production of all foods necessarily contributes some GHGs but livestock production is agreed to be the main source. This has become a difficult issue for policy makers. Every country's agriculture ministry wants to protect its national interests. Other estimates of how the production of different foods impact on GHG have been done, for example in Sweden, where it has been calculated that 1 kg of GHG emissions is associated with yields of 162 g protein from wheat, 32 g from milk, and only 10 g from beef.

Changes in climate have many impacts on the environment including increased evaporation and ocean storm surges, greater numbers of gales, floods, rains, and cyclones, as well as drought and reduced rainfall in other areas. Predicted outcomes for food supply are mostly through the impacts on agriculture: poor crop yields, increased and new plant and animal diseases, damage to habitats of some species, increase in pests, and destruction of crops through loss of land, fires, floods, drought, and storm damage.

There are a number of ways in which climate change impacts on agriculture will alter food availability and this may be in both the quantity and quality of food produced. A reduced availability of some main staple foodstuffs will lead to increased prices and this would have major implications for

food security in many areas of the world. Those most at risk of inadequate nutrition through food shortages would be the most economically disadvantaged, but higher food prices also impact on the quality as well as the quantity of foods available for many, and this has potential health consequences. For example, poorer weight gain in livestock may lead to lower quality meat, lower nitrogen in wheat crops may make it less suitable for bread and pasta making, and poorer quality fruit and vegetables may have reduced storage capacity and be more vulnerable to pest damage.

26.3.2 Water

Pure, safe water is essential for public health. In Africa already, an estimated 340 million people currently lack access to safe drinking water, and many populations around the world offer free, safe water to a minority of their population. About 70% of the planet is water, but this is mostly salty and food systems require salt-free water. Agriculture is the greatest user of water worldwide, accounting for an estimated 70% of potable water use, with livestock playing a significant part in that. About 30–40% of global agricultural production comes from non-renewable water, from sources which are increasingly difficult to extract. Considerable food production relies on aquifers (natural underground reservoirs) for irrigation and watering which are not being replenished. Seventy-one countries are now experiencing some stress on 'blue water' sources (sources of high-grade potable water). Nearly two-thirds of these experience moderate-to-severe stress. The United Nations' (UN) Environment Programme estimated in 2007 that by 2025, 1.8 billion people will be living in regions with absolute water scarcity, and by 2050, 54 countries will be in absolute stress, affecting 40% of the future population.

Hidden or 'virtual' water in food products is called embedded water and calculating the amount of embedded water in different foods and drinks has been used to illustrate the high water use of many foods typically consumed in western diets. Dutch water scientists calculated that one cup of black coffee represents 140 litres of pure water to create it: on the farm, processing, packing, and finally in the delivery to the customer. If the coffee was a milky one, the embedded water rose to 200 litres. A 150 g burger has 2400 litres of embedded water. This stems from crop water use for grain and grass, water drunk by the animal, and used by services for the animal (cleaning etc). Life-cycle analyses show considerable disparities in products (Table 26.1).

Water use surveys show how water flows across borders via the food system. Of the UK's total water footprint, 62% was embedded in agricultural commodities and products imported from other countries; only 38% is used from domestic water resources, making the UK a net importer of water, with some of this coming from countries who are under water stress.

26.3.3 Biodiversity

The planet has a wealth of species on which food systems rely and trade and culture have spread food plants far from their origins. Although historically 7000 plant species and several thousand animal species have been used as human food, a study of 146 countries found that 103 species provided 90% of world's plant food supply. Anthropological studies of traditional peoples highlight how far lifestyles have changed for urbanized mass populations. While 5 million pre-historic hunter-gatherers had about 25 square kilometers per person and drew on around 4000 plants, mid-twentieth-century humans had 1/25th the space per person and ate from around 150 plants worldwide, with the majority of energy requirements coming from just 15 plants.

Table 26.1 Embedded water in some common products

Product	Size or weight	Embedded water (L)
Glass beer	250 mL	75
Glass milk	200 mL	200
Glass wine	125 mL	120
Glass apple juice	125 mL	190
Cup coffee	125 mL	140
Cup of tea	125 mL	35
Slice of bread	30 g	40
Slice of bread with cheese	30 g (bread) + cheese (10 g)	90
1 potato	100 g	25
1 bag of potato crisps	200 g	185
1 egg	40 g	135
1 hamburger	150 g	2400
1 cotton T-shirt (medium)	500 g	4100
1 sheet A4 paper	80 g/m²	10
1 pair of shoes (bovine leather)	800 g	8000
1 microchip	2 g	21

Source: Chapagain, A.K., and Hoekstra, A.K. (2004) *Water Footprints of Nations*, vols. 1 and 2. UNESCO-IHE Value of Water research report series no. 16. Paris, UNESCO; Williams, E.E., Ayres, R.U., and Heller, M. (2002) The 1.7 kilogram microchip: Energy and material use in the production of semiconductor devices. *Environ Sci Technol*, **36**, 5504–10.

The gene pool within individual crops has also declined. A survey of 75 US crop species found that 97% varieties listed in old government-approved catalogues are now extinct. The FAO has estimated that approximately three-quarters of the genetic diversity of agricultural crops was lost in the twentieth century. Rice varieties grown in Asia have dropped from thousands to a few dozen. In Thailand, the 16 000 known varieties has shrunk to 37, and 50% of rice production there now uses just two varieties.

Awareness of the rapid reduction of biodiversity has, until relatively recently, engendered a split between conservation and farming perspectives and policies, separating biodiversity protection from food production. But as the destruction continues, conservationists are turning to food arguments to preserve that biodiversity.

As the FAO has stated: 'when natural diversity is lost, so is irreplaceable genetic material, the essential building blocks of the plants and animals on which agriculture depends'. Low-impact traditional food production systems can be seen as important sources of knowledge about how humans can manage dietary diversity, and diets rich in indigenous vegetables can be rich in micronutrients. Wild foods can play a significant role for forest people, for instance through consumption of insects.

26.3.4 Soil

The link between soil and nutrition has an important place in nutrition history, and increasing science knowledge and investment has increased agricultural productivity, notably through application of manufactured fertilizers, agrichemicals, plus minerals to compensate for soil deficiencies. Interest in soil–nutrition links has, however, narrowed to one of how plants grow rather than the wider ecological links to human health.

In the second half of the twentieth century, an estimated 1035 million hectares of land with food growing potential was affected by human-induced soil degradation. This has been mostly due to wind erosion (45%) and water erosion (42%), but also chemical damage (10%). According to the UN's Global Environment Facility and International Fund for Agriculture and Development, 12 million hectares are lost to desertification every year, enough to grow 20 million tonnes of grain. Between 1957 and 1990, in China, the area of arable land was reduced by an area equal to all the crop land in Denmark, France, Germany, and The Netherlands combined, mainly because of land degradation (Table 26.2).

26.3.5 Land use

As populations get wealthier, patterns of food consumption alter, and higher meat and dairy consumption is usually observed, with a direct impact of this on land use. Meat consumption in China has more than doubled since the 1990s for example, and is projected to double again by 2030. Shifts in consumption patterns reshape land use. Destruction of forest and ploughing up of long-term grassland for crop production (much of which is for animal feed) is agriculture's major source of CO_2 emissions, because it leads to a 50% loss of carbon embedded in the soil. Ploughing deforested land continues the carbon loss. Developed countries have mostly gone through this process in the past but the conversion of forests to farming, mainly in developing countries, is now estimated to account for 80% of CO_2 emissions through land-use change and forestry.

Table 26.2 Regions affected by land degradation

Region affected	Area affected (million hectares)
Asia: Pacific	550
Africa	500
Latin America	300
North America	95
Europe	157

Source: GEF and IFAD (2002) Tackling land degradation and desertification. Washington, DC: Global Environment Facility and International Fund for Agricultural Development. p. 2.

26.3.6 Energy and non-renewable fossil fuels

An estimated 75% of the global fossil energy used annually is expended by developed country populations. About 17% of that unequal share goes on the production, processing, and packaging of food products. On farms, the availability of cheap and plentiful petroleum has been a key factor in the twentieth-century rise of productivity. The internal combustion engine and oil-driven machinery replaced animals as motive power, releasing not just horses and oxen but humans from hard labour. The number of horses and mules on US farms, for instance, dropped from 12 million in 1945 to 2 million in 1960, while the number of tractors doubled. The energy input from fertilizers is considerable. One US study showed how in 1945–85, energy inputs in the form of fertilizers for maize crops grew from 974 to 15,650 MJ/hectare, a far greater growth in energy input than for machinery. It is now estimated that 20% of energy used on US farms is through fertilizers and 19% on water systems. With pressures on oil supplies, price rises, and technical advances, greater efficiencies in fossil fuel use can be and have been achieved. In the USA, for instance, whereas in 1973, 33 gallons of fuel were used to produce 1 tonne of grain, by 2005 that tonne could be achieved from 12 gallons of fuel use.

26.3.7 Sociocultural issues

Urbanization UN Habitat estimates that by 2030, 5 billion people, 60% of the planet, will be urbanized. Half of humanity already is. Developing world cities gain 5 million residents every month. By 2050, Asia alone will host 63% of the world's urban population, 3.3 billion people. Africa's 1.2 billion town people will be nearly a quarter of the world urban total.

In 2007, the world population was 6.7 billion, and this is projected to rise by over 25% by 2050. This increase of 2.5 billion is equivalent to the total size of the world population in 1950, and it will occur mostly in less-developed regions, whose population is projected to rise, according to the UN Population Division, from 5.4 billion in 2007 to 7.9 billion in 2050. In contrast, the population of the more-developed regions is expected to remain largely unchanged at 1.2 billion, and would have declined were it not for the projected net migration from developing to developed countries, which is expected to average 2.3 million persons annually.

With such projections, some analysts paint a neo-Malthusian future of food shortages. Such conclusions tend to underplay existing let alone future maldistribution of nutrients. In the last half-century, world food production has risen remarkably. But difficulties lie ahead, unless ambitious redistribution schemes are created. There will be an increasing burden on remaining rural populations to feed the urban masses and increasing inequalities in food distribution among urban populations highly reliant on price-sensitive food commodities.

Waste A significant amount of food can be lost at each stage of production, processing, distribution, and domestic use. Spoilage, pests, and consumers all account for food waste. The International Rice Research Institute has estimated that rice is lost during harvest (1–3%), handling (2–7%), threshing (2–6%), drying (1–5%), storage (2–6%), and transport (2–10%), totalling 10–37% of all rice grown. Losses later in retailing and by consumers add to the picture.

According to the United Nations Environment Programme (UNEP), Indian losses for cereals and oil seeds are 10–12%. In some African countries, 25% of cereals are lost post harvest, and for more perishable crops such as fruits, vegetables, and roots, post-harvest losses can be 50%. Dairy sector losses due to spoilage and waste in East Africa are also considerable: in Tanzania over 16% of dry season production and 25% of the wet season's, while in Uganda milk losses are an estimated 27% of all milk produced.

Developed countries also have high food wastage. In the USA, 25% of all food, worth US$48.3 billion annually is wasted after purchase. In the UK, consumers threw away 6.7 million tons of food in 2007, valued at £10.2 billion, and a quarter of the food they purchased that could have been eaten was thrown away. Whereas in developing countries waste may be due to inefficiencies along the supply chain, in the UK, avoidable waste occurs due to a combina- tion of factors such as excess purchasing, marketing, and price incentives to buy more than is needed, obeying sell-by-dates, large portion sizes, plate waste, and poor food skills in using leftovers wisely.

26.4 Defining sustainable diets

Many organizations now are working to create sus- tainable diets, bringing together notions of public health, environment, and social justice under the single term 'sustainable diets', but there remains no clear single definition of what a healthy sustainable diet is. Many nongovernmental organizations (NGOs) have been championing localism as the key criterion for sustainable diets. In Vancouver, a citi- zen's group called for Canadians to eat the majority of their food from products grown within 100 miles

Table 26.3 The evolution of international calls to define sustainable diets

Date	Event	Organization	Content
2000	Millennium Development Goals	UN	Goal 1: to halve the proportion of people experiencing hunger Goal 7: to ensure environmental sustainability
2006	Cross-Cutting Initiative on Biodiversity	Convention on Biological Diversity; FAO; Bioversity International (CGIAR)	Identifies contribution of agricultural biodiversity for food and nutrition
2009	World Summit on Food Security	FAO	FAO 'will actively encourage the consumption of foods, particularly those available locally, that contribute to diversified and balanced diets, as the best means of addressing micronutrient deficiencies and other forms of malnutrition, especially among vulnerable groups'
2009 (Dec)	Call for Action from the Door of Return for Food Renaissance in Africa	5th Afrofoods meeting in Dakar, Senegal	Calls for return to 'local foods and traditional food systems [as] a prerequisite for conservation and sustainable use of biodiversity for food and nutrition'
2010	Symposium on Biodiversity Sustainable Diets	FAO & Bioversity International (CGIAR)	Draft Definition of Sustainable Diets with Call for Action, based on linking nutrition with eco-system support

CGIAR, Consultative Group on International Agricultural Research; FAO, Food and Agriculture Organization; UN, United Nations.

Table 26.4 How environmental issues might reframe simple nutrition advice

Food	Nutrition health issues	Possible environmental issues	Potential dietary advice implications	Societal and policy implications
Meat	Positive: Good source of iron, zinc, protein Negative: High in saturated fat, links to cancer and cardiovascular diseases	Negative: High water use; land use for feed production and grazing; high GHG emissions Positive: Use of some land for grazing unsuitable for other crops	**Eat less in total** Eat more grass-fed meat rather than cereal-fed; eat the whole animal Eat more meat alternatives	Changing patterns of farming Impact on livelihoods during transition Impact on trading and exports Impact on cultural and family eating patterns
Fish	Positive: Oil-rich fish contain essential fatty acids, iodine, vitamin D Negative: Some fish contain high levels of contaminants	Negative: Over-fishing is leading to some stock collapse and considerable pressure on many fish stocks	**Eat oil-rich fish once a week and only from sustainable sources**	Changing consumer advice can be confusing Fish linked to culture and food patterns for many Potential loss of livelihoods for some fishing communities Possible increase in fish farming and fish imports Sustainable fishing communities may be protected
Fruit and vegetables	Positive: Fruit and vegetables are low-energy foods, providing vitamins and minerals and other substances linked to reduction in wide range of diseases	Positive: Fruit and vegetable growing can be local for many and use low-energy production methods Negative: Some modes of production use considerable resources, land use, air freight, and cold storage add to climate impact; pesticide contamination; high use of fertilizers	**Eat at least five portions of fruit and vegetables a day sourced locally in season or use frozen local produce out of season**	Consumers used to year-round fruit and vegetable intakes without seasonal restrictions Freezing local produce uses energy Trade implications of more localized purchasing has both positive and negative implications Requires skills and labour for local growing

of home; and in central Scotland, another group has run a project to eat only from within the area of Fife. The World Wildlife Fund (WWF), the international conservation organization, has developed a set of criteria by which consumers can estimate whether their diet is a 'One Planet Diet'. Food companies are also increasingly aware of the need to improve their environmental performance, whether to deliver profitability, ensure long-term viability, or reduce the chance of future litigation. Experiments in presentation of advice to consumers are emerging.

Governments have been slow to link nutrition advice with environmental food advice, but some government bodies, usually arms-length advisory ones, have begun to propose such advice. These recommendations are primarily based on food commodity choices and are informed by national eating patterns as well as by local food production and its importance for trade. Meanwhile, a process has emerged through international bodies for a definition (Table 26.3).

Policy makers and politicians are wary about constraining consumer choice. Yet a review by the UK's Sustainable Development Commission suggested considerable overlap between public health nutrition and environmental goals. It concluded that on some core issues such as meat, dairy, fruit, and vegetables, there was less need for government to be wary of defining sustainable diets or giving nutrition-related advice to decrease (meat and dairy) or increase (fruit and vegetable) intake. Advice on fish consumption remains an exception, with health advice typically recommending greater intakes than at present, and environmental advice suggesting there would be a total collapse of world fish stocks if even current consumption rates persist. A review of climate change and nutrition concluded that benefits come from:

* reducing overall intake of meats and dairy foods and replacement with lower GHG footprint foods;
* reducing intake of sugary foods and drinks, and of tea, coffee, and chocolate;
* reducing food waste, and composting what food waste we cannot avoid;
* reduction in the air freighting of foods.

Table 26.4 outlines some of the issues for even potentially simple health messages which consider environmental implications.

26.5 The role of nutritionists

The role of nutritionists in promoting sustainable diets and looking at nutrition through an environmental lens is not new but has new urgency. Dietary guidelines for sustainability were proposed 25 years ago by Gussow and Clancy and the term eco-nutrition was used over 20 years ago by Wahlqvist and Specht. More recently, nutrition scientists have played active roles in defining statements such as the 2009 World Federation of Public Health Associations' Istanbul Declaration that 'human health and well-being depend on and are inseparable from the health, welfare and maintenance of the living world and the biosphere'.

Governments are under pressure to consider how to join environmental issues with public health nutrition concerns. Public procurement strategies are one immediate opportunity, bringing environmental messages alongside nutrition in food-purchasing advice where food is bought for hospitals, schools, the armed forces, or other public institutions, for example. Most countries have scientific committees that advise government departments on consumer advice and national public health strategies and these organizations must now also encourage more sustainable diets. Currently, there are few practical examples of how people can meet their nutrition needs in a range of different eating patterns whilst also eating a sustainable diet, and most advice is more general (e.g. cut down on milk and dairy foods, eat more locally). This is an area in which nutritionists have a key role to play and small changes across populations could potentially have a large impact on GHG emissions. In addition, third-sector and campaigning groups remain important in harnessing public opinion and offering practical solutions around key issues and these groups may be pivotal in many areas in terms of pushing the sustainable diet agenda.

Further Reading

1. **Beauman, C., Cannon, G., Elmadfa, I., et al.** (2005) The Giessen Declaration. *Public Health Nutr,* **8**(6A), 117–20.

2. **Boccaletti, S.** (2008) Environmentally responsible food choice. *OECD Journal;* General Papers (2), 117–53.

3. **Chapagain, A.K. and Hoekstra, A.K.** (2004) *Water Footprints of Nations,* vols. 1 and 2. UNESCO-IHE Value of Water research report series no. 16. Paris, UNESCO.

4. **FAO** (2008) *Expert consultation on nutrition indicators for biodiversity: 1 Food Composition.* Rome, Food and Agriculture Organization.

5. **Garnett, T.** (2008) *Cooking up a storm: Food, greenhouse gas emissions and our changing climate.* Guildford. Food and Climate Research Network, University of Surrey.

6. **GEF and IFAD** (2002) *Tackling land degradation and desertification.* Washington, DC: Global Environment Facility and International Fund for Agricultural Development. p. 2.

7. **Global Footprint Network** (2010) *Living Planet Report 2010: Biodiversity, biocapactity and development.* Gland, London and Oakland, WWF, Institute of Zoology, Global Footprint Network.

8. **Lang, T., Barling, D., and Caraher, M.** (2009) *Food policy: Integrating health, environment and society.* Oxford: Oxford University Press.

9. **Millennium Ecosystem Assessment (Program)**, *Ecosystems and human well-being: Synthesis.* The Millennium Ecosystem Assessment series. 2005, Washington, DC, Island Press.

10. **Millward, D.J. and Garnett, T.** (2010) Plenary lecture 3: Food and the planet: Nutritional dilemmas of greenhouse gas emission reductions through reduced intakes of meat and dairy foods. *Proc Nutr Soc,* **69**, 103–18.

11. **Steinfeld, H., Gerber, P., Wassenaar, T.D., et al.** (2006) *Livestock's long shadow: Environmental issues and options.* Rome, Food and Agriculture Organization.

12. **Sustainable Development Commission** (2009) *Setting the table: Advice to government on priority elements of sustainable diets.* London, Sustainable Development Commission.

13. **UN Habitat** (2008) *State of the world's cities 2008/2009—harmonious cities.* Nairobi, UN Habitat.

14. **WRAP** (2008) *The food we waste.* Banbury, Waste and Resources Action Programme.

Useful Websites

To see topical and scientifically robust updates on nutrition associated with this textbook and web links to many of the journals in the Further Reading sections, please see the dedicated Online Resource Centre at **http://www.oxfordtextbooks.co.uk/orc/mann4e/**

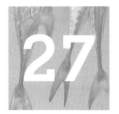

27 Food toxicity and safety

Peter Williams

Until recently, eating food in modern industrialized countries has usually been regarded as a low-risk activity, but several highly publicized food safety scares have raised consumer concerns about the safety of our food supplies (Table 27.1).

Very few of the foods that we commonly eat have been subject to any toxicological testing and yet they are generally accepted as being safe to eat. However, all chemicals, including those naturally found in foods, are toxic at some dose. Laboratory animals can be killed by feeding them glucose or salt at very high doses and some nutrients such as vitamin A and selenium are hazardous at intakes only a few times greater than normal human requirements. Even very common foods such as pepper have demonstrated carcinogenic activity. Toxicity testing of a food or ingredient can tell us what the likely adverse effects are and at what level of consumption they may occur, but by itself this does not tell us whether it is safe to eat in normally consumed amounts.

'Risk' is the probability that the substance will produce injury under defined conditions of exposure. The concept of risk takes into account the dose and length of exposure, as well as the toxicity of a particular chemical and is a better guide to the safety of a food. Consequently, any attempt to

Table 27.1 A chronology of recent food scares

1986	First cases of mad cow disease in Britain
1990	Benzene in Perrier mineral water in France
1996	Salmonella in peanut butter in Australia
1997	Contagious swine fever in The Netherlands
1999	Contaminated Coca-Cola in Belgium
1999	Pollen from genetically modified maize reported to kill Monarch butterflies
2001	Foot-and-mouth disease all over Europe
2002	Acrylamide found in starchy foods cooked at high temperature
2003	Outbreak of bird flu in Asian poultry
2004	Warnings about mercury in shark, mackerel, and swordfish in the USA
2008	Melamine contamination of baby milk formula in China

examine the safety of the food supply should not be based on the question 'Is this food or ingredient toxic?' (the answer is always 'yes'), but rather by finding out if eating this substance in normal amounts is likely to increase the risk of illness significantly, i.e. 'Is it safe?'

27.1 Hazardous substances in food

Three general classes of hazards are found in foods: (1) microbial or environmental *contaminants*; (2) naturally occurring toxic *constituents*; and (3) those resulting from intentional *food additives* or *novel foods or ingredients*. The most dangerous contaminants are those produced by infestations of bacteria or moulds in food, which can produce toxins that remain in the food even after the biological source

Table 27.2 Potential hazards in foods

Hazards	Examples
Microbial contamination	
Pathogenic bacteria	Toxins from *Clostridium botulinum*
Mycotoxins	Aflatoxin from mould on peanuts
Environmental contamination	
Heavy metals and mineral	Arsenic and mercury in fish
Criminal adulteration	Aniline in olive oil
Packaging migration	BPA from plastics
Industrial pollution	PCB, radioactive fallout
Changes during cooking or processing	Carcinogens produced in burnt meat
Natural toxins	
Inherent toxins	Cyanide in cassava
Produced by abnormal conditions	Ciguatera poisoning from fish
Enzyme inhibitors	Protease inhibitors in legumes
Antivitamins	Avidin in raw egg white
Mineral-binding agents	Goitrogens in brassica vegetables
Agricultural residues	
Pesticides	DDT
Hormones	Bovine somatotrophin
Intentional food additives	
Artificial sweeteners	Cyclamate
Preservatives	Sodium nitrite

BPA, Bisphenol A; DDT, dichlorodiphenyltrichloroethane; PCB, polychlorinated biphenyl.

has been destroyed. Other contaminants, such as pesticide residues or heavy metals, are usually well controlled in modern food supplies but can be significant hazards in particular localities. Naturally occurring toxic constituents are usually present in doses that are too small to produce harmful effects when foods are eaten normally, except in the cases of atypical consumers who may be sensitive to individual ingredients. Food additives or novel foods are generally the least dangerous hazards because their toxicology is well studied and the conditions of use are tightly controlled. Table 27.2 summarizes the types of hazardous substances that may be present in food.

The US Food and Drug Administration (FDA) has ranked the relative importance of health hazards associated with food in the following descending order of seriousness:

1 Microbiological contamination.

2 Inappropriate eating habits.

3 Environmental contamination.

4 Natural toxic constituents.

5 Pesticide residues.

6 Food additives.

This list is very different from that found in public opinion polls, which show that most people rate food additives as one of their major concerns about the safety of the food supply.

27.2 Microbial contamination

27.2.1 Pathogenic bacteria

Outbreaks of acute gastroenteritis caused by microbial pathogens are usually called food poisoning. They can be caused by foodborne *intoxication* (where microbes in food produce a toxin that produces the symptom) or foodborne *infection* (where the symptoms are caused by the activity of live bacterial cells multiplying in the gastrointestinal system). Table 27.3 lists the most common bacterial causes of food poisoning, in order of the rapidity of onset of symptoms. In general, the intoxications have a more rapid onset.

The most important pathogens are *Clostridium botulinum*, *Staphylococcus aureus*, *Salmonella* species and *Clostridium perfringens*. The last three organisms account for about 70–80% of all reported outbreaks of foodborne illness, but there are also many others, as well as some viral and protozoan agents. The four most frequently identified factors contributing to food-poisoning incidents are: improper cooling of food, lapses of 12 hours or more between cooking and eating, contamination by food handlers, and contaminated raw foods or ingredients.

The reported incidence and cost of foodborne illness in most countries is increasing, although it is difficult to measure this exactly. It is estimated that less than 1% of cases are captured in existing notification schemes. Some of the reasons for increasing rates of foodborne illness are: new and emerging pathogens, changes in the food supply (including more intensive animal husbandry and longer shelf life fresh-chilled products), aging populations, and a greater proportion of food eaten away from home. Around 60–80% of foodborne illness arises from the food service industry.

27.2.2 Control of food poisoning

The trend in all countries today is to require more formal training of all food handlers and the development of food safety plans wherever food is prepared and served to the public, based on the principles of Hazard Analysis of Critical Control Points (HACCP). HACCP is a preventative approach to quality control, used worldwide in all segments of food production, from primary production to food manufacture

Table 27.3 Common bacterial food-poisoning organisms

Organism	Symptoms	Time after food	Typical food sources
Toxins			
Staphylococcus aureus	Vomiting, diarrhoea, abdominal pain	1–6 hours (mean 2–3 h)	Custard and cream-filled baked goods, cold meats
Clostridium perfringens	Diarrhoea and severe pain, nausea	8–24 hours (mean 8–15 h)	Meat products incompletely cooked or reheated
Bacillus cereus	a) nausea, vomiting b) abdominal pain, watery diarrhoea	a) 1–5 hours b) 6–16 hours (mean 10–12 h)	Rice dishes, vegetables, sauces, puddings
Clostridium botulinum	Dry mouth, difficulty swallowing and speaking, double vision, difficulty breathing. Often fatal	2 h–8 days (mean 12–36 h)	Home canned foods (usually meat and vegetables), and inadequately processed smoked meats
Infection			
Vibrio parahaemolyticus	Diarrhoea, abdominal cramp, nausea, headache, vomiting	4–96 hours (mean 12 h)	Fish, crustaceans
Salmonella spp.	Diarrhoea, fever, nausea, vomiting	8–72 hours (mean 12–36 h)	Undercooked poultry, reheated food, cream-filled pastries
Yersinia enterocolytica	Fever, abdominal pain, diarrhoea	24–36 hours	Raw and cooked pork and beef
Escherichia coli	Fever, cramps, nausea, diarrhoea	8–44 hours (mean 26 h)	Faecal contamination of food or water
Shigella spp.	Diarrhoea, bloody stools with mucus, fever	1–7 days (mean 1–3 d)	Faecal contamination of food
Campylobacter jejuni	Fever, abdominal pain, diarrhoea	1–10 days (mean 2–5 d)	Raw milk, poultry, eggs, meat
Listeria monocytogenes	Septic abortion, septicaemia, meningitis, encephalitis. Often fatal	1–7 weeks	Milk and dairy products, raw meat, poultry and eggs, vegetables and salads, seafood

and food service settings. It is based on seven principles:

- Identify all potential *hazards* at each step in the food chain and possible preventative actions.

- Determine the *critical* points in the operation where the hazards must be controlled.

- Establish *limits* at each critical control point: examples of control procedures are washing hands, sanitizing food preparation surfaces and tools, cooking food to specific temperature, maximum food storage times.

- Set up procedures to *monitor* each critical control point.

- Plan the *corrective actions* to be taken if a critical limit is exceeded.

- Establish a *recording system* to document performance of the process.

- *Verify* that the HACCP process is working.

Table 27.4 outlines an example of some parts of a HACCP plan for a commercial food product sold as ready-to-eat.

27.2.3 Mycotoxins

Moulds, or fungi, are capable of producing a wide variety of chemicals that are biologically active.

Table 27.4 An example of six steps from a HAACP plan for chilled chicken salad

Step	1. Growing and harvesting	2. Raw material processing	3. Supply storage temperatures	4. Ingredient assembly	5. Bagging	6. Labelling
Hazard	Chemicals, antibiotics	Chemical, microbiological	Microbiological	Microbiological	Microbiological	Incorrect dates, traceability
Control	Raw material specifications	Certified supplier	Raw material specifications	Temperature control specs	Correct seal settings	Legible, correct dates and codes
Limit	Regulatory approved residues	Free of pathogens and foreign material	Chicken < −12°C, vegetables < 4°C	Food < 4°C	Upper tolerance limit on sealer	Use proper labels
Monitoring	Certificate of compliance	Monitor supplier HACCP program	Check cool room records daily	Check temperature once per shift	Check setting every 15 min.	Each batch at changeover
Action if limit exceeded	Reject lot	Reject as supplier	Investigate time/temp abuse	Report to supervisor	Examine all packages	Destroy incorrect labels
Responsibility	Receiving operator	Purchaser	Store person	Cook	Seal inspector	Packer

Source: Adapted from Microbiology and Food Safety Committee of the National Food Processors Association (1993) HACCP implementation: a generic model for chilled foods. *J Food Prot*, **56**, 1077.

Humans have used some of these as effective antibiotics, but there are also a number of diseases resulting from accidental exposure to fungal products that contaminate food. Some examples are as follows.

Aflatoxins These are a group of highly toxic and carcinogenic compounds from the common *Aspergillus* fungus species. They are stable to heat and survive most forms of food processing. Aflatoxin contamination can occur whenever environmental conditions are suitable for mould growth, but the problem is more common in tropical and semitropical regions. Aflatoxins were first recognized in the 1960s in peanuts. On a worldwide basis, maize is the most important food contaminated with aflatoxin.

Patulin is an antibiotic that is produced by the mould *Penicillium caviforme*. It has been implicated as a possible carcinogen from one study in rats, although other studies have not confirmed this. Patulin is primarily associated with the apple-rotting fungus and so apple juices and some baked goods with fruit can contain patulin.

Fumonisins are carcinogenic mycotoxins from the *Fusarium* fungus associated with maize. These were first characterized in 1988 and are known to be potent inhibitors of sphingolipid synthesis. Ingestion of fumonisin-affected corn has been shown to be carcinogenic in rats. In 1990 it was reported that use of mouldy corn with high levels of fumonisins to make beer in the Transkei of South Africa was associated with a very high incidence of oesphageal cancer.

27.2.4 New foodborne diseases

Three of the most serious food pathogens today (*Campylobacter*, *Listeria*, and enterohemorrhagic *Escherichia coli*) were unrecognized as causes of illness 30 years ago. Some of the more important new organisms are described here.

Campylobacter jejuni was a well-known bacterium in veterinary medicine before it was identified as a human pathogen in 1973. It is now recognized as one of the most important causes of gastroenteritis in humans, of similar importance to *Salmonella*. It is present in the flesh of cattle, sheep, pigs, and poultry and can be introduced wherever raw meat is handled.

Listeria monocytogenes is a bacterium widely distributed in nature but is unusual in that it grows at refrigeration temperatures (down to 0°C). Listeriosis can cause abortions as well as death in the elderly and those with compromised immune systems, such as people with AIDS. Listeria has been linked to the consumption of contaminated pâtés, milk, soft cheese, and undercooked chicken, and is often found in pre-prepared chilled food.

Escherichia coli 0157:H7 is a bacterium that can damage the cells of the colon, leading to bloody diarrhoea and abdominal cramps. Raw or undercooked hamburger meat was a major vehicle of transmission in a number of well-publicized outbreaks in the USA in 1993 and contaminated metwurst was responsible for a major outbreak of illness in Australia in 1995.

Salmonella typhimurium is a multidrug-resistant strain that has become a major pathogen in the UK in the 1990s. As well as being highly virulent it can survive at low pH and be infectious in very low numbers.

Norwalk virus is found in the faeces of humans, and illness is caused by poor personal hygiene among infected food handlers. Symptoms include nausea, vomiting, diarrhoea, abdominal pain, and fever. Because it is a virus, it does not reproduce in food, but remains active until the food is eaten.

'Mad cow disease' (or BSE, bovine spongiform encephalopathy) is a slowly progressive and ultimately fatal neurological disorder of adult cattle that results from infection by an unique transmission agent called a prion. Prions seem to be modified forms of normal cell surface proteins. BSE was first confirmed in Britain in 1986, but has now spread to cattle in other countries of Europe, Japan, and North America. The same infective agent is also responsible for variant Creutzfeldt Jakob Disease (vCJD), a fatal disease of humans, mostly affecting young adults. By October 2009, it had killed 166 people in Britain and 44 elsewhere, with the number expected to rise because of the disease's long incubation period. Three principal controls have been put in place to keep infected meat out of the food chain: banning slaughter of beef aged over 30 months (before the age at which BSE typically develops), removal of parts of the body with the highest levels of infection (e.g. nervous and bone tissue), and a ban on feeding meat and bonemeal to any farmed livestock. Milk and gelatine products from beef do not appear to be affected.

27.3 Environmental contamination

27.3.1 Heavy metals and minerals

Selenium is one of the most toxic essential trace elements. The level of selenium in foods usually reflects the levels in the soil and in a few high-selenium areas, such as North Dakota and parts of China, excessive selenium intake has been associated with gastrointestinal disturbances and skin discolouration.

Mercury Fish can contain 10–1500 mg/kg of organic mercury, and even higher levels when mercury wastes are released into lake waters. Serious poisonings from mercury in fish have occurred in Japan, the most famous being that in Minamata Bay (from 1953 to 1960). Another example of widespread mercury intoxication occurred in Iraq in 1971/72 as a result of bread made from wheat treated with mercury-based pesticides. Most countries have now established maximum permitted levels on mercury in fish in the range of 0.4–1.0 mg/kg.

Cadmium is a toxic element that accumulates in biological systems. Chronic exposure at excessive levels can lead to irreversible kidney failure. Plants readily take up cadmium from the soil, and there has been a slow increase in the cadmium levels in soils due to the use of phosphate fertilizers and the affect of air and water pollution. The average food-based cadmium intake is now approximately 10–50 µg per day, which is approaching the provisional tolerable weekly intake. Measures to control cadmium contamination include controls on waste disposal and developing new crops that accumulate less cadmium.

27.3.2 Criminal adulteration

Modern food regulations began in the nineteeth century when there were widespread examples of adulteration of foods to increase profits. Milk was diluted with water, cocoa with sawdust, and butter with borax. Today standards in the food industry are much higher and risks from illegal adulteration are rare. However, there are still some notorious instances.

In Spain in 1981 there was an outbreak of an apparently new disease characterized by fever, rashes, and respiratory problems. Many thousands were hospitalized and over 100 people died. The agent responsible was identified as cooking oil that had been fraudulently sold as pure olive oil but in fact was mostly rapeseed oil intended for industrial uses, which was contaminated with aniline. In China in 2008, at least six children died of acute kidney failure and nearly 300 000 fell ill after consuming tainted infant formula. Melamine, a synthetic nitrogenous product found in many industrial goods, was found to have been illegally added to milk-based foods to make them appear higher in protein than they really were.

27.3.3 Packaging migration

The materials used to package food can sometimes contaminate the food itself. At one time, the lead used in the solder of metal cans was a significant source of contamination of infant formulae, but this problem has been eliminated by the introduction of non-soldered cans. Bisphenol A (BPA) is an industrial chemical used as the starting material for the production of polycarbonate plastics and synthetic resins. BPA is found in containers that come into contact with foodstuffs such as drinking vessels, baby bottles, and the internal coating on cans for tinned food. BPA belongs to a group of substances that can act in a similar way to some hormones, and studies in laboratory animals suggest that low levels may have an effect on the reproductive system. In 2010, the FDA released a report on the safety of BPA, which raised concern about its potential effects on the brain, behaviour, and prostate gland in fetuses, infants, and young children. Subsequently manufacturers of baby bottles around the world have agreed to move to BPA-free bottles as soon as possible.

27.3.4 Industrial pollution

Throughout the industrial era, many potentially hazardous substances have been released into the environment and are now widely distributed in the food chain. Among the most important are the polychlorinated biphenyls (PCBs). PCB is a generic term for a wide range of highly stable derivatives of biphenyl that have been used in a vast number of products, including plastics, paints, and lubricants. Although manufacture has now ceased, their stability and lipid solubility has meant that they accumulate in fatty tissue and they have become widespread, particularly in seafood. They can be found at low levels now even in human milk. The health effects of PCBs are not well established, although they are thought to be mild carcinogens. In one incident in Japan in 1978 when rice oil was contaminated with 2000–3000 ppm PCB, growth retardation occurred in young children and the fetuses of exposed mothers.

27.3.5 Radioactive fallout

The most important dangerous radioisotopes in fallout are strontium-90 and caesium-137, with half-lives of 28 and 30 years, respectively. Strontium is absorbed and metabolized like calcium and stored in bones. Because it is concentrated in milk it is particularly dangerous for infants and children. Since the Nuclear Test Ban Treaty of 1963, the level of radioactive contamination from atmospheric dust has markedly declined, but accidental exposure can still occur, such as that after the Chernobyl disaster, and lead to dangerous food contamination over widespread areas.

27.3.6 Changes during cooking or processing

Food is frequently exposed to high temperatures during cooking. In roasting and frying, localized areas of food may be subjected to temperatures that lead to carbonization and under these circumstances any organic substance is likely to give rise to carcinogens. The major compounds are polycyclic aromatic hydrocarbons (PAH), produced mainly by burning of fats, and heterocyclic amines (HCA), produced from amino acids. Char-broiling or barbecuing is particularly likely to lead to carcinogen formation.

Acrylamide In 2002 the Swedish National Food Authority announced that acrylamide could be found in starch-containing foods cooked at high temperatures, such as fried or roasted potato products, and cereal-based products, including sweet biscuits and toasted bread. In 2010 a World Health Organization (WHO) expert committee determined that there is evidence that acrylamide can cause cancer in laboratory animals and, while there is currently no scientific evidence which links acrylamide with cancer risk in humans, all food regulatory agencies around the world are encouraging new technological strategies aimed at reducing its formation.

Irradiation can be used to sterilize foods, control microbial spoilage, eradicate insect infestations, and inhibit undesired sprouting. Despite the great potential of the technology, there has been substantial opposition from consumer groups concerned about the process producing toxic chemicals in foods. Extensive studies have shown that the products formed are no different from those produced in normal cooking and over 1300 studies have consistently found no adverse effects from feeding irradiated food to animals or humans. Food irradiation is approved by the WHO and currently more than 30 countries allow some form of use.

27.4 Natural toxins

Many plant species contain hazardous levels of toxic constituents. Intoxications from poisonous plants usually result from the misidentification of plants by individuals harvesting their own foods, but many ordinary foods also contain potential toxicants at less harmful levels. numerous detoxification systems, mainly enzymes in the liver, to deal with any toxins we do ingest. So we can still happily eat nutmeg and sassafras, even though both contain the naturally occurring carcinogen safrole.

27.4.1 Inherent natural toxins

There are many examples of potentially dangerous toxins in natural food products: cyanogenic glycosides in plants such as almond kernels, cassava, and sorghum, alkaloids in herbal teas and comfrey, and lathyrus toxin in chickpeas. In Japan the puffer fish, which contains a potentially fatal neurotoxin, is considered a delicacy and is consumed to produce a tingling sensation. However, natural toxicants are a generally accepted hazard because the foods that contain them have been eaten in traditional diets for many generations. We are protected from their harmful effects in three ways: avoidance, removal, and detoxification.

First, traditional knowledge has been passed down about which foods are safe and which are not. Thus we know it is safe to eat certain mushrooms and not others. Second, traditional preparation methods have evolved to reduce harmful effects. Specialist chefs prepare puffer fish to remove the parts with the highest toxin concentration. People in South America and Africa use complex chopping and washing procedures in their preparation of cassava that removes much of the cyanide naturally found in the raw product. Third, the body has

27.4.2 Abnormal conditions of the animal or plant used for food

Some foods only become hazardous during particular conditions of growth or storage.

Ciguatera poisoning This is serious human intoxication, caused by eating contaminated fish, causing gastrointestinal disorders, neurological problems and, in severe cases, death. There are over 400 species of fish that may become ciguatoxic, but almost all of the fatal cases are attributable to barracuda. The poisoning is particularly insidious because it occurs in tropical and subtropical fish that are normally safe to eat, but not so when they have been feeding on certain dinoflagellates that produce toxins that accumulate in the flesh.

Paralytic shellfish poisoning It has been known for many centuries that shellfish can occasionally become toxic. Symptoms include numbness of the lips and fingertips and ascending paralysis, which can lead to death within 24 hours. The poisoning, which primarily affects mussels and clams, occurs when dinoflagellates undergo periods of rapid growth ('blooms', or 'red tides') in areas where the shellfish grow. The toxin cannot be removed by washing or destroyed by heat.

Glycoalkaloids in potatoes Solanine is one of a range of heat-stable glycoalkaloid compounds found in the green parts of the potato plant that are toxic above concentrations of 20 mg/100 g. In normal peeled potatoes there is about 7 mg solanine/100 g. Solanine synthesis can be induced by exposing the tubers to light and also by simple mechanical injury. In very green potatoes, the levels can reach up to 100 mg/100 g. These glycoalkaloids possess anticholinesterase activity which can produce gastrointestinal and neurological disorders, and deaths have occasionally been reported from consumption of excessive amounts of green potatoes.

27.4.3 Enzyme inhibitors

Protease inhibitors Substances that inhibit digestive enzymes are widespread in many legume species, and trypsin inhibitors are found in oats and maize as well as Brussels sprouts, onion, and beetroot. These inhibitors are proteins and therefore are denatured and inactivated by cooking. Thus, for humans, these substances are not a problem, although feeding raw legumes to animals can result in pancreatic enlargement.

27.4.4 Antivitamins

One of the best known antivitamins is the biotin-binding protein, avidin, in raw egg white. Biotin deficiency induced by eating raw egg white is rare because biotin is well provided in most human diets. The few cases that have been reported involved abnormally large amounts of raw egg white, so the occasional raw egg is perfectly safe. Avidin is inactivated when heated. Other antivitamins, such as the pyridoxine antagonist amino-D-proline in flax seeds and a tocopherol oxidase in raw soybeans, are only of importance in animal feeding.

27.4.5 Mineral-binding agents

Goitrogens There is a number of glucosinolate and thiocyanate compounds in foods that interferve with normal utilization of iodine by the thyroid gland and can result in goitres. Goitrogens are widely distributed in cruciferous vegetables such as cabbage, brussel sprouts, and broccoli. The average intake of glucosinolates from vegetables in Great Britain is 76 mg per day and clinical studies have found that intakes of 100–400 mg per day may reduce the uptake of iodine by the thyroid. There is no evidence that normal consumption of these foods by humans is harmful, but it is possible that eating large amounts of brassica plants might contribute to a higher incidence of goitre in areas where dietary iodine intake is low.

Phytate In wholemeal cereals, phytate can bind minerals and make them less available for absorption. In leavened bread, phytases in the yeast break down the phytate, but in some parts of the Middle East, where unleavened bread is a dietary staple, phytate has been reported to be the cause of zinc deficiency.

Oxalate Certain plants, including rhubarb, spinach, beetroot, and tea, contain relatively high levels of oxalate. Oxalate can combine with calcium to form an insoluble complex in the gut that is poorly absorbed and high intakes can lower plasma calcium levels. Kidney damage and convulsions can accompany oxalate poisoning. However, the average diet supplies only 70–150 mg oxalate per day which could theoretically bind 30–70 mg calcium. Since calcium intakes are usually 10 times this amount, food oxalates do not normally have any detrimental effect on mineral balance.

Tannins (polyphenols) These are present in tea, coffee, and cocoa, as well as broad beans. Tannins inhibit the absorption of iron and in Egypt, in children with low iron intakes, regular consumption of stewed beans has been associated with anaemia. High levels of tea consumption may contribute to low iron status in people with marginal iron intakes.

27.5 Agricultural residues

27.5.1 Pesticides

The most common agricultural chemicals found in foods are pesticides, albeit at very low levels. The chlorinated organic pesticides (such as dichlorodiphenyltrichloroethane (DDT) and chlordane) were among the first modern pesticides to be used. In general they have low toxicity to mammals and are highly toxic to insects. However, they are very stable compounds, which persist in soils, and they are stored in the fat tissue of animals. Because of concern about their effect on the reproduction of certain birds and possible carcinogenic activity, use of these compounds has been restricted. Surveys of foods show that the levels of organochlorine compounds have been declining in recent years. Alternative insecticides now in use, such as organophosphates, do not accumulate in the environment. No food poisonings have ever been attributed to the proper use of insecticides on foods, but in 1997 there were 60 cases of food poisoning in India attributed to indiscriminate organophosphate spraying in a kitchen.

27.5.2 Fungicides and herbicides

Most fungicides and herbicides show very selective toxicity to their target plants and therefore present very little hazard to humans. In addition, most do not accumulate in the environment.

27.5.3 Hormones

The use of hormones, such as bovine somatotrophin (BST), to improve yields of meat and milk has been controversial in many countries. Although low levels of BST can be detected in the milk of treated cows, the hormones in humans are digested and inactivated in the stomach when consumed in food. The FDA approved the commercial use of BST in 1993 and later reviews by Canadian authorities and Codex Alimentarius have agreed that there are no health risks to humans. However, in several countries, BST use is not permitted on animal welfare grounds.

27.6 Intentional food additives

27.6.1 Approval process for food additives

Each country has its own legislation to control the approval of additives in foods, but most follow the same general principles that are used by the two main international bodies of experts organized by WHO and the Food and Agriculture Organization (FAO): the Joint Expert Committee on Food Additives (JECFA), and the Codex Alimentarius Committee on Food Additives and Contaminants.

The aim of the evaluation of a food additive is to establish an acceptable daily intake (ADI). The ADI is usually expressed in mg/kg of body weight and is defined as the amount of a chemical that might be ingested daily, even over a lifetime, without appreciable risk to the consumer. The evaluation process consists of a number of steps:

1 Toxicity testing is carried out in experimental animals—usually mice and rats, but other species may also be employed. Three types of testing are

performed: (a) acute toxicity studies at high doses to determine the range of possible toxic effects of the chemical, (b) short-term feeding trials at various doses, and (c) long-term studies of 2 years or more to examine the effect of exposures over several generations.

2 From the feeding trials, the level of additive at which observed health effects do not appear in the animals is determined. This is called the 'no observed effect level' (NOEL).

3 The lowest NOEL is divided by a safety factor to derive an exposure level that is regarded as acceptable for humans, the ADI. Most commonly a safety factor of 100 times is used, but for some substances factors of up to 1000 have been used. This safety factor allows for possible differences in susceptibility between experimental animals and humans and also the differences in sensitivity of individual people.

Not all additives have been evaluated for safety using modern testing procedures. Some have been used for many years without apparent harm and in the USA ingredients not evaluated by prescribed testing procedures can be classified as generally recognized as safe (GRAS). This list includes common ingredients such as salt, sugar, seasonings, and many food flavourings.

While the 100-fold safety factor is accepted for most additives, in the USA the Delaney Clause prohibits the use in *any* amount of substances known to cause cancer in animals or humans. When the bill was introduced in 1958, chemicals could be detected down to 100 parts per billion; anything less was considered zero. Improved analytical techniques can now detect substances at parts per trillion and there might be only trivial risks from such minute quantities. The FDA has now changed the interpretation of the clause so that if a food additive increases the chance of developing cancer over a lifetime by less than one case per million of cancer, the threat is considered too small to be of concern.

Ames has ranked the level of carcinogenic risk associated with a variety of chemicals we may be commonly exposed to. The Human Exposure/ Rodent Potency Index (HERP) expresses the typical human intakes as a percentage of the dose required to produce tumours in 50% of rodents. The values in Table 27.5 show that the risk from the alcohol in a glass of wine is almost 100 times higher than that from the saccharin in a can of diet cola, and more than 10 000 times the hazard from the residues of the pesticide ethylene dibromide. That the risks from wine appear more acceptable to most consumers seems to relate to the fact that benefit is easily perceived, that wine is seen as 'natural', and because the risk is voluntary. Although the risks from other additives and contaminants may be far smaller, they arouse suspicion because they are risks that people generally cannot control.

27.6.2 Artificial sweeteners

Saccharin is one of the oldest artificial sweeteners, having been used in foods since the twentieth century. Studies in rats have linked very high doses (7.5% of the diet by weight) of saccharin with bladder cancer and because of this there have been attempts to ban its use in human foods. However, at lower doses, such as 1%, no adverse effects are found and large epidemiological studies of diabetics who have had lifetime exposure to saccharin have found no increased incidence of cancer in humans.

Cyclamate Dietary cyclamate appears to promote bladder cancer and induce testicular atrophy in rats, although carcinogenicity testing in mice, dogs, and primates have all been negative. The US FDA banned the food use of cyclamate in 1969, but in over 50 other countries it is still a permitted sweetener, and there is no good evidence from mutagenicity testing or epidemiological studies that it is a health risk to humans.

Aspartame is a dipeptide of two amino acids, phenylalanine and aspartic acid. Aspartame is metabolized to phenylalanine and therefore carries a risk for people with phenylketonuria, but for the

Table 27.5 Rankings of possible carcinogenic hazards

Daily human exposure	Carcinogen and dose per 70 kg person	Index of possible hazard (HERP, %)
Natural dietary toxins		
Wine (250 mL)	Ethyl alcohol, 30 mL	4.7
Basil (1 g of dried leaf)	Estragole, 3.8 mg	0.1
Peanut butter (32 g, one sandwich)	Aflatoxin, 64 ng	0.03
Cooked bacon (100 g)	Dimethylnitrosamine, 0.3 µg	0.003
Food additives		
Diet cola (1 can)	Saccharin, 95 mg	0.06
Pesticides		
DDE/DDT (daily diet intake)	DDE, 2.2 µg	0.0003
EDB (daily diet intake)	EDB, 0.42 µg	0.0004

EDB, ethylene dibromide; DDE, dichlorodiphenyldichloroethylene; DDT, dichlorodiphenyltrichloroethane; Reprinted with permission from Ames, B.N., Magaw, R., and Gold, L.S. (1987) Ranking of possible carcinogenic hazards. *Science*, **236**, 271–80. *Science* Copyright 1987. American Association for the Advancement of Science.

normal population it is an extremely safe sweetener that is digested like any other protein.

27.6.3 Preservatives

Preservatives are used in foods as antioxidants and to prevent the growth of bacteria and fungi. Most pose no toxicological problems, but a few have generated some concerns.

Sodium nitrite is used as an antimicrobial preservative that is very effective in preventing the growth of *Clostridium botulinum,* as well as acting as a colour-fixing agent (to preserve the red colour) in cured meat products such as bacon and ham. Nitrite reacts with primary amides in foods to produce N-nitroso derivatives, many of which are carcinogenic. However, the risk to human health from dietary nitrite is difficult to assess. While food additive nitrites are significant, a substantial amount is also produced by bacterial reduction from naturally occurring nitrate in vegetables. In recent years, manufacturers have worked to reduce the levels of nitrite used in cured meats and have added agents such as ascorbic acid, which help to prevent the formation of nitrosamines in the stomach.

Sulphur dioxide and its salts (sulphites) are commonly used as inhibitors of enzymic browning, dough conditioners, antimicrobials, and antioxidants. Although sulphites have been used for many centuries, with no adverse effect for most consumers, 1–2% of asthmatics are sensitive to sulphites and in those individuals the reaction can be fatal.

27.6.4 Colours and flavours

All colours and flavours approved for use in foods are rigorously evaluated before being approved for use.

Red No 2 (amaranth) In the early 1970s, data from Russian studies raised questions about Red No 2's safety. The FDA Toxicology Advisory Committee evaluated numerous reports and decided that there was no evidence of a hazard but concluded that feeding it at a high dosage results in a statistically significant increase in malignant tumours in female rats. The FDA ultimately decided to ban the colour, but it is still found in foods in Canada and Europe.

Tartrazine (E102) Food sensitivity to tartrazine can be experienced by a small number of individuals, but claims related to clinical problems such as asthma and hyperactivity are not well supported by scientific studies. Tartrazine is still a permitted additive, but its presence has to be declared in ingredient lists so sensitive individuals can avoid it.

Monosodium glutamate (MSG) The flavour enhancer MSG is a sodium salt of glutamic acid, one of the most common amino acids. It is present in virtually all foods and found in high levels in toma-toes, mushrooms, broccoli, peas, cheese, and soy sauce. Chinese restaurant syndrome has been claimed to be caused by foods with a lot of added MSG, but most controlled studies have not demonstrated this effect.

Traditional methods for evaluating the safety of colours have not usually considered their potential behavioural effects. New research published in 2007 in the *Lancet*, using a mixture of six permitted colours (sunset yellow, tartrazine, carmoisine, ponceau, quinoline yellow, and allura red) at relatively high doses, concluded that there was limited evidence that these colours could affect the activity and attention of children in the general population. However, the European Food Safety Authority concluded that uncertainties in the study meant that there was insufficient evidence to change current permissions for use of these colours.

27.7 Novel foods

Technology now allows the development of many new ingredients or whole foods that do not have a history of traditional use in the human food supply. Many of these novel foods have been developed to have improved nutritional quality. Recent examples include genetically modified foods, artificial fat substitutes for energy-reduced foods, new algal sources of omega-3 fatty acids, and phytosterols to reduce cholesterol.

27.7.1 Approval process for novel foods

There are significant practical difficulties in assessing the long-term safety of modified whole foods or ingredients. Unlike additives, which can be fed at very high doses to assess their toxic effects, it is not possible to feed large amounts of one single food to animals without making their diet nutritionally unbalanced. Animals also prefer a mixture of foods and are likely to refuse to eat if offered a single food in large amounts. These difficulties, and welfare concerns about the use of animal studies that were unlikely to result in meaningful information, led to the development of the concept of 'substantial equivalence', particularly for the assessment of genetically modified (GM) foods. This type of assessment does not quantify the safety or risk of a food, but aims to determine whether novel foods are as safe as traditional counterparts. For GM foods the process involves assessment and comparison of a wide range of factors, including:

- source and nature of any new protein;
- stability of any genetic changes;
- potential toxicity of the new protein;
- levels of naturally occurring and newly introduced allergens;
- nutritional composition;
- levels of antinutrients;
- ability of the food to support normal growth and wellbeing;
- potential unintended environmental consequences.

27.7.2 Genetically modified (GM) foods

Modern biotechnology now allows specific individual genes to be identified, copied, and transferred into other organisms in a much more direct and controlled way. For example, genes for the enzyme chymosin from beef have been inserted into yeast, and the GM chymosin from these organisms has now widely replaced natural rennet from animals in cheese making. Genetic modification can also allow individual genes to be switched on or off: the gene that controls fruit softening can be repressed to maintain a higher solids content in tomatoes designed for use in tomato paste.

In 2009, 134 million hectares of GM crops were planted worldwide and 77% of all soy is now grown from GM varieties. Most plants have been modified for agricultural purposes: herbicide-tolerant soy and canola and insect-resistant corn and cotton now make up the bulk of those crops in North America. There are many future uses planned that will bring more direct consumer benefits: oils with improved fatty acid profiles, rice with higher levels of vitamins (Golden rice), nuts with lower levels of allergens, and potatoes that absorb less fat during frying. However, concern has been expressed about the environmental impacts and safety of these novel foods, in particular related to the issues of allergenicity, toxicity of transgenic food, and possible transfer of antibiotic resistance.

Genetic modification usually requires the introduction of the selected gene together with a marker gene. The marker genes are often antibiotic resistance genes that allow selection of the plants that have successfully integrated the new selected gene. Many have expressed concern that when the modified food is eaten the resistance gene might be transferred to bacteria in the gut and acquire resistance to clinically useful antibiotics. Although the chances of this occurring are extremely small, the use of this marker method is now being phased out.

Most countries have now established stringent approval processes for GM foods, including mandatory labelling to inform consumers when foods include GM-modified ingredients. Assessments to date have usually found GM foods to be as safe as their normal counterparts and there are likely to be increasing numbers of GM foods in the marketplace in the future.

27.7.3 Fat substitutes

There are a number of fat substitutes now in use, including *Simplesse* (microcapsules of milk proteins or egg white), *Splendid* (derived from pectin), and *N-oil* (derived from tapioca). In the USA, *Olestra*, a mixture of heat-stable sugar polyesters, that are not digested and yield no energy, has been controversial because it can reduce the absorption of fat-soluble vitamins. The FDA approved use of Olestra in a limited range of foods in 1996, but required addition of vitamins A, D, and K as well as further monitoring of the health impacts and warning labelling that it may cause abdominal cramping and loose stools. In 2003, after a scientific review of several post-market studies, the FDA concluded that the warning statement was no longer warranted. Olestra is not yet approved in the UK, Europe, or Australasia.

27.7.4 Phytosterols

In many countries, plant sterols are now approved to be added to a range of foods to help lower blood cholesterol. They reduce the absorption of cholesterol from the gut, but have a side effect of also lowering absorption of carotenoids. A typical daily dose of 2–3 g per day can reduce serum β-carotene levels by 20–25%. Safety reviews have concluded that since there is no evidence of reduction in serum retinol levels, this effect is not a significant health concern and that advice to maintain adequate fruit and vegetable intakes can ensure adequate carotene intakes.

27.7.5 Nanotechnology

Nanotechnologies comprise a range of technologies, processes, and materials that involve manipulation of substances at sizes in the nanoscale range (from 1 nm to 100 nm). Food and drinking water naturally comprises particles in the nanometre scale. Humans ingest many millions of organic and inorganic nanoscale particles every day in their food and it is estimated that people inhale around 10 million nanometre scale particles in every breath. Generally, proteins in foods are globular structures 1–10 nm in size and the majority of polysaccharides and lipids are linear polymers with thicknesses in the nanometre range. Milk is an example of an emulsion of fine fat droplets of nanoscale proportions.

It has been claimed that some of the nanomaterials now being used in foods and agricultural products introduce new risks to human health because they may be absorbed more easily. For example, nanoparticles of silver, titanium dioxide, zinc, and zinc oxide materials now used in nutritional supplements and food packaging. However reviews have concluded that safety cannot be determined from the size alone, and it is novelty and not size which raises concern and has to be considered in undertaking risk assessments.

27.8 Regulatory agencies

Although all regulators use similar processes to evaluate scientific evidence and assess the safety of foods, the management of food safety legislation varies between countries.

The Codex Alimentarius Commission (Codex) was created in 1963 by the FAO and WHO to develop international standards, guidelines, and codes of practice related to food composition and safety, with the aim of harmonizing food regulations between countries. Over 165 countries are members of Codex. While not legally binding on individual countries, Codex standards are very influential and form benchmarks for key World Trade Organization agreements, such as those on the Application of Sanitary and Phytosanitary Measures and Technical Barriers to Trade, which make it increasingly difficult for countries to adopt food standards that are significantly different from Codex.

In the USA, the FDA develops standards for food composition, quality, and safety as well as being responsible for approval of therapeutic drugs and cosmetics. It also has food inspection and monitoring responsibilities nationally. The work of the FDA, such as the GRAS listings, is influential internationally because of the high quality and resourcing of the many expert scientific staff.

In Australasia, the binational authority, Foods Standards Australia New Zealand, sets standards for all manufactured foods for both countries, including standards for additives and contaminants, and assesses the safety of novel foods. Primary food production and food service safety standards are set separately in each country. In Australia compliance is the responsibility of individual state governments, not the national standard setting agency.

In Britain, an independent food safety watchdog, the Food Standards Agency, was established in 2000 to protect the public's health and consumer interests after concerns raised by the BSE outbreak. The FSA provides advice and information to the public and government on food safety from farm to fork, nutrition, and diet. It also protects consumers through effective food enforcement and monitoring.

In Europe, the European Food Safety Authority (EFSA) was created in 2002 to provide independent scientific advice on all matters linked to food and feed safety. EFSA principally deals with requests for risk assessments from the European Commission, Parliament, and Council and plans to take on a wider brief from other European institutions in the near future.

One of the key roles of all regulatory agencies is risk assessment and management.

Risk assessment is a scientific process consisting of four steps:

1 Hazard identification (biological, chemical, or physical agents capable of causing adverse health effects)

2 Hazard characterization (qualitative and quantitative evaluation of the hazards, including dose–response effects)

3 Exposure assessment (the likely intake of the risk factor from food, taking into account typical dietary patterns)

4 Risk characterization (estimating the probability and severity of potential adverse effects).

Risk management is the process of weighing policy options in the light of the risk assessment results and selecting appropriate control measures. Control options can include prohibiting certain substances in foods entirely (some carcinogenic herbs, for example), setting maximum permitted levels in foods (e.g. additives or agricultural residues), through the development of codes of good manufacturing practice, labelling requirements (e.g. warnings about allergens), and public education about safe use of foods (e.g. in relation to mercury in fish).

Risk communication is the process of making the risk management information comprehensible to food producers, policy makers, and consumers.

Key points

- Despite the many potential health risks associated with foods, in practice the degree of risk associated with the modern food supply is extremely low.

- By far the most important hazards of significance are those from biological agents: pathogenic bacteria, viruses, fungi, and a few toxic seafoods.

- Trends to larger-scale production, longer distribution chains in the food supply, increased eating away from the home, and the emergence of new pathogens mean foodborne illness continues to be a significant public health issue.

- Assessment of the safety of food additives is led internationally by JECFA, but each individual country still develops and determines their own local regulations and food standards.

- The ADI is defined as the amount of a chemical that might be ingested daily, even over a lifetime, without appreciable risk to the consumer.

- Genetically modified foods, novel foods, and nanomaterials pose new challenges for traditional safety assessment processes but, as the food supply becomes increasing global, food regulations about food safety are becoming more harmonized internationally.

Further Reading

1. **Ames, B.N., Magaw, R., and Gold, L.S.** (1987) Ranking of possible carcinogenic hazards. *Science*, **236**, 271–80.

2. **Barlow, S.** (2009) Scientific opinion of the scientific committee on a request from the European Commission on the potential risks arising from nanoscience and nanotechnologies on Food and Feed Safety. *EFSA J*, **958**, 1–39.

3. **Barlow, S. and Schlatter, J.** (2010) Risk assessment of carcinogens in food. *Toxicol Appl Pharmacol*, **243**, 180–90.

4. **Blackburn, C.D. and McClure, P.J.** (eds) (2010) *Foodborne pathogens: Hazards, risk analysis and control*, 2nd edition. Cambridge, UK, Woodhead Publishing.

5. **Branen, A.L., Davidson, P.M., Salminen, S., and Thorngate, J.H.** (eds) (2002) *Food additives*, 2nd edition. New York, Marcel Dekker.

6. **Fischer, A.R., De Jong, A.E., Van Asselt, E.D., De Jonge, R., Frewer, L.J., and Nauta, M.J.** (2007) Food safety in the domestic environment: An interdisciplinary investigation of microbial hazards during food preparation. *Risk Anal*, **27**, 1065–82.

7. **Food Standards Australia New Zealand.** (2005) *Safety assessment of genetically modified foods*. Canberra, FSANZ.

8. **Jackson, L.S.** (2009) Chemical food safety issues in the United States: Past, present, and future. *J Agric Food Chem*, **57**, 8161–70.

9 **McCann, D., Barrett, A., Cooper, A. *et al.*** (2007) Food additives and hyperactive behaviour in 3-year-old and 8/9-year-old children in the community: A randomised, double-blinder, placebo-controlled trial. *Lancet* **370**, 1560–7.

10. **Microbiology and Food Safety Committee of the National Food Processors Association** (1993) HACCP implementation: A generic model for chilled foods. *J Food Prot*, **56**, 1077.

11. **Nyachuba, D.G.** (2010) Foodborne illness: Is it on the rise? *Nutr Rev*, **68,** 257–69.

12. **Omaye, S.T.** (2004) *Food and nutritional toxicology*. Boca Raton, FL, CRC Press.

13. **Shibamoto, T. and Bjeldanes, L.F.** (eds) (2009) *Introduction to food toxicology*, 2nd edition. Burlington, MA, Academic Press.

14. **Stevenson, K.E.** (2006) *HACCP: A systematic approach to food safety*, 4th edition. Washington, DC, Food Producers Association.

Useful Websites

 To see topical and scientifically robust updates on nutrition associated with this textbook and web links to many of the journals in the Further Reading sections, please see the dedicated Online Resource Centre at **http://www.oxfordtextbooks.co.uk/orc/mann4e/**

Some Key Food Safety Websites

World Health Organization: http://www.who.int/foodsafety/en/
US Food and Drug Administration: http://www.cfsan.fda.gov/list.html
European Food Safety Authority: http://www.efsa.europa.eu/
Food Standards Australia New Zealand: http://www.foodstandards.gov.au/
Codex Alimentarius Commission: http://www.codexalimentarius.net/web/index_en.jsp
Joint Expert Committee on Food Additives: http://www.who.int/ipcs/food/jecfa/en/index.html

28 Functional foods

Martijn B. Katan

This textbook teaches you who needs to eat which nutrients and in what amounts. But translating this knowledge into foods and meals is no simple task. Armies, hospitals, and nursing homes employ dietitians to translate nutritional recommendations into diets and meals, so that soldiers, patients, and residents receive the nutrients they need, and in the right amounts. However, most people do not have access to a dietitian. Also, the variety of food keeps increasing, as does the number of potentially beneficial food ingredients. And last but not least, many persons—whether healthy or sick—would like to decide for themselves which foods are good for them, without the advice of a professional.

All this has created a market for new foods that promises to increase the wellbeing or health of the consumer. Functional foods are part of that market. This chapter reviews typical functional foods, their ingredients, and their efficacy in improving health. It will also review health claims and their regulation—or lack of regulation.

28.1 What is a functional food?

The definition of a functional food is a contentious issue. The International Food Information Council, which is supported primarily by food, beverage, and agricultural industries, defines functional foods as 'foods that provide health benefits beyond basic nutrition' (Box 28.1). That definition is unsatisfactory because it leaves the status of foods without a brand name (such as fruits, vegetables, or low-fat cheese) up in the air. Even tap water would meet this definition because a liberal intake of water prevents cystitis, kidney and bladder stones, and possibly bladder cancer, but no one would call tap water a functional food.

A more concrete definition is provided by the Institute of Medicine of the US National Academy of Sciences. The Institute of Medicine defines functional foods as 'those foods in which the concentrations of one or more ingredients have been manipulated or modified to enhance their contribution to a healthful diet'. Functional foods are indeed specifically created to promote health, but the Institute of Medicine definition still omits one aspect that is central to functional foods—namely the commercial aspect. In the reality of the marketplace, the term 'functional foods' is almost exclusively attached to branded products that claim or suggest to improve health.

Therefore, functional food is defined here as:

'A branded food that claims explicitly or implicitly to improve health or wellbeing'.

An example may clarify the central role of branding and health claims. Polyunsaturated oils such as sunflower or soybean oil reduce plasma cholesterol and the risk of coronary heart disease, but few people would call a generic bottle of sunflower oil a functional food. However, if a manufacturer developed a proprietary brand of sunflower oil and marketed it with a cholesterol claim, then that oil could well be called a functional food. Box 28.2 emphasizes the role of marketing in creating a functional food.

The active ingredients of functional foods, such as vitamins, plant sterols, lactic acid bacteria, or herbal extracts, can also be packaged into a capsule or tablet instead of a food, and such products are not called foods but dietary supplements. The terms 'nutraceutical' and 'nutriceutical' have been used both for foods and for supplements; there is no consensus on what these words mean. Some products are halfway between foods and supplements, e.g. candies or sweets with added vitamins.

28.2 Typical ingredients of functional foods

28.2.1 Established nutrients

Many functional foods employ ingredients that are also available from regular foods. You can get lycopene from special drinks and supplements, but the same lycopene is found in tomatoes or tomato ketchup. The newness of such functional foods is in the way in which known ingredients are incorporated into a palatable and attractive food that can be patented and marketed. That is also the benefit of functional foods from a nutritional point of view— they may provide nutrients in a form that is more attractive or convenient for the consumer than

Table 28.1 Examples of established nutrients that are used as functional food ingredients, and the evidence for the efficacy of these ingredients in maintaining health and preventing disease. Whether the food itself is efficacious depends on the amount and bioavailability of the ingredients

Ingredient	Examples of products	Health claim	Strength of evidence in humans
Folic acid	Cereals	Protects against neural tube defects	++
Dietary fibre	Drinks	Relieves constipation	++
Low in sodium and/or high in potassium	Drinks, soups, margarine	Reduces blood pressure	++
Unsaturated fatty acids	Spreads, cookies	Reduces risk of heart disease	++
Sugar alcohols	Chewing gum	Reduce caries risk	++
Soluble fibre from whole oats or *Psyllium* husk	Cereals, cookies	Reduces cholesterol and risk of heart disease	++ For cholesterol reduction
Soy protein	Drinks, bars	Reduces cholesterol and risk of heart disease	+– For cholesterol lowering +– For reduction of heart disease
Calcium	Cereals, fruit juices, milk products, spreads	Protects against osteoporosis, helps maintain bone density	+ For consumers with a low calcium intake
Folic acid + vitamin B$_6$ (pyridoxine)	Cereals	Decreases homocysteine and risk of cardiovascular disease	++ For homocysteine – For cardiovascular disease
Vitamin E	Supplements	Antioxidant; prevents cardiovascular disease	– For cardiovascular disease
Zinc	Sweets, lozenges	Prevention/cure of common cold	+–
Vitamin C	Drinks, sweets	Protects against cardiovascular disease	+– In observational studies – In clinical trials

Evidence was graded according to the Australia New Zealand Food Authority criteria for levels and kinds of evidence for public health nutrition. The evidence consisted of randomized trials in humans, unless indicated otherwise.

++, Proven efficacy, consistent effect seen in multiple high-quality studies; +, reasonable evidence for efficacy, effect seen in a limited number of studies, or some inconsistency between studies; + –, evidence for no effect, absence of an effect evident from a limited number of studies; –, proven not to work, absence of an effect evident in multiple high-quality studies.

Source: References may be found in Katan and De Roos (2004).

regular foods that contain the same nutrients. Thus, people who do not like to eat vegetables may be persuaded to buy vegetable drinks that supposedly provide the same benefits.

Table 28.1 lists established nutrients typically found in functional foods, and the quality of the evidence for the efficacy of these ingredients. Whether the food itself is efficacious also depends on the amount and form of the ingredient; thus, 'whole-wheat cookies' may contain too little wheat bran to affect defecation, or the bran may have been ground to a powder, which is less active than coarse bran.

The health claims for some of these ingredients are well substantiated, as indicated by the 'Evidence' column of the table. For other ingredients, the evidence is weaker.

Intakes of vitamins and minerals from functional foods, but especially from supplements, may be much higher than from regular foods, and the adverse effects of such high intakes are a cause for concern. For example, megadoses of vitamin B_6 cause peripheral neuropathy, and some authors have listed concerns over excessive intakes of calcium.

28.2.2 Novel ingredients

Table 28.2 lists some more novel or exotic ingredients of functional foods. Most of the claims for benefits of novel or 'exotic' ingredients have not been substantiated in clinical trials. However, a few have been well investigated and show some promise, such as the following examples.

Sterols and stanols Margarines and other foods can be enriched with plant stanols or sterols, which lower low-density lipoprotein (LDL)-cholesterol. The effect on LDL has been documented in many well-controlled trials in humans, and no major adverse effects have been noted. However, long-term safety and clinical efficacy have not been evaluated in clinical trials. Sterols and stanols act by blocking cholesterol absorption. The new drug Ezetimibe also lowers plasma cholesterol by blocking cholesterol absorption, but in clinical trials it failed to produce the expected improvement in atherosclerosis. This highlights the need for a similar test of the clinical efficacy of sterols and stanols.

Pre- and probiotics Probiotics are viable bacteria that survive passage through the gastrointestinal tract and exert beneficial effects on the consumer. Probiotic bacteria provide a novel approach to diet and health and, unlike most food ingredients, probiotics can be patented because each bacterial strain is unique. That makes probiotics attractive to industry, but documented beneficial effects of probiotics are still scarce. Some foods with lactic acid bacteria may reduce the severity of certain types of diarrhoea, but results of trials of probiotics and atopic eczema are contradictory, and there is little evidence for other claimed effects including cancer prevention and lowering of serum cholesterol. Prebiotics are non-digestible carbohydrates that selectively stimulate growth of beneficial bacteria. Inulin and fructo-oligosaccharides are examples of compounds marketed as prebiotics. Health effects of prebiotics appear to be limited to improved bowel function; no adequate scientific support exists for other proposed health effects such as cancer prevention, lipid lowering, and prevention of diarrhoeal diseases.

Polyphenols High intakes of tea rich in catechins and other flavonoid polyphenols have been associated with a reduced risk of coronary heart disease. A clinical trial to evaluate these effects would be justified. Whether polyphenols explain the so-called 'French paradox' is questionable, as foods typically eaten in France are not particularly rich in polyphenols. For example, red wine and olive oil are lower in phenolic compounds than tea or coffee.

28.2.3 Herbs and herbal extracts

Herbal ingredients are used both in supplements and in foods, but amounts in foods are much lower. Safety is a concern, as exemplified by herbal teas with *Aristolochia*, which causes renal cancer, and products with *ephedra*, which causes hypertension, strokes, and seizures. The efficacy of herbal supplements is hotly debated, but most of the popular herbal remedies have not been shown to be safe and effective by pharmaceutical standards.

Table 28.2 Newer functional food ingredients and their efficacy

Ingredient	Product examples	Health effect or claim	Evidence in humans
Plant stanols and sterols	Margarine, yoghurt, cereal bars	Lower cholesterol and risk of coronary heart disease	++ For LDL cholesterol lowering + – For coronary heart disease No data on coronary heart disease
Lactobacillus GG bacteria	Yoghurt	Reduce diarrhoea	+ For rotavirus-induced diarrhoea in infants + For antibiotic-induced infections
Lactobacillus GG bacteria	Yoghurt	Reduce risk of early atopic disease	+ – Results of trials contradictory
Other 'probiotic' live bacteria, plus fermentable sugars ('prebiotics')	Yoghurt	Enhance immunity	+ – Some effects on biomarkers but none on disease
Isoflavones (phyto-oestrogens)	Soy products	Reduce menopausal symptoms, osteoporosis, cardiovascular disease	– For hot flushes + – For osteoporosis and heart disease
Catechins	Tea	Reduce cardiovascular risk	+ – Some epidemiological evidence No trial data
Conjugated linoleic acid (CLA)	Supplements (small amounts occur naturally in milk, beef, and lamb)	Reduces body weight, protects against cancer	– Minimal effects on body weight in humans No data on cancer in humans – For blood lipids in humans

++ , Proven efficacy, consistent effect seen in multiple high-quality studies; +, reasonable evidence for efficacy, effect seen in a limited number of studies, or some inconsistency between studies; +– , evidence for no effect, absence of an effect evident from a limited number of studies; –, proven not to work, absence of an effect evident in multiple high-quality studies; LDL, low-density lipoprotein.

28.3 How to prove efficacy and safety

28.3.1 Types of evidence: food versus pharma

The health benefits of a functional food should be supported by solid scientific evidence. But should we require the same level of evidence for functional foods as for new drugs?

This author believes not, because pharmaceutical research produces *new* molecules while nutrition deals with molecules that have been eaten for many centuries. Associations between diet and disease provide important clues about efficacy and safety, and such epidemiological studies are a vital source of evidence for diet that is not available for drugs. However, epidemiology has its limitations, and therefore other types of research need to be combined with epidemiology to show that a functional food is effective—and safe. Table 28.3 lists the types of research applied in nutrition and their strengths and weaknesses.

28.3.2 Cell studies

A true understanding of the effect of a nutrient on health requires insights at the molecular level, and such comprehension remains the ultimate goal of nutrition science. However, as phrased by Willett (1998), 'our understanding of biological mechanisms remains far too incomplete to predict confidently the ultimate consequences of eating a particular food or nutrient' and therefore cell and molecular studies cannot by themselves establish efficacy and safety of a food ingredient.

28.3.3 Animal research

Animal feeding trials have been a prime source of knowledge about nutrition and health, from the thiamin-deficient chickens that helped Eijkman and Grijns to discover the cause of beri-beri (see Chapter 13), down to recent findings on the anti-arrhythmogenic effects of n-3 polyunsaturated fatty acids in marmosets. However, the existence of such an effect in animals does not prove that the same effect exists in humans, because animal 'models' are often expressly constructed to reflect a hypothetical effect of a nutrient on a disease. For instance, a mouse strain may be made sensitive to a nutrient by deleting a gene or by giving it drugs. The nutrient will be effective in this model because that is what it was built to do, but extrapolation to man is uncertain.

Table 28.3 Types of research used to investigate the relation between diet and disease, and the strengths and weaknesses of the various approaches

Type	Strengths	Limitations
(Sub)cellular studies	Mechanistic insights	Extrapolation to entire human organism uncertain
Animal feeding trials	Long term Hard endpoints Show cause and effect	Extrapolation to humans uncertain Conditions often extreme and unphysiological
Hereditary diseases	Human Long term Hard endpoints Show cause and effect	Mutation may act through other paths than the one of interest (pleiotropic mutations) Effects involved are often extreme
Randomized trials with surrogate endpoints	Human Controlled Show cause and effect	Short duration Validity of surrogate endpoints uncertain
Epidemiological observations	Long term Hard endpoints Applicable to general populations	Confounding Associations do not prove causality
Randomized clinical trials	Hard endpoints Show cause and effect	Duration sometimes too short Selected groups

28.3.4 Hereditary diseases

The role of a metabolite or pathway in disease causation can often be deduced by studying genetic polymorphisms that produce unusual levels of the metabolite in people who carry a certain mutation. Such 'Mendelian randomization' studies (Davey Smith *et al.*, 2005) do not suffer from the confounding that plagues conventional epidemiology, because such genetic variants usually do not cause people to smoke, exercise, or eat differently. An example is familial hypercholesterolaemia—once the nature of the mutation in this disease was cleared up, the conclusion that high levels of LDL-cholesterol caused coronary heart disease became inescapable. However, even these 'experiments of nature' are not foolproof, because a mutation may act through another pathway than the one suspected, or through several pathways. Also, patients with inborn errors of metabolism often represent extremes, and extrapolation to milder conditions is not automatically justified.

28.3.5 Trials with surrogate endpoints

Trials with surrogate endpoints measure the effect of diet on an intermediate disease marker such as blood pressure or insulin sensitivity. Such trials are valuable because they allow causal conclusions about the effects of diet in humans. However, even established markers can lead us astray. For instance, high-carbohydrate, low-fat diets lower total serum cholesterol, and this was long equated with lowering of the risk of coronary heart disease. The distinction between 'bad' and 'good' cholesterol came only later, and then it became clear that high-carbohydrate, low-fat diets lower both the harmful LDL and the beneficial high-density lipoprotein (HDL)-cholesterol. If both are taken into account, the predicted effect on coronary heart disease risk becomes nil.

Thus, even changes in established markers cannot be automatically equated with changes in the disease that they predict. Also, there are few validated markers outside the cardiovascular field; thus, one can measure the effect of diet on hundreds

of variables involved in immune response, but the relevance of each of them to prevention of infection is uncertain. Therefore, we still need experiments in which disease and death are outcome variables.

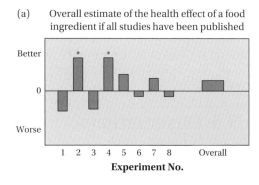

(a) Overall estimate of the health effect of a food ingredient if all studies have been published

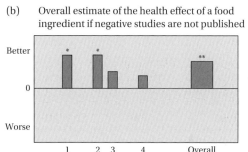

(b) Overall estimate of the health effect of a food ingredient if negative studies are not published

Fig. 28.1 Hypothetical representation of the effect of publication bias on the perceived health effect of a food ingredient. The vertical axis plots the effect of a food ingredient on some risk indicator for disease. Each bar represents the mean outcome of one experiment. All experiments measured the effect of the same ingredient on the same risk factor; the differences between outcomes are due to chance and biological variability. (a) If all experiments are published, then the mean overall effect in a meta-analysis would be small and not significantly different from zero. (b) If experiments with nil or negative outcomes are kept secret, then the mean overall effect in a meta-analysis becomes significant, and the effect of the ingredient appears favourable.

* = $P < 0.05$; ** = $P < 0.01$.

Finally, selective publication is an issue. A study that fails to support a health effect may not be published (Fig. 28.1). Alternatively, emphasis may be put on a secondary outcome when the primary outcome shows no benefit. As a result, the scientific literature may offer a biased view of what a food or ingredient really does. This explains why meta-analysis of small studies may show beneficial effects while large studies do not; small negative studies may end up in a drawer, but large studies are usually published, even if the results are negative.

28.3.6 Observational epidemiology

Epidemiology is the prime source of information on the effects of foods on disease, but an epidemiological association is not enough to prove causality unless the association is very strong, and, unfortunately, relative risks in nutritional epidemiology are typically weak. When associations are weak, confounding becomes a problem; someone who eats lots of vegetables may also exercise more, smoke less, and do other healthy things, and even the best computer programs cannot completely separate these factors. When epidemiological findings are consistent with other forms of evidence, a causal link becomes more probable. That is why a causal role of *trans*-fat in heart disease is highly likely; the association between *trans*-fatty acids intake and coronary heart disease in epidemiological studies is corroborated by the adverse effects of *trans*-fatty acids on blood lipids in metabolic trials.

Selective publication and 'data-dredging' is also a problem in epidemiology, because hundreds of associations may be tested but only the 'statistically significant' ones may get published. The validity of such selected associations is much more doubtful than suggested by the P-values. Therefore, associations should be observed in multiple cohorts, preferably from different societies.

28.3.7 Randomized clinical trials

Randomization eliminates confounding. Therefore, randomized clinical trials with hard endpoints—disease and death—are the gold standard in biomedical research, and they offer a level of confidence that no other type of research can match.

Randomized clinical trials also have their weaknesses. Chief of these is that they last too short a time. Many benefits of diet may not be reaped within the 3–5 years of a randomized clinical trial, and a negative outcome is thus less than definitive, especially if contradicted by the outcomes of observational epidemiological studies.

28.3.8 Conclusion

The costs of establishing properly that a functional food promotes health is huge, and understandably there is pressure from industry to adopt *in vitro* and 'functional' tests as substitutes for more expensive and lengthy studies. However, the history of β-carotene—which seemed to prevent cancer *in vitro* but actually may have caused cancer in clinical trials—shows the risks of relying on soft evidence.

28.4 Health claims

Functional foods are more expensive than 'ordinary' foods, and the price is justified by the claimed beneficial effect on health. Unlike taste or convenience, the health effect of a food cannot be perceived directly by the consumer, which is why it is communicated in the form of a health claim.

28.4.1 Soft and hard claims

The demands of the market put pressure on manufacturers to document health claims rapidly without the excessive costs of proving that a food really prevents disease. The alternative preferred by many food producers is a claim for a 'functional' effect. The 'function' can be a surrogate marker for disease, but it can also be something as simple as showing that an added ingredient reaches the circulation, thus: 'Vitamin C is an essential nutrient. Product "X" increases the level of vitamin C in your bloodstream'. Even though such 'function' claims are legally distinct from health claims, they can still be used to suggest an effect on health. The reason is that consumers do not recognize the subtle legal distinctions between soft and hard claims; to them the phrases 'rich in calcium' and 'prevents fractures' mean essentially the same (Williams, 2005). The message that every claim tries to convey is: 'Buy this product. It will make you healthier and feel better'. Present regulations offer producers room for suggestive claims, competition forces them to exploit this room, and a whole industry has sprung up of consultants, seminars, and conferences that teach food manufacturers how to express unsubstantiated health effects of foods without breaking the law.

28.4.2 Health claims and the law

The trustworthiness of health claims is largely dependent on government regulation. Consumers often assume that claims have been approved by government authorities, but many countries does not require that the health benefits claimed or suggested for functional foods be supported by proper scientific evidence. As a result there is now a plethora of foods that carry a suggestion of a health benefit that has not been proven scientifically. In the USA, food supplements are an extreme case: they can be marketed without proof that they work or that they are safe.

However, the climate for health claims may be changing. The European Union recently introduced legislation which puts strict demands on nutrition and health claims. Claims must be substantiated by proper scientific evidence, and should be clearly intelligible to consumers. Candidate claims are evaluated by independent scientific experts of the European Food Safety Agency (EFSA). At the time of writing, most claims proposed by industry have failed to pass EFSA evaluation. This includes claims for antioxidants, for pre- and probiotics and for improvement of immune function.

This is a worrying development for manufacturers who wish to develop new functional foods. Meeting the EFSA standards for proof will require huge investments in research, with no promise of success. If the European Union maintains its hard line, then prospects for new functional foods in Europe are limited. However, manufacturers might also turn to true-and-tried healthy ingredients as outlined in Table 28.1. That is economically less attractive because such ingredients cannot be patented, but it could be of great benefit to European consumers.

Further Reading

1. **Aggett, P.J., Antoine, J.M., Asp, N.G.,** *et al*. (2005) PASSCLAIM: Consensus on criteria. *Eur J Nutr*, **44** (Suppl. 1), 15–30.
2. **American Dietetic Association** (1999) Position of the American Dietetic Association: Functional foods. *J Am Diet Assoc*, **99**, 278–85.
3. **Davey Smith, G., Ebrahim, S., Lewis, S., Hansell, A.L., Palmer, L.J., and Burton, P.R.** (2005) Genetic epidemiology and public health: Hope, hype, and future prospects. *Lancet*, **366**, 1484–98.
4. **Harper, A.E.** (ed.) (2000) Physiologically active food components. Proceedings of the 17th Ross Conference. *Am J Clin Nutr*, **71**, 1647S–1743S.
5. **Jacobson, M.F. and Silverglade, B.** (1999) Functional foods: Health boon or quackery? *BMJ*, **319**, 205–6.
6. **Katan, M.B.** (2004) Editorial: Health claims for functional foods. *BMJ*, **328**, 180–1.
7. **Katan, M.B. and De Roos, N.M.** (2004) Promises and problems of functional foods. *Crit Rev Food Sci Nutr*, **44**, 369–77.

8. **McClements, D.J., Decker, E.A., Park, Y., and Weiss, J.** (2009) Structural design principles for delivery of bioactive components in nutraceuticals and functional foods. *Crit Rev Food Sci Nutr*, **49**, 577.

9. **Verhagen, H., Vos, E., Francl, S., Heinonen, M., and van Loveren, H.** (2010) Status of nutrition and health claims in Europe. *Arch Biochem Biophys*, **501**, 6–15.

10. **Willett, W.C.** (1998) Nutritional epidemiology, 2nd edition. New York, Oxford University Press.

11. **Williams, P.** (2005) Consumer understanding and use of health claims for foods. *Nutr Rev*, **63**, 256–64.

Useful Websites

To see topical and scientifically robust updates on nutrition associated with this textbook and web links to many of the journals in the Further Reading sections, please see the dedicated Online Resource Centre at **http://www.oxfordtextbooks.co.uk/orc/mann4e/**

The European Food Safety Authority provides expert opinions on the health effects of many functional foods and their ingredients. See EFSA > Nutrition and Health Claims > Scientific Documents: **http://www.efsa.europa.eu/en/topics/topic/nutrition.htm**

The Linus Pauling Institute's Micronutrient Information Center provides clear and reliable information on vitamins, minerals, and plant constituents (phytochemicals), and their effects on health: **http://lpi.oregonstate.edu/infocenter/index.html**

Part 5

Nutritional assessment

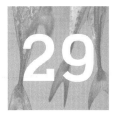

29 Food analysis, food composition tables, and databases

Philippa Lyons-Wall

Food composition tables or databases are designed to describe the composition of the foods in the country of origin. They contain data on foods eaten on a regular basis by the population and generally include some less widely consumed foods that are unique to the culture or eaten on special occasions. The values for nutrient and nonnutrient constituents are based on chemical analyses, sometimes performed by the compiler of the tables (or databases) or in an associated laboratory. Some food composition values may be 'borrowed' from a major overseas food table, or represent estimated averages from reports in the literature. Alternatively, they may be imputed from analytical values existing for a similar food or derived from the ingredients of a mixed food. The origins of the nutrient composition values should be specified, although in practice this is not always done. The UK food composition tables (*McCance and Widdowson's: The composition of foods*) and the US data (*USDA Handbook, No. 8*) are widely used reference sources. The US data are also available as a nutrient database at the USDA internet site, which is updated regularly.

When compiling food composition data, there are two important considerations. First, food items must be relevant; sampling of an individual food should be representative of the types commonly consumed by the population on a year-round, nationwide basis and should be pertinent to the current food supply. Second, the food composition data must be of high quality; analyses of the foods should be conducted in a rigorous, scientific environment so that values are precise and accurate. Well-established food composition tables have evolved over many years and often combine old and new analytical methods from a variety of different sources. Clear and detailed documentation of sampling and analytical procedures at all stages is as critical as the choice of the analytical procedure itself, so that compilers of tables, faced with the challenge of inevitable changes in the food supply, can continue to evaluate the relevance of the item and quality of the data.

29.1 Sampling

How does one sample foods that are truly representative of a particular food item? Does the analyst just go out to the corner shop nearest the laboratory and buy some food or try to include the varieties of that food across the nation? Foods are ultimately based on parts of plants or animals that vary naturally according to many factors. For example, varieties of sweet potato differ widely in β-carotene content according to whether the flesh is orange, yellow, or white in colour. Seasonal variation can markedly influence water and vitamin content, and fruits and vegetables tend to increase their concentration of sugars as they ripen, a process that is highly temperature dependent. Fat depots in animal foods are also extremely variable according to degree of exercise, type of feed, and age of the animal. Guidelines for sampling protocols that take these variations into account are detailed by Greenfield and Southgate (2003). In general, the greater the natural variation in a particular food the larger the number of samples required. National food production figures may also indicate the types of foods most widely consumed and therefore most representative of the population.

When the food arrives in the laboratory for analysis, it must first be unambiguously identified with both scientific and local names. Full descriptions are required for the part of the animal or plant used, and its stage of maturity, size, shape, and form (Table 29.1). Any cooking or processing methods used in preparing the item must be documented and the edible portion must be carefully separated from inedible refuse. Analyses may then proceed in one of two directions. Individual samples of the same food from different locations can be analysed separately in order to provide information on the variation between samples as well as their average nutrient content. This approach, however, may be a luxury that many laboratories cannot afford. Alternatively, a composite sample can be prepared by pooling several individual subsamples of a food from many locations to give a single sample for analyses. Often, a weighting scheme is used to ensure that those varieties and/or locations where the food item is consumed more frequently are proportionately represented in the final composite. Whether derived from an individual or composite sample, the edible portion must be homogenized or ground thoroughly to ensure that the aliquot taken for analysis is representative of the original sample. For trace minerals, it is also important that the sample is not exposed to adventitious sources of contamination during the collection, homogenization, sample preparation, and analytical stages. Similarly, care must be taken that vitamins and other susceptible organic components are not degraded by air or light, for example.

29.2 Analysis

The ultimate aim of food tables or databases is to provide nutrient information on food components that are of nutritional importance to the health of the population, over their lifetime and in different disease states (Table 29.2). Some of the more common methods used to analyse food components are described below. It is important to document the accuracy and precision of all analytical methods and to use reference materials of a similar matrix to the food sample and certified for the nutrient of interest. Reference materials can be obtained from the US National Institute for Standards and Technology, Washington, DC, and the International Atomic Energy Agency, Vienna.

29.2.1 Moisture

Moisture (water) is the first component to be analysed in a food, and it is probably the single most important piece of food composition data.

Table 29.1 INFOODS guidelines for describing foods

Name and identification	Name of food in national language of the country
	Name in local language or dialect
	Nearest equivalent name in English, French, or Spanish
	Country or area in which sample of food was obtained
	Food group and code in database used in the country
	Food group and code for food in regional nutrient database
	Codex Alimentarius or INFOODS food indexing group
Description	Food source (common and scientific name)
	Variety, breed, strain
	Part of plant or animal
	Manufacturer's name and address
	Other ingredients (including additives)
	Food processing and/or preparation
	Preservation method
	Degree of cooking
	Agricultural production conditions
	Maturity or ripeness
	Storage conditions
	Grade
	Container and food contact surface
	Physical state, shape, or form
	Colour

Source: Truswell, A.S., Bateson, D.J., Madafiglio, K.C., Pennington, J.A.T., Rand, W.M., and Klensin, J.C. (1991) INFOODS guidelines for describing foods: A systematic approach to describing foods to facilitate international exchange of food composition data. *J Food Comp Anal*, **4**, 18–38.

Underestimation of water content will lead to an overestimation of other components that are subsequently determined in the dried food. Water can be gained or lost during the cooking process, with changes in the apparent content of an array of nutrients, as well as energy. Water content is an important preliminary consideration when comparing the nutrient content of similar items in tables from different countries, as may happen if a specific food is not available in the local database. Furthermore, a high moisture content, typical of many fresh fruits and vegetables, indicates a low-energy value, while the reverse is true for items of low-moisture content.

The moisture content in foods is determined by simply evaporating off the water and calculating the difference in weight at the beginning and end. Different methods are used. Water may be driven off in an oven at temperatures around its boiling point, provided the sample itself does not decompose or oxidize or contain other volatiles that would

Table 29.2 Food components of nutritional importance

Basic components[a]
Moisture
Energy
Protein, fat, and carbohydrate
Up to 13 vitamins, and 10 or more minerals or trace elements
More detailed profiles[b]
Fatty acid profile (up to 37 fatty acids)
Amino acid profile (around 18 amino acids)
Carbohydrate components (sugars, starches)
Dietary fibre and components (soluble, insoluble)
Alcohol
Optional components[c]
Cholesterol
Vitamin A-inactive carotenoids (lycopene, lutein, zeaxanthin, and others)
Organic acids (malic, citric, lactic, formic, oxalic, and salicylic acids)
Biologically active components (e.g. flavonoids and isoflavonoids)
Glycaemic index

[a]Essential for growth and maintenance of body tissues and always listed in food tables.

[b]Useful for research into diet and disease risk and usually included in well-established tables.

[c]Not essential nutrients but may influence nutritional status indirectly by exerting physiological effects. Not routinely listed in food tables but may be cited in appendix sections.

contribute to the weight loss. Alternatively, evaporation can be achieved at lower temperatures by vacuum drying under reduced pressure, or by freeze-drying. In practice, a wide range of methods varying in temperature, time interval, and sample preparation have evolved to optimize this apparently simple process.

29.2.2 Protein and amino acids

Protein in foods is determined indirectly by measuring the content of amino-nitrogen, an essential constituent of the amino acid units that combine to form proteins. For the amino-nitrogen assay, the food sample is digested in hot concentrated sulphuric acid to convert the nitrogen into ammonium ion, which is then quantified by either distillation and titration in the classic *Kjeldahl method* or by *spectrophotometric analysis*. The protein content in the original food is then estimated by multiplying the total nitrogen value by specific conversion factors for different foods, as shown in Table 29.3 (based on their amino acid composition). Alternatively, the general conversion factor of 6.25 is used because nitrogen is assumed to represent about 16% of the protein content.

From a nutritional viewpoint, the importance of a particular dietary protein lies in its ability to sustain growth or replenish tissues, functions that depend more on the quality of the protein (or pattern of content of indispensable amino acids) than the total amount (see Chapter 5). Gelatin, for example, is a food that comprises over 80% protein, one of the highest values listed in food composition tables, yet as the sole protein source it cannot sustain life no matter how much is eaten because it is deficient in the indispensable amino acid tryptophan. *Amino acids* are measured by hydrolysing the protein with strong acid or alkali to break down the peptide bonds, followed by separation and measurement of the free amino acids using ion-exchange chromatography. Food tables may list the amino acid composition of major foods in addition to the total amount of protein, either in the main tables or in an appendix. The profile of indispensable amino acids can then be compared with that of a reference protein, such as hen's egg (a protein known to be utilized very efficiently) for adults, or human milk for babies, to develop a measure of the protein quality, referred to as the amino acid score or chemical score. Table 29.4 shows the indispensable amino acids in two common food proteins compared with those in hen's egg.

Table 29.3 Sample calculations of protein content from nitrogen

Item (100 g)	Total nitrogen (g)		Conversion factor[a]		Protein (g)
Rump steak	3.02	×	6.25	=	18.9
White rice	1.23	×	5.95	=	7.3

[a]Conversion factors for converting nitrogen in foods to protein: milk and milk products, 6.38; eggs, meat, fish, 6.25; rice, 5.95; barley, oats, rye, whole wheat, 5.83; soybeans, 5.71; peanuts, brazil nuts, 5.46; almonds, 5.18.

Table 29.4 Content of indispensable amino acids in food proteins (mg amino acid per g of protein)

	Hen's egg	Cheese	Wheat flour
Isoleucine	54	67	42
Leucine	86	98	71
Lysine	70	74	20[a]
Methionine + cysteine	57	32	31
Phenylalanine + tyrosine	93	102	79
Threonine	47	37	28
Tryptophan	17	14	11
Valine	66	72	42

The nutritive value of a dietary protein can be estimated by comparing its pattern of indispensable amino acids with those in a reference protein such as hen's egg. The amino acid score is the content of the most limiting (inadequate) amino acid, as a percentage of the reference value for this amino acid.

[a]For wheat flour, the most limiting amino acid is lysine and the amino acid score is 20/70 or 28%. In real life, however, wheat flour (as bread) is frequently eaten with another protein (e.g. cheese) that has even more lysine than egg, so the amino acid score of whole meals is usually much higher than for individual foods. The limiting amino acid in an equal mixture of wheat and cheese protein is methionine + cysteine and the amino acid score is 55%.

29.2.3 Fat

A characteristic property of fats is their solubility in organic solvents such as *n*-hexane, petroleum ether, or chloroform. Estimation of fat in foods involves extraction with one of these solvents followed by evaporation of the solvent and weighing of the final fat residue.

The accuracy of this estimation depends on the type of fat as well as the mix of other components in the food. The traditional *Soxhlet method* tended to underestimate fat that was bound to other food components such as protein. To overcome this problem, the sample is now predigested in concentrated acid or alcoholic ammonia to release the bound portion before extraction. The fat residue may be further analysed in various ways. Thin-layer chromatography can separate the fat into lipid classes, including triglycerides, phospholipids, and sterols. If lipids are hydrolysed to liberate their fatty acids, these can be separated by gas–liquid chromatography. Fatty acid profiles of major foods are provided in several comprehensive food tables such as the *USDA Handbook, No. 8* and the New Zealand Food Composition Tables. Total saturated fatty acids (including branched-chain acids), monounsaturated (*cis* and *trans* together) and polyunsaturated fatty acids are given in a supplement to the UK's *McCance and Widdowson's: The composition of foods*.

The presentation of the fat content of foods differs among food tables. In addition to providing the total fat content, compilers may sum the individual fatty acids into groups: polyunsaturated, monounsaturated, and saturated, and list each class separately, or they may present these as a ratio of polyunsaturated and monounsaturated fatty acids to that of saturated fatty acids, termed the PMS ratio. Alternatively, they may list each fatty acid according to its chain length and degree of saturation. The PMS ratio provides a crude estimate of overall atherogenic risk; the higher the proportion of unsaturates, the more favourable the ratio. For research purposes, however, the content of individual fatty acids is more useful because each may exert independent effects. (Chapters 4 and 21 discuss further the role of individual fatty acids in health and disease.)

29.2.4 Carbohydrates

Food composition tables vary widely in the methods used to measure carbohydrate. One approach is to estimate 'by difference', which defines carbohydrate as the difference between 100 and the sum of the weight percentages for protein, fat, water, and ash. However, inaccuracies arise using this approach because of the summation of the errors in estimating these four constituents. In addition, such values are of limited use because they do not distinguish between different carbohydrates, especially those that are available to the body (i.e. digested, absorbed, and utilized) and those that are unavailable. More accurate methods quantify the available and unavailable carbohydrate by direct measurements.

Available carbohydrate includes sugars (monosaccharides and disaccharides) and starches and dextrins (which are polysaccharides). Individual sugars can be extracted with aqueous alcohol and measured by high-performance liquid chromatography or using specific enzymatic colorimetric tests. Starches and dextrins, which are glucose polymers, are measured in the same way after an initial hydrolysis step to liberate free glucose. Food tables that report carbohydrate by direct analysis may list the monosaccharide equivalents because this is the form in which the carbohydrate is estimated. To obtain the actual values for disaccharides and starch (polysaccharide) in the food, these values should be divided by 1.05 and 1.10, respectively. A published

database is also available for the glycaemic index (GI), which ranks carbohydrate-containing foods according to the degree of rise in blood glucose immediately after the food is consumed, compared with that of a standard food—either glucose or white bread (Atkinson et al., 2008). The GI data are derived from studies in which human subjects are fed a range of carbohydrate-containing foods and, therefore, provide a qualitative biological rather than quantitative chemical measure of carbohydrate intake.

Unavailable carbohydrate or dietary fibre is the mixture of plant components that are resistant to digestive enzymes in the human small bowel. With advances in food technology, the term has been expanded to include chemically synthesized, and also extracted fibre components; these components can be added for functional purposes to nonplant foods, such as dairy products, but are not usually listed as a separate nutrient in food composition databases. The chemical diversity of fibre makes it a very challenging and elusive component to analyse in the laboratory. Accordingly, a number of methods have evolved. All begin with the defatted, dried food sample but each method measures a different chemical fraction. The Englyst method is the most sensitive and perhaps the most useful from a nutritional perspective because it can distinguish between soluble and insoluble fibres, both of which have physiologically distinct effects in the body in relation to chronic diseases such as diabetes, heart disease, and cancer. In the Englyst method, starch is initially removed by digestion with strong amylases and then the constituent sugars of dietary fibre are measured directly after acid hydrolysis to produce the free sugars. This yields estimates of both soluble (pectin, gums, mucilages, and hemicelluloses) and insoluble (cellulose and other hemicelluloses) fibre components, collectively called nonstarch polysaccharides (NSPs). Lignin escapes detection because it is not a carbohydrate but a polymeric phenolic compound. The older Southgate method gives a higher value for dietary fibre content as it measures lignin, as well as NSPs.

Other methods are less precise because they measure fibre 'by difference' but they involve less analytical work and so are more economical. In the widely used procedure of the *Association of Official Analytical Chemists* (AOAC), developed by Prosky *et al.* (1984), starch is first removed by enzymatic hydrolysis and the undigested residue is weighed, analysed for nitrogen, and then ashed. Protein and ash contents are then subtracted from the residue weight. *Van Soest's neutral detergent fibre* method measures only the insoluble cellulose and lignin, and not the soluble fibre; hence, this method underestimates total dietary fibre. The *crude fibre* method is the least accurate, involving rigorous treatment with boiling acid and alkali, which removes much of the dietary fibre itself.

A further complication in the analysis of dietary fibre is the recognition that a variable but small proportion of the dietary starch found in beans, wholegrains, potatoes (especially if eaten cold), or unripe bananas is not completely digested and is unavailable to the body for absorption. This starch, termed 'resistant starch', escapes digestion because it is physically inaccessible to the enzymes and, instead, it is probably fermented in the colon, thus behaving like soluble dietary fibre. Current values for dietary fibre in food tables do not include separate values for resistant starch, although the AOAC and Southgate methods include some of the resistant starch in the fibre value.

Different analytical methods can result in severalfold variations in the estimate of fibre for the same item, as shown in Table 29.5. Most food tables, however, are internally consistent in their choice of analytical method(s) and these should be stated clearly in the introductory section or in the main tables alongside the nutrient values. Special care should be taken when comparing carbohydrate values from different food composition tables. For reasons outlined above, values from those tables in which total carbohydrate is analysed by difference (i.e. including dietary fibre) are not compatible with others in which carbohydrate constituents are analysed directly.

29.2.5 Energy

The total energy of a food is measured by *bomb calorimetry* in which a sample of the food is burned with oxygen in a sealed chamber until completely oxidized. The heat released corresponds to the chemical or gross energy of the food. Food energy is reported in kilojoules (kJ) or kilocalories (kcal), where 1 kJ = 0.24 kcal or 1 kcal = 4.187 kJ. When a food is eaten, however, the energy-yielding components—protein, fat, carbohydrate, and (where present) alcohol—are oxidized by enzymatic processes within the body to provide energy, but not with 100% efficiency. Some energy is lost into the faeces as not all food components are fully absorbed from the digestive tract. Further energy is lost into urine since dietary protein, unlike carbohydrate and fat, is not completely oxidized by the body and its excretory product, urea, still retains some of the chemical energy from the original protein. The eminent American physiologist Atwater measured the energy losses into faeces and urine by a series of meticulous experiments in humans fed a mixture of foods. In his experiments, 92% of protein, 95% of fat, and 97% of carbohydrate were absorbed by the body, but for every gram of protein ingested, about one-quarter of its gross energy was lost into the urine.

Atwater's experiments, conducted at the turn of the nineteenth century, represent landmark studies from which the energy content of foods in today's food composition tables are derived. Atwater developed a system of four conversion factors, which represent the energy available in: (1) protein (17 kJ/g, 4 kcal/g); (2) fat (37 kJ/g, 9 kcal/g); (3) carbohydrate (16 kJ/g, 4 kcal/g); and (4) alcohol (29 kJ/g, 7 kcal/g), taking into account the estimated energy losses into faeces and urine. The value is slightly higher for starch (due to lower hydration) than that given for all carbohydrates, and slightly lower for sugars. These factors provide values for food energy as it is utilized by the body (i.e. metabolizable energy). The energy content of each food is calculated by first multiplying the weight of each component by its Atwater conversion factor, and second, summing the energy from each component to give a grand total for the food, as shown in Table 29.6. Note that the total weight of each nutrient is obtained by direct analysis of the food, as described previously (see also Chapter 5).

Table 29.5 Dietary fibre content of dried red kidney beans estimated by five different methods

Method	Fibre content (g/100 g)	Fibre components
Englyst[a]	15.7	Soluble + insoluble fibre (not lignin or resistant starch)
Southgate[a]	23.4	Soluble + insoluble fibre, lignin
AOAC (Prosky and Asp)[b]	21.5	Soluble + insoluble fibre, lignin
Neutral detergent fibre (Van Soest)[c]	10.4	Insoluble fibre only
Crude fibre[c]	6.2	Part of the insoluble fibre

Red kidney beans contain both soluble and insoluble dietary fibre. AOAC, Southgate, and Englyst methods measure total dietary fibre, but Englyst fibre is lower because it does not measure lignin or resistant starch. Neutral detergent fibre is lower because it does not measure soluble fibre. AOAC, Association of Official Analytical Chemists.

Sources: [a]Food Standards Agency (2002) *McCance and Widdowson's: The composition of foods*, 6th summary edition. Cambridge, Royal Society of Chemistry; [b]Food Standards Australia New Zealand (2007). *NUTTAB 2006 Australian food composition tables.* Canberra: Food Standards Australia New Zealand; [c]USDA (1986) *Composition of foods: Legumes and legume products.* Handbook No. 8–16. Washington, DC, US Department of Agriculture.

The biggest variable is the carbohydrate value and whether this includes fibre, because Atwater factors are applied to the total carbohydrate content irrespective of whether this is analysed directly or by difference. In practice, the value for energy is somewhere between the two extremes of 16 kcal/g for available carbohydrate and 0 kJ/g for unavailable carbohydrate. This is because a proportion of dietary fibre is fermented in the colon to short-chain fatty acids, which can be absorbed from the large bowel and oxidized for energy. Livesey (1991) has estimated that about half the dietary fibre can

Table 29.6 Calculation of metabolizable energy content in raw soy bean using Atwater conversion factors

Component	Weight (g/100 g)		Atwater factor (kJ (kcal)/g)		Energy content (kJ (kcal)/100 g)
Water	8	–	–	=	–
Protein	31	×	17 (4)	=	527 (124)
Fat	20	×	37 (9)	=	740 (180)
Available carbohydrate	7	×	16 (4)	=	112 (28)
Dietary fibre	20	–	Not *usually* included	=	–

The energy content of individual components is then summed to give a grand total of 1379 kJ/100 g or 332 kcal/100 g.

be utilized by the body in this way and proposed an average energy conversion factor of 8 kJ/g (2 kcal/g) for unavailable carbohydrates, about half the value for available carbohydrate. Estimates of the energy from fibre are included in some more recent databases, such as the Australian Food and Nutrient Database (Food Standards Australia New Zealand, 2008).

The energy conversion factors used today vary somewhat from Atwater's original factors. The German, British, Australian, and New Zealand food composition tables, for example, apply the same four factors to all foods, whereas the US and East Asian tables use a range of slightly differing conversion factors, rather lower for components in plant foods than in animal foods, reflecting Atwater's initial observation that the energy from plants was less available. The conversion factors selected to calculate energy should be specified in the introduction or appendix section of all food composition tables and the reader is referred to these for more in-depth information.

29.2.6 Inorganic nutrients and vitamins

The range of inorganic nutrients in foods including calcium, iron, magnesium, zinc, copper, manganese, potassium, and sodium can be determined by *flame atomic absorption spectrophotometry* (AAS), a method whereby a solution of the ashed or acid-digested food sample is sprayed into the flame of an atomic absorption spectrophotometer and quantified by the degree of absorption at a specified wavelength. For selenium, direct AAS with a Zeeman background correction is required. Graphite-furnace AAS is used for analysing the ultratrace elements, such as chromium, nickel, and manganese. Alternatively, all the minerals can be measured in the one sample using inductively coupled plasma spectrophotometry or X-ray fluorescence. Minerals are a very stable component of foods and these procedures can be highly accurate provided any interfering substances such as plant pigments or organic constituents have first been

removed. This is achieved by reducing the food sample to a dry ash by thorough heating in a muffle furnace or by breaking down and oxidizing the organic components by wet ashing with boiling concentrated acids. For trace element analysis, precautions must be used to avoid adventitious contamination by the use of ultrapure acids, acid-washed glassware, plastic materials for sample preparation and analysis, and high-grade deionized water.

In contrast to the minerals, many of the vitamins in foods are not very stable. Riboflavin and vitamin A are sensitive to light; thiamin, folate, and vitamin C are sensitive to heat; and vitamin E to oxidation. Vitamins are either analysed by the traditional but more time-consuming microbiological methods or by newer, faster chemical techniques. *Microbiological assays* are conducted with a culture of organisms that have a specific growth requirement for the particular vitamin. The assumption is made, however, that the microorganism reacts in the same way as the human organism. Such methods are available for a wide range of B vitamins including thiamin, niacin, riboflavin, vitamins B_6 and B_{12}, folate, biotin, and pantothenic acid and have the advantage of estimating the total biological potential of the vitamin. Alternative chemical methods, such as *high-performance liquid chromatography* (HPLC), can be used for most of the vitamins. They require an initial extraction step to remove other components in the food, but are useful for separating and quantifying different chemical forms of the vitamin. It should be borne in mind that many of the existing values for vitamins, as well as minerals, in food tables were obtained with older, less specific colorimetric methods that may now be obsolete.

Values in food composition tables represent the total content of each mineral or vitamin in the food and do not address the complex problem of bioavailability, defined as the proportion of a nutrient that is actually absorbed from the food and utilized. When a vitamin exists in two or more forms that are utilized differently in the body, some food composition tables tabulate each form separately. Vitamin A, for example, has two major components obtained from quite different food sources: preformed vitamin A (retinol), which is found in many animal products, and the provitamin A carotenoids derived from plants. The compiler may further attempt to calculate the overall potency of the vitamin in the body by summing the different forms, taking into account their relative biological activities. Some of the assumptions and calculations made in food tables regarding the different forms of niacin, folate, and vitamins A, C, D, and E are shown in Table 29.7.

29.2.7 Nonnutrient biologically active constituents

In addition to the nutrient components, such as protein, fat, carbohydrate, vitamins, and minerals, plant foods in particular contain an abundant array of chemical constituents or 'phytochemicals'. Examples of nutritional importance include the flavonoids, isoflavonoids, and nonvitamin A carotenoids. Although

Table 29.7 Presentation of different vitamin forms in food composition tables

Vitamin	Main forms	Unit of total vitamin activity
Niacin[a]	1. Preformed in foods (nicotinic acid + nicotamide) 2. Derived from tryptophan	Niacin equivalents (NE)
Folate[b]	1. Food folates 2. Folic acid enrichment	Dietary folate equivalents (DFE)
Vitamin A[c]	1. Retinol 2. Provitamin A carotenoids	Retinol equivalents (RE) or Retinol activity equivalents (RAE)
Vitamin C[d]	1. Ascorbic acid 2. Dehydroascorbic acid	Vitamin C
Vitamin D[e]	1. Vitamin D (cholecalciferol) 2. 25-Hydroxyvitamin D	Total vitamin D activity
Vitamin E[f]	1. Tocopherols ($\alpha, \beta, \gamma, \delta$) 2. Tocotrienols ($\alpha, \beta, \gamma, \delta$)	α-Tocopherol equivalents

[a]Because approximately 1% of protein is tryptophan and 1/60th tryptophan is converted to niacin in the body: NE (mg) = preformed niacin (mg) + dietary protein (g) × 0.16.

[b]Bioavailability of folate from food is about 50% from foods, 85% from fortified foods or as a supplement (consumed with food), or 100% as a supplement (on an empty stomach) (Institute of Medicine, 2006): 1 µg DFE = 1 µg food folate = 0.6 µg folic acid (taken with meals) = 0.5 µg folic acid (on empty stomach).

[c]Vitamin A can be expressed as RE, where β-carotene has one-sixth the activity of retinol and other carotenoids have one-twelfth the activity of retinol. To acknowledge lower reported availability from vegetable sources, some databases (e.g. Agricultural Research Service, 2010) now express vitamin A as RAE, where β-carotene has only one-twelfth the activity of retinol (Institute of Medicine, 2006): RAE(µg) = retinol (µg) + β-carotene (µg)/12 + (α-carotene + β-cryptoxanthin (µg)/24.

[d]Both forms have equal activity and are summed to give total vitamin C.

[e]Vitamin D in food is measured as natural cholecalciferol (or ergocalciferol) and 25-hydroxyvitamin D (an active circulating form in animals, and hence meats), which has about five times the activity of cholecalciferol (Food Standards Agency, 2002): total vitamin D activity = sum of cholecalciferol + 5 × 25-hydroxycholecalciferol (in meats).

[f]α-Tocopherol is the most abundant form, with over twice the activity of other tocopherols and tocotrienols. Activities of individual vitamin forms are cited in Food Standards Agency (2002).

not classed as essential nutrients in terms of preventing a specific nutritional deficiency, these constituents are biologically active in the body and are thought to contribute to optimal health and longevity (see Chapter 16).

Phytochemicals occur in relatively small mg or μg quantities per 100 g food. While precise HPLC assays are available for quantification, it is often difficult to estimate levels in foods accurately. For example, the concentration of isoflavonoids in soybeans, a rich natural source, shows up to six-fold variation. This reflects genetic differences and also the fact that isoflavonoids, unlike more stable structural components, such as proteins, are part of the plant's natural response to stress. Insect infestations or climatic considerations, including low temperature and high soil moisture, can trigger dramatic increases in isoflavonoid content. This natural variability means that the isoflavonoid content in the same variety of soybean or soy product available in local retail outlets could vary several-fold between different batches. Despite certain limitations, the identification and quantification of biologically active substances in plants is an area of intense current research. Databases for isoflavonoids and a range of other special-interest constituents have been collated by the Nutrient Data Laboratory at the US Department of Agriculture, and are available at the USDA internet site http://www.ars.usda.gov/nutrientdata

29.3 Compilation of food composition data

Compilation of food composition data either in the form of tables or computerized databases is a very large task. It requires painstaking inspection of a wide range of sources that use a variety of sampling and analytical procedures. Data analysed outside the compiler's laboratory must frequently be traced back to its source and any items without clear documentation discarded because there is no way to evaluate their quality. Values from different sources must be compared and statistical calculations made to provide a meaningful average for the nutrient content of a food. As food patterns within a population are constantly changing and evolving, data must also be scrutinized to determine its relevance in the current food supply.

Not only should data be accurate and relevant, but also the format must be clear so that the user may easily understand the data. Food items are listed alphabetically and usually grouped according to food groups with similar nutritional properties (e.g. vegetables, fruits, grains, meats, and dairy products) or by product use (e.g. snacks, desserts, and breakfast cereals). In cases where foods are collected or prepared with inedible matter, the percentage edible portion, sometimes expressed indirectly as percentage refuse, is also given. However, irrespective of the proportion of edible matter or the accustomed serving size, nutrient values for items are always presented in terms of 100 g edible portions. Consequently, this does not include the core or stone in fruit, or the bones in meat and chicken, but it does include optional materials such as certain vegetable skins and trimmable meat fat, unless specified otherwise. Most food tables cite both scientific and local names for each item, and some specify the number of food items analysed and whether a single or composite sample was used for analysis. Rarely do tables include the natural variation around the mean value, but rather provide a single mean representative value. The German (Souci *et al.*, 2008) and the US (Agricultural Research Service, 2009) tables are exceptions, citing the range (i.e. highest and lowest values known) or the standard error of the mean, respectively, in addition to the mean value.

Ideally, food composition tables or databases should include analyses for all food components of nutritional relevance to the potential user, whether this be a dietitian/nutritionist prescribing advice to a client, a research worker investigating certain nutrients in relation to disease risk, or a food manufacturer seeking accurate nutrient information on their products for the purposes of marketing and food legislation. In practice, however, inclusion is determined more by the analytical resources and public health priorities of the country concerned. A wealth of analytical and descriptive information on food habits and customs already exists within different cultures. Yet, many of these data are not widely accessible outside the country, often because local names are idiosyncratic or culture-specific, making it difficult to identify the food. In this regard, the INFOODS guidelines (Table 29.1) were established to ensure that foods are named and described in a standardized manner with a view to facilitating interchange of food composition data at the international level.

Further Reading

1. **Agricultural Research Service** (2010) *USDA National nutrient database for standard reference, release 22, Nutrient data laboratory.* Washington, DC, US Department of Agriculture.

2. **Atkinson, F.S., Foster-Powell, K., and Brand-Miller, J.C.** (2008) International table of glycaemic index and glycaemic load values. *Diabetes Care*, **31**, 2281–3.

3. **Food Standards Agency** (2002) *McCance and Widdowson's: The composition of foods*, 6th summary edition. Cambridge, Royal Society of Chemistry.

4. **Food Standards Australia New Zealand** (2008) *AUSNUT 2007: Australian food, supplement and nutrient database for estimation of population nutrient intakes.* Canberra, Food Standards Australia New Zealand.

5. **Lesperance, L. et al.** (2009) *The concise New Zealand food composition tables*, 8th edition. Palmerston North NZ, Crop and Food Research Ltd; Wellington, NZ, Ministry of Health.

6. **Greenfield, H. and Southgate, D.A.T.** (2003) *Food composition data. Production, management and use*, 2nd edition. Rome, Food and Agricultural Organization.

7. **Institute of Medicine** (2006) *Dietary reference intakes: The essential guide to nutrient requirements.* Washington, DC, The National Academies Press.

8. **Livesey, G.** (1991) Calculating the energy values of foods: Towards new empirical formulae based on diets with varied intakes of unavailable complex carbohydrates. *Eur J Clin Nutr*, **45**, 1–12.

9. **Prosky, L., Asp, N.G., Furda, I., De Vries, J.W., Schweizer, T.F., and Harland, B.F.** (1984) Determination of total dietary fibre in foods, food products and total diets: Interlaboratory study. *J Assoc Off Anal Chem*, **67**, 1044–52.

10. **Souci, S.W., Fachmann, W., and Kraut, H.** (2008) *Food composition and nutrition tables*, 7th revised and completed edition. Stuttgart, Medpharm Scientific Publishers.

11. **Truswell, A.S., Bateson, D.J., Madafiglio, K.C., Pennington, J.A.T., Rand, W.M., and Klensin, J.C.** (1991) INFOODS guidelines for describing foods: A systematic approach to describing foods to facilitate international exchange of food composition data. *J Food Comp Anal*, **4**, 18–38. Available online at http://www.fao.org/infoods/.

12. **USDA** (1986) *Composition of foods: Legumes and legume products.* Handbook No. 8–16. Washington, DC, US Department of Agriculture.

13. **Wu Leung, W.T., Butrum, R.R., Chang, F.H., Rao, M.N., and Polacchi, W.** (1972) *Food composition table for use in East Asia.* Rome, Food and Agricultural Organization.

Useful Websites

To see topical and scientifically robust updates on nutrition associated with this textbook and web links to many of the journals in the Further Reading sections, please see the dedicated Online Resource Centre at **http://www.oxfordtextbooks.co.uk/orc/mann4e/**

US Department of Agriculture, Nutrient Data Laboratory home page: http://www.ars.usda.gov/ba/bhnrc/ndl

Souci-Fachmann-Kraut online database: http://www.sfk-online.net/cgi-bin/sfkstart.mysql?language=english

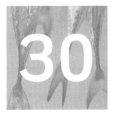

30 Dietary assessment

Jim Mann and Sheila Bingham*

Dietary assessment is one of the specialized interests of nutritionists, used in surveillance of populations, nutritional epidemiology, clinical assessment, and experimental research. There are two basic approaches to estimating food intake: one principally concerned with determining the intake of populations, the other with assessing the diets of individuals. These approaches are not mutually exclusive, since methods for assessing dietary intake of individuals may be used for estimating intake of populations as happens in most national nutrition surveys which generally involve individual 24-hour recalls. This chapter describes the various methods used in the different contexts in which knowledge of food and nutrient intakes are required.

Methods used for assessing dietary intake in carefully controlled experimental studies will differ appreciably from those required in large, epidemiological studies. The chapter also considers the reliability of the various methods, taking into account the conflict between the need for accuracy to establish exactly where an individual lies within the overall distribution of foods and nutrients and the logistics of doing so when very large populations required for epidemiological studies are investigated.

30.1 Population estimates

Population estimates are needed principally for surveillance, for example, to assess intakes of a particular food or nutrient in relation to reference nutrient intakes (RNIs) and to determine changes over time. Such information would also be used during emergencies when food is in short supply, to make recommendations concerning usual diet, and in considering the case for fortification of foods on a national basis. Population estimates of dietary intake have also been compared with disease rates in different countries or populations or within the same country over time to identify clues as to possible nutritional causes of the disease. Population estimates may be derived from food balance sheets, household food surveys, national nutrition surveys, and, potentially, supermarket records.

Food balance sheets are based on national statistics of food produced, imported, and exported with factors for wastage included. The Food and Agricultural Organization (FAO) of the United Nations (http://faostat.fao.org/) collates these and they have been used extensively for monitoring changes in consumption and for population comparisons, linking, for example, population

*deceased

Food consumption at the national level is also called food moving into consumption, food disappearance data, and apparent food consumption. The food supply is calculated from estimates of domestic food production plus imports minus exports. Potential food diverted for farm animal feed, nonfood industrial use, and wastage at wholesale level are subtracted. The total is divided by the estimated population each year. These statistics are useful for monitoring changes in consumption of commodities and comparing countries' food habits. FAO food balance sheets are based on these statistics and available each year from some 175 countries. For many countries, these are the only regular measures of food intakes. However, these are macro figures. The calorie and nutrient numbers are around 25% (or more) above what individuals actually eat and drink, because there is wastage of food in homes and catering establishments, and food is fed to tourists and pets. They give no idea of distribution of food resources among regions, socioeconomic groups, or within the family.

estimates of fat and cardiovascular disease rates and population estimates of meat and fat and bowel and breast cancer rates (Box 30.1).

Household surveys are records kept by the householder of all food available to the family over 1 week, and the total food entering the household is divided by the number of people living there. This approach has been used in the UK in the National Food Survey, which has been running continuously for over 50 years as a combined food consumption and expenditure survey and which in recent years has taken into account food eaten away from home (http://www.defra.gov.uk/statistics/foodfarm/food/familyfood/nationalfoodsurvey/). From this, regional comparisons and secular trends in consumption are available, for example the trend towards a lower saturated fat composition of the diet in the UK.

When using data derived from food balance sheets or household surveys, it is not possible to compare the intake of food or nutrients in different age and sex groups with differential trends in disease incidence or risk factors, nor for individual data to be assessed. This is because the findings relating to, for example, children, the elderly, or males and females cannot be separated out from the overall population average data. Potentially, computerized supermarket records of sales or loyalty cards could be used to obtain regional information on nutritional consumption (Robertson *et al.*, 2004).

Typically the 24-hour recall (see Section 30.2 and Box 30.2) is used in *national nutrition surveys*. Although the information is derived from individuals, the aim is to describe the nutritional intake of the population. This requires the study of large numbers of people who are representative of the

National nutrition surveys estimate food intake of individuals and may involve clinical examination and blood tests to further assess nutritional status. Although based on the intakes of individuals, such surveys provide the average and range intakes of foods and nutrients of different age and sex subgroups relating to the population from which the individuals are drawn. Examples are NHANES in the USA, National Diet and Nutrition Surveys in the UK, National Nutrition Survey in Australia (1995), and the National Nutrition Survey in New Zealand (2009). They have all been somewhat different. They identify nutrients for which intakes are lower than recommended on the one hand and frequency of overweight/obesity on the other. They also gather information about food usage as a basis for formulating and evaluating health policy and regulatory needs. The food intake method used has to be a 24-hour recall or food record because of the need to know the exact types of food people are eating.

population of interest in order to be reasonably confident that the survey yields an unbiased estimate of the usual mean intake of nutrients of interest.

National nutrition surveys often involve a repeat 24-hour recall on a subsample of participants.

30.2 Individual methods

Several methods are available for measuring the dietary intake of individuals. They generally consist either of the collation of observations from a number of separate days' investigations, as in records, checklists, and 24-hour recalls, or attempts to obtain average intake by asking about the usual frequency of food consumption, as in the diet history and food frequency questionnaires (FFQs). In all methods of dietary assessment, some estimate of the quantity of food consumed is required, and for the determination of nutrient or other food component intake, either an appropriate description that can be matched with an entry in the food tables or an aliquot for chemical analysis (Box 30.3). Each of the methods is described briefly below and further details regarding equipment, protocols, uses, and limitations are available in the references in Further reading. Detailed examples of methods used in particular studies are shown on the web sites given.

30.2.1 Food records

Food records involve subjects being taught to describe and either weigh or estimate the amount of food immediately before eating and to record leftovers. Records are generally completed by the participant on sheets or booklets, which, in the case of estimated records, may include photographs to facilitate estimation of portion size. Cups, spoons, rulers, and scales may be provided to aid accurate description. Verbal records, with descriptions of amounts recorded on tape cassettes, have also been used, as have records incorporating bar codes from purchased foods. As this method is a record kept at the time of eating and does not involve participants attempting to remember if or how often a food has been eaten, it is generally regarded as providing the most reliable information regarding the dietary intake of individuals, provided sufficient days' observations are collected on each individual

---

BOX 30.3 Estimating individual food intake

Basically, four types of method are used to estimate individual food intakes:

- **Food diary or record** 'Please write down (and describe) everything you eat and drink (and estimate the amount) for the next 3 (4 or 7) days.' Amounts are usually recorded in household measures, but for more accuracy subjects can be provided with quick-reading scales to weigh food before it goes on the plate (and any leftovers).
- **24-hour recall** 'Tell me everything you had to eat and drink in the last 24 hours.' This is less subject to wishful thinking about what the subject feels they ought to have eaten. The weakness is that yesterday may have been an unusual day; 24-hour recalls can, however, be repeated.
- **Food frequency questionnaire** 'Do you eat meat/fish/bread/milk, etc. on average more than once a day, two or three times a week, once a week, once a month, etc.?' (usually filling in 100 to 150 lines on a questionnaire form) (Fig. 30.2).
- **Dietary history** 'What do you eat on a typical day and how does your food intake vary?' This requires a skilled and patient interviewer. Food models, cups, plates, and spoons are used to estimate portion sizes.

(see Section 30.4.2). In the past, it has been used for the purpose of validating other methods of dietary assessment, but this approach is now recognized to underestimate the extent of measurement error (see Section 30.4.6). Respondent burden is higher than with other methods, but the approach has been used in multicentre cross-sectional comparisons of representative population samples in which instructions to participants have been standardized among different centres (e.g. the Key's study of coronary heart disease (see Chapter 21) and other epidemiological settings such as the very large prospective studies of diet and health, for example a study of 25 000 people in the European Prospective Investigation of Cancer in Norfolk (EPIC Norfolk; see http://www.srl.cam.ac.uk/epic/nutmethod/). Fig. 30.1 shows an example from this website. Weighed records have also been used in surveillance procedures; for example, records from representative population samples have been routinely obtained by the UK Government National Diet and Nutrition Survey (http://www.food.gov.uk/science).

30.2.2 Twenty-four-hour recalls

This method is also a report of daily habits, but interviewed or written information about the previous day's intake, the 24-hour recall, is obtained. The participant has to remember the actual foods consumed and give information on portion weights from memory. Some information may be forgotten and descriptions of portion size are more difficult to supply, though the interviewers will often use food models or photographs as memory aids and to assist in quantifying portion size. Although the 24-hour recall may consist of a very simple written list completed by the participant, most 24-hour recalls have several stages or multiple passes, in which data are checked and verified by a skilled interviewer, and each recall may take about 40 minutes. The respondent burden for a single 24-hour recall is less than for several days of food records and the method is typically used for determining average usual intakes of a

large population or group, for example in national nutrition surveys. For details of methods used in the USA NHANES survey, see http://www.cdc.gov/nchs/nhanes.htm. National nutrition surveys are typically based on a single 24-hour recall, sometimes with a repeat recall being undertaken on a subsample. However, when attempting to assess the diet of individuals using this method, multiple 24-hour recalls may be needed, with a subsequent increase in respondent burden, depending on the level of precision required and nutrient to be studied (see Section 30.4).

30.2.3 Food frequency questionnaires

FFQs are designed to assess long-term habits, over months or years, and may either comprise a relatively small list of foods that are the major sources of a limited group of nutrients of interest, or a longer list if a full dietary assessment is required. Participants usually complete the FFQ themselves, generally after receiving the FFQ in the post with detailed instructions regarding completion of the questionnaire. The length of the list of foods generally does not exceed 150 items. Various methods to assess portion sizes may be used, for example fitting average portion weights derived from other data to the respondents' chosen food and frequency selections. To assess the frequency of food consumption, accompanying the food list is a multiple response grid in which respondents attempt to estimate how often selected foods are eaten. Up to ten categories ranging from never or once a month or less, to six times per day is a usual format. Fig. 30.2 shows an example of a FFQ taken from EPIC Norfolk. Because responses are standardized, FFQs can be analysed in comparatively short periods of time so that large numbers of individuals can be investigated relatively inexpensively. The FFQ has been widely used in large epidemiological cohort studies to classify participants according to quantiles of intake of nutrients and disease incidence in each quantile examined, to identify food patterns associated with excessive or inadequate

DATE 2 3 1 0 1 9 9 3 **DAY OF WEEK** SATURDAY

BEFORE BREAKFAST

Food/drink	Description and preparation	Amount
Orange Squash	Robinsons whole orange-sweetened	1 Glass

BREAKFAST

Food/Drink	Description and Preparation	Amount
Beef Patty with onion	Homebaked cold Salt added	3a
Tea	Typhoo	1 Cup
Milk	S/Skimmed	1 Dessertspoon
Sugar	White	1½ Teaspoon

MID MORNING – between breakfast time and lunch time

Food/Drink	Description and Preparation	Amount
Coffee	Maxwell House, Instant ½ Water/½ S/Skimmed milk	1 Mug
Sugar	White	1½ Teaspoons
Cake	Homemade Date Cake	16a

LUNCH

Food/drink	Description and preparation	Amount
Gammon Steak	Microwaved	6oz
Chips	Deep Fried in Oil (Crisp & Dry)	7a
Peas	Birds Eye (Frozen)	12a
Bread	Local Bakery White unsliced	½ Slice ½ Thick
Apple Pie	Homemade	3B
Sugar	White-sprinkled on	1 Teaspoon
Custard	Birds-made with S/Skimmed milk	Small Fruit Dish

TEA – between lunch time and the evening meal

Food/Drink	Description and Preparation	Amount
Tea	Typhoo-tea bag	1 Mug
Milk	S/Skimmed	1 Dessertspoon
Sugar	White	1½ Teaspoons
Biscuit	Chocolate Digestive Fox's	1

Fig. 30.1 Example of a food diary.

Source: Reproduced with permission from EPIC Norfolk (http://www.srl.cam.ac.uk/).

PLEASE PUT A TICK (✓) ON EVERY LINE

FOODS AND AMOUNTS	AVERAGE USE LAST YEAR								
DRINKS	Never or less than once/month	1–3 per month	Once a week	2–4 per week	5–6 per week	Once a day	2–3 per day	4–5 per day	6+ per day
Tea (cup)								✓	
Coffee, instant or ground (cup)						✓			
Coffee, decaffeinated (cup)	✓								
Coffee whitener, eg. Coffee-mate (teaspoon)	✓								
Cocoa, hot chocolate (cup)						✓			
Horlicks, Ovaltine (cup)	✓								
Wine (glass)	✓								
Beer, lager or cider (half pint)	✓								
Port, sherry, vermouth, liqueurs (glass)	✓								
Spirits, eg. gin, brandy, whisky, vodka (single)	✓								
Low-calorie or diet fizzy soft drinks (glass)	✓								
Fizzy soft drinks, eg. Coca cola, lemonade (glass)						✓			
Pure fruit juice (100%) e.g. orange, apple juice (glass)	✓								
Fruit squash or cordial (glass)							✓		
FRUIT (1 fruit or medium serving) **For very seasonal fruits such as strawberries, please estimate your average use when the fruit is in season**									
Apples				✓					
Pears				✓					
Oranges, satsumas, mandarins		✓							
Grapefruit	✓								
Bananas			✓						
Grapes			✓						
Melon	✓								
Peaches, plums, apricots				✓					
Strawberries, raspberries, kiwi fruit						✓			
Tinned fruit		✓							
Dried fruit, eg. raisins, prunes	✓								
	Never or less than once/month	1–3 per month	Once a week	2–4 per week	5–6 per week	Once a day	2–3 per day	4–5 per day	6+ per day

Please check that you have a tick (✓) on EVERY line

Fig. 30.2 Example of a food frequency questionnaire. This is one of several different pages that have to be filled in.

Source: Reproduced with permission from EPIC Norfolk (http://www.srl.cam.ac.uk/).

intakes of nutrients, and to obtain descriptive information on usual intakes of foods. Although their use is increasing, some doubt has been expressed regarding the ability of FFQs to detect associations between diet and disease using this method (Kristal *et al.*, 2005).

30.2.4 Diet histories

The diet history is usually conducted by trained interviewers who record a 24-hour recall followed by more detailed information on usual foods consumed, portion sizes, recipes, and frequency of food consumption over the recent past. This method is less commonly used in epidemiological research due to the necessity for face-to-face interviews of up to 90 minutes, and consequent costs, but it is the most frequently used method for the assessment of diet by dieticians in the clinical context (see Gibson, 2005).

30.2.5 Checklists

The checklist is a record, to be completed for 7 days or more. However, the checklist method is a printed list of representative foods in which participants are asked to check off at the end of each day which foods they have eaten. This means that participants do not have to estimate how often the food is eaten, thus avoiding problems in the estimation of the frequency of food consumption that occur in the FFQs. Like the FFQs however, the foods can be precoded for rapid data entry and computerized linkage to food tables. In one published version, the checklist took the form of a booklet, which comprised one page of instructions, one of an example, and seven pages (one for each day over 1 week) of the checklist. When selecting foods, participants were asked to count half for a small portion and two for a large portion. A space was left to record foods not present on the printed list, but otherwise the list was precoded for nutrient analysis. The list of 160 foods was that used for a FFQ and, where possible, 'units' (slices, cups, etc.) were specified (Bingham *et al.*, 1994). This method has been further developed more recently (Lillegaard and Andersen, 2005).

30.2.6 Duplicate diets

If there is inadequate food table information, 'precise weighing' of duplicate diets may be necessary, for example if food composition tables with values for cooked foods are not available, in carefully controlled experiments when precise knowledge of nutrients and energy intake is required or if exposure to phytochemicals and contaminants are being investigated. Raw ingredients, the cooked food, meal, or snack, plus the individual portions are generally prepared in duplicate, one for consumption, the other for weighing and chemical analysis if required. Amounts not consumed are taken into account. This method is very labour-intensive compared with the records outlined above and it is usual for skilled field-workers to carry out this survey, rather than the subjects themselves (Bingham, 1987).

30.2.7 Retrospective assessment

Methods that are designed to assess recent past diet (the 24-hour recall, FFQs, and diet history) can in theory also be used to assess distant past diet, for example in case–control investigations where dietary habits before the onset of symptoms (and possible change in diet) are required. However, there is evidence to suggest that individuals cannot remember past diet and instead report present diet (Friedenreich *et al.*, 1992). This may introduce bias into case–control studies if dietary habits have changed as a result of the symptoms of the disease in question. For this reason, more weight is placed on results of prospective studies than retrospective case–control studies in nutritional epidemiology.

30.3 Calculation of nutrient intake

Once the primary data concerning foods consumed are obtained, the information is converted to nutrient intake using tables of food composition. In the past, this was generally done manually, perhaps with the assistance of a calculator, and the information obtained was generally restricted to a narrow range of nutrients, for example energy and macro-nutrient consumption. Computerized databases of food composition revolutionized the amount of information that could be obtained, but in some data entry systems the matching of the description of the food consumed to the correct computer code has to be done manually, which leads to errors. In present-day surveys, necessitated partly by the growth in the variety of foods consumed, this proce-dure is now usually entirely computerized, usually by the investigators themselves. Programs are more expensive to run and develop for record or 24-hour recall methods than for FFQs, since at least 150 000

different food items are available in Westernized food supplies, all of which require estimation of por-tion size and individual computer coding (see http://www.srl.cam.ac.uk/epic/nutmethod/). Furthermore, most investigators will incorporate some means of calculating nutrient intake from individual recipes used in home cooking, since these can have a marked effect on some nutrients, for example on specific fatty acids. The checklist and FFQ methods require much simpler methods and considerably less coding time by the investigator, although much information on actual foods con-sumed is lost.

30.4 Measurement error in dietary assessments

Methods of measuring diet are associated with both random and systematic error. Both types of error can arise in the assessment of portion size, daily variation, frequency of food consumption, and fail-ure to report usual diet, either because of changes in habits while taking part in an investigation or misre-porting of food choice or amount. Error may also result from the use of food tables.

30.4.1 Assessment of portion size

Information about the weight of food consumed may be obtained either by asking subjects to weigh out individual items of food onto the plate as it is being served (weighed records), or requiring that portions of food be described in terms of household meas-ures, volume models, photographs, average por-tions, units, or pack sizes (estimated records, diet histories, and 24-hour recalls). Errors are reduced when weights are obtained, but participants need to be given a set of scales accurate to 1–2 g with a capac-ity of 2 kg. Digital scales are now usually used and have replaced spring balances used in older surveys. Participants need instruction on the use of the scales and on the detail of information required, including description of recipes used (see Further reading).

Estimated records are much easier for participants to complete, but conversion of descriptions of food into weights requires considerable investment by the investigator and may necessitate the determination of density of separate foods, as well as a detailed database of weights of foods equivalent to the photo-graphs, models, package sizes, and household meas-ures used. On balance, there appears to be little or no systematic bias in group averages of nutrients obtained by records with estimates of food, com-pared with group averages obtained by weighed die-tary records. Nevertheless, despite the absence of overall bias in a population, the estimation of por-tion size rather than direct weighing is associated with imprecision at the individual level. In general, this is in the order of 50% (coefficient of variation) for foods, but less, about 20%, for nutrients, probably due to cancellation of error from the use of food tables. Models and photographs may incur less error in the estimation of portion weights, at least when compared with estimations from household meas-ures and dimensions.

30.4.2 Daily variation

Individuals do not consume the same food from day to day and substantial error is introduced when diet is assessed from a single day's dietary investigation in records or 24-hour recalls. Thus, daily variation is one of the main factors in reducing precision of individual estimates in either of these methods of assessing diet. The variability from day to day is closely related to the nutrient under study. The early descriptions of record techniques specified that subjects should be observed for 7 days, and this practice has been followed for over 60 years. Nevertheless, when only the average intake of a group of individuals is required for cross-sectional studies, it is difficult to justify gathering this amount of data, even for the more variable nutrients such as cholesterol or polyunsaturated fatty acids. A 1-day record or 24-hour recall collected from a large number of subjects may suffice for the assessment of group means, although it is generally more useful to undertake the assessment on at least 2 days in order to be able to estimate the within-subject component error.

Seven days is generally accepted as the minimum length of time required to gain precision in observations on each individual, although shorter periods of time with correction for the within-subject component error are under investigation. The actual number of records required to classify individuals in any specific population according to quantiles of nutrient intake will depend on the ratio of the average within-person daily variation and the between-person variation. Thus, whereas a 7-day record is probably sufficient to classify into thirds of the distribution for energy and energy-yielding nutrients, longer periods are necessary for items such as some vitamins and minerals and cholesterol.

30.4.3 Frequency of food consumption

Overestimation, compared with records of food consumption, particularly of vegetables but also of energy and energy-yielding nutrients, is a usual finding with FFQs. The cause of this is uncertain, but may result from the use of lists. Restriction of the choice of food into a comparatively short list of around 150 foods or fewer, means that error associated with estimation of amounts of single items is more likely to be biased than when the full variety of foods is analysed, as occurs, for example, in a 24-hour recall or record of food consumption. Participants using the FFQ may also have difficulty in choosing the correct category of how often food is consumed, so that overestimation occurs of the number of times foods are eaten over a defined period of time. FFQs routinely overestimate intake of fruits and vegetables.

30.4.4 Under-reporting

The term 'under-reporting' particularly applies to methods that attempt to assess total energy intake. This problem has been demonstrated by comparing the group average intake of energy from diet assessment methods with group energy expenditure estimated from body weight, or, more accurately, the doubly labelled water technique (see Section 30.5). Under-reporting has been documented with all methods of dietary assessment, including 24-hour recalls, weighed records, diet histories, and FFQs designed to assess total diet. Overweight individuals in particular are likely to under-report the amount they eat. Table 30.1 is an example showing that some but not all nutrients and foods are under-reported: protein, sugars, and fat, and foods such as cakes and sweets, tend to be under-reported but nutrients such as carotene, nonstarch polysaccharides and vitamin C, and vegetables are not.

The problem of under-reporting is particularly difficult when mean intakes are to be compared with reference nutrient intakes for surveillance and clinical work, or amounts of nutrients eaten by a different population or group (such as obese compared with lean individuals). Cut-offs based on estimated energy expenditure calculated from body weight have been devised, but they are imprecise when used in the absence of information on energy expenditure. Ideally, all dietary studies should include independent measures of validity (see Section 31.6 and Black, 2000).

30.4.5 Energy adjustment

Energy adjustment can be carried out by a variety of methods, including expressing results for

Table 30.1 Intakes of energy and macronutrients expressed as reported and after energy adjustment in individuals who under-reported dietary intake and those who did not, as judged by the urine to dietary nitrogen ratio

Nutrient	Valid records $n = 126$ (mean ± SE)	Under-reporters $n = 33$ (mean ± SE)	P-value
Reported intakes			
MJ	8.14 ± 0.04	6.65 ± 0.23	<0.001
Protein (g)	71 ± 0.2	60 ± 1.7	<0.001
Fat (g)	80 ± 0.3	62 ± 2.5	<0.001
Carbohydrate (g)	231 ± 4.3	191 ± 8.2	<0.001
Energy adjusted intakes			
Protein (g)	69 ± 0.8	67 ± 1.4	>0.05
Fat (g)	77 ± 0.9	75 ± 0.9	>0.05
Carbohydrate (g)	223 ± 2.7	225 ± 4.0	>0.05

nutrients as a percentage of the total energy, or using regression techniques (Willett, 1997). One reason for attempting to correct for energy intake in dietary assessments is to reduce extraneous variation from the general correlation of nutrients with total energy intake, brought about by differences in body size and hence (in sedentary populations) energy expenditure. In addition, the correlation between results from one method and another is sometimes improved by energy adjustment. Furthermore, although there are significant differences in absolute macronutrient intake between individuals who give valid records and those who do not, these differences are substantially reduced after energy adjustment, although the overall mean within a population is not altered. Table 30.1 shows reported and energy-adjusted intakes of fat, carbohydrate, and protein in a group of women. Differences between under-reporters and those who gave valid records were no longer significant after energy adjustment.

The effect of energy adjustment depends on the correlation between the nutrient concerned and energy intake, and also on the correlation between the errors of measurement for these two quantities.

The latter is heavily dependent on the dietary method used. Hence, the relation between nutrient intakes derived from FFQs and weighed records can be much improved by energy adjustment, but to a lesser extent between nutrient intakes derived from weighed records and 24-hour recalls. Energy adjustment is inappropriate (and without effect) if there are zero correlations between energy intake and the nutrient concerned, for example in the case of some vitamins. More details of techniques for energy adjustment are given in Willett (1997).

30.4.6 Effects of measurement error

Measurement error is a serious problem in dietary assessment. The effect of measurement error may be to introduce bias, so that, for example, group mean intakes may be over- or underestimated when population intakes are investigated for comparison against recommended levels (see Section 30.4.4). In epidemiological research, individuals may be misclassified in the distribution of nutritional intakes so that a null or attenuated relationship may be obtained and the true effect between diet and disease missed. For example, in a prospective study relating diet to breast cancer risk, diet was assessed using both a FFQ and a detailed 7-day diary of food and drink in 13 070 women in 1993–97. By 2002, there were 168 incident breast cancer cases for analysis. When their baseline dietary intake was compared with matched controls (four for each of the breast cancer cases), the hazard ratio for breast cancer for each quintile increase of energy-adjusted fat was strongly associated with saturated fat intake measured using the food diary (1.219 (95% CI 1.061–1.401), $P = 0.005$). However, with saturated fat measured using the FFQ, the comparable ratio was 1.100 (0.941–1.285, $P = 0.229$) (Bingham et al., 2003).

Different methods of dietary assessment have different types of error structure, so that the magnitude of the error varies according to the method and may not always be predictable in different populations. In large prospective epidemiological studies, it is now common practice to correct for measurement error in the assessment of relative risk by regression calibration when the correction factors are derived by comparison of the method in use, such as a FFQ, with a 'reference' method, such as a record. This 'relative validation' relies on the assumptions that errors in the reference instrument are not correlated

with both 'true' intake and errors in the method in use. However, errors associated with the method under investigation may be correlated with those of the reference method, so that correction for regression dilution is substantially underestimated (Day et al., 2001; Schatzkin et al., 2003). For example, an individual who under-reports using one dietary assessment method such as a food record will also do so with another, such as a FFQ. The validity of dietary assessment methods for determining intake of 15 priority micronutrients and n-3 fatty acids has recently been reviewed by the EURopean micronutrient RECommendations Aligned Network of Excellence (EURRECA) (Willett, 2009). The conclusion of this substantial report generally supports the view that in epidemiological studies, FFQs provide reasonable estimates of intake when their preference is compared with a presumed superior method or biomarker. Most correlations were regarded as being in the acceptable to good range ($r = 0.30$–0.70). Whether such correlations are acceptable and whether it is appropriate to compare one dietary intake method with another will continue to be debated. It is generally accepted that wherever possible and appropriate, biomarkers rather than 'relative validation studies' should be used to validate methods for assessing dietary intake.

30.5 Biomarkers

True estimates of food consumption can only be obtained by actually observing the activities of participants, or by developing some other independent way of assessing food intake. This has become possible with the advent of biological markers in biological specimens, such as blood, urine, or hair, that reflect intake sufficiently closely to act as objective indices of true intake (Bingham, 2002).

30.5.1 Types of biomarkers

There are four main classes of biomarkers used for assessment of the accuracy of dietary methods (Bingham, 2002). The most important are recovery

biomarkers. These biomarkers have been tested under controlled conditions, usually in a metabolic suite, and have been shown to reflect an individual's intake of energy or of a particular nutrient with a high degree of accuracy. Thus, they provide a true gold standard against which another method of dietary assessment may be compared. Few such biomarkers of dietary intake have been identified; they include doubly labelled water as a measure of energy intake, used for example in the OPEN study (Schatzkin et al., 2003) and markers of potassium and nitrogen in 24-hour urine collections (Bingham et al., 1995; Bingham, 2002). A recent new category has been the predictive biomarker of 24-hour urinary sucrose and fructose, which is closely correlated with intake of sugars, despite the very small fraction of intake that is present in urine collections (Tasevska *et al.*, 2005).

Several *concentration biomarkers* (including serum levels of some vitamins such as vitamin C and carotenoids) are available to compare with estimates of dietary intake. Concentration biomarkers cannot be related directly to absolute levels of intake but concentrations do correlate with intakes of corresponding foods or nutrients, although correlation coefficients are much lower (usually equal to less than 0.6) than that expected for recovery biomarkers. Results from a dietary intake method that agreed most closely with these biomarkers would be expected to yield more reliable estimates of intake than one that did not. Finally, *replacement biomarkers* may be used if databases of food composition for certain items are not available or considered to be inaccurate, for example iodine, aflatoxins, and phyto-oestrogens. As it is not usually possible to measure added salt or salt used in cooking, and as a consequence salt intake cannot be measured by dietary methods, 24-hour urine sodium is also an example of a replacement biomarker.

30.5.2 Validation of dietary methods with biomarkers

Biomarkers have been used to validate methods used for dietary assessments in both large-scale epidemiological studies designed to establish the nutritional aetiology of non-communicable diseases and in national nutrition surveys intended to evaluate population nutrient intakes. For example, in the UK National Diet and Nutrition Survey, pilot studies were carried out before the main survey in order to compare intakes of energy from the dietary assessment method and energy expenditure from doubly labelled water (see http://www.ons.gov.uk/ons/search/index.html?pageSize=50&newquery=enery+expenditure+and+doubly+labelled+water). In the USA, doubly labelled water has been used to assess 24-hour recalls and FFQ methods used in epidemiological studies (Schatzkin *et al.*, 2003). To assess the validity of several different methods of dietary assessment in UK cohorts of the EPIC study, 160 women were asked to complete 16 days of weighed-food records over 1 year, as four repeated 4-day records. The volunteers were also asked to provide eight 24-hour urine collections, as four repeated 2-day collections, and completeness of the urine collections was assessed using a specially developed marker. Correlations were greater between the biomarker 24-hour urine nitrogen and estimates of nitrogen intake from records ($r = 0.7$) than from estimates of intake from other methods, including FFQs ($r = 0.4$). A similar pattern was evident with the urinary potassium biomarker (Bingham *et al.*, 1995). This study showed that the 7-day food diary was associated with less measurement error and, consequently, estimates of diet from the 7-day food diary as well as a FFQ were obtained in the full cohort of 25 000 people in EPIC Norfolk (Black, 2000; Bingham *et al.*, 2001).

30.5.3 Calibration

Another way to reduce measurement error is to increase the heterogeneity of the population and pool results from different populations with diverse dietary practices so that it becomes easier to correctly classify intake of individuals in the distribution of food and nutrient intake. This was the approach adopted in the largest epidemiological study of diet, cancer, genetic factors, and health in the European Prospective Investigation of Cancer (EPIC). However, as diet was measured by country-specific questionnaires designed to capture local dietary habits and to provide high compliance, it was also necessary to calibrate results. A second dietary measurement was taken from an 8% random sample (36 000 individuals) of the cohort using a computerized, 24-hour diet recall method (EPIC SOFT) in order to calibrate the questionnaires. A total of 1103 volunteers of both genders from 12 centres also provided complete 24-hour urines for biomarker analysis, and the high, sex-partial Spearman correlation of 0.72 between mean urinary and dietary nitrogen suggests that confidence can be placed in the validity of the calibration method used. When dietary intake was related to disease risk, calibration of the main method against the more detailed method strengthened associations considerably. Examples of the effect of calibration include the reduced risk of colorectal cancer associated with dietary fibre consumption and increased risk associated with red and processed meat consumption (Bingham and Riboli, 2004; Norat et al., 2005).

Conclusion

Dietary assessment methods have enabled nutritional surveillance, facilitated clinical management of patients, and demonstrated powerful and sometimes causal associations between diet and disease which have led to nutrition recommendations with important public health implications. However, the limitations of the methods have not always been appreciated.

Many lessons about the ability to obtain accurate data have been learnt from incorporating appropriate statistical, biomarker, and epidemiological techniques into nutritional assessment. Use of biomarkers has shown that substantial attenuation of diet effects and loss of statistical power can

occur in epidemiological studies in homogeneous populations when relatively inaccurate methods of dietary assessment are used. There has even been a suggestion that FFQs should be abandoned in large epidemiological studies (Kristal et al., 2005). Attenuation and loss of power, together with genetic variation in response, could account for the inability of existing studies to show causal links between diet and chronic disease. Caution in the interpretation of null results from the epidemiological literature should be exercised. Failure to do so may account for some of the potentially misleading interpretation of the findings from cohort studies suggesting that saturated fatty acids may not be strongly related to coronary heart disease, as was previously believed to be the case. (Siri-Tarino et al., 2010). This may also be the case in other types of research and in clinical studies. Some of this measurement error can be overcome by studying populations whose dietary habits are more heterogeneous than single populations, but biomarker studies suggest that improved, more detailed, and novel methods of dietary assessment will be necessary if further causal associations between diet and disease are to be established with any degree of certainty in future investigations.

Further Reading

1. **Bingham, S.A.** (1987) The dietary assessment of individuals: Methods, accuracy, new techniques and recommendations. *Nutr Abstracts Rev*, **57**, 705–42.
2. **Bingham, S.A.** (2002) Biomarkers in nutritional epidemiology: Key note lecture. *Publ Hlth Nutr*, **5**, 821–8.
3. **Bingham, S. and Riboli, E.** (2004) Is diet important in cancer pathogenesis? The European Prospective Investigation of Cancer (EPIC). *Nat Rev Canc*, **4**, 206–15.
4. **Bingham, S.A., Gill, C., Welch, A. et al.** (1994) Comparison of dietary assessment methods in nutritional epidemiology. *Br J Nutr*, **72**, 619–42.
5. **Bingham, S.A., Cassidy, A., Cole, T., et al.** (1995) Validation of weighed records and other methods of dietary assessment using the 24-hour urine nitrogen technique and other biological markers. *Br J Nutr*, **73**, 531–50.
6. **Bingham, S.A., Welch, A., McTaggart, A., et al.** (2001) Nutritional methods in the European Prospective Investigation of Cancer in Norfolk. *Publ Hlth Nutr*, **4**, 847–58.
7. **Bingham, S.A., Luben, R., Welch, A., et al.** (2003) Fat and breast cancer: Are imprecise methods obscuring a relationship? Report from the EPIC Norfolk prospective cohort study. *Lancet*, **362**, 212–14.

8. **Black, A.E.** (2000) The sensitivity and specificity of the Goldberg cut-off for EI: BMR for identifying diet reports of poor validity. *Eur J Clin Nutr*, **54**, 395–404.

9. **Day, N.E., McKeown, N., Wong, M.Y.,** *et al.* (2001) Epidemiological assessment of diet: A comparison of a 7-day diary with a food frequency questionnaire using urinary markers of nitrogen, potassium and sodium. *Int J Epidemiol*, **30**, 309–17.

10. **Friedenreich, C.M., Slimani, N., and Riboli, E.** (1992) Measurement of past diet: Review of previous and proposed methods. *Epidemiol Rev*, **14**, 177–96.

11. **Gibson, R.S.** (2005) *Principles of nutritional assessment*, 2nd edition. New York, Oxford University Press.

12. **Kristal, A.R., Peters, U., and Potter, J.D.** (2005) Is it time to abandon the food frequency questionnaire? *Cancer Epidemiol Biomarkers Prev*, **14**, 2826–8.

13. **Lillegaard, I.T. and Andersen, L.F.** (2005) Validation of a pre-coded food diary with energy expenditure, comparison of under-reporters versus acceptable reporters. *Br J Nutr*, **94**, 998–1003.

14. **Margetts, B.M. and Nelson, M.** (1997) *Design concepts in nutritional epidemiology*, 2nd edition. Oxford, Oxford Medical Publications.

15. **Norat, T., Bingham, S., Ferrari, P.,** *et al.* (2005) Meat, fish, and colorectal cancer risk: The European Prospective Investigation into Cancer and Nutrition. *J Natl Canc Inst*, **97**, 906–16.

16. **Robertson, C., Best, N., Diamond, J., and Elliott, P.** (2004) Tracing ingestion of 'novel' foods in UK diets for possible health surveillance—a feasibility study. *Publ Hlth Nutr*, **7**, 345–52.

17. **Schatzkin, A., Kipnis, V., Carroll, R.J.,** *et al.* (2003) A comparison of a food frequency questionnaire with a 24-hour recall for use in an epidemiological cohort study: Results from the biomarker-based OPEN study. *Int J Epidemiol*, **32**, 1054–62.

18. **Siri-Tarino, P.W., Sun, Q., Hu, F.B.,** *et al.* (2010) Meta-analysis of prospective cohort studies evaluating the association of saturated fat with cardiovascular disease. *Am J Clin Nutr.* **91**, 535–46.

19. **Tasevska, N., Runswick, S.A., McTaggart, A.,** *et al.* (2005) Urinary sugars as biomarkers for sugars consumption. *Canc Epidemiol Biomarkers Prevent*, **14**, 1287–94.

20. **Willett, W.** (1997) *Nutritional epidemiology*, 2nd edition. New York, Oxford University Press.

21. **Willett, W.** (2009) Foreword. The validity of dietary assessment methods for use in epidemiological studies. *BMJ*, **102** (Suppl 1), S1–2.

Useful Websites

To see topical and scientifically robust updates on nutrition associated with this textbook and web links to many of the journals in the Further Reading sections, please see the dedicated Online Resource Centre at **http://www.oxfordtextbooks.co.uk/orc/mann4e/**

http://www.cdc.gov/nchs/nhanes.htm
http://www.ons.gov.uk/ons/search/index.html?pageSize=50&newquery=energy+
expenditure+and+doubly+labelled+water
http://faostat.fao.org/
http://www.srl.cam.ac.uk/epic/nutmethod/
http://www.defra.gov.uk/statistics/foodfarm/food/familyfood/nationalfoodsurvey/

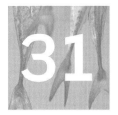

31 Assessment of nutritional status and biomarkers

Stewart Truswell

31.1 Nutritional status versus dietary intake

Dietary intake estimation, described in the preceding chapter, cannot always prove that an individual or community is well nourished or poorly nourished—or overnourished. This has to be confirmed or established by one or more methods of examination.

Food intake can be distorted by intrusion of investigators; intake over a day or a few days may not represent intake over time. It is difficult to relate mixed dishes to lines in the food tables. Nutrients in food tables are only averages, often from another country and an earlier time. Not all nutrients are in the food tables. Nutrient reference intakes (recommended dietary intakes) may not be enough for everyone, especially if they have an illness. Then is an intake below the recommended dietary intake serious or covered by safety factors? Health professionals cannot rely on the history of quantity and type of food when assessing a patient's state of nourishment. You cannot diagnose obesity, overnutrition, from someone's dietary history, and undernourished people may not be able to tell you what they have and have not eaten for a variety of reasons.

Food intake measurement—really estimation—is ultimately *subjective*. It depends on the memory, cooperation, and honesty of individuals. Assessment of nutritional status is, by contrast, ultimately *objective*. A person's weight, height, and chemical concentration in blood or urine is measured by an outside observer and if a second and third observer repeats the measurement, they should obtain about the same result.

BOX 31.1 Nutritional status

Nutritional status is a multidimensional concept, a jargon term used by nutrition professionals. It ultimately means whether a person has functioning in their body enough, but not too much of all the nutrients, from calories down to the micronutrients. Nutritional status can be obvious, with wasting or obesity or only discovered with high technology chemical methods on samples of body fluids or a biopsy. Different aspects of nutritional status are the focus for hospital dietitians and clinicians, for public health workers and epidemiologists, and for nutrition researchers.

31.2 Uses of nutritional assessment

31.2.1 Evolution of assessment methods: looking for malnutrition

The scientific methods of assessing nutritional status were put together after World War II when there was widespread malnutrition across Europe. They were used to detect people who were poorly nourished. Nutrition surveys were done in communities considered at risk by nutrition specialists from Britain and North America.

In the 1950s, these methods were applied in the rest of the world, especially in less-developed countries (where kwashiorkor (Chapter 19) was rediscovered in 1952). The US Interdepartmental Committee for Nutrition in National Defense carried out surveys of military personnel and civilians between 1956 and 1967 in 26 countries that had alliances with the USA, each as a separate operation with its own report. The standardized methods for the nutritional surveys (national food supply, sampling, clinical examination, biochemical studies, and dietary data) were published in a manual in 1963. This enabled investigators to compare results between communities, to plan applied nutrition programmes, and to advise on national food and nutrition policy.

In the same year, the World Health Organization (WHO) Expert Committee on Medical Assessment of Nutritional Status commissioned Derek Jelliffe to prepare a standard guide for nutrition surveys everywhere in the world. He consulted 25 top nutrition experts in various countries and wrote a WHO monograph, *The assessment of the nutritional status of the community (with special reference to field surveys in developing regions of the world)* in 1966. This classic of nutrition literature is the foundation of examining people systematically to see whether they are malnourished.

Since the 1960s, the biggest change is that most of the 50 clinical signs of malnutrition in Jelliffe's book are little used today. They are rare in industrial countries, require experienced medical personnel to diagnose, and many have other causes as well as

malnutrition. Pallor (anaemia), oedema, sore lips, inflamed tongue, and enlarged liver can all be due to poor nutrition, but other causes are more common in most countries. A small number of clinical signs are important in nutrition work but it depends where you are. Hair changes of kwashiorkor in a toddler suggest protein deficiency in deprived parts of Africa but not in the developed world. Bitôt's spots or the skin changes of pellagra are reliable signs of vitamin A deficiency or niacin deficiency, respectively, in places where these deficiencies are known to occur and when observed by an experienced clinician. Thyroid enlargement in teenagers (likely to be endemic goitre from iodine deficiency) and mottled teeth (likely to indicate mild excess of fluoride in early life) are reliable signs of nutritional status and so are some of the signs of rickets (enlarged radial epiphysis, beading of costochondral junction).

The two main types of methods used today for nutritional assessment are anthropometry, measuring weights and heights and other body measurements, and biochemical tests, usually on blood, sometimes on urine. These are described in detail in Sections 31.3 and 31.6. Professional staff have to be trained and paid to do accurate anthropometry and each particular biochemical measurement has a cost, so nutritional assessments can only be done where there is sufficient funding.

31.2.2 Parenteral and enteral nutrition (see Chapter 42)

Modern formulae for total parenteral nutrition, including balanced amino acids and safe intravenous lipid preparation, have been available and approved since 1977. Special nutrition support teams have been set up in major hospitals and there are international societies for the nutritional speciality of enteral and parenteral nutrition (ASPEN in America, ESPEN in Europe). For assessing and monitoring hospital patients' nutritional status, clinical teams use selections from the general methods for nutritional assessment. Rapid biochemical tests are available for monitoring, but critically ill patients lying in bed with lines and tubes attached cannot be weighed so other anthropometric measurements have to be used. Chapter 42 discusses nutritional support for the hospitalized patient in more detail.

31.2.3 Overnutrition

With the increase of overweight and obesity in the last decade, there has naturally been a focus on reliable and accessible indicators of the amount and effects of a person's excess accumulated calories. The two established simple anthropometric measures are: (1) body mass index (BMI), where:

BMI = weight/height^2 (see Section 31.3.3)

where weight is in kg and height is in metres; and (2) waist circumference (either alone or expressed against hip circumference). Reference numbers have been derived for different ages and nations for BMI and for men and women (for the waist measurement). Along with these physical measurements,

biochemical tests can indicate if overweight is accompanied by metabolic abnormalities. The most usual are plasma low-density and high-density lipoprotein cholesterol, fasting triglycerides, and fasting or postprandial glucose.

31.2.4 Biomarkers to check, support, or replace some food intake estimates

Some biochemical tests are increasingly being used for this purpose in human nutrition experiments and epidemiological studies. Not many are suitable, but four good examples are:

- for checking protein intake (and hence roughly energy intake)—24-hour urinary nitrogen;
- to support change of type of fat—plasma fatty acid pattern, especially 18:2 ω-6;
- more reliable than estimating salt intake—24-hour urinary sodium;
- the only way to gauge iodine intake (because it varies greatly among foods)—urinary iodine.

31.3 Anthropometric assessment

The basic anthropometric measurements are simple, straightforward, inexpensive, and safe and anyone can do them. For research purposes, weight and height are measured more precisely and for clinical work some other measurements are made.

31.3.1 Body mass (body weight)

In affluent communities, most people know their body weight and many weigh themselves regularly on an electronic bathroom scale. These are not as accurate as health professionals require in a clinic or consulting room. The best weighing machines are beam balances with non-detachable weights

(Fig. 31.1), but these are bulky and difficult to move. They should stand on a level, hard surface and be checked with a known weight regularly. People should be weighed to the nearest 0.1 kg, wearing minimal clothing. If changes in body weight are being followed, the measurement should if possible be made at the same time of day because meals, drink, a full bladder, and bowel action can all affect the reading. When people in a steady state are weighed repeatedly, the day-to-day fluctuation can be ±1.0 kg.

Nutritionists are very interested in the measurement of body weight and its interpretation, whether someone is overweight or underweight, and whether their weight is increasing or going down. They want as well to estimate what components

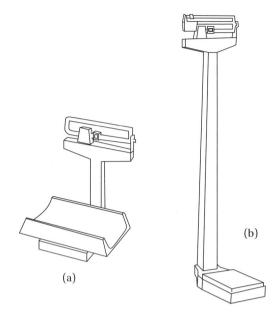

Fig. 31.1 Measurement of weight. (a) Paediatric scale for infants, and (b) beam balance for a child or adult.

Source: Gibson, R.S. (2005) *Principles of nutritional assessment*, 2nd edition. Oxford, Oxford University Press.

average person is fat and the rest is fat-free mass. Women have more fat and less muscle than men. Of the fat-free mass, part is muscle (about 40% of total body weight), part is bones, and the rest is all the other organs, in descending order of weight, skin, blood, gut, liver, brain, lungs, heart, and so on. Chemically, the largest component is water, then there are about equal amounts of protein and fat (each around 20%) and the rest is bone mineral. In adults, weight gain is nearly all fat; weight loss from negative energy balance is of fat, but some fat-free mass, i.e. protein is lost as well.

When total body mass has been measured, we need to judge whether it is in the healthy range or whether he/she is too thin or too fat. First, an adjustment has to be made for size. A lean giant must weigh more than a dwarf. Weight has to be considered in terms of height (or stature). Different indices have been proposed and tested. Of all the possibilities, weight/height^2 has been found the most generally useful (Cole, 1991) as a direct measure of over- or underweight. It only requires two measurements, weight and height, and a simple calculation. This BMI is expressed in kg (for weight) and metres (for height), i.e. in SI units. Quite different numbers would be obtained if height were in centimetres. The Belgian mathematician Quetelet first recommended this index.

inside the body make up the weight and the change in weight.

Fig. 31.2 shows the different compartments in an average, healthy weight adult. About 20% of this

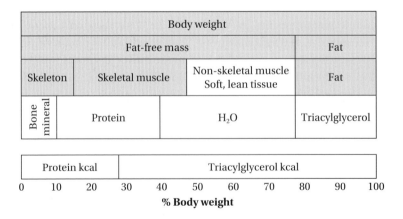

Fig. 31.2 Compartments of the body. Relationship between anthropometry (shaded), body composition, and energy reserves.

Source: Heymsfield, S.B. (1984) Anthropometric assessment of adult protein-energy malnutrition. In: Wright, R.A., Heymsfield, S.B., and McManus, C.B. (eds) *Nutritional assessment*. Boston, Blackwell Scientific.

31.3.2 Measurement of height (stature)

Height is more difficult to measure than weight. Consequently, people's heights are seldom measured and often not accurately remembered. For adults and children, a level floor and straight wall are needed (Fig. 31.3). The subject has to stand straight with buttocks, shoulders, and back of the head touching the wall, with heels flat and together, shoulders relaxed, and arms hanging down. The head should be erect and look straight forward, the lower border of the orbit in line with the external auditory meatus (the Frankfurt plane). The headpiece (a metal bar or wooden block) is lowered gently, pressing down the hair. Ideally, this headpiece should be on a sliding scale but if a loose object is used, such as a firm book, this must be kept horizontal. In practice, two people can better manage an accurate reading. For research work, a specially designed stadiometer can be obtained. There is a circadian variation in height. People are taller in the morning by 1–2 cm. Then, during the day, the intervertebral discs get somewhat compressed.

For very young children that cannot yet stand properly, their length is best measured lying supine on a specially designed measuring board. Two examiners are needed to position the infant correctly and comfortably.

For adults who are deformed (e.g. with scoliosis) or bedridden, estimates of what their height would be if they could stand straight can be made from *knee height* or *arm span* (right fingertips outstretched to tips of left fingers) or *demispan* (from sternal notch to webspace between middle and ring fingers). These measurements are used in geriatrics. Equations to give estimated height differ for gender and ethnic group.

31.3.3 Interpretation of body mass index

WHO and government health departments of the major countries have all adopted BMI as the

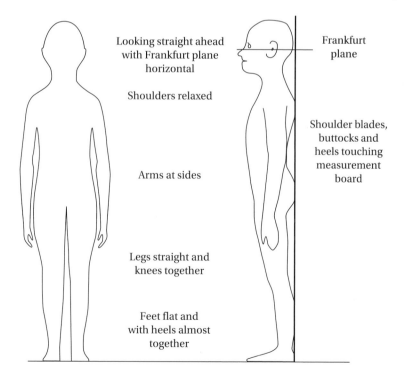

Fig. 31.3 Positioning of person for height measurement.

Source: Gibson, R.S. (2005) *Principles of nutritional assessment.* Oxford, Oxford University Press.

standard way of diagnosing overweight and obesity. With the same cut-offs for men and women, this is much simpler than the earlier tables of desirable weights for height, with different numbers for frame size and for gender. For those who are put off by, say,

$$65 \text{ (kg)} \div (1.73 \times 1.73 \text{ (metres)}) \to 21.67 \text{ kg/m}^2$$

graphs like Fig. 31.4 are available.

Increased BMI indicates increased adiposity, but the correlation is not, of course, 100%. People with broad frame and weight lifters (with big muscles) can have a high BMI for their present body fat. In older people (see Chapter 35), muscle bulk declines and percentage of body fat increases. As BMI increases above 25 kg/m², mortality increases gently at first and then (above BMI 30 kg/m²) more steeply (Fig. 31.5).

WHO classifies adults according to BMI:

- Underweight = <18.50 kg/m²
- Normal range = 18.5–24.99 kg/m²
- Overweight = 25.00–29.99 kg/m²

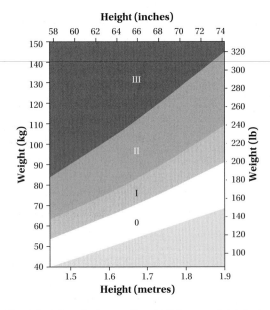

Fig. 31.4 Graph for reading BMI from weight (in kg or lb) and height (in metres or inches). Obesity grades I, II, and III have a BMI (kg/m²) of 25–29.9, 30–40, and over 40, respectively.

Source: Garrow, J.S. (1981) *Treat obesity seriously.* Edinburgh, Churchill Livingstone.

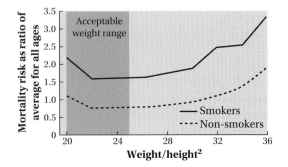

Fig. 31.5 Variations in mortality by body mass index (BMI) among 750 000 US men and women.

Source: Lew, E.A. and Garfinkel, L. (1979) Variations in mortality by weight among 750,000 men and women. *J Chron Dis*, **32**, 563–7.

- Obese = >30.00 kg/m²
- Severely obese = >35.00 kg/m²
- Very severely obese = >40.00 kg/m².

The value of these BMI levels probably has to be adjusted for ethnic groups because of differences in body composition and proportions. At a given BMI, South Asians and Indonesians have relatively more body fat, while Polynesians tend to have more muscle.

Assessing adult undernutrition, below a BMI of 18.5 kg/m², Ferro Luzzi *et al.* (1992) suggest that severity of chronic energy deficiency is moderate down to 17.0 kg/m², severe down to 16.0 kg/m², and very severe below this.

In children, the BMI that corresponds to start of overweight in adults (i.e. 25 kg/m²) is lower. From surveys in different countries, Cole *et al.* (2000) estimate it should be 17.3 kg/m² at age 5, 19.9 kg/m² at age 10, and 23.6 kg/m² at age 15.

31.3.4 Waist circumference

The metabolic complications of overweight and obesity (see Chapter 17) have been found to be more likely if some of the adipose tissue is specially concentrated inside the abdomen (in the omentum, mesentery, etc.). This abdominal or visceral obesity can be estimated with a simple tape measure around the waist. Waist circumference correlates quite closely with BMI. Some authorities prefer measurement of the waist/hip ratio to allow for people with a heavy frame, but it is more complicated to do and does not seem to have better predictive value.

Table 31.1 gives the WHO recommendations for Caucasians. The identification of risk using waist circumference is population-specific and depends on the levels of obesity and other risk factors for cardiovascular diseases and diabetes in the ethnic group.

31.3.5 Measuring children's growth

The primary index of growth, used universally, is *weight for age*. At any particular age, the infant's or the child's weight (unclothed) is compared against a reference, a sort of standard to see if its weight is at, below, or above the average. If it is far off the average, percentile lines on the reference graph will show how it compares with the reference population.

The most used weight-for-age set for older children is probably the US Centers for Disease Control and Prevention growth reference. Graphs for boys and girls aged 2–20 years are reproduced in Chapter 34.

For boys and girls from birth to 5 years there is a new WHO child growth standard (WHO, 2006). Infants are weighed more frequently, so a broader horizontal scale is needed; infants' stature is measured lying down and length is 1.0–2.0 cm longer than height. The reference subjects were healthy and included all ethnic groups, excluding those who had very low birth weights.

In Britain, the current weight-for-age reference (Freeman *et al.*, 1995) is based on measurements of 25 000 white children between 1978 and 1990. These references replace earlier standards because more infants are now breast-fed and children have fewer infections and grow taller.

In weight-for-age graphs, the average is the 50th percentile, i.e. median of the reference sample. An individual's difference up or down from this median can be read firstly from the *percentile lines*. A second way used for distance from the median is the *standard deviation* or *Z-score* above or below the median. One SD below the median is a Z score minus one (–1). A third indicator used for undernutrition is not percentile of the reference children but *percentage of the median*, i.e. of the 50th percentile, the international standard. Below 80% of the median, a child is 'underweight'; this weight is near the 3rd percentile line and near a Z-score of –2. A child under 60% of the median is seriously underweight and has marasmus.

In developing countries, a simplified version of the weight-for-age graph; a 'Road to Health' card, can be kept by the mother for her child and brought back to the clinic on each visit (see Chapter 19).

There is little difference in weight for age of modern children of the privileged class between different countries and ethnic groups. The reference data can thus be used internationally. If a child is somewhat heavy for age (say 80th percentile) or light (say 20th percentile), this does not mean overnutrition or undernutrition. The child may be larger (taller) or smaller (shorter) than average. The weight has to be judged against the height (or length).

Length-for-age (for infants) and *stature-for-age* references will show if a child's longitudinal growth is taller or average, or shorter than the reference population. In developing countries, *stunting* is an important measure of poor nutrition and/or other adverse environment. It is usually defined as 2 standard deviations below the international median reference height for age, i.e. a Z-score of –2.

Excessive thinness or *wasting* is recognized anthropometrically from *weight-for-height* of 2 standard

Table 31.1 WHO recommendations for Caucasians		
Risk of metabolic complications	Waist circumference (cm)	
	Men	Women
Increased	≥94	≥80
Severely increased	≥102	≥88

deviations below the median for age, i.e. a Z-score of −2.

Prevalence of wasting, stunting, and underweight (as defined by WHO) in preschool children in different countries are given in Table 31.2. This shows the value of simple anthropometry in monitoring the nutrition situation in the world's young children.

In adolescence, the growth references have to be used cautiously because there is a growth spurt around the time of puberty followed by slowing of growth, and some girls mature early and some late, with about 5 years between their peaks (see Fig. 34.1). There is the same sort of range in peak height velocity in boys.

Table 31.2 Wasting, stunting and underweight in 0–5-year-old children, 2000–2006 (%)			
	Wasting	Stunting	Underweight
Afghanistan	7	54	39
Bangladesh	13	43	48
Brazil	2	11	6
China	–	11	7
Cuba	2	5	4
Ethiopia	11	47	38
Guatemala	2	49	23
India	20	48	43
Kenya	6	30	20
South Africa	3	25	12
USA	0	1	2

Wasting, <2 SD below international reference median (WHO/NCHS) weight for height.

Stunting, <2 SD below reference median height-for-age.

Underweight, <2 SD below reference median weight-for-age.

Source: UNICEF (2008) *The state of the world's children.* New York, United Nations Children's Fund.

31.4 Estimating body composition: simple methods

The methods available that anyone can do measure body fat or muscle at one or more sites and from these total body fat and/or muscle can be estimated approximately. The following methods are used by clinical nutritionists.

31.4.1 Skinfold thickness

With special precision callipers (Fig. 31.6), a pinch of subcutaneous fat is gently taken up and the width measured. Caught between the jaws of the callipers is a double layer of fat and skin. This fold is measured in mm. Skinfolds could be measured at many sites, but the best established are:

- *triceps skinfold*: over the triceps muscle midway down the back of the upper arm;
- *biceps skinfold*: measured as a vertical fold midway down the front of the upper arm, over the biceps muscle;

(a) (b)

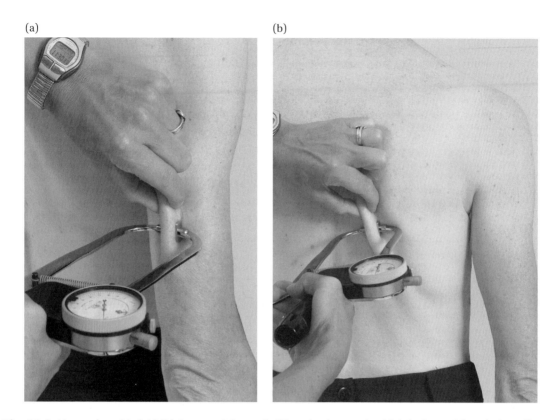

Fig. 31.6 Measuring skinfold thickness—triceps (left) and subscapular (right) sites with Holtain callipers.
Source: Truswell, A.S. (2003) *ABC of nutrition.* London, BMJ Books.

- *subscapular skinfold*: a vertical fold taken just below and lateral to the inferior angle of the scapular, with shoulder and arm relaxed;
- *suprailiac skinfold*: in the mid-axillary line immediately above the iliac crest, grasped obliquely.

The skinfold is first picked up between finger and thumb, clean away from the underlying muscle before closing the callipers on the fold.

Reference tables are published for triceps and subscapular skinfolds (see Gibson, 2005).

The above four skinfold sites are most commonly used partly because they are easily accessible and reference tables are available, partly because they were chosen by Durnin and Womensley (1974), who measured total body fat from body density by underwater weighing in 480 white men and women ranging in age and fatness. They then derived different equations to predict total body fat from the sum of four skinfolds in men and women at different ages. These were all arm or trunk skinfolds but the British Olympic Association recommends that addition of the anterior thigh skinfold improves the estimate of percentage body fat. In very fat people, skinfolds at some trunk sites are not practicable as it is impossible to take up and measure a fold or the fold is too large for the callipers.

31.4.2 Limb circumferences

By simply measuring the circumference of an arm or leg and skinfolds at the same level, it is possible to calculate the circumference or the cross-sectional area of the limb's muscle. An assumption for the area of bone inside the muscle section improves the muscle area for estimating total muscle in the body.

Mid-upper arm is the usual site. The other two sites are mid-thigh and mid-calf. The arm is not always accessible. Heymsfield and Baumgartner (2006) found that the sum of limb muscle area for arm, thigh, and calf predicted quite well the skeletal muscle measured by whole-body magnetic resonance imaging:

$$\text{Limb muscle circumference} = C - \pi \times SF$$

$$\text{Limb muscle area} = \frac{[C - \pi \times SF]^2}{4\pi}$$

where C is a limb circumference (upper arm, thigh, or calf) and SF is the skinfold taken at the same level.

The uncorrected mid-upper arm circumference reflects muscle and fat in the limb and is used for screening preschool children in the field where no weighing scales are available. A tape is used, marked at 12.5 and 13.5 cm. From 12 to 60 months of age, the arm circumference of healthy children, boys and girls, stays the same. A circumference over 13.5 cm is normal, between 12.5 and 13.5 cm suggests mild undernutrition, and under 12.5 cm indicates definite malnutrition.

31.5 High-technology methods for body composition

Total body water by isotope dilution
This method uses a tracer dose of water, labelled with deuterium ^2H, tritium ^3H, or ^{18}O. After time for equilibration, the concentration of the label is measured in serum or urine.

Bone mineral density by DEXA
Dual energy X-ray absorptiometry (DEXA) scanning is usually of the lumbar spine and hip with X-rays at two energies. There is relatively more attenuation of the lower voltage rays by more dense tissue (i.e. bone mineral). Results are related to average bone mineral density for age. All major hospitals have this equipment. DEXA can also be used to quantify fat versus other tissue in regions of the body.

Underwater weighing using Archimedes principle
The subject is weighed in air (i.e. in the usual way) and again when completely submerged in water in a large tank. Body volume is given by the apparent loss of body weight in water (i.e. the difference between weight in air and in water), which corresponds to the displaced water. Weight (in air)/volume gives body density. Knowing that the density of fat is 0.90, the percentage body fat can be calculated. Adjustments have to be made for residual air in the lungs.

Bioelectrical impedance
Relatively inexpensive equipment is used to measure the impedance of an electrical current (typically 800 microamps) passed between an electrode on the right foot and another on the right wrist, where there is a voltage sensor. The fat-free mass is a good conductor of electricity, while fat is not. The voltage drop between foot and wrist is greater in subjects with more fat. A computer calculates fat-free mass and fat when data on weight, height, age, gender, and level of physical activity are entered. A number of factors, including hydration state, meals, and length of limbs affect the reliability of the results.

Total body potassium, by counting ^{40}K
This depends on the fact that 0.012% of potassium everywhere (and in our bodies) is the γ-emitting isotope ^{40}K. The amount of this can be counted in a whole-body counter from which background radiation has been screened with thick steel or lead. Potassium occurs in the body almost exclusively inside the cells so that from total body potassium the body's cell mass can be calculated.

Total body nitrogen by in vitro neutron activation analysis
This is an ingenious method for determining total body nitrogen and hence total protein in the body (N × 6.25). The patient is

'bombarded' while lying on a special table with a low neutron flux from a neutron source (such as californium-252). This converts a proportion of the nitrogen, ^{14}N, to a very short-lived state of ^{15}N, which emits a γ-ray at 10.83 MeV. This is counted with a gamma counter as the neutron source is moved over the subject's body on a motorized bed. The method is very expensive; only a few institutions can use it, and it gives a significant radiation dose.

Ultrasound This is harmless, not expensive, and has some uses, e.g. in quantifying the size of the thyroid gland.

Magnetic resonance imaging and computed tomography These have also been used for some research studies on body composition. Both use very expensive, bulky equipment.

31.6 Biochemical methods

A person may be ill from a qualitatively inadequate diet and yet their body measurements can be within normal limits. The right biochemical test would show the deficiency. Anthropometry mostly reflects undernutrition or overnutrition, too little or too much food energy. Biochemical tests are needed to demonstrate micronutrient status. On the other hand, there is no biochemical test on a body fluid that gives a measure of carbohydrate or total fat intake. Biochemical methods are an essential part of nutritional assessment. There are many more biochemical tests than anthropometric measurements. Each test costs money, for collecting the blood or urine, for the equipment, chemicals, and the skilled laboratory worker's time, and for reporting and interpreting the test. So tests have to be selected, based on the situation and the subject, so that they are likely to yield useful results.

31.6.1 Different situations for laboratory tests

Biochemical methods for nutritional assessment are used for several different purposes:

- to recognize acute malnutrition for which the clinical signs are non-specific, e.g. potassium deficiency;
- to confirm the clinical diagnosis of a deficiency disease, e.g. xerophthalmia, scurvy, beri-beri, rickets, Wernicke's encephalopathy, kwashiorkor;

- for monitoring nutritional management in intensive care, with parenteral nutrition and/or tube feeding;
- in haematological diagnosis, e.g. iron, folate, and vitamin B_{12} estimations;
- in community nutrition surveys, to detect subclinical micronutrient deficiency, e.g. iodine deficiency, iron deficiency;
- for checking validity of food intake measurement: 24-hour urinary nitrogen indicates protein intake in people with stable dietary pattern; carotenoids reflect fruit and vegetable intake;
- for reliability and convenience: biomarkers, for some nutrients, are more reliable and convenient than food intake estimations (e.g. 24-hour urinary sodium is better than trying to work out dietary salt);
- to demonstrate objectively the response to a nutrition education programme, e.g. reduction of plasma cholesterol or of urinary sodium;
- for biochemical confirmation of alcoholism;
- to diagnose nutritional supplement overdosing (e.g. with vitamin A, pyridoxine).

31.6.2 Stages of nutrient deficiency

When absorbed intake of a nutrient is less than the requirement, i.e. less than losses from metabolism and excretion, the depletion goes through four stages:

1 reduced excretion of the nutrient, e.g. reduced urinary excretion, but body pool maintained;

2 body pool smaller but no disturbance of function;

3 biochemical signs of impaired function: reduced activity of an enzyme or cell depletion;

4 morphological changes and clinical signs of deficiency disease.

Obviously, many more people are found at stage 1 than are found with obvious classic deficiency disease. In other words, biochemical tests usually show *subclinical* nutritional deficiency; the subject may or may not be ill and an illness may or may not be due to the nutritional depletion.

31.6.3 Which biochemical tests

The principal biochemical tests for nutritional status are shown in Table 31.3. Most clinical biochemical laboratories are set up for only some of the methods in the table as a routine, but others could be set up in special circumstances, or alternatively a laboratory specializing in nutrition research could be asked. It is usually easy to find methods reflecting recent intake. Good methods for nutritional dysfunction or tissue depletion are not available for all nutrients. To estimate stores of a nutrient, the only method generally available is serum ferritin for iron stores.

31.6.4 Some problems with biochemical tests

Instability of the nutrient in vitro Vitamin C is the outstanding example. Plasma should be acidified with metaphosphoric or trichloracetic acid and analysed the same day or kept for a few days at −80°C.

Chemical specificity of the method Older methods were often not specific for the nutrient, e.g. DCIP or DNPH methods for vitamin C.

Other influences Non-nutritional influences can significantly raise or lower plasma concentrations of most, if not all, nutrients. Plasma albumin goes down (without protein deficiency) with inflammatory disease or trauma. The liver switches to synthesis of 'acute-phase' plasma proteins and albumin may move to the extravascular space.

The relation between intake and plasma concentration This shows important differences among nutrients (Fig. 31.7). Plasma selenium increases in the expected linear fashion but serum calcium is homeostatically maintained the same over the range of usual calcium intakes. Plasma retinol also stays the same over most vitamin A intakes but it does go down at very low intakes, so this test is useful in low-income communities. Vitamin C concentration plateaus at intakes of about 150 mg/day (see Chapter 14), so it is no higher in people who take megadoses than in those who eat a moderate amount of fruit.

Blood and urine tests cannot show calcium status Calcium is not in Table 31.3. To estimate body calcium requires measurements of bone mineral.

Biochemical tests for zinc are also unreliable. Serum zinc is affected by age, gender, acute inflammation, time of day, fasting status, oral contraceptives, storage, haemolysis, zinc contamination of collecting tube, or anticoagulant. It therefore needs careful technique and interpretation.

31.6.5 Methods used

A previous edition of this book contained a table that gave the names of the methods then likely to be used for the different nutrients. However, such methods are constantly evolving, and the three main questions the nutritionist can ask the laboratory are: Is this specific for the nutrient? Is it a standard method? Is the laboratory experienced with using it?

Urine tests These should if possible be made on 24-hour urine collections. This may be inconvenient

Table 31.3 Biochemical methods for diagnosing nutritional deficiencies

Nutrient	Indicating reduced intake	Indicating impaired function (IF) or cell depletion (CD)	Supplementary method
Protein	Urinary nitrogen	Plasma albumin (IF)	Fasting plasma amino acid pattern
Vitamin A	Plasma β-carotene	Plasma retinol	Relative dose–response
Thiamin	Urinary thiamin	Red cell transketolase and TTP effect (IF)	
Riboflavin	Urinary riboflavin	Red cell glutathione reductase and FAD effect (IF)	
Niacin	Urinary N'-methyl nicotinamide or 2-pyridone, or both	Red cell NAD/NADP ratio	Fasting plasma tryptophan
Vitamin B_6	Urinary 4-pyridoxic acid	Plasma pyridoxal 5'-phosphate	Urinary xanthurenic acid after tryptophan load
Folate	Plasma folate	Red cell folate (CD)	
Vitamin B_{12}	Plasma holotranscobalamin II	Plasma vitamin B_{12} Plasma methylmalonate	Schilling test
Vitamin C	Plasma ascorbate	Leukocyte ascorbate (CD)	Urinary ascorbate
Vitamin D	Plasma 25-hydroxy-vitamin D	Raised plasma alkaline phosphatase (bone isoenzyme) (IF)	Plasma 1,25-dihydroxy-vitamin D
Vitamin E	Ratio of plasma tocopherol to cholesterol + triglyceride	Red cell haemolysis with H_2O_2 *in vitro* (IF)	
Vitamin K	Plasma phylloquinone	Plasma prothrombin (IF)	Plasma des-γ-carboxy-prothrombin
Sodium	Urinary sodium	Plasma sodium	
Potassium	Urinary potassium	Plasma potassium	Total body potassium by counting ^{40}K
Iron	Plasma iron and transferrin	Plasma ferritin (CD)	Free erythrocyte protoporphyrin
Magnesium	Plasma magnesium	Red cell magnesium (CD)	
Iodine	Urinary (stable) iodine	Plasma thryroxine (IF)	Plasma TSH
Zinc	Plasma zinc	Red cell zinc	
Selenium	Plasma selenium	Red cell glutathione peroxidase	Toenail selenium
Fluoride	Urinary fluoride	Plasma ionic fluoride	(Bone fluoride)

^{40}K, natural radioactive potassium; FAD, flavin adenine dinucleotide; NAD, nicotinamide adenine dinucleotide; NADP, NAD phosphate; TPP, thiamin pyrophosphate; TSH, thyroid-stimulating hormone.

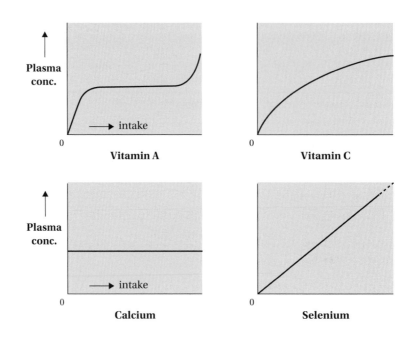

Fig. 31.7 Difference in relation of serum concentrations to intake of four nutrients: vitamin A, vitamin C, calcium, and selenium.

for the subjects; they have to carry a 2-litre bottle with them during the day. As second best, an early morning sample can be collected at home and the nutrient concentration related to the creatinine concentration, because creatinine excretion (in health) is assumed to be more or less constant from day to day. However, within subjects the coefficient of variation of 24-hour creatinine is 10% or more and it is larger between subjects because it depends on muscle mass and is increased after eating meat.

Hair is unreliable Researchers have sent hair samples from the same subjects for trace element analysis to several commercial laboratories and have received widely differing results. It is difficult to remove the many environmental contaminants that adhere to hair and the distribution of inorganics may not be uniform. Hair analysis may have some value in forensic work or detecting toxic exposure to heavy metals, but for nutritional work urine analysis is more reliable.

Further Reading

1. **Cole, T.J.** (1991) Weight-stature indices to measure underweight, overweight and obesity. In: Himes, J.H. (ed.) *Anthropometric assessment of nutritional status.* New York, Wiley-Liss. pp. 83–111.
2. **Cole, T.J., Bellizzi, M.C., Flegal, K.M., and Dietz, W.H.** (2000) Establishing a standard definition for child overweight and obesity worldwide: International survey. *BMJ,* **320,** 1240–3.
3. **Durnin, J.V.G.A. and Womersley, J.** (1974) Body fat assessed from total body density and its estimation from skinfold thickness: Measurements on 481 men and women aged from 16 to 72 years. *Br J Nutr,* **32,** 77–97.
4. **Eston, R.G., Rowlands, A.V., Charlesworth, S., Davies, A., and Hoppitt, T.** (2005) Prediction of DXA-determined whole body fat from skinfolds: Importance of including skinfolds from the thigh and calf in young, healthy men and women. *Eur J Clin Nutr,* **59,** 695–702.

5. **Ferro-Luzzi, A., Sette, S., Franklin, M., and James, W.P.T.** (1992) A simplified approach to assessing adult chronic energy deficiency. *Eur J Clin Nutr*, **46**, 17–86.

6. **Freeman, J.V., Cole, T.J., Chinn, S., Jones, P.R.M., White, E.M., and Preece, M.A.** (1995) Cross sectional stature and weight reference curve for the UK. *Arch Dis Child*, **73**, 17–24.

7. **Garrow, J.S.** (1981) *Treat obesity seriously*. Edinburgh, Churchill Livingstone.

8. **Gibson, R.S.** (2005) *Principles of nutritional assessment*, 2nd edition. Oxford, Oxford University Press.

9. **Heymsfield, S.B.** (1984) Anthropometric assessment of adult protein-energy malnutrition. In: Wright, R.A., Heymsfield, S.B., and McManus, C.B. (eds) *Nutritional assessment*. Boston, Blackwell Scientific.

10. **Heymsfield, S.B. and Baumgartner, R.N.** (2006) Body composition and anthropometry. In: Shils, M.E. (ed.) *Modern nutrition in health and disease*. Philadelphia, Lippincott Williams, and Wilkins. pp. 751–70.

11. **Jelliffe, D.B.** (1966) *The assessment of the nutritional status of the community (with special reference to field surveys in developing regions of the world)*. WHO Monograph Series No. 53. Geneva, World Health Organization.

12. **Kukzmarski, R.J., Ogden, C.L., Grummer-Strawn, L.M., *et al*.** (2000) CDC growth charts: United States. *Adv Data*, **314**, 1–27.

13. **Lew, E.A. and Garfinkel, L.** (1979) Variations in mortality by weight among 750,000 men and women. *J Chron Dis*, **32**, 563–7.

14. **Sauberlich, H.E.** (1999) *Laboratory tests for the assessment of nutritional status*, 2nd edition. Boca Raton, FL, CRC Press.

15. **Steindel, S.J. and Howanitz, P.J.** (2001) The uncertainty of hair analysis for trace metals. *J Am Med Assoc*, **285**, 83–5.

16. **Truswell, A.S.** (2003) *ABC of nutrition*. London, BMJ Books.

17. **UNICEF** (2008) *The State of the World's Children*. New York, United Nations Children's Fund.

18. **WHO** (2000) *Obesity: Preventing and managing the global epidemic*. Report of a consultation. Technical Report Series 894. Geneva, World Health Organization.

19. **WHO** (2006) *WHO Child Growth Standards. Length/height-for-age, weight-for-age, weight-for-length, weight-for-height and body mass index-for-age. Methods and development*. Geneva, World Health Organization.

Useful Websites

To see topical and scientifically robust updates on nutrition associated with this textbook and web links to many of the journals in the Further Reading sections, please see the dedicated Online Resource Centre at **http://www.oxfordtextbooks.co.uk/orc/mann4e/**

Part 6

Life stages

Pre-pregnancy, pregnancy, and lactation

Annie S. Anderson

32.1 Pre-pregnancy

The lifelong nutritional status of a mother, from her own conception and throughout her life to the birth of her baby, will impact on the health and wellbeing of that baby. In addition, the particular importance of the mother's nutrition in the months before conception is now recognized. Here the emphasis is on the achievement of appropriate body weight and optimal nutritional status (and stores) for the months ahead. In addition, pre-pregnancy nutrition takes account of the needs of the very early stages of pregnancy (embryogenesis) when the woman may not be sure she is pregnant.

Maternal nutrition has a profound effect on all aspects of reproduction, including fertility. When energy stores are low, menarche may be delayed, and if energy stores are diminished after menarche, menses are likely to become irregular, infrequent, and possibly stop. Amenorrhoea has been well described in excessive weight loss and in anorexia nervosa. It is estimated that where body fat is less than 22% of body weight, ovulation is unlikely. Healthy, fertile young women have an average body fat proportion of 28%. Menarche can be delayed by athletic training or eating disorders and accelerated by excessive nutrient consumption. It is thought this is due to a requirement for a certain energy store to be present to permit reproduction to occur. In natural settings where energy has been acutely restricted (e.g. due to famine) prior to pregnancy, ovulation is likely to fail.

Obese women are commonly infertile but simple weight reduction of at least 5–10% body weight is thought to bring about return of ovulation, menstruation, and fertility. It is estimated that approximately 30% of sub-fertile couples are overweight or obese. Women with a high body mass index (BMI) also have a lower live birth rate after assisted conception, as well as an increased miscarriage rate.

While there has been considerable speculation about the role of pre-conceptual nutrition and malformation, the only strong evidence relates to the benefit of folic acid supplements in minimizing neural tube defects (NTDs) (spina bifida, anencephaly, and encephalocele). NTDs are the most common congenital malformations of the central nervous system. The highest rates in the Western world are found in Ireland and Scotland (9.9 per 10 000 pregnancies). The neural tube, which will develop into the brain and spinal cord, starts as the neural fold, under the ectoderm along the back of the embryo. Between days 21 and 28 after conception, it closes into a tube, the neural tube. If folate is inadequate, the tube may not close fully and spina bifida may result or the brain may not develop at all. It is thought that NTDs arise from a combination of genetic and environmental components, both of which must be triggered for the defects to occur. An MRC trial demonstrated that a daily 4-mg folic acid supplement given around the time of conception to women at high risk (those who had already had one affected NTD pregnancy) was shown to prevent the disease in most women (MRC Vitamin Study Research Group, 1991). From the MRC trial it was concluded that folic acid should be given to all women with a previous affected pregnancy and that public health measures (e.g. supplement and/or food fortification) should be available to all women of childbearing age. In the UK, folic acid supplements (400 μg/day) are recommended to all women prior to conception so that folate status is adequate during the early embryonic stages. Surveys suggest that about 55% of women do take this action, but as around a half of all pregnancies are unplanned, universal supplementation is unlikely to be achieved. Low pre-conception folic acid use is associated with low levels of formal education, young maternal age, lack of a partner, immigrant status, and unplanned

pregnancy. A higher-dose supplement (5 mg) is recommended for women if they (or their partner) have a neural tube defect, have had a previous baby with a NTD, or have a family history of NTDs or have diabetes.

Mean (± SD) daily intakes of folate in non-pregnant women from dietary sources in the UK is 290 ± 500 μg, which is lower than that provided by supplement use (400 μg) and likely to be insufficient to meet the requirements of women at risk of having an NTD-affected pregnancy. It should be noted that the bioavailability of natural folates found in food is approximately half that of pure folic acid. Some countries (USA and Canada) now have mandatory fortification of key staple foods with folic acid e.g. bread and cereals, and recent data from the USA associates this action with the decreasing spina bifida rates of 14% per year between 1991 and 2002. In other countries, there has been voluntary fortification of some processed foods with folic acid.

32.2 Pregnancy

Pregnancy is a period of rapid growth and development of the fetus, with high physiological, metabolic, and emotional demands on the mother. Adequate nutrition during pregnancy is important to enable the fetus to grow and develop physically and mentally to full potential. It is widely believed that fetal nutrition plays a key role in the wellbeing of the newborn infant and further influences health during childhood and adulthood, with possible effects into the next generation. In addition to fetal nutrient needs, food intake during pregnancy needs to be free from food safety hazards and contribute to the health and wellbeing of the mother. Nutrition during pregnancy is especially important in adolescent mothers who have not yet completed their own growth.

Fetal growth is divided into three stages: the 2-week blastogenesis stage, where the fertilized ovum rapidly develops and implants itself into the endometrial lining of the uterus; the critical embryonic stage where the rudiments of all the principal organs and membranes develop (lasts for 6 weeks);

and the fetal stage, which extends to term (40 weeks). During the embryonic stage, all the tissues and organs are defined. The fetus is particularly vulnerable to retarded development or abnormality at this stage if necessary nutrients are absent.

32.2.1 Regulation of nutrient supply to the fetus

The relationship between fetal nutrition and maternal food intake is indirect. In addition to the quantity, quality, and balance of maternal dietary intake, nutrient supply to the fetus will be influenced by a number of adaptive physiological processes that occur during pregnancy. These include increased maternal absorption of some nutrients (e.g. iron), increased bone turnover (facilitating calcium needs), an increase in circulating blood volume resulting in haemodilution of red cells (as plasma volume increases), and an accompanying fall in haemoglobin concentration. In general, maternal plasma levels of water-soluble vitamins fall with a relative rise in fat-soluble vitamins. The placenta is responsible for the exchange of nutrients between the mother and fetus, and nutrient supply will be influenced by an expanding uteroplacental blood flow (up to 800 mL/min at term), placental transfer mechanisms (by diffusion, facilitated diffusion, and active transport), and fetal uptake. Thus, mothers have many protective mechanisms that will help to moderate the effect of poor diet and lifestyle (alcohol, activity, smoking), but these do not provide universal protection or guarantee life-long health.

32.2.2 The energy cost of pregnancy

Researchers who have investigated energy economics in pregnancy have found big differences between women in developing countries, who tend to be smaller and have to do more physical work, and well-nourished women in developed countries. In both settings individual women vary considerably in their pre-pregnant size, in how much fat they put on during the pregnancy, in changes of basal metabolic rate, and in reduction of their physical activity.

Recommendations for average energy intake are based on energy expenditure for women within the healthy weight category. In pregnancy, this is estimated from (i) the energy value of the fetus and placenta and the extra maternal tissues: uterus, breasts, and adipose tissue; plus (ii) any extra energy expenditure (basal metabolic rate plus physical activity for the heavier body) at the different stages of pregnancy. The total energy cost of pregnancy is then distributed into the trimesters and it is agreed that there is little or no extra energy need in the first trimester. It is estimated that the *average* energy cost of pregnancy for a woman who gains 12 kg weight works out to 325 MJ. From this, the expert committees in North America and Australasia both recommend an extra 1.5 MJ/day in the second trimester and 1.9 MJ/day in the third trimester (Table 32.1).

However, many measurements of energy intake throughout pregnancy in women in 10 different

Table 32.1 Extra energy recommendations in pregnancy for the average woman (MJ/day)

	North American 2002 and Australasian 2006	WHO 2004	UK 1991
First trimester	0	+0.375	0
Second trimester	+1.4	+1.2	0
Third trimester	+1.9	+1.95	+0.8

countries (nearly 1000 women in all) found that most of them ate less than one extra MJ/day and the average was +0.3 MJ/day. This finding forms the basis of the 1991 UK recommendation of 0.8 MJ extra/day (only) in the third trimester (Table 32.1), but women who are underweight at the beginning of pregnancy and women who do not reduce activity may need more, the report stated.

Weight gain throughout pregnancy is thought to average 11, 47, and 42% of the total in the first, second, and third trimesters. Table 32.2 shows the

Table 32.2 The distribution of maternal weight gain at 40 weeks' gestation

	Weight gain distribution (g)
Fetus	3300–3500
Placenta	650
Increase in blood volume	1300
Increase in uterus and breasts	1300
Amniotic fluid	800
Fat stores and additional fluid retention	4200–6000
Total	11 550–13 550

distribution of maternal weight gain at birth. Increase in maternal tissue (i.e. uterine and breast tissue), blood and other body fluids, and adipose tissue occurs mainly in the second trimester, while growth of the fetus, placenta, and amniotic fluid occurs mainly in the third.

Adequate maternal weight gain during pregnancy is the principal means of ensuring adequate fetal growth and, hence, infant birth weight. Excessive gain is associated with large infants (>4200 g), increased likelihood of caesarean delivery, and postpartum obesity. Because of the wide variation in weight gain among women who give birth to optimally grown infants, a range of weight gains is regarded as acceptable for each BMI. A normal weight gain for most healthy women is between 11–15 kg, averaging about 12.5 kg. The US Institute of Medicine guidelines, which are based on observational data, indicate that healthy American women who are a normal weight for their height (BMI 18.5–24.9 kg/m^2) should gain 11.5–16 kg (25–35 pounds) during pregnancy. Overweight women (BMI 25–29.9 kg/m^2) should gain 7–11.5 kg (15–25 pounds) and obese women (BMI > 30 kg/m^2) should only put on 5–9 kg (11–20 pounds). However, these figures are not recommended by NICE (UK), who note that there are no evidence-based guidelines from the UK government or professional bodies on what constitutes appropriate weight gain during pregnancy.

Maternal anthropometry differs between ethnic groups and separate guidelines should be used for other ethnic groups, such as Chinese and Polynesians.

32.2.3 Birth weight: the effect of maternal age, maternal weight, and energy intake

Birth weight is regarded as one of the best indicators of overall nutritional status of the infant and its wellbeing. The normal birth weight range is considered to be between 2500 and 4200 g.

Low-birth-weight (LBW), i.e. babies weighing less than 2500 g, is a major cause of infant mortality and has been linked with long-term morbidity, including deficits in growth and cognitive development in childhood and diabetes and heart disease in adult life.

UNICEF estimates that around 19 million newborns each year in the developing world weigh less than 2500 g at birth, and more than half of them are born in South Asia. India has the highest number of LBW babies each year: 7.4 million.

In Australia, babies born to indigenous (aboriginal) women in 2007 were twice as likely to be LBW (12.5%) as those born to non-indigenous women (5.9%). LBW is caused by preterm birth, intrauterine growth retardation, or both.

Adolescents who are still growing are one population subgroup at greater risk of having LBW babies. Even when their own weight gain is sufficient to ensure adequate fat stores, they do not appear to mobilize these stores to enhance fetal growth late in pregnancy. Consequently, their nutritional requirements are greater, and this is reflected in higher recommended energy intakes for younger pregnant women in the UK. Low maternal body weight is also associated with LBW. However, in the developed world, current evidence suggests that chronic low maternal energy intakes does not significantly contribute to LBW, and attempts to increase birth weight through energy supplements have had negligible effects. One (positive) potential nutritional influence on birth weight is a diet rich in long-chain ω-3 polyunsaturated fatty acids (LCP), and randomized control trials have shown an increase in gestation (6 days) with LCP supplements, although overall the effects are rather modest. A wide range of nutrients has been examined in an attempt to influence birth outcomes (including iron, folate, zinc, vitamin D) but these have had little effect. Supplementation with magnesium from the 25th week of gestation has been shown to result in fewer preterm and LBW deliveries, but these results did not differ significantly from placebo groups. It should be noted that protein supplements have a negative effect on birth weight.

32.2.4 Obesity in pregnancy

Recent data (2007) from England show that maternal obesity has doubled from 7.5% to 15.6% over 19 years. In addition, around a quarter of all women in the first trimester are in overweight category. Women who are obese when they become pregnant have higher health risks, including impaired glucose tolerance and gestational diabetes, miscarriage, pre-eclampsia, thromboembolism, and maternal death. Additionally, it has been observed that even a relatively small gain of 1–2 BMI units (kg/m^2) between pregnancies may increase the risk of gestational hypertension and gestational diabetes. Obese women are more likely to have an induced or longer labour, instrumental delivery, caesarean section, or postpartum haemorrhage. Reduced mobility during labour can result in the need for more pain relief and possibly general anaesthesia with its associated risks. Babies born to obese women also face health risks, including a higher risk of fetal death, stillbirth, congenital abnormality, shoulder dystocia, macrosomia (large baby), and subsequent obesity. However, in the absence of trial data on the impact of weight modification during pregnancy, obstetricians remain cautious and recommend that dieting for weight loss during gestation should be discouraged, as this may result in LBW infant if there is serious caloric restriction in the third trimester.

In the UK, the National Institute for Health and Clinical Excellence (NICE) (2010) advises that during pregnancy the key message is to ensure that the myth to 'eat for two' is dispelled. Professionals should be clear that extra calories (above nonpregnant intake) are required, but only during the last trimester, and it is also important to communicate that slimming is not appropriate during pregnancy. For women with a BMI > 30 kg/m^2, weight loss during pregnancy is not recommended. Personalized guidance on healthy eating (with appropriate assessment) and ways to become more physically active are advised. In terms of starting to increase activity, women should begin with no more than 15 min of continuous exercise, 3 times a week, increasing gradually to daily 30 min sessions.

Encouragement should be given to lose weight after pregnancy.

32.2.5 Fetal nutrition, birth outcome, and health in later life

An increasing body of evidence suggests that early nutritional status (as indicated by birth weight and other parameters) modifies the risk of disease (notably cardiovascular) in later life. Birth weight has been used as a proxy measure of fetal nutrient exposure, although it may not be a sensitive enough measure to describe inadequate or unbalanced maternal nutrition. The hypothesis for the relationship between nutrition and early origins of disease is based on the concept that in fetal life the tissues and organs of the body go through periods of rapid development, termed critical periods. Critical periods may coincide with periods of rapid cell division. Thus, if the fetus is deprived of nutrients or oxygen at such times, it may adapt by slowing the rate of cell division, especially in tissues undergoing critical periods. Even brief periods of undernutrition may permanently reduce the numbers of cells in particular organs. It is postulated that fetal undernutrition may change or programme the body with respect to distribution of cell types, hormonal feedback, metabolic activity, and organ structure.

Extensive research by David Barker and colleagues (Barker, 1994) has related causes of adult mortality and morbidity to fetal and infant life. These observational studies have related LBW to adverse health outcomes in adulthood, including hypertension, type 2 diabetes, and coronary heart disease. Variations in newborn ponderal index (kg/m^3) and placenta weight/birth weight ratios have also been related to subsequent hypertension. These observations have led to the fetal origins hypothesis, which states that fetal undernutrition in middle-to-late gestation leads to disproportionate fetal growth and programmes the later development of several diseases which are common in affluent societies and other groups undergoing rapid acculturation.

This hypothesis has been challenged by a number of researchers. Other studies only show a direct association between small size in early life and later adult health outcomes if body size at some intermediate period has been adjusted for. Researchers have suggested that this finding implies that it is probably the change in size across the whole time interval (postnatal centile crossing), rather than fetal biology, that is implicated. Thus, it remains to be resolved whether people who are small in early life and then grow rapidly are more at risk than those who remain small.

32.2.6 Nutrient requirements during pregnancy

Energy Women do not eat or need to eat for two (see Section 32.2.2), but they do need to eat a high-quality nutritious diet to ensure that they obtain their extra requirements for several essential nutrients.

Protein A summary of recommended intakes for protein and other nutrients for a number of countries is presented in Table 32.3. Additional protein is

Table 32.3 Recommended daily nutrient intakes during pregnancy

	USA[a]			Australia/ NZ[b]	UK
	Women NOT pregnant 2005	Change for pregnancy	Pregnant 2005	Pregnant 2006	Pregnant 1991
Protein (g)	46	+54%	71	60	51
Vitamin A (µg)	700	+10%	770	800	700
Vitamin D (µg)	5	0	5	5	10
Vitamin E (mg)	15	0	15	7	–
Vitamin C (mg)	75	+13%	85	60	50
Thiamin (mg)	1.1	+27%	1.4	1.4	0.9
Riboflavin (mg)	1.1	+27%	1.4	1.4	1.4
Niacin (NE) (mg)	14	+29%	18	18	13
Folate (µg)	400	+50%	600	600	300[c]
Vitamin B$_{12}$ (µg)	2.4	+8%	2.6	2.6	1.5
Calcium (mg)	1000	0	1000	1000	700
Magnesium (mg)	310	+13%	350	350	300
Iron (mg)	18	+50%	27	27	15
Zinc (mg)	8	+38%	11	11	7
Iodine (µg)	150	+47%	220	220	140

[a]Numbers for USA are recommended daily allowances (RDAs) from dietary reference intake (DRI) recommendations for females 19–50 years.

[b]These recommendations are RDIs 2004, except for vitamin D and vitamin E, which are adequate intakes.

[c]A supplement of 400 µg/day folic acid is now advised.

NE, niacin equivalents.

required during pregnancy to provide for the synthesis of fetal, placental, and maternal tissue. Maternal and fetal growth accelerates in the second month of pregnancy and continues to increase until just before term. The need for protein follows this growth. However, the extra amount is relatively small (6–10 g/day) and is usually readily provided in a normal pre-pregnant Western diet.

Folate Pregnancy is a period characterized by extra cell division and growth. This increases folate requirements more than for any other nutrient. Folate requirement is increased in the first 12 weeks (see Section 32.2.6) and supplements are recommended preconceptually and in early pregnancy. Increases in dietary intakes of folates are also recommended throughout pregnancy to avoid megaloblastic anaemia in late pregnancy or the puerperium. Differences in recommended dietary intakes by country (Table 32.3) have arisen due to differences in primary indicators of status.

Calcium Around two-thirds of the calcium in the fetus is deposited during the last 10 weeks of gestation, mostly in the fetal skeleton. Alterations in maternal calcium metabolism, including a substantial increase in the absorption of dietary calcium, occur early in pregnancy to facilitate this increase in fetal demand. There has been concern that inadequate dietary intake of calcium during pregnancy was compensated by mobilization of skeletal calcium, leading to an increased risk of osteoporosis in later life. However, recent evidence suggests that the adaptation in calcium metabolism that occurs in pregnancy is sufficient to maintain fetal growth, even if dietary calcium is not increased. Current guidance promotes an adequate calcium intake throughout life, rather than increasing dietary intake during the gestation period. A Cochrane review on calcium supplementation during pregnancy for preventing hypertensive disorders and related problems (Hofmeyr et al., 2006) has reported that calcium supplementation appears to be beneficial for women at high risk of gestational hypertension and in communities with low dietary calcium intake, although optimum dosage requires further investigation.

Iron The demand for iron is not evenly distributed throughout gestation. During the first trimester, requirements are minimal, as iron is no longer lost during menstruation. Iron absorption increases as pregnancy progresses, from an absorption rate of around 7% at 12 weeks' gestation to 66% at 36 weeks. Many women enter pregnancy with low iron stores or even frank iron-deficiency anaemia (IDA). Maternal IDA may increase the risk of preterm delivery, resultant LBW, and perinatal mortality. As well, evidence is accumulating that maternal IDA reduces infant iron stores postpartum, leading to the possibility of impaired development in the infant. There remains considerable debate on the use of iron supplements during pregnancy with respect to whether this is an attempt to alter a natural physiological process that in some way enhances nutrient supply. Dietary guidance in the UK suggests that no dietary changes to iron intake are required due to physiological changes, although women with poor iron status at the time of obstetric booking may need iron supplements. The WHO recommend a cut-off of 110 g/L for anaemia throughout pregnancy and in the UK NICE recommends that iron supplementation should be considered for women with haemoglobin concentrations below 110 g/L in the first trimester and 105 g/L at 28 weeks.

Zinc Zinc is necessary for DNA and RNA synthesis. Maternal zinc deficiency may be responsible for growth retardation, preterm delivery, and abnormality in the fetus, and birth complications in the mother. Factors that limit the absorption of zinc such as high intakes of dietary phytate, calcium, and iron supplements may cause secondary zinc deficiency. Recently published dietary recommendations include an increase of zinc intake in pregnancy. The extra zinc should come from foods (see Section 11.1.5). It is possible that iron supplements could reduce zinc intake.

Iodine Iodine deficiency during pregnancy remains a major public health problem in many areas of the world. Cretinism, caused by severe lack of iodine during fetal development, is characterized by both mental and physical retardation. Millions of babies are born each year at risk of mental impairment due to iodine-deficient diets. Iodization of salt is commonly used to prevent deficiency. In areas where there is cretinism and extensive goitres, expectant mothers should be given an injection of iodized oil, preferably before conception (see Section 11.3.5). However, overt iodine deficiency is not seen in developed countries among pregnant women.

Vitamin A

Vitamin A Vitamin A deficiency, seen mostly in some developing countries, may be associated with blindness, depressed immune function, and increased morbidity and death from measles and other infectious diseases, as well as increased mother-to-child transmission of AIDS. Encouraging foods rich in this vitamin (see Chapter 12) is the most appropriate approach to ensuring adequacy. But in pregnancy, intakes above the RDI (> 3000 µg retinol daily) resulting from the use of supplements, excessive intakes of fortified foods, and, occasionally, high intakes of liver can be teratogenic, causing central nervous and heart defects. High levels of vitamin A have been detected in the liver of farmed animals in the UK (due to the composition of animal feedstuffs); thus, all pregnant women are advised to avoid liver, liver products, vitamin supplements, and fish oil supplements that are high in retinol. In developing countries where appropriate foods are not readily available, supplementation may be considered (700 µg/day).

Vitamin D

Vitamin D Populations at risk for vitamin D deficiency are those whose skin exposure to sunlight is low, particularly dark-skinned women living in northern climates such as ethnic minority groups in the UK. The infants born in such populations have low vitamin D stores. Vitamin D insufficiency during pregnancy is associated with lower maternal weight gain, neonatal tetany, and biochemical evidence of disturbed skeletal homeostasis in the infant. In extreme situations, reduced bone mineralization, radiologically evident rickets, and fractures may occur. In the UK, it is recommended that all pregnant women take a vitamin D supplement (10 µg/day), and this has been reinforced recently following cases of rickets.

Vitamin C

Vitamin C It appears that the fetus concentrates vitamin C at the expense of maternal stores and circulating vitamin levels. Accordingly, it is recommended that dietary intake of foods rich in vitamin C are increased during pregnancy.

In summary, while mineral requirements increase during pregnancy, most of the extra nutrients can be attained through physiological adaptation rather than dietary change (in the well-nourished). With respect to vitamins, extra dietary intakes of vitamin C and vitamin A are required, which may mean increasing intakes by rich dietary sources (but not by supplements). Increasing intakes of folate and vitamin D should be met by increasing dietary sources, as well as by supplements.

32.2.7 Lifestyle factors that impact on pregnancy outcome

Alcohol Heavy drinkers have a greatly increased risk of inducing the fetal alcohol syndrome, with characteristic underdevelopment of the mid-face, small body size, and mental retardation. Any effect of alcohol is likely to be greatest in the first few weeks after conception, the embryogenesis stage. Women who intend to become pregnant should not have multiple alcoholic drinks whatever the occasion; they could already be 2 or 3 weeks pregnant. Once pregnancy is established, the rule should be no more than one standard drink a day to be sure of avoiding minor effects, chiefly growth retardation.

Smoking Smoking causes retardation of fetal growth, thereby increasing the risk of producing a LBW baby. The older the mother and the more cigarettes smoked, the greater the effect. A decrease in birth weight of approximately 200–250 g is usually found in infants of mothers who smoke more than 20 cigarettes a day. Smoking also increases the risk of spontaneous abortion, preterm delivery, and sudden infant death.

Exercise Most recent studies show that moderate exercise during pregnancy does not harm the fetus and benefits the mother. Benefits can include reduced fat gain, lower risk of gestational diabetes, maintenance of aerobic fitness, shorter labour, quicker delivery, and fewer surgical interventions. However, high-impact exercise or hard physical work can affect fetal development and often results in LBW babies and a higher frequency of obstetric complications.

32.2.8 Other diet and health concerns

Coffee Caffeine freely crosses the placenta. The risk of spontaneous abortion and LBW appears to increase with high maternal caffeine intake during pregnancy. It is sensible to limit caffeine consumption in pregnancy and current guidelines suggest pregnant women have no more than 200 mg of caffeine a day (approximately 2 mugs of instant coffee or 4 cups of tea). Some women develop aversion to coffee when they are pregnant.

Oil-rich fish Due to contaminants such as mercury, which may be stored in high concentrations in fatty fish, pregnant women are recommended to restrict intake of oily fish. These recommendations will vary by region. In the UK, pregnant women are advised not to eat marlin, shark, or swordfish, to limit tuna to four cans per week, and not to exceed oily fish consumption above two portions per week. However, it is considered beneficial to consume at least one portion of oil-rich fish, e.g. herring, salmon, and sardines, weekly during pregnancy.

Food safety Pregnant women are unusually susceptible to infection with *Listeria monocytogenes*, which can contaminate uncooked foods. After an incubation period of 2–6 weeks, infection can result in a mild chill or more severe illness, premature birth, or stillbirth. There can also be effects in the newborn, including meningitis. Listeriosis responds to antibiotics when it is diagnosed. In the UK, the incidence is estimated at 1 in 30 000 live and stillbirths. The department of health recommends that

pregnant women avoid certain ripened soft cheeses, such as Brie, Camembert, and blue-veined cheese, and any type of paté.

Salmonella, toxoplasma and food poisoning more generally also needs to be avoided with greater care during pregnancy than at other times.

32.2.9 Physiological effects of pregnancy that impact on dietary intake

Nausea and vomiting It is hypothesized that nausea and vomiting are part of the maternal system to protect against toxins. In support of this hypothesis, a comprehensive review reported that: (i) symptoms peak when embryonic organogenesis is most susceptible to chemical disruption (weeks 6–18); (ii) women who experience morning sickness are less likely to miscarry than women who do not; (iii) women who vomit suffer fewer miscarriages than those who experience nausea alone; and (iv) many pregnant women have aversions to alcoholic and non-alcoholic (mostly caffeinated) beverages and strong-tasting vegetables, especially during the first trimester.

There is no generally effective remedy for morning sickness and, given the vulnerability of the fetus in the early stages of development, it is important to find alternatives to drug therapy.

Changes in eating habits such as small, frequent meals and avoidance of strong food odours appear to help some women. A recent Cochrane review using data from six double-blind randomized controlled trials with a total of 675 participants and a prospective observational cohort study indicated that ginger was effective in relieving the severity of nausea and vomiting episodes with no significant side effects or adverse effects on pregnancy outcomes. The authors concluded that more observational studies are needed to confirm this encouraging preliminary data on ginger.

Hyperemesis gravidarum (HG) is a condition that causes severe nausea and vomiting in early pregnancy, often resulting in hospital admission. The incidence of HG varies from 0.1 to 1% and appears higher in multiple pregnancies, hydatidiform mole, and other conditions associated with increased pregnancy hormone levels. Both the aetiology and pathogenesis of HG remain unknown, although a range of pregnancy hormones (progesterone, oestrogen, and human chorionic gonadotrophin) and other hormones have been implicated. Infants from HG pregnancies have significantly lower birth weight, younger gestational age, and a greater length of hospital stay. The persistent vomiting can lead to Wernicke's encephalopathy (also see 13.1.4) so it is important that thiamin is given with replacement intravenous fluids.

Cravings and aversions Some change in liked and disliked foods is common in pregnancy. There can be cravings or aversions. Food cravings are popularly believed to be related to the nutritional needs of the mother, to have symbolic value, or to be related to sensory or physiological causes. Food aversions have been defined as 'a definite revulsion against food and drink not previously disliked'. Typical examples are tea, coffee, and alcohol. The explanation for these cravings and aversions is incomplete. They may relate to changes in olfactory and taste sensitivity during pregnancy.

Constipation Around 40% of women report having been constipated some time during pregnancy. Its aetiology is complex and includes depressed gut mobility in pregnancy, increased fluid absorption from the large intestine, decreased physical activity, and dietary changes. However, an increase in fibre, from an average intake of about 18 g/day to 27 g/day, has shown to be effective in treating constipation.

32.3 Lactation

The decision to breastfeed is influenced by psycho-biological and psychosocial factors, which vary between and within cultures. The proportion of babies who were ever breastfed varies widely, as does the duration of exclusive feeding. Across Europe, less than 70% of babies in France and Ireland to around 100% in Denmark, Norway, and Sweden initiate breastfeeding. In Australia in 2005, around 88% of mothers started breastfeeding but only 17% were exclusively breastfeeding at 6 months. In the UK around 78% of mothers initiate breastfeeding but less than 3% are still exclusively breastfeeding at 6 months.

This compares with Rwanda and North Korea, where 88% and 65% are still exclusively breastfeeding at 6 months. In most countries, initiation and duration of breastfeeding are positively associated with maternal education status, maternal income, and marital status.

The physiology of lactation is complex, but may be briefly summarized as follows: the suckling infant stimulates the mother's pituitary gland to release prolactin, a hormone required for the synthesis of breast milk. Milk-producing cells synthesize most of the protein and some of the fats and sugars, which combine with other nutrients derived from the mother's circulation. A second pituitary hormone, oxytocin, is responsible for releasing the milk from the cells into the ducts that carry the milk to the nipples.

32.3.1 Composition of breast milk and implications for maternal nutrition

Human milk feeding is adequate as the sole source of nutrition for up to age 6 months providing that the maternal diet and stores are adequate and the milk is successfully transferred to the infant. The composition and volume of breast milk progressively changes with the stage of lactation and can be influenced by maternal nutritional factors. Current evidence indicates that infant demand is the major determinant of the quantity of milk produced. The nutritional demands of lactation on the mother are directly proportional to volume and duration of milk production.

The daily milk volume varies over the duration of lactation but is fairly consistent except in extreme maternal malnutrition or severe dehydration. Breast milk intake among healthy infants averages 750–800 g/day and ranges from 450 to 1200 g/day. The composition of milk will be influenced by time of day, gestational age (prematurity versus term), stage of lactation, parity, month (i.e. seasonal food intake), nutritional status of mother, and maternal dietary intake. Lipids are the most variable constituent in human milk. In the first week after birth, colostrum is produced, which has a fat content of 2.6 g/100 mL. This is followed by transitional milk between days 7 and 14, and then finally mature milk, which has a fat content of 4.2 g/100 mL.

32.3.2 Maternal nutrient requirements to support lactation

During pregnancy, the mother's body prepares for lactation by storing some nutrients and energy. It is difficult to determine precise nutrient requirements for lactation since there is variation in nutritional status before and during pregnancy, and limited knowledge about utilization of maternal nutrient stores and adaptations of maternal metabolism during lactation.

The total energy cost of lactation is derived from the energy content of the milk plus the energy required to produce it. The energy value of breast milk is between 2.7 MJ/L and 3.1 MJ/L. The ratio between the energy content of milk and the total energy cost of lactation is the efficiency of milk production. Current estimates for exclusive breastfeeding suggest that the energy cost of lactation is around 2.625 MJ/day (625 kcal) based on a mean milk production of 750 g/day with an energy density of milk of 2.8 kJ/g and energetic efficiency of 0.80. In well-nourished women, this will be partially met by energy mobilization from fat tissues of about 0.65 MJ/day (for weight reduction of 0.5 kg fat/month), resulting in a net increment of around 2.0 MJ/day (480 kcal)) over non-pregnant, non-lactating energy requirements. This assumes the ideal situation where the new mother gradually uses up the extra 2–5 kg fat put on during pregnancy over 6 months of breastfeeding. The value will vary when complementary feeding is introduced or the baby becomes only partially breastfed. Women who exclusively breastfeed for 6 months may require as much as 2.4 MJ extra/day.

32.3.3 Other nutrients

Table 32.4 shows recommended nutrient intakes for five countries. The North American recommended nutrient intakes were published between 1998 and

Table 32.4 Recommended daily nutrient intakes during lactation

Nutrient	USA	USA and Canada, Australia/NZ[a]	USA and Canada	UK 1991
	NPNL women	Lactating	% Increase	Lactating
Protein (g)	46	67	+46	56
Vitamin A (µg)	700	1300 (1100)	+86	950
Vitamin D (µg)	5	5	0	10
Vitamin E (mg)	15	19 (11)	+27	–

(Continued)

Table 32.4 Recommended daily nutrient intakes during lactation (*Continued*)

Nutrient	USA	USA and Canada, Australia/NZ[a]	USA and Canada	UK 1991
	NPNL women	Lactating	% Increase	Lactating
Vitamin C (mg)	75	120 (80)	+60	70
Thiamin (mg)	1.1	1.4	+ 27	1.0
Riboflavin (mg)	1.1	1.6	+45	1.6
Niacin (NE) (mg)	14	17	+21	15
Folate (µg)[b]	400	500	+25	260
Vitamin B_{12} (µg)	2.4	2.8	+17	2.0
Calcium (mg)	1000	1000	0	1250
Iron (mg)	18	9[c]	−50	15
Zinc (mg)	8	12	+50	13
Iodine (µg)	150	290 (270)	+93	140

[a]Where the Australasian RDI is different, it is shown in brackets.

[b]These are RDIs for dietary folate equivalents in USA, Australia, and NZ.

[c]For first 6 months of lactation; assumes menstruation not restarted.

NPNL = not pregnant, not lactating.

2002 and the Australasian in 2005–2006. The British recommendations date from 1991. In developed countries, there is sufficient protein and most other nutrients in usual diets so that the average extra 2.0 MJ of food per day will cover the extra nutrient needs with two exceptions. In the northern winter, a vitamin D supplement is advisable, and vegans must take a vitamin B_{12} supplement (these are available from microbiological, i.e. non-animal, sources). Although some 260 mg of calcium are secreted per day in mother's milk, epidemiological studies have found no increase in osteoporosis or fracture in women who have breastfed compared with those who did not.

The US Institute of Medicine sums it up:

'The loss of calcium from the maternal skeleton that occurs during lactation is not prevented by increased dietary calcium, and the calcium lost appears to be regained following weaning. There is no evidence that calcium intake in lactating women should be increased above that of non-lactating women.'

Some nutrients in the breast milk are increased if there is more of them in the mother's diet: water-soluble vitamins, vitamin A, and polyunsaturated fatty acids. Most other constituents in the milk—protein, lactose, total fat, and calcium—do not appear to be influenced by maternal intake.

It is now no longer considered necessary to advise mothers with a family history of allergy to avoid peanuts or peanut butter during pregnancy and lactation. After a cup of coffee or glass of wine, the concentration of caffeine or alcohol in the milk is about the same as in the mother's plasma; the infant gets a lower dose per kg than the mother but has less metabolizing capacity.

Adequate fluid intake (especially water) should be advised for breastfeeding mothers. The exact amount required is unknown but 6–8 glasses is generally sufficient. The nutrient reference values for Australia and NZ (2005) recommend 2.6 litres per day during lactation (2.3 L during pregnancy).

32.3.4 Lactation and maternal obesity

Pregnancy is a risk factor for obesity. Some women put on more than the standard 2–5 kg of fat. The question arises whether milk production and the baby will suffer if the lactating mother restricts her food intake. Lovelady *et al.* (2000) tested this out in a randomized controlled trial in overweight (not obese) women. They lost approximately 0.5 kg per week between 4 and 14 weeks postpartum from moderate food restriction and exercise: their infants gained the same weight and length as the controls, but some of the control mothers put on weight. Overall, current evidence (reviewed by NICE, 2010) suggests that weight management interventions (addressing diet and physical activity) during lactation have little or no adverse effects on breastfeeding outcomes, including milk volume, infant intake, and time and frequency of feeding.

Further Reading

1. **Allan, L.H.** (2005) Multiple micronutrients in pregnancy and lactation: An overview. *Am J Clin Nutr*, **81** (Suppl.), 1206S–12S.

2. **Anderson, A.S. and Wrieden WL** (2010) Teenage pregnancies. In Symonds ME and Ramsey MM (eds) *Maternal-fetal nutrition during pregnancy and lactation*. Cambridge, Cambridge University Press.

3. **Barker, D.J.P.** (1998) *Mothers, babies and disease in later life*. London, UK, BMJ Books.

4. **Bartley, K.A., Underwood, B.A., and Deckelbaum, R.J.** (2005) A life cycle micronutrient perspective for women's health. *Am J Clin Nutr*, **81** (Suppl.), 1188S–93S.

5. **Butte, N.F. and King, J.C.** (2005) Energy requirements during pregnancy and lactation. *Publ Hlth Nutr*, **8**, 1010–27.

6. **Hofmeyr, G.J., Atallah, A.N., and Duley, L.** (2006) Calcium supplmentation during pregnancy for preventing hypertensive disorders and related problems. *Cochrane Database Syst Rev*, CD000145.

7. **Lovelady, C.A., Garner, K.E., Moreno, K.L., and Williams, J.P.** (2000) The effect of weight loss in overweight lactating women on the growth of their infants. *New Engl J Med*, **343**, 449–53.

8. **MRC Vitamin Study Research Group** (1991) Prevention of neural tube defects: Results of the Medical Research Council Vitamin Study. *Lancet*, **338**, 131–7.

9. **NICE** (2008) *Guidance for midwives, health visitors, pharmacists and other primary care services to improve the nutrition of pregnant and breastfeeding mothers and children in low income households*. London, National Institute of Health and Clinical Excellence. http://guidance.nice.org.uk/PH11.

10. **NICE** (2010) *Dietary interventions and physical activity interventions for weight management before, during and after pregnancy*. London, National Institute of Health and Clinical Excellence. http://guidance.nice.org.uk/PH27.

11. **Ramachenderan, J., Bradford, J., and McLean, M.** (2008) Maternal obesity and pregnancy complications: A review. *Aust NZ J Obstet Gyneacol*, **48**, 228–35.

12. **Scholl, T.O.** (2005) Iron status during pregnancy: Setting the stage for mother and infant. *Am J Clin Nutr*, **81** (Suppl.), 1218S–22S.

13. **Scientific Advisory Committee on Nutrition** (2005) *Folate and disease prevention*. London, Food Standards Agency. http://www.sacn.gov.uk/reports_position_statements/reports/report_on_folate_and_disease_prevention.html

14. **Scientific Advisory Committee on Nutrition** (2011) *The influence of maternal, fetal and child nutrition on the development of chronic disease in later life.* London, Food Standards Agency. http://www.sacn.gov.uk/reports_position_statements/index.html

Useful Websites

 To see topical and scientifically robust updates on nutrition associated with this textbook and web links to many of the journals in the Further Reading sections, please see the dedicated Online Resource Centre at **http://www.oxfordtextbooks.co.uk/orc/mann4e/**

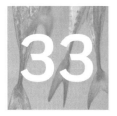

33 Infant and toddler feeding

Vishal Avinashi, Donna Secker, and Stanley Zlotkin

Interest in infant and toddler feeding centres around two principal objectives: the promotion of normal growth and brain development, and the prevention of illness during the first years of life. Infants and toddlers grow and develop rapidly in the first 2 years, making them particularly vulnerable to nutritional inadequacies. Breastfeeding, followed by the introduction of a wide variety of solid foods, provides the best opportunity for optimal growth and health during infancy. After 1 year of age, the infant should be consuming a variety of foods from the adult diet to ensure a nutritionally balanced intake.

Decades of animal experiments as well as studies evaluating the growth of human infants under varying environmental conditions suggest that early infant nutrition and postnatal growth are important factors for long-term health. Researchers have hypothesized that nutritional deficits occurring during fetal life predispose or programme an individual towards a tendency to develop chronic diseases in later life. The original fetal origins hypothesis by Barker, also known as the thrifty phenotype, proposed an association between low birth weight, accelerated postnatal growth, and adult heart disease. This hypothesis has since been expanded to include chronic diseases such as hypertension, insulin resistance, and obesity. More recently, researchers have proposed a postnatal programming hypothesis (the Lucas hypothesis), implying that it is early postnatal nutrition and growth that influences later health, rather than prenatal life. It has been suggested that limiting caloric intake and subsequently the rate of weight gain in infancy could reduce the risk of developing these chronic conditions. However, providing evidence to support this claim is nearly impossible given the multiple confounders and differing genetic backgrounds and exposures, as well as the great difficulty and cost following up such a cohort. Restriction of nutrition during infancy is not recommended, especially as undernutrition adversely affects brain growth.

33.1 Milk diet

33.1.1 Breastfeeding

Human milk is specifically composed to meet the nutritional requirements of the human infant and is considered the optimal nutrition source for healthy newborns (Box 33.1). Breastfeeding provides immunological protection, which is greatest

BOX 33.1 Benefits of breastfeeding	
Short-term benefits	Possible long-term benefits
Low cost	Decreased obesity
Increased bonding	Decreased type 1 diabetes
Immunological benefit	Increased cognitive benefits
Decreased infections— diarrhoeal and respiratory	
Decreased SIDS	

during the early months, but increases with the duration and exclusiveness of breastfeeding. The psychological benefit of early and prolonged physical contact contributes to the development of a strong mother–infant bond. Other benefits include convenience, safety, and low cost, in addition to the benefits gained by the mother, such as delayed resumption of ovulation, increased postpartum weight loss, and decreased risk of breast cancer. With the exception of vitamins D and K, breast milk produced by adequately nourished mothers provides all the nutrients needed by a normal, healthy, full-term infant for the first 6 months of life. Water or other fluid supplementation is unnecessary in the otherwise-healthy infant in the first 6 months of life. The water requirements of infants in a hot, humid climate can be provided entirely by the water content in human milk. When it is hot, infants may just nurse more often.

Recent studies have provided good evidence that, even in developed countries, breastfeeding protects against gastrointestinal and respiratory infections, reduces the risk of otitis media, and reduces the incidence of sudden infant death syndrome. Breastfeeding also decreases the incidence of atopy (clinical forms of inherited hypersensitivity) in infants, with some evidence to suggest that the protection is extended into childhood.

On the longer-term basis, there is some evidence suggesting that breastfeeding may play a role in preventing type 1 diabetes (insulin-dependent diabetes mellitus). Breastfed children have been shown to have a lower prevalence of obesity later in life than formula-fed infants, even after adjusting for key factors such as energy intake, screen time, physical activity, and mothers' body mass index. In addition, there is documentation that the mean values for cognitive development in populations of children who were breastfed are slightly higher compared with bottle-fed infants from similar environments.

Breastfeeding is rarely contraindicated. Exceptions include infants with galactosaemia and mothers who have untreated active tuberculosis, active herpetic breast lesions, or human T-lymphotropic virus type I infection, or are receiving ongoing radiation therapy or certain chemotherapeutic agents. Neither smoking nor environmental contaminants are necessarily contraindications to breastfeeding. Moderate, infrequent alcohol ingestion, the use of most prescription and over-the-counter drugs, and many maternal infections do not preclude breastfeeding.

Although maternal-to-child transmission of HIV through breast milk is a known route of transmission, avoidance of breastfeeding is not practical in settings where formula feeding is not available, affordable, sustainable, or safe. Lessons learned have shown that in the context of an HIV-positive mother, if one cannot provide appropriate infant formula feeds consistently, there will be less viral transmission if the infant is breastfed exclusively until 6 months compared to infants who are receiving a mix of formula and breast milk.

33.1.2 Formula feeding

When a mother chooses not to breastfeed, the only acceptable alternative is a commercial infant formula. Manufacturers continue to modify their products in an effort to emulate human milk and, although they provide less than the optimal benefits of human milk, they are nutritionally adequate for the first year of life. The standard formula choice is a formula based on cow's milk, containing skimmed milk powder, lactose, and a variable blend of oils. These formulas are available in two versions: low iron (similar amounts to human milk, but with much lower bioavailability) or iron-fortified (10–12 mg/L elemental iron). Use of low-iron formulas is one of several risk factors implicated in the incidence of iron-deficiency anaemia, the most common nutritional deficiency among infants and toddlers. To provide the best guarantee of normal iron status, the use of iron-fortified formulas is recommended.

Soy-based formulas made from soy protein, vegetable oils, and glucose polymers (with or without sucrose) are available for infants of vegetarian families, infants with galactosaemia, confirmed lactose intolerance, or infants with confirmed IgE-mediated allergy to cow's milk protein. Soy formulas are not indicated for low-birth-weight infants, prevention or management of colic, prevention of allergy or food intolerance, routine treatment of gastroenteritis, or treatment of infants with non-IgE-mediated allergy to cow's milk protein (i.e. enteropathy or enterocolitis). Since the distinction between IgE- and non-IgE-mediated allergy to cow's milk protein is not easily made or practical, it is safer not to use soy formula for the treatment of cow's milk protein allergy.

Recent concerns with respect to the safety of soy formulas are related to their content of phyto-oestrogens. Since phyto-oestrogens have oestrogen-like activity, it has been suggested that adverse effects on the developing endocrine system may occur in infants fed soy protein-based formulas. The presence of phyto-oestrogens in human infants does not necessarily mean that they are biologically or clinically active. Soy-based formulas have been used for almost 40 years without evidence of hormone-related adverse effects and term infants fed soy-based formula have grown and developed normally. The only caution should be in infants with congenital hypothyroidism, as abnormal thyroid function has been described in those infants consuming soy-based formula.

Studies provide conflicting evidence about the importance of providing preterm and full-term infant formula supplemented with long-chain polyunsaturated fatty acids. Long-chain polyunsaturated fatty acids (docosahexanoic acid in particular) accumulate in the brain and eye of the fetus, especially during the last trimester of pregnancy, and some studies suggest that infants, in particular preterm infants, may benefit from direct consumption. Infants receiving breast milk or infant formula supplemented with docosahexanoic acid and arachidonic acid have higher levels of these fatty acids in the blood, brain, and retina than infants fed regular formula. These higher levels are thought to have benefits related to visual acuity, growth, and psychomotor and mental development. Despite the widespread availability of infant formulas supplemented with long-chain polyunsaturated fatty acids and their use in research settings for nearly a decade, there is limited evidence of long-term benefit to term and preterm populations.

Lactose-free cow's milk-based formulas are also available for infants; however, routine use is not recommended. 'Follow-on' or transition formulas are designed for the second 6 months of life and although nutritionally superior to cow's milk, they provide no nutritional advantages over regular iron-fortified infant formulas. Home-made formulas from evaporated milk are nutritionally incomplete and are not recommended. Formulas containing pre- and probiotics have gained popularity in recent years. While prebiotics have been shown to increase the number of bifidobacteria and lactobacilli in infant stools and probiotics have been shown to likely help prevent infectious diarrhoea in the short term, long-term clinical benefits have not been shown. Until research can promote their standardization (strain and dose) and long-term effects, caution should be taken in promoting such formula.

Specialized infant formulas are available for the small number of infants who are allergic to, or unable to digest, intact proteins. These products, which come as extensively hydrolysed formulas and free amino-acid formulas, have been heat-treated and enzymatically hydrolysed to produce peptides of various lengths and/or free amino acids. The more the proteins are broken down, the more unpalatable and expensive the products become. Partially hydrolysed formulas should not be considered 'hypoallergenic', nor should they be used for the purposes of allergy treatment. Some formulas contain medium-chain triglycerides; these formulas are designed for infants with fat malabsorption.

33.1.3 Vitamin and mineral supplementation

With the exception of vitamins D and K, human milk from well-nourished mothers provides all the nutrients required for approximately the first 6 months of life. Routine administration of intra-muscular vitamin K at birth has eliminated vitamin K deficiency. Commercial infant formulas are forti-fied with vitamins and minerals; therefore, supple-ments are unnecessary.

Vitamin D The amount of vitamin D in human milk is insufficient to prevent rickets. Although vita-min D can be produced from exposure of the skin to sunlight (ultraviolet B rays), with increasing use of sunscreen and avoidance of sun exposure due to the risks of sunburn and skin cancer, both mothers and infants are at risk of vitamin D deficiency and indeed, the incidence of vitamin D deficiency is ris-ing in many countries. Hence, in Canada and the USA, a daily vitamin D supplement is recommended for breastfed infants, beginning at birth and contin-uing until vitamin D intake from other dietary sources meets their recommended intake. Few foods contain significant amounts of naturally occurring vitamin D (e.g. liver and oily fish), whereas only milk and margarine are fortified with vitamin D in some countries. Infants at the highest risk for vitamin D deficiency and the development of nutritional rick-ets are those who are born to vitamin D-deficient mothers, dark-skinned, exclusively breastfed, living at high northern or southern latitudes, or weaned to vegan diets. There is an increasing amount of research being done on vitamin D status throughout the lifespan which extends far beyond bone health to include multiple sclerosis, autoimmune condi-tions, cardiovascular diseases, and cancer. The con-servative recommended dose of vitamin D for infants who are breastfeeding is between 200 and 400 IU/day. Recently, the American Academy of Paediatrics has suggested that all infants, children, and adolescents have a minimum daily intake of 400 IU (10 µg) per day.

33.2 Transition to solids

33.2.1 Introduction of solids

At some point in time, exclusive breastfeeding no longer meets a growing infant's energy and nutrient needs and complementary foods must be added. These additional foods are not intended to replace or interfere with breastfeeding. The timing and type of complementary foods is variable, reflecting the numerous cultural practices of soci-ety, as well as the child's developmental matura-tion. Recommendations that breast milk should be given exclusively for the first 6 months and that complementary food should be introduced after this time are based on issues related to nutri-tional need, physiological maturation, behavioural and developmental aspects of feeding, immuno-logical safety, and environmental influences. Most evidence suggests that introduction before

4 months or later than 6 months has more risks than benefits. Individual infants may have unique needs or feeding behaviours that may require introduction of complementary foods as early as 4 months of age.

Scientific evidence in support of traditional rec-ommendations for the order and progression of introducing solids is limited. Infants should be introduced to nutrient-rich solid foods, and because they require a good source of iron around 6 months of age, the most commonly used first food has been iron-fortified infant cereal. Iron-rich meat is also a good choice. Gluten, one of the more common allergens, is found in wheat, rye, oats, and barley, but not rice or maize. Therefore, for theoretical reasons, rice cereal has been consid-ered the most appropriate first food. Because each new food constitutes a potential allergic challenge, the introduction of one new food every 2–3 days has been advised, using single rather than mixed foods initially. This is primarily important for infants at high risk for allergies, who are generally introduced to new foods more cautiously. Puréed or finely mashed vegetables and fruits, meats, poultry, tofu, legumes, and lentils are generally introduced after infant cereals. Although not evidence-based, highly allergenic foods such as fish, seafood, and eggs are commonly introduced later. While it can be common practice in developed countries to offer bland foods, there is no evidence to suggest that infants are unable to tolerate spices or strong flavours. When an infant begins to make lateral motions of the jaw, chewing should be encouraged by increasing the texture of foods to include mashed table foods. An infant who is not encouraged to chew at this time may have trouble later accepting anything but fluids and purees. Between 9 and 12 months of age, finger foods should be introduced to encourage self-feeding. The size, shape, and texture of the food should be considered because they influence the infant's ability to chew and swallow safely without choking (Table 33.1).

Feeding a toddler The second year of life involves infants becoming more involved with their own feeding, which gives them a sense of control and independence. With more teeth and the advancement in fine motor skills and oral coordination, infants can successfully use feeding utensils and move towards different foods with firmer textures. A transition from bottle feeding should be encouraged to promote drinking from a cup. As infants gain mobility and are more active, food intake does not always increase correspondingly. With increasing age, toddlers' likes and dislikes can be intensified, which certainly involves having strong and sometimes limited food preferences. Efforts must be made to continue to offer a wide variety of foods, allow toddlers to play with their food, and make eating an enjoyable experience for the parents and the child.

33.2.2 Safety issues around feeding

Infants are less immune to bacteria in the digestive tract than older children and adults. The risk of choking on foods with the potential for aspiration and asphyxia is highest for infants and toddlers. Therefore, foods provided to infants must be free of pathogens, appropriate in size and texture, nutritionally wholesome, and fed safely (Box 33.2).

The greatest risk of choking and aspiration on food occurs in children under the age of 4 years, with a significant peak in the 12–24-month age group. Small, round, smooth foods such as sausages, hotdogs, grapes, nuts, peanuts, candies, raisins, seeds, peas, kernel corn, and popcorn are the most dangerous, as they can slip prematurely into the pharynx and with a quick gasp for breath be drawn downward and become lodged in the airway. These foods are not recommended before 3–4 years of age unless they are cut into pieces. Highly viscous foods, such as peanut butter, can plug the airway and should not be served by themselves. In addition to the shape and texture of foods, environmental factors such as distractions or inadequate supervision during eating increase the risk of food asphyxiation.

33.2.3 Iron deficiency

Iron deficiency is most common among infants between the ages of 6 and 24 months. The major risk factors for iron-deficiency anaemia in infants relate to socioeconomic status and include the early consumption of cow's milk, use of non-iron-fortified infant formula, inadequate funds for appropriate foods, and poor knowledge of nutrition. Other high-risk groups include low-birth-weight and premature infants and older infants who drink large amounts of milk (>1 L/day) or juice and eat little solid food. The importance of preventing rather than treating anaemia has been accentuated by findings that iron-deficiency anaemia is a risk factor for developmental delays in cognitive function and that this delay is irreversible with iron therapy and persists into early childhood (Box 33.3).

Table 33.1 Development of feeding skills and introduction of appropriate foods

Age	Oral–motor skills	Self-feeding	Foods to introduce
Birth–6 months	Well-developed sucking and rooting reflexes facilitate intake of human milk or formula Extrusion reflex causes tongue to protrude when solid food or spoon is put in mouth	Sees breast or bottle and becomes excited	Human milk or iron-fortified infant formula is all the infant needs
6 months	Sits up alone or with support Holds head up on own Indicates desire for food by watching spoon, opening mouth and closing lips over spoon, and swallowing Indicates disinterest in food or satiety, by leaning back, keeping mouth closed, and turning head away Extrusion reflex decreases Able to depress the tongue and transfer semi-solids from spoon to back of mouth for swallowing Smacks lips	Pats or puts hands on breast or bottle	Iron-fortified infant cereal or puréed meat to introduce a supplementary source of iron
6–9 months	Teething starts Lips begin to move while chewing Begins chewing up and down Jaw and tongue move up and down Lip closure achieved	Plays with spoon May help spoon find mouth Holds bottle Feeds self crackers, toast, cookies, etc. Feeds from cup with help	Cooked, puréed, or mashed vegetables to add new flavours and textures Soft, puréed, or mashed fruits Puréed, minced, or finely chopped meat, poultry, cooked egg yolk, cooked mashed legumes, lentils, tofu to provide additional iron, protein and B vitamins Grains, toast, crackers, and dry unsweetened cereals to provide opportunity for self-feeding Limited amounts of unsweetened fruit juices offered in a child-sized cup

Table 33.1 (*Continued*)

Age	Oral–motor skills	Self-feeding	Foods to introduce
			Yoghurt, cheese, and cottage cheese
9–12 months	Rotary chewing movement develops Rhythmic biting movements begin Licks food from lower lip Fine motor skills improve	Can hold own bottle well Can hold cup but may spill contents Picks up foods in fingers or palms Puts food in mouth	Soft, bite-sized pieces of vegetables, mashed potatoes, fruits, meats, and alternatives; soft breads, rolls, plain muffins, rice and noodles to enhance chewing skills Finger foods: soft-cooked vegetables, cut into bite-sized pieces; soft, ripe, peeled fresh fruit, or canned fruits; strips of tender meat; soft, whole legumes or lentils; diced tofu to enhance motor skills and encourage self-feeding

BOX 33.2 Guidelines for feeding infants safely

- Unpasteurized milk, or unpasteurized food should not be fed to infants as they can introduce pathogens such as *Escherichia coli* 0157:H7, *Salmonella*, or *Cryptosporidium*, which cause diarrhoea or other more serious infections.
- To prevent botulism, infants under 1 year of age should not be fed honey.
- To prevent *Salmonella* poisoning, raw eggs and foods containing raw eggs should not be fed to infants.
- Infant cereal or other solids should not be added to human milk or formula in a bottle as it may put the infant at risk for choking and aspiration.
- To avoid burns to an infant's palate or face, formula or food warmed in a microwave should be shaken or stirred thoroughly, and the temperature tested, before serving.
- Avoid hard, small and round, smooth, and sticky solid foods, which may cause choking and aspiration.
- Avoid feeding an infant using a 'propped' bottle.
- Ensure that infants are always supervised during feeding.

33.2.4 Fruit juice

Infants may drink excessive amounts of fruit juice for a variety of reasons, including taste; however, juice overall plays a minimal role in providing nutrients to the infant or toddler. If juice consumption decreases the infant's appetite for solid foods, energy and nutrient intakes (e.g. fat, protein, calcium, vitamin D, iron, zinc) can be inadequate, leading to poor weight gain, nutrient deficiencies, and failure to thrive. While 100% pure juice can be a good source of vitamin C, it can also cause problems by displacing the intake of milk and whole foods, including fruits. It can also cause diarrhoea due to the osmotic effect of carbohydrates such as fructose and sorbitol. If juice is given, it should always be offered in a cup (not a bottle) and the amounts should not exceed 120 mL. Fruit drinks should be avoided.

33.2.5 Cow's milk

The use of unmodified cow's milk before 9–12 months of age is not recommended. In comparison with human milk and iron-fortified formula, cow's milk is higher in nutrients such as protein, calcium, phosphorus, sodium, and potassium and significantly lower in iron, zinc, ascorbic acid, and linoleic acid (Table 33.2). Nutrients in solid foods emphasize these excesses and deficiencies, so that infants fed cow's milk receive a higher renal solute load and are at greater risk of eating an unbalanced diet. In particular, the risk for iron depletion and iron-deficiency anaemia is higher because the iron content of cow's milk is low and not readily bioavailable, and its absorption may be impaired by the high concentrations of calcium and phosphorus and low concentration of ascorbic acid. In addition, intestinal loss of (blood) iron in the stool is associated with cow's milk-feeding in the first 6 months of life. Whole cow's milk (3.3% butterfat) continues to be recommended for the second year of life. Two per cent milk may be an acceptable alternative provided that the child is eating a variety of foods and growing at an acceptable rate; there is, however, a theoretical risk of growth faltering and essential fatty deficiency when partially skimmed milk provides a significant component of the infant's daily intake.

Cow's milk and diabetes The aetiology of type 1 diabetes appears to require both genetic predisposition to an autoimmune destructive process and exposure to environmental triggers. Several infant-feeding practices have been investigated as possible environmental factors for genetically predisposed individuals, including early exposure to cow's milk protein (or early termination of breastfeeding) and the timing of solids with a focus on gluten ingestion. The evidence supporting these specific foods as triggering antigens remains inconclusive. Modification of current infant-feeding practices to avoid the disease is not warranted.

33.2.6 Goat's milk

Pasteurized goat's milk is not an appropriate milk choice for infants before 9–12 months of age. Like cow's milk, it contains a high renal solute load with large amounts of sodium and protein. When goat's milk is used after this age, a product with added vitamin C, vitamin D, and folic acid should be chosen.

Table 33.2 Nutrient content of human milk, formula, and cow's milk (per litre)

Nutrient	Human milk mature	Formula			Cow's milk 3.3% fat
		Cow's milk[a]-based	Soy-based[b]	Follow-on[b]	
Energy (kcal)	680	670	670	670	640
Protein (g)	10	15	19	17	32
Fat (g)	39	36	37	33	36
Carbohydrate (g)	72	72	69	79	48
Sodium (mmol)	8	8	11	10	22
Potassium (mmol)	14	18	19	23	40
Chloride (mmol)	12	13	13	15	27
Vitamin D (µg)	<0.5	10	10	10	9[d]
Iron (mg)[c]	0.4	2.3/12	12	12	0.4

[a]Average value of seven brands.
[b]Average value of four brands.
[c]Non-fortified/iron-fortified.
[d]If fortified.

Infants who are allergic to cow's milk protein should not try goat's milk as they are also likely to have an allergic reaction to goat's milk. Unmodified (raw) goat's milk is never an appropriate feeding choice.

33.2.7 Other beverages and herbal teas

Soy, rice, and other vegetarian beverages, whether or not they are 'fortified', are inappropriate alternatives to breast milk or infant formula or to pasteurized whole cow's milk in the first 2 years. There are no minimum requirements for total fat or protein content of these products, and if used as a whole or major source of nutrition, they may result in malnourishment and failure to thrive. Herbal teas are of no known benefit to an infant and may be harmful; toxic effects of herbal teas have been reported in infants fed herbal tea, as well as breastfed infants whose mothers were drinking large amounts of herbal tea.

33.3 Common feeding-related problems

33.3.1 Food allergies

Adverse food reactions are divided into two general categories: food intolerance and food allergy. A true allergic reaction to a food involves the body's immune system. In the paediatric population, estimates of food allergy range from 1–8%, with the highest frequency in the first year of life. There is general agreement that the prevalence is increasing with time. The risk of developing food allergies is largely related to genetic predisposition and the age at which the food is introduced, with the chance of sensitization greatest in the first year of life. Young infants are especially prone because their immature intestinal system is more permeable to absorption of food allergens and lacks local immunity defences. Most allergens are proteins of large molecular size. Therefore, food allergy commonly presents in infancy with the intake of milk, egg, or peanuts. Along with soy, fish, nuts, and wheat, these foods are responsible for about 95% of food allergies in infants and toddlers.

The issue of preventing allergy is controversial. There is good evidence that when there is a family history of atopic disease, exclusive breastfeeding for at least 6 months decreases the risk of food allergy. It is no longer believed that maternal elimination diets during pregnancy and lactation play a role in decreasing the incidence of food allergies. Prebiotics and probiotics have also not proven to be effective in allergy prevention. There is no scientific evidence that anyone without a close family history of allergic disease should make changes to the normal introduction of solid foods. In at-risk infants, there is not agreement about the benefits of delaying introduction of, or the age at which to introduce, commonly allergenic foods. Avoidance of allergenic foods can postpone the development of allergic disease in individuals at risk, but not prevent it. Traditionally, parents have been advised to delay the introduction of allergenic foods such as peanuts and nuts until 1 year of age (Box 33.4). Management of food allergies involves strict avoidance of the allergenic food and requires careful reading of food labels to detect hidden sources. Sensitivity to many foods disappears within a few years; therefore, retesting and rechallenging with the offending food should occur at regular intervals in a controlled and supervised manner. Allergies to peanuts, nuts, fish, and seafood are the most severe and tend to be lifelong. Follow-up should take place particularly in the context of multiple allergies to ensure that infants ingest adequate macro- and micronutrients and achieve appropriate growth while on their elimination diet.

33.3.2 Allergy to cow's milk protein

Cow's milk protein is the most important trigger of food allergy in infancy, with estimations of prevalence ranging from 1 to 5%. If the child is formula fed, the decision of which formula to use should include consideration of the type of allergic reaction to cow's milk protein. Studies have revealed that 8–60% of milk-sensitive infants also react to soy. Although soy formulas are not hypoallergenic, they may be tolerated by infants with IgE-associated symptoms of cow's milk protein allergy (e.g. urticaria, wheezing, rhinitis, vomiting, eczema, anaphylaxis). In infants at high risk for allergy, identified by a strong family history of allergies, who are unable to be breastfed completely, there is no evidence that feeding with a soy formula compared with a cow's milk formula reduces allergies, whereas there is evidence that prolonged feeding with a hydrolysed formula compared with cow's milk formula reduces infant and childhood allergy including cow's milk protein allergy. Goat's milk has some similar antigens to cow's milk and is not recommended. Newer formulas with partially hydrolysed protein are less expensive and more palatable than the hypoallergenic hydrolysed formulas;

BOX 33.4 Strategies for reducing the incidence and severity of allergy in high-risk infants

- Exclusive breastfeeding until 6 months
- Use of protein hydrolysate formulas in at-risk non-breast-fed infants
- Delayed introduction of solids until at least 4 months, and preferably 6 months, especially for foods that are hyperallergenic

however, they contain a significant percentage (approximately 20%) of peptides in the allergenic range and therefore should not be used as treatment. The partially hydrolysed formulas have also not been shown to prevent milk allergy as much as extensively hydrolysed formulas. Rare reactions to extensively hydrolysed formulas have been reported in highly allergic infants who are then fed formulas based on free amino acids.

33.3.3 Lactose intolerance

The majority of adverse reactions to foods do not involve the immune system and are known as food intolerance. The most common food intolerance in humans is lactose intolerance, from lack of the lactase enzyme that normally splits lactose in the intestine. Congenital lactase deficiency is extremely rare, while primary lactase deficiency is very common in the general population due to a normal developmental decrease in lactase activity with increasing age. It is uncommon for infants under the age of 2 to have primary lactase deficiency, and, as a result, other conditions should be excluded prior to treatment. Certain ethnicities are more affected, including Blacks, Ashkenazi Jews, Chinese, and North American Aboriginal people. Lactose intolerance that develops in infants as a result of intestinal mucosal damage caused by infectious gastroenteritis, malnutrition, cow's milk protein enteropathy, coeliac disease, giardiasis, bacterial overgrowth, inflammatory bowel disease, or drugs is called secondary lactase deficiency. Common symptoms include gas, cramps, and diarrhoea. Diagnosis can be obtained by performing a non-invasive breath-hydrogen test in older children or through intestinal biopsies with enzyme activities; however, on a more practical level, diagnosis is confirmed clinically by a trial of a lactose-free diet. Infants under the age of 12 months with lactose intolerance should be changed from a cow's milk formula to either a lactose-free cow's milk formula or a soy formula. Infants beyond 9–12 months of age can be given cow's milk treated with β-galactosidase (LactAid) or a soy formula. Soy milks, even those fortified

with calcium and vitamin D, are inadequate in the first 1–2 years of life due to their low fat and energy content. Infants and children with primary lactase deficiency may be able to tolerate small amounts of lactose-containing foods such as yoghurt and cheese, particularly if taken in small amounts and spaced out. Special attention should be paid to ensure affected infants have an adequate calcium intake. Following secondary lactase deficiency, reintroduction of small amounts of lactose should be tried at regular intervals to return to a balanced diet as soon as possible.

33.3.4 Dietary management of acute diarrhoea

In developed countries, the typical infant with acute diarrhoea is well nourished, presents with mild to moderate dehydration, and has a viral-induced diarrhoea with low stool electrolyte losses. In developing countries, children with acute diarrhoea are more likely to be malnourished and severely dehydrated with a viral or bacterial-induced diarrhoea with high stool electrolyte losses. Oral rehydration therapy, which combines the use of oral electrolyte solutions with early refeeding, has proven to be safe and efficacious for restoring and maintaining hydration and electrolyte balance in infants with mild and moderate dehydration, including those with vomiting. Oral rehydration therapy has been shown to decrease childhood mortality from diarrhoeal diseases. Infants with severe dehydration should receive intravenous rehydration. Oral electrolyte solutions containing specific concentrations of carbohydrate, sodium, potassium, and chloride promote fluid and electrolyte absorption, whereas fluids such as juices, soft drinks, tea, jelly, or broth do not. Human milk is well tolerated during diarrhoea and may reduce its severity and duration; therefore, breastfeeding should continue throughout the diarrhoeal illness with additional fluids given as oral electrolyte solutions.

Early and rapid refeeding should occur as soon as rehydration is achieved and vomiting stops (ideally within 6–12 h of beginning treatment) as infants treated with oral rehydration therapy and early refeeding have reduced stool output, shorter duration of diarrhoea, and improved weight gain. Routine change to lactose-free or diluted feedings is unnecessary in well-nourished infants with mild to moderate gastroenteritis. Factors that appear to increase the risk of developing lactose intolerance include younger age, malnutrition, bacterial diarrhoea, prolonged diarrhoea before treatment, and a greater degree of dehydration on assessment. Infants and toddlers who were fed solid food before the onset of the diarrhoea should continue to receive their usual diet once rehydration occurs. The use of age-appropriate, nutrient-dense mixtures of common foods is recommended. These foods should be nutritious, easily digested and absorbed, and culturally acceptable, and should not have a deleterious effect on the illness. Although not based on strong science, starchy foods are generally well tolerated as the initial foods for refeeding. Use of a low-residue diet (commonly called the BRAT diet: bananas, rice, apple sauce or apple juice, and tea or toast) can theoretically worsen the clinical state as it supplies less than one-half of an infant's daily energy and protein needs.

Newer interventions for the control of diarrhoea Administration of certain strains of probiotic bacterium (e.g. *Lactobacillus* GG) can be given to patients with acute diarrhoea (regardless of the cause) with the intent of modifying intestinal flora. When given at the beginning of the illness, probiotics have been shown to be safe and to shorten recovery of acute diarrhoea managed by oral rehydration therapy and early refeeding. The probiotic may even decrease viral shedding.

In the context of malnourished children, it has been demonstrated that zinc supplements given during an episode of acute diarrhoea reduce the severity and duration of the episode and reduce the incidence of diarrhoea during the following 2–3 months. The WHO currently recommends 10–20 mg zinc/day for 10–14 days (10 mg for infants under 6 months of age) at the start of an episode of diarrhoea.

33.3.5 Constipation

There is wide variation in the stooling patterns of infants, ranging from a bowel movement after each feed to one every few days. Stool frequency and consistency are influenced by the infant's volume and type of feeding (e.g. human milk or formula, introduction of solid foods, and transition from puréed foods to table foods). Bowel frequency decreases with age as a result of the maturing gut's ability to conserve water. After 3–4 years of age, the frequency of bowel movements does not change. Breastfed and non-breastfed infants receiving an adequate diet are rarely constipated. Although an infant may appear to be straining, it is normal for an infant to grimace or have a red face when having a bowel movement. Educating parents about the wide variation in stooling patterns is important for avoiding overtreatment of normal stooling habits. Hard and painful bowel movements, abdominal distension, or blood in the stool may be signs of true constipation.

Approximately 90–97% of infants and children with constipation have idiopathic non-organic constipation, most often due to a conscious or unconscious decision to delay defecation after experiencing a painful or frightening evacuation (e.g. due to an anal fissure). This is known as *functional* constipation, or withholding constipation. Functional constipation is uncomfortable but not dangerous, and therefore is considered benign. An infant of less than 6 months who is believed to be truly constipated should be referred to a physician for investigation of organic causes. The earlier constipation occurs, the greater the chance of an underlying problem (e.g. Hirschsprung's disease). Common recommendations regarding therapy for constipation in infants are based on theory, not scientific evidence. Practices such as adding sugar or corn syrup to formula to cause osmotic diarrhoea, or increasing free fluid intake by giving additional water, are generally safe but without scientific support in the literature. Fruit juices such as prune, apple, and pear are also commonly suggested because of their high sorbitol content. However, there is no evidence to support the use of dietary factors to alleviate chronic constipation once stool withholding and stool retention have become a problem. In a small, select population of infants, chronic constipation can be a manifestation of intolerance or allergy to cow's milk. For children with constipation who do not respond to laxatives and dietary modifications, a trial of cow's milk elimination may be considered.

33.3.6 Infant obesity

With an increasing prevalence of preschool children who are overweight and obese, increased attention is being paid towards modifiable risk factors such as infant growth and feeding practices. The first protective risk factor is breastfeeding, which has a true effect even after correcting for relevant factors such as parental obesity, maternal smoking, and social class. Other infant risk factors that have been linked with obesity include being a large infant (weight for height) and prolonged bottle use. One study showed delayed introduction of solid foods was protective against obesity; a decade later, however, the timing of food introduction was earlier than present-day recommendations. In recent years much attention is being drawn to early rapid weight gain in the first few months and first year of life as a predictor of obesity in adolescence. While the issue of childhood obesity should not be oversimplified to focus solely on infant feeding, it does increase the awareness that obesity is a lifelong condition. Infants should never be overfed and attention should be paid to follow their cues of being full.

Fat intake Dietary fat modifications recommended for adults are not applicable to infants. In contrast, a high-fat diet (approximately 50% of energy from fat) helps to meet the infant's requirements for energy and fatty acids. Restricting dietary fat may lead to inadequate energy intake and jeopardize growth and development. There is no consistent evidence that use of a fat-reduced, cholesterol-lowering diet in infancy decreases the risk of atherosclerosis in adulthood.

33.3.7 Early childhood caries

The cause of extensive tooth decay in infants is multifactorial and should be considered a preventable infectious condition. Acids produced by bacteria (*Streptococcus mutans*) ferment dietary carbohydrate and attack the teeth, eventually causing demineralization and cavitation, particularly during sleep, when salivary secretions are decreased. Infection or severe tooth decay may warrant tooth extraction. One modifiable aspect of early childhood caries involves decreasing the amount (and frequency) of carbohydrate exposure, particularly sucrose. Feeding practices such as not putting an infant to bed with a bottle of milk or formula, avoiding the use of pacifiers dipped in sugar, syrup, or honey, avoiding bottle-feeding past 12 months of age, and limiting juice intake and other sugary items can all help in decreasing early caries. Bedtime bottles are unnecessary, but if used should contain only plain water.

Fluoride Fluoridation of the water supply has proven to be the most effective, cost-efficient means of preventing dental caries. In areas with low fluoride levels in the water source, fluoride supplements are recommended. The increased availability of fluoride (fluoridated water, foods, or drinks made with fluoridated water, toothpaste, mouthwashes, vitamin and fluoride supplements) has resulted in an increasing incidence of mild forms of dental fluorosis in both fluoridated and non-fluoridated communities. This is relevant to infants as the first year of life has been shown to be the most important period in the development of fluorosis. This sign of excess fluoride intake has led to modifications in fluoride recommendations, including later introduction and lower doses of fluoride supplements, and caution to parents of children to use small amounts and to discourage the swallowing of toothpaste. Mild dental fluorosis has not been shown to pose any health risks and, while there may be mild cosmetic effects, the teeth remain resistant to caries.

33.3.8 Vegetarianism

The past decade has seen an increased interest and acceptance of vegetarian diets. The focus has switched from questions about nutritional adequacy to studies demonstrating benefits for disease prevention. Whether the beneficial effects observed in adults take root in infants and toddlers raised on vegetarian diets has not been investigated.

Although the low saturated fat and high-fibre content of vegetarian diets offers advantages to the health of adults, their bulky nature and low energy density can restrict the amount of food energy that infants (with their limited stomach capacity and higher needs for accelerated growth) can consume. Vegetarian infants fed adequate amounts of breast milk or commercial infant formula and a balanced, varied diet grow similarly to non-vegetarian infants. However, the risk of nutritional deficiencies increases if the variety of foods making up the diet is very restrictive (e.g. macrobiotic, Rastafarian, fruitarian, raw diets) and/or if supplementation and medical supervision is avoided. Key nutrients include energy, protein, fibre, vitamin B_{12}, iron, vitamin D, calcium, zinc, and n-3 fatty acids. Because dietary practices among vegetarians are variable, assessment of dietary intake is important to determine whether fortified foods or supplements are needed to meet recommendations for individual nutrients.

Most vegetarians will continue breastfeeding well into the second year of life. Problems of nutritional inadequacy in the infant (e.g. vitamin B_{12})

are likely to occur if the mother's diet is very restricted, if prolonged breastfeeding is not supplemented around 6 months of age, or if infants are weaned prematurely on to an unsuitable breast-milk substitute. While some still advocate that infants should not be fed vegan diets, vegan infants who are weaned from the breast before 1 year of age should receive a commercial soy formula until 1–2 years of age.

In infants consuming a macrobiotic diet, a clear relationship has been demonstrated between diet, nutrient intake, and physical and biochemical evidence of deficiency for several nutrients, including iron, vitamin B_{12}, vitamin D, and riboflavin. Slower growth rates (peaking between 6 and 18 months), slower psychomotor development, and higher incidence of nutritional diseases such as rickets, kwashiorkor, and anaemia have been reported. Macrobiotic diets consist of unpolished rice, pulses, and vegetables with small additions of fermented foods, nuts, seeds, and fruits; animal products are generally not consumed but some types of fish may be accepted for occasional use. Even less restricted vegetarian diets typically have a high content of phytates and other modifiers of mineral (e.g. iron, zinc, calcium) absorption, which are associated with a higher prevalence of rickets and iron-deficiency anaemia.

33.4 Assessing nutritional adequacy

In general, it is assumed that an infant or toddler's nutritional status is normal, and nutritional needs are being met, if he or she has a normal rate of growth, drinks adequate amounts of breast milk (or suitable formula or milk for age), and eats a variety of age-appropriate foods from each of the food groups. When nutritional status or growth is questionable, the infant or toddler's intake should be evaluated in comparison with established standards such as growth charts and recommended nutrient intakes or allowances.

33.4.1 Energy and nutrient requirements

Due to their rapid rate of growth and higher metabolic rate, energy requirements for infants and toddlers are higher than at any other time of life. Recent studies have facilitated measurements of total energy expenditure of infants and toddlers. Evidence from these studies resulted in lower energy requirements than previously predicted, starting from 110 kcal/kg/day in the first month of life down to 80 kcal/kg/day at one year of age. During the second year of life, energy requirements stay stable on a per-kilogram basis but the overall amount of calories required does increase.

When an infant or toddler's energy requirements are met from a well-balanced diet the risk of other nutrient deficiencies is minimized. Intakes of individual nutrients that fall between 70% and 100% of recommended levels do not necessarily indicate a deficiency, as recommendations (with the exception of energy) are set at the mean requirement, plus two standard deviations, to ensure that the needs of almost all infants and toddlers are met.

33.4.2 Monitoring growth

Postnatal growth and development of the central nervous system are most rapid during the first year of life. The typical infant doubles his or her birth weight during the first 4–5 months, triples it in the first year, and quadruples it by 2 years of age, by which time a child has grown to half of their adult height. Plotting serial measurements of length-by-age and weight-by-length can be used to compare growth with normative values for healthy infants.

International in scope, the new WHO growth charts reflect the growth of children from six developed and developing countries around the world who were raised under favourable conditions for supporting optimal growth. Based on the growth pattern of breastfed infants, the charts now reflect current international guidelines for optimal feeding of infants and toddlers and, as such, are considered growth *standards,* rather than growth *references.*

In most children, height and weight measurements follow consistently along a channel (i.e. on or between the same centile(s)). Normal growth is indicated by weight-for-length and length-for-age tracking along similar percentiles or growth channels; however, it is common for infants to shift percentiles for both length and weight in the first 2–3 years of life, with the majority settling into a channel towards the 50th percentile (i.e. regression towards the mean), rather than away. When length-for-age and weight-for-length percentiles are disproportional or weight and/or height measurements are on a downward or upward trend, investigation of potential nutritional imbalances is indicated.

Summary

- Nutrition during infancy is an important determinant of overall health.
- Breastmilk is the only nutrition a healthy infant needs for the first six months and it carries many benefits over formula.
- The evidence for the importance of vitamin D in all infants and toddlers is growing.
- At six months, texture-appropriate foods should be introduced one at a time. Efforts should be made to choose iron-rich sources of food in order to prevent iron deficiency anaemia.
- By 9–12 months the infant can begin drinking whole cow's milk and should be eating a wide variety of foods.
- Adequate nutritional intake can be monitored by infant and toddler growth charts.

Further Reading

1. **No authors listed** (2009) Concerns for the use of soy-based formulas in infant nutrition. *Paediatr Child Health*, **14**, 109–18.
2. **Agostoni, C., Decsi, T., Fewtrell, M., *et al.*,** (2008) Complementary feeding: A commentary by the ESPGHAN Committee on Nutrition. *J Pediatr Gastroenterol Nutr*, **46**, 99–110.
3. **Agostoni, C., Braegger, C., Decsi, T., *et al.*** (2009) Breast-feeding: A commentary by the ESPGHAN Committee on Nutrition. *J Pediatr Gastroenterol Nutr*, **49**, 112–25.

4. **American Academy of Pediatrics** (2001) The use and misuse of fruit juice in pediatrics. *Pediatrics*, **107**, 1210–13.

5. **Basnet, S., Schneider, M., Gazit, A., *et al.*** (2010) Fresh goat's milk for infants: Myths and realities—a review. *Pediatrics*, **125**, e973–77.

6. **Butte, N.F.** (2005) Energy requirements of infants. *Public Health Nutr*, **8**, 953–67.

7. **Christie, L., Hine, R.J., Parker, J.G., *et al.*** (2002) Food allergies in children affect nutrient intake and growth. *J Am Diet Assoc*, **102**, 1648–51.

8. **Craig, W.J. and Mangels, A.R.** (2009) Position of the American Dietetic Association: Vegetarian diets. *J Am Diet Assoc*, **109**, 1266–82.

9. **Dietitians of Canada, Canadian Paediatric Society, The College of Family Physicians of Canada and Community, Health Nurses of Canada** (2010) *Promoting optimal monitoring of child growth in Canada: Using the new WHO growth charts. A collaborative public policy statement.* Toronto, Dietitians of Canada and Canadian Paediatric Society. http://www.dietitians.ca/growthcharts

10. **Gartner, L.M., Morton, J., Lawrence, R.A., *et al.*** (2005) Breastfeeding and the use of human milk. *Pediatrics*, **115**, 496–506.

11. **Halken, S., Hansen, K.S., Jacobsen, H.P., *et al.*** (2000) Comparison of a partially hydrolyzed infant formula with two extensively hydrolyzed formulas for allergy prevention: A prospective, randomized study. *Pediatr Allergy Immunol*, **11**, 149–61.

12. **Heine, R.G. and Tang, M.L.** (2008) Dietary approaches to the prevention of food allergy. *Curr Opin Clin Nutr Metab Care*, **11**, 320–8.

13. **Heyman, M.B.** (2006) Lactose intolerance in infants, children, and adolescents. *Pediatrics*, **118**, 1279.

14. **Ismail, A.I. and Hasson, H.** (2008) Fluoride supplements, dental caries and fluorosis: A systematic review. *J Am Dent Assoc*, **139**, 1457–68.

15. **Joeckel, R.J. and Phillips, S.K.** (2009) Overview of infant and pediatric formulas. *Nutr Clin Pract*, **24**, 356–62.

16. **King, C.K., Glass, R., Bresee, J.S., *et al.*** (2003) Managing acute gastroenteritis among children: Oral rehydration, maintenance, and nutritional therapy. *MMWR Recomm Rep*, **52**, 1–16.

17. **Loening-Baucke, V.** (2005) Prevalence, symptoms and outcome of constipation in infants and toddlers. *J Pediatr*, **146**, 359–63.

18. **Lozoff, B., De Andraca, I., Castillo, M., *et al.* T.,** (2003) Behavioral and developmental effects of preventing iron-deficiency anemia in healthy full-term infants. *Pediatrics*, **112**, 846–54.

19. **North American Society for Pediatric Gastroenterology, Hepatology and Nutrition.** (2006) Evaluation and treatment of constipation in infants and children. *J Pediatr Gastroenterol Nutr*, **43**, e1–13.

20. **Oddy, W.H.** (2009) The long-term effects of breastfeeding on asthma and atopic disease. *Adv Exp Med Biol*, **639**, 237–51.

21. **Owen, C.G., Martin, R.M., Whincup, P.H., *et al.*** (2005) Effect of infant feeding on the risk of obesity across the life course: A quantitative review of published evidence. *Pediatrics*, **115**, 1367–77.

22. **Rao, S., Srinivasjois, R., and Patole, S.** (2009) Prebiotic supplementation in full-term neonates: A systematic review of randomized controlled trials. *Arch Pediatr Adolesc Med*, **163**, 755–64.

23. **Sandhu, B.K.** (2001) Practical guidelines for the management of gastroenteritis in children. *J Pediatr Gastroenterol Nutr*, **33** Suppl 2, S36–9.

24. **Seach, K.A., Dharmage, S.C., Lowe, A.J., *et al.*** (2010) Delayed introduction of solid feeding reduces child overweight and obesity at 10 years. *Int J Obes (Lond)*, **34**, 1475–9.

25. **Simmer, K., Patole, S.K., and Rao, S.C.** (2008) Longchain polyunsaturated fatty acid supplementation in infants born at term. *Cochrane Database Syst Rev* (**1**), CD000376.

26. **Simpson, M.D. and Norris, J.M.** (2008) Mucosal immunity and type 1 diabetes: Looking at the horizon beyond cow's milk. *Pediatr Diabetes*, **9**, 431–3.

27. **Singhal, A. and Lucas, A.** (2004) Early origins of cardiovascular disease: Is there a unifying hypothesis? *Lancet*, **363**, 1642–5.

28. The use of fluoride in infants and children. (2002) *Paediatr Child Health*, **7**, 569–82.

29. **Trumbo, P., Schlicker, S., Yates, A.A., et al.** (2002) Dietary reference intakes for energy, carbohydrate, fiber, fat, fatty acids, cholesterol, protein and amino acids. *J Am Diet Assoc*, **102**, 1621–30.

30. **Van Niel, C.W., Feudtner, C., Garrison, M.M., et al.** (2002) Lactobacillus therapy for acute infectious diarrhea in children: A meta-analysis. *Pediatrics*, **109**, 678–84.

31. **Wagner, C.L. and Greer, F.R.** (2008) Prevention of rickets and vitamin D deficiency in infants, children, and adolescents. *Pediatrics*, **122**, 1142–52.

32. **World Health Organization**. (2008) *HIV transmission through breastfeeding: A review of available evidence—2007 update.* http://www.who.int/nutrition/publications/hivaids/9789241596596/en/index.html

Useful Websites

To see topical and scientifically robust updates on nutrition associated with this textbook and web links to many of the journals in the Further Reading sections, please see the dedicated Online Resource Centre at **http://www.oxfordtextbooks.co.uk/orc/mann4e/**

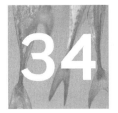

34 Childhood and adolescent nutrition

Anne-Louise Heath and Rachael Taylor

Introduction

Childhood and adolescence are periods of rapid growth, learning, and development. Nutritional needs are high and differ in many respects from those of adults. Ensuring adequate food intake remains the challenge for many of the world's children. In contrast, for most children in the developed world, making more appropriate food choices and maintaining healthy eating habits is paramount. Most of this chapter refers to both childhood (age 2–12 years), and adolescence (age 13–18 years). The final section (34.8) covers issues that predominantly relate to adolescents.

34.1 Dietary recommendations

Dietary recommendations for children and adolescents are expressed in two very different but complementary formats: dietary guidelines (providing advice on food intake and related behaviours in a way that is accessible to members of the general public), and nutrient intake values (levels of nutrient intake calculated to minimize the risk of deficiency or disease).

Ideally, each country should develop its own dietary guidelines to ensure that the food- and nutrient-related health concerns of the country are addressed in the context of customary dietary patterns. However, the dietary guidelines for children shown in Table 34.1 are fairly typical.

Nutrient intake values such as dietary reference intakes (in Canada and the USA), dietary reference

Table 34.1 Dietary guidelines for children and adolescents in Australia

Encourage and support breastfeeding
Children and adolescents need sufficient nutritious foods to grow and develop normally
• Growth should be checked regularly for young children
• Physical activity is important for all children and adolescents
Enjoy a wide variety of nutritious foods
Children and adolescents should be encouraged to:
• Eat plenty of vegetables, legumes, and fruits
• Eat plenty of cereals (including breads, rice, pasta, and noodles), preferably wholegrain
• Include lean meat, fish, poultry, and/or alternatives
• Include milks, yoghurts, cheese, and/or alternatives
– Reduced-fat milks are not suitable for young children under 2 years, because of their high energy needs, but reduced-fat varieties should be encouraged for older children and adolescents
• Choose water as a drink
– Alcohol is not recommended for children
and care should be taken to:
• Limit saturated fat and moderate total fat intake
– Low-fat diets are not suitable for infants
• Choose foods low in salt
• Consume only moderate amounts of sugars and foods containing added sugars
Care for your child's food: prepare and store it safely

values (in the UK), and nutrient reference values (in Australia and New Zealand) provide specific information on nutrient requirements and safe upper limits of intake. Nutrient requirements alter so rapidly during childhood and adolescence that three age bands are usually reported for children (1–3 years, 4–8 years, 9–13 years), and one for adolescents (14–18 years). A typical set of nutrient intake values is shown in Table 34.2.

34.2 Growth

34.2.1 Growth and body composition

The rapid growth period of infancy sees a tripling of birth weight during the first year, growth then slows during childhood, and is relatively consistent and predictable, with annual increments typically ranging from 6–7 cm in height and 2–3 kg in weight. Body proportions also change over this time, from that in infancy, where the head and trunk predominate, to a more adult profile resulting from considerable

Table 34.2 Dietary reference intakes for children and adolescents

Nutrient	Age group (years) and gender					
	Children		Boys		Girls	
	1–3	4–8	9–13	14–18	9–13	14–18
Protein (g/day)						
EAR	10	15	27	45	28	38
RDA	13	19	34	52	34	46
Calcium (mg/day)						
EAR	500	800	1100	1100	1100	1100
RDA	700	1000	1300	1300	1300	1300
Iron (mg/day)						
EAR	3.0	4.1	5.9	7.7	5.7	7.9
RDA	7	10	8	11	8	15
Vitamin C (mg/day)						
EAR	13	22	39	63	39	56
RDA	15	25	45	75	45	65
Vitamin A (μg/day)						
EAR	210	275	445	630	420	485
RDA	300	400	600	900	600	700

EAR, estimated average requirement; RDA, recommended dietary allowance.

Source: Dietary reference intake documents prepared for the USA and Canada by the Food and Nutrition Board and Institute of Medicine (2000, 2001, 2002) available at http://www.nap.edu. Calcium values are from the revised 2010 report.

lengthening of the limbs and a reduction in the size of the head relative to the rest of the body. The onset of puberty signals a second accelerated phase in growth, typically lasting 2 or so years, with a younger onset in females. Although the age of onset can vary considerably (Fig. 34.1), males typically gain around 20 kg of weight and 20 cm in height and females 16 kg and 16 cm.

Marked age and sex differences in body composition are apparent between birth and the end of adolescence. Children are relatively lean at birth (approximately 15% body fat), but increase steadily in adiposity during the first year of life. Adiposity tends to decline during the preschool years and reach a nadir at approximately 5–6 years of age,

before increasing again through later childhood. This phenomenon is known as the adiposity rebound (AR) and has received considerable attention over recent years as a potential 'critical period' in the development of childhood obesity. Children who undergo AR at an early age are more likely to be overweight in later adolescence and early adulthood. During adolescence, males gain approximately twice as much lean tissue as females, with a rapid acceleration during the peak growth spurt and much smaller increments in body fat. By contrast, gains in lean tissue mass appear more consistent during growth in females and body fat continues to be laid down until late adolescence/early adulthood.

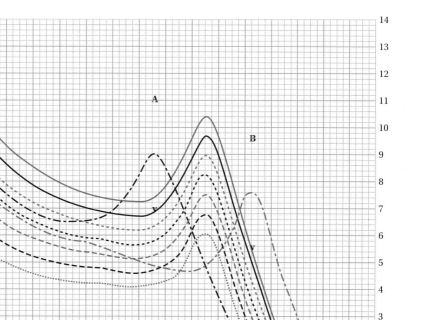

Fig. 34.1 Height velocity for girls. The outlying peaks are an early (A) and a late (B) maturer.

Source: Tanner, J., and Davis, P.S.W. (1985) Clinical longitudinal standards for height and weight velocity for North American children. *J Pediatr*, **107**, 317–29.

34.2.2 Assessment of growth and body composition

An accurate record of growth remains one of the most useful tools for the assessment of both under- and overnutrition. Serial measurements at multiple time points reveal more information about a child's health than single measurements because of individual variation in growth and development. Anthropometric indices such as height and weight can most usefully be interpreted by plotting them on reference growth charts. These provide a reference for an individual child's growth, rather than the absolute standard that each child should achieve. The most commonly used are the Centers for Disease Control and Prevention (CDC) 2000 growth charts (http://www.cdc.gov/growthcharts) which are based on breast-fed and formula-fed American children (Fig. 34.2).

Given known differences in growth between breast-fed and formula-fed infants, the World Health Organization (WHO) published the WHO Child Growth Standards (http://www.who.int/childgrowth/en/) in 2006, created from the Multicentre Growth Reference Study which followed approximately 8500 breast-fed infants from widely different ethnic backgrounds and cultural settings from birth to 5 years. These are expressed (separately) both as centiles and as Z scores (see Chapter 31).

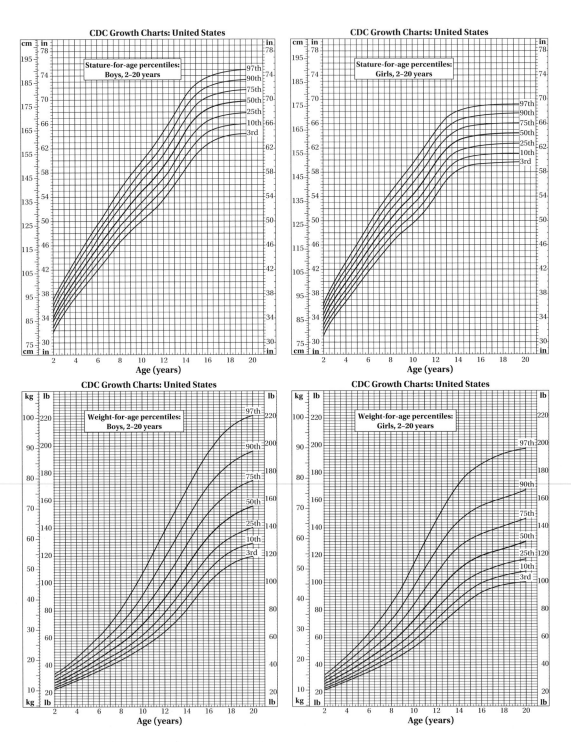

Fig. 34.2 CDC growth charts for boys and girls aged 2–20 years: stature (height) for age and weight for age, with percentile lines.

Source: National Centre for Health Statistics (NCHS)/National Center for Chronic Disease Prevention and Health Promotion (CDC), USA (2000).

> **BOX 34.1** Measuring the child's growth
>
> 1 Regular measurement of weight is the best way of assessing undernutrition or obesity.
> 2 Growth reference charts for use should be based on current CDC or WHO charts.
> 3 Growth trends give more information than one measurement.
> 4 A child who is approximately the same percentile for height and weight and whose height and weight track over time is unlikely to have a serious nutrition or chronic health problem.
> 5 A child crossing the 90th or 10th percentiles should be assessed.
> 6 Referral for growth hormone treatment should only be made if the child is consistently below the 3rd percentile and there is no other cause to be found.
> 7 Dietary guidelines provide advice on consuming a healthy, varied diet that will enable the nutrient reference values to be met.

Although the accurate assessment of body composition (fat and fat-free masses) (see Chapter 31) provides considerable additional information about the health and wellbeing of a child, in most instances the use of anthropometry (height, weight, body circumferences, and skinfold thicknesses) remains the most commonly used way to monitor growth (Box 34.1).

34.3 Undernutrition/failure to thrive

Failure to thrive occurs when a child of normal height and head circumference has a weight-for-age below the 3rd percentile (or a Z-score of minus 2). As well as this absolute definition, a child who was previously growing well who stops growing and drops through several percentile lines should also be included in this group. In developing countries, the same children are usually called 'undernourished'.

In the developed world about half of the cases are due to non-organic causes, including psychosocial problems in carers (e.g. depression) or simply an inadequate diet due to lack of knowledge, neglect, or a very restrictive dietary regime. Organic causes of failure to thrive are numerous and include chronic renal, cardiorespiratory, and endocrine diseases. Gastrointestinal causes include coeliac disease, cystic fibrosis, and Hirschsprung's disease.

More than half of the children diagnosed as 'failure to thrive' in primary care have a relatively simple nutrition problem—not enough food to meet their needs. For example, a child may be thought to have an 'allergy' and may have been placed on a very restrictive diet, or because the adults in the families are placed on a low-fat diet, the child may also be eating the same diet. Many chronic diseases cause growth retardation. In the absence of other symptoms or signs, it is usually appropriate to undertake a trial of improved nutrition rather than going immediately to further investigation. Referral for investigation of growth hormone deficiency is not necessary unless the child is consistently below the lowest percentile line and no other disease is present.

Children may develop food fads and be described by their parents as 'difficult eaters'. Prevention depends on the whole family eating a healthy diet and the children naturally falling into a pattern of good nutrition. The use of food, snacks, and sweets in reward and punishment systems for inappropriate behaviour may lead to poor eating habits.

34.4 Childhood overweight and obesity

34.4.1 Prevalence and health effects

Overweight or obesity in childhood is generally defined as having a body mass index (BMI) value greater than certain age- and sex-specific reference standards, typically the 85th and 95th percentiles, respectively. The CDC and WHO growth standards (see Section 34.2.2) are widely used. In 2000, Cole *et al.* published BMI criteria for defining overweight and obesity in children and adolescents created from a dataset of children from six countries (Brazil, Great Britain, Hong Kong, the Netherlands, Singapore, and the USA); the criteria are often referred to as the International Obesity Taskforce (IOTF) cutoffs. These BMI values were created from determining the percentiles corresponding to a BMI of 25 kg/m^2 (overweight) and 30 kg/m^2 (obesity) at 18 years of age. Use of the IOTF cutoffs (Table 34.3) is advantageous for international comparisons of the prevalence of overweight and obesity. However, the CDC or WHO growth charts are more useful for tracking weight status in individual children over time, as exact percentiles or Z-scores can be calculated.

In most developed countries, childhood overweight and obesity represents a major health issue, with national estimates indicating that 25–40% of children are heavier than is desired for their health. Much of the recent focus has been on the rapid increase in prevalence that has been observed in many countries. Recent data, however, offer promise that these increases in prevalence appear to be abating, at least in some countries. Regardless of the trends over time, the fact remains that too many of our children are carrying excess body weight, with resultant implications for health. In young children, this translates to deleterious effects on psychosocial health in terms of bullying and impaired self-esteem, and the increased risk of transition to an overweight state as an adult, with all the accompanying health effects. In older children and adolescents, other physical health risks become more apparent including, but not limited to, an increased risk of type 2 diabetes, high blood pressure, high cholesterol, and bone and joint problems, especially fractures of the forearm.

34.4.2 Causes

Obesity is a result of excessive food intake in relation to energy requirements, and may arise due to

Table 34.3 Body mass index levels (kg/m^2) to diagnose overweight and obesity in children

Age (years)	Overweight		Obesity	
	Boys	Girls	Boys	Girls
2	18.41	18.02	20.09	19.81
3	17.89	17.56	19.57	19.36
4	17.55	17.28	19.29	19.15
5	17.42	17.15	19.30	19.17
6	17.55	17.34	19.78	19.65
7	17.92	17.75	20.63	20.51
8	18.44	18.35	21.60	21.57
9	19.10	19.07	22.77	22.81
10	19.84	19.86	24.00	24.11
11	20.55	20.74	25.10	25.42
12	21.22	21.68	26.02	26.67
13	21.91	22.58	26.84	27.76
14	22.62	23.34	27.63	28.57
15	23.29	23.94	28.30	29.11
16	23.90	24.37	28.88	29.43
17	24.46	24.70	29.41	29.69
18	25	25	30	30

Source: Adapted from Cole, T.J., Bellizzi, M.C., Flegal, K.M., *et al.* (2000) Establishing a standard definition for child overweight and obesity worldwide: International survey. *BMJ*, **320**, 1240–3.

imbalance from either (or both) sides of the energy balance equation. Genetics also plays a major role in determining weight, and susceptibility to weight gain, although very few cases of obesity are a result of an endocrine disorder, chromosomal abnormality, or genetic disorder. Children in affluent countries live in an 'obesogenic' environment, which discourages physical activity and promotes the consumption of nutrient-poor energy-dense foods.

Dietary factors While there is general acceptance that a high consumption of energy-dense foods is an important cause of obesity, there is little certainty regarding the role of individual foods, drinks, or nutrients. High intakes of sugar-sweetened beverages has been fairly consistently shown to be associated with increased weight or weight gain in children. However, the few randomized controlled trials in which advice to reduce intake of such drinks has been the key intervention have not provided convincing evidence of benefit, perhaps because of poor compliance. 'Fast foods' and 'snack foods' have also been implicated but the fact that most such foods are high in sugars and fats and therefore energy-dense, is the most likely explanation for their contribution to an energy intake which exceeds output.

Activity factors The extent to which physical activity has reduced in recent years and thus contributed to the 'epidemic' of childhood obesity is uncertain. However, a number of studies have shown a fairly strong association between television viewing and excess body weight accumulation in young children. This might result, as much if not more, from consumption of energy-dense snack or fast foods while watching television as from lost opportunities for physical activity during prolonged periods of inactivity. The use of computers, computer games, and labour-saving devices and reduction of the use of active transport and school-based physical education are other examples of the obesity-promoting environment which characterize Western and some other affluent societies.

Other behaviour factors Poor sleeping habits have been related to excessive weight gain, especially in young children. This might simply be due to having more opportunities to eat or less time for exercise but changes in several hormones (including cortisol, ghrelin, leptin, and growth hormones) involved in body weight regulation have been observed, suggesting the possibility of more complex mechanisms. Family environment, role modelling, and parental support are also considered as potential determinants of excessive weight gain. Some of the behavioural and societal factors which have been implicated in the development of childhood obesity are listed in Table 34.4.

34.4.3 Prevention and treatment of overweight and obesity

Changes in the obesogenic environment are essential if the prevalence of overweight and

Table 34. 4 Behavioural and societal factors implicated in the development of childhood obesity

Larger portion sizes	Television viewing
Sweetened beverages	Computer use
Fast foods	Video games
Inappropriate snack choices	Labour-saving devices
Food advertising	Built environment
Skipping breakfast	Community access to resources
Reduced sleep	Declines in active transport (cycling or walking to school)
Family environment	Reduced physical education in schools
Parenting styles	Less school recess time
Poverty	Parental work commitments

obesity in children and adolescents is to be reduced (see Chapter 17). This will not be achieved without commitment from relevant opinion leaders and policy makers including governments, local and education authorities, media, food industries, and health professionals. Voluntary as well as legislative measures are required. Abolition or limiting of television advertisements promoting inappropriate foods to children, provision of opportunities for physical activity, and increasing availability of affordable healthy food choices are but three of the many measures which require implementation.

Treating overweight children should in theory be relatively straightforward, since only small changes to eating and/or activity behaviour should be required for most overweight children to successfully reduce their weight over time, given that the energy imbalance is relatively small on a daily basis. Such children need to 'grow into'

their weight by restoring the rate of excessive weight gain to a more appropriate level while maintaining linear growth. The fact that so many children are now overweight or obese and that the health consequences are generally not immediately apparent have led to parents often failing to recognize overweight in their children. Furthermore, health professionals finding it difficult to initiate appropriate management, which principally involves the promotion of physical activity and appropriate food choices. For children who are obese, the level of intervention will depend upon severity and duration of obesity. Some form of behavioural theory, including expert dietary advice, given within the context of the family environment is usually regarded as an essential component (see Chapter 38). Management of the overweight and obese child is made all the more difficult by the existence of the obesity-promoting environment.

34.5 Some critical micronutrients

34.5.1 Iron

In adults, iron status reflects the balance between iron losses and iron intake.

In children, iron intakes also need to be sufficient to support growth. In addition to their increased requirements for growth, adolescent girls need to absorb 0.45 mg of iron a day to cover menstrual losses once they reach menarche. This is equivalent to approximately 2.5 mg a day of additional dietary iron. Some girls will require considerably more than this as losses can be three times higher than the median. The age at which this increased requirement starts varies from child to child.

Although the iron status of school-age children is usually adequate, 4% of preschool children in the 2003–06 US National Health and Nutrition Examination Survey (NHANES) were iron-deficient.

In the UK and the USA, there are higher rates of iron deficiency amongst the poor, immigrants, and non-Caucasian populations. The rates of iron deficiency are much higher for adolescent girls, with NHANES 2003–06 estimating that 9–16% of girls aged 12 to 19 years are iron-deficient. Approximately 4% of adolescent girls have the severe form of iron deficiency—iron deficiency anaemia.

Iron deficiency anaemia is associated with poorer mental, motor, and behavioural development in young children, and fatigue and poorer cognitive function (especially verbal learning and memory) in adolescents. The effects of non-anaemic iron deficiency are less clear, but probably include subtle negative effects on cognitive function and fatigue. It is important that non-anaemic iron deficiency is treated, because it increases the risk of developing iron deficiency anaemia with rapid growth or onset of menstruation.

Dietary measures may play a role in preventing and treating non-anaemic iron deficiency, although supplementation is required to treat iron deficiency anaemia. Red meat, a rich source of haem iron, is an effective way to boost intake, noting that processed food such as sausages contain much less iron than meat such as lean meat. Beans, peas, lentils, and iron-fortified foods are useful sources of non-haem iron. Absorption of non-haem iron is enhanced by ascorbic acid found in many fresh fruits and vegetables and a yet-to-be identified factor (MFP factor) in meat, fish, and poultry. Phytates and polyphenols (including tannins) are inhibitors of non-haem iron absorption. Wholegrains, nuts, and legumes are sources of phytates but valuable sources of many nutrients. Wholemeal products which are leavened with yeast (e.g. wholemeal bread) and legumes soaked with water discarded before cooking have less phytate. Tea and coffee, rich sources of tannins, should be discouraged. If dietary measures are unable to achieve satisfactory iron status, iron supplements may be necessary.

Iron deficiency and its prevention and treatment are covered more fully in Chapter 10.

34.5.2 Vitamin D

Although severe vitamin D deficiency is now uncommon amongst children in relatively affluent countries such as the UK, Europe, USA, Australia, and New Zealand, clinicians have recently reported a concerning increase in the number of cases of rickets, particularly amongst children with darker skin and from cultures in which the skin is kept covered. Rickets is described in Chapter 15. It has also become apparent that less severe vitamin D insufficiency is common amongst children and adolescents, even in countries such as the USA that have widespread fortification programmes in place. In the US NHANES 2000–04, suboptimal serum 25-hydroxyvitamin D concentrations (defined as serum <50 nmol/L) were present in almost 10% of preschoolers and more than 30% of adolescent girls. Interestingly, supplementation trials in unselected

adolescent girls in Lebanon and Finland both reported increased bone mineral density on supplementation with vitamin D even in the absence of rickets. There is some evidence to suggest that low vitamin D status also increases susceptibility to infection and increases the risk of type 1 diabetes; however, these effects have only been investigated in observational studies to date.

Factors that increase the risk of vitamin D deficiency in children and adolescents include darker skin pigmentation (children with dark skin pigmentation may need 5–10 times longer in the sun to generate the same amount of vitamin D), lack of sunlight exposure (including use of sunscreen or concealing clothing), obesity, and clinical conditions resulting in fat malabsorption (e.g. cystic fibrosis) or requiring medication that alters vitamin D metabolism (e.g. anticonvulsants).

A number of foods including milk, margarine, and juice are fortified with vitamin D in the USA, but children and adolescents would need to consume 1 L of milk a day to get the 400 IU currently recommended by the American Academy of Paediatrics. The alternative is daily supplementation with vitamin D, but given the large numbers of people of all ages who have low vitamin D status, a more sustainable solution that is less reliant on individual compliance may be needed should it be determined that the year-round vitamin D status of the population is suboptimal for health.

34.5.3 Iodine

Although severe iodine deficiency is principally seen in the developing world, lesser degrees of iodine deficiency sufficient to influence aspects of cognition have been reported in a number of European countries, Australia, and New Zealand. The problem was believed to have improved with the introduction of iodized salt, but it appears to have recurred at least in some countries to the extent that iodine fortification has been proposed. Iodine is discussed in Chapter 11.

34.6 Other matters related to diet

34.6.1 Dental caries

Dental caries (tooth decay) is the second most common infectious disease after the common cold and is one of the more expensive diet-related health problems. It is also preventable. In the USA, by the age of 5–9 years, more than half of children have had at least one cavity or filling, and by 17 years of age, 78% have had tooth decay. The consequences include pain and infections.

Dental decay is an interaction between three factors: sugars, oral bacteria, and the tooth. Sugars (glucose and fructose, as well as sucrose) are fermented by oral bacteria (particularly *Streptococcus mutans*) that produce acids which demineralize the enamel and may eventually break down the tooth. All three factors are required for dental decay, although in treating and preventing dental caries, multiple strategies are likely to be more successful than attempting to eliminate any one single factor.

It is the frequency of exposure to sugars, rather than the amount of sugar that predicts caries risk. In practice, this means that:

- Sugars can be consumed with meals (especially if children are encouraged to brush their teeth afterwards), but should not be consumed between meals.

- Sticky carbohydrate foods (such as hard sweets, muesli bars, fruit roll-ups, honey, and even dried fruit such as raisins) are particularly bad for teeth because they remain on the tooth surface for longer.

- Children should be encouraged to drink plain water rather than sugar-containing beverages (including fruit juice and sports and energy drinks). The practice of using sugar-containing beverages to settle children to sleep at night is particularly risky because the beverage bathes the teeth for a prolonged period—at a time when production of protective saliva is low.

The sugars contained in the cellular structure of foods (such as the intrinsic sugars of fresh fruits and vegetables) have little cariogenic potential so these are good food choices for snacks.

Bacterial numbers are controlled by twice-daily tooth brushing with a fluoride toothpaste (supervised by an adult until the child is at least 8–9 years of age). Fluoride in the saliva of children who consume fluoridated water or supplements inhibits bacterial growth and the enamel is made more resistant to decay by ingestion of fluoride. In many countries, fluoridation of water supplies and the use of fluoridated toothpaste have resulted in dramatic declines in average levels of dental decay (see Section 11.5).

34.6.2 Food allergies and intolerances

Food allergy in the narrow, technical sense is an abnormal reaction to a food by a mechanism that involves a specific immunoglobulin E in the plasma.

The most common food allergies in young children are to cow's milk, eggs, peanuts, tree nuts, sesame seeds, soy, and wheat. Peanuts, tree nuts, and shellfish are the foods most commonly associated with life-threatening anaphylaxis. Most children who are allergic to cow's milk, soy, wheat, or eggs have grown out of their food allergy by the time they are 5 years of age.

Symptoms of food allergy include hives (urticaria) and/or swelling around the mouth, vomiting, cough, wheeze, a runny or blocked nose, stomach pains, or diarrhoea. Food allergy may also result in gastro-esophageal reflux and eczema.

The three most widely accepted tests used to confirm or exclude potential food triggers are: skin prick allergy tests, blood tests for immunoglobulin E (IgE) specific to the allergen (RAST), and a closely supervised temporary elimination diet followed by food challenges with the suspected food. Currently, it is considered that food allergies are best managed by identifying and avoiding the food.

A *food intolerance* is a reaction to a food that does not involve immunoglobulins (e.g. urticaria in response to consumption of certain food additives such as tartrazine). Other adverse reactions to food (i.e. reactions other than allergy and food intolerance) include wind and diarrhoea in response to milk in children who have lactase insufficiency; and coeliac disease, an autoimmune enteropathy triggered by sensitivity to wheat gluten.

Diagnosis of food intolerance and other non-immune adverse food reactions is usually based on clinical history and response to removal of the food from the diet, although in some cases a strictly supervised temporary elimination diet followed by food challenges is also used diagnostically.

It is important to avoid unorthodox testing and treatments that can be expensive, and harmful if they delay effective treatment or result in a nutritionally inadequate diet (either because major foods such as milk or wheat have been removed from the diet without appropriate replacement, or because the diet becomes so unpalatable that the child's energy intake is compromised).

34.6.3 Vegetarianism and meat avoidance

There are many different types of vegetarianism, but most vegetarians are either lacto-ovo-vegetarian (avoid meat, poultry, and fish but consume dairy products and eggs) or, less commonly, vegan (no animal products are consumed). Some children are raised as vegetarians within vegetarian families, but many more become vegetarian through personal choice, particularly during adolescence. Reasons for becoming vegetarian include concerns about animal exploitation, the environment, and health. However, adolescents with disordered attitudes to eating may use vegetarianism as a socially acceptable way to restrict their food intake. Many more children and adolescents are meat reducers, consuming small amounts of meat (or poultry or fish only)

infrequently, and presumably experiencing health benefits and risks that are intermediate between those of vegetarians and non-vegetarians.

In 2005, 4% of 8–18-year-old US children described themselves as vegetarian or vegan, but this masks what are likely to be higher rates in certain sectors of the population, particularly amongst teenage girls. In the UK, approximately 10% of girls aged 15–18 years describe themselves as vegetarian or vegan.

The nutrient of greatest concern in vegetarian diets is vitamin B_{12}, particularly for vegans who have no natural sources of the vitamin in their diets (foods such as spirulina contain inactive analogues). It is essential, therefore, that vegan children and adolescents either use foods fortified with vitamin B_{12}, or take vitamin B_{12} supplements. Recommended iron intakes are 80% higher for vegetarians; however, studies in adults suggest that while vegetarians have lower iron stores, they do not have a higher risk of iron deficiency anaemia than their non-vegetarian counterparts, perhaps in part because they tend to have higher total iron intakes. Zinc may also be a concern, particularly because of the high phytate content of foods traditionally consumed by vegetarians such as legumes, nuts, and wholegrain cereals. In the past there was some concern that protein intakes might be inadequate in diets that avoided meat, but it is now known that as long as a variety of protein-containing foods are consumed each day, and energy intake is sufficient, protein needs are easily met.

Vegetarian diets are associated with a number of potential benefits. In particular, vegetarians tend to have a healthier body mass index, their saturated fat intake can be lower (as long as meat is not replaced with high-fat dairy products such as cheese), they have a higher fibre intake, and fruit and vegetable intake tends to be greater. They have been noted to have lower cholesterol and blood pressure levels than nonvegetarians and in the long term, vegetarianism is associated with a lower risk of death from ischaemic heart disease. It is uncertain whether these health benefits are due to meat avoidance or the other potentially health-promoting attributes of the diets of most vegetarians.

A vegetarian dietary pattern is certainly consistent with good health in children and adolescents provided it is well planned so that it includes a wide variety of nutritious foods. Some young people remove meat from their diet without ensuring appropriate replacements.

34.7 Developing countries

34.7.1 Introduction

Even in a country that is poor, poverty is not experienced equally across all members of the population. It may not be experienced equally within a family—it is common for children and women to have more limited access to resources, including food, than men. Growing up in a developing country may mean that there is less food and that the nutritional quality of the food is lower. In many cases access to clean water, health care, education, and good sanitation is limited or absent. These factors all have an impact on access to food and on nutritional status.

In 2005–07, 830 million people in developing countries, many of them children, were estimated by WHO to be undernourished and with the recent economic crisis, the rate may exceed 1 billion in 2009. Young children are particularly vulnerable, so that one in four children under the age of 5 is underweight, i.e. 146 million children in developing countries. Childhood undernutrition increases mortality such that it has been estimated that 60% of childhood deaths in developing countries are associated with malnutrition. Malnutrition stunts physical growth, increases the risk of infections (gastroenteritis, pneumonia, tuberculosis) and of serious obstetric complications. Malnourished children are less able to benefit from education, hence there is lower economic productivity, and slowed socioeconomic development.

In developing countries, and poor communities in other countries, childhood malnutrition is due to a complex interaction of factors including insufficient or poor quality food and poor sanitation and health services leading to an increased risk of infection (Fig. 34.3).

Children may not get sufficient food because of: crop failure; conflict which makes it unsafe to plant, tend, or harvest the crops; and, in some cases, poor care and feeding practices. Displacement because of natural disasters such as drought, or conflict and persecution also affects the lives of millions of children (see Chapter 20). The classic protein-energy malnutrition conditions marasmus and kwashiorkor are discussed in Chapter 19.

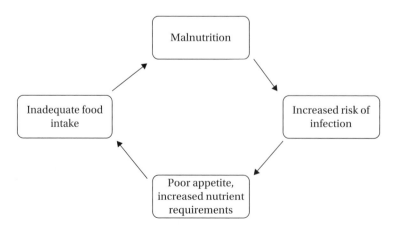

Fig. 34.3 The cycle of malnutrition and infection seen in children living in developing countries.

Consumption of poor-quality food with low nutrient content has been described as the 'hidden hunger' of micronutrient deficiency. In the 2002 World Health Report the World Health Organization identified iodine (Chapter 11), iron (Chapter 10), vitamin A (Chapter 12) and zinc (Chapter 11) deficiencies as being amongst the most serious global health risks.

Key anthropometric indices used as measures of nutritional and health status in children in developing countries are:

- weight-for-age: measures weight relative to that of a healthy reference population of the same age (used to identify 'underweight');
- height-for-age: measures *long-term growth faltering* (used to identify 'stunting');
- weight-for-height: measures *acute growth disturbance* (used to identify 'wasting').

The terms 'underweight', 'stunting', and 'wasting' are used when a child's measurement is two or more standard deviations below the median reference standards for the index.

34.7.2 The Millennium Development Goals

The Millennium Development Goals were adopted by United Nations member states in 2001 and are a set of specific measurable goals for the international community to support developing countries to achieve by 2015. They are all relevant to children and adolescents (Table 34.5). Targets and indicators under these goals with specific nutrition implications are in Table 34.6.

There has been mixed progress towards achieving the Millennium Development Goals. Positive gains have been made in terms of poverty reduction, getting more children into school, and immunization, but some of the nutrition targets are proving more resistant to change. The number of people in developing regions who were undernourished increased from 817 million to 830 million between 1990–92 and 2005–07. Disparities within countries have continued, or in some countries worsened. In Southern

Table 34.5 The Millennium Development Goals

- Goal 1: Eradicate extreme poverty and hunger
- Goal 2: Achieve universal primary education
- Goal 3: Promote gender equality and empower women
- Goal 4: Reduce child mortality rate
- Goal 5: Improve maternal health
- Goal 6: Combat HIV/AIDS, malaria, and other diseases
- Goal 7: Ensure environmental sustainability
- Goal 8: Develop a global partnership for development

Table 34.6 Millennium Development Goals targets and indicators with special relevance to nutrition

- *Target 1C: Halve the proportion of people who suffer from hunger*
  - Prevalence of underweight children under 5 years of age
  - Proportion of population below minimum level of dietary energy consumption
- *Target 4A: Reduce by two-thirds, between 1990 and 2015, the under-5 mortality rate*
- *Target 5B: Achieve, by 2015, universal access to reproductive health*
  - Reduce the adolescent birth rate
- *Target 7C: Halve, by 2015, the proportion of people without sustainable access to safe drinking water and basic sanitation*

Asia, for instance, 60% of children in the poorest areas are underweight, compared to 25% in the richest areas.

34.7.3 Interventions for childhood malnutrition

The main dietary approaches to addressing childhood malnutrition in developing countries include supplementation with specific nutrients (e.g. iron supplementation of children identified with anaemia), fortification of a commonly consumed food vehicle (e.g. the iodization of salt), and dietary change (e.g. increasing the intake of animal foods or encouraging processing methods such as fermentation that decrease the phytate content of unrefined cereals and legumes). Deworming can also markedly decrease iron requirements in children who have hookworm or other gastrointestinal parasites. Less direct approaches such as vaccination, improved sanitation, and education on good feeding practices are also important.

Much work has been done in recent years to develop and test home or 'point-of-use' fortification strategies. Two such products being used in programmes for preschool children and school meals are:

- micronutrient sprinkles: these are pre-packaged micronutrients that are sprinkled onto food before it is eaten;
- lipid-based nutrient supplements: these are products that contain vitamins and minerals, protein, and essential fatty acids in a palatable form. One example is 'nutributter', which is based on peanut, milk powder, and flavouring such as cocoa.

The advantage of these home fortification approaches is that the amount of nutrient provided is not dependent on the child's energy intake, and that the nutrients are targeted to the person who needs them.

34.7.4 Emerging issues

HIV continues to place many children in developing countries at extreme nutritional risk. The risk to children lies not only in contracting the condition, but also if one or both their parents are infected (see Chapter 41). It has been estimated that in 2008 alone, 17.5 million children and adolescents lost at least one parent to AIDS. These children are more likely to be malnourished, unwell, or subjected to exploitation and discrimination than children orphaned for other reasons. In addition, the increasing success of programmes to prevent the transmission of HIV from mother to child means that there are now substantial numbers of HIV-exposed uninfected (HIV-EU) children. In some countries in sub-Saharan Africa, up to one in four babies born may be HIV-EU.

Over the past decade there has been increasing concern about the 'double burden of disease' in developing countries, the coexistence of undernutrition and overnutrition in the same country. It is assumed that the substantial changes in traditional diets (to foods that are more energy-dense but micronutrient-poor) and lifestyles (with less physical activity) that have occurred in recent decades are responsible, particularly in urban settings. The problem may be more widespread than is currently thought because the use of weight-for-age to identify malnutrition can incorrectly identify many overweight stunted children as normal or even underweight.

34.8 Special issues in adolescents

Adolescents represent a significant proportion of the total population. It is a time of rapid physical and psychological growth, with numerous pressures and influences resulting from the transition from a dependent childhood state to independent living in some societies. While many of the nutritional problems that affect children also apply in this age group, adolescents also face additional nutrition-related issues.

34.8.1 Pregnancy

More than 13 million children are born annually to teenage mothers, the vast majority to women in developing countries. For these women, young motherhood may be common, but complications from pregnancy and childbirth also form the leading cause of mortality in girls aged 15–19 years. In developed countries, considerable social stigma can be associated with teenage pregnancy. Teenage mothers are more likely to be unmarried and live in poverty, and most teenage pregnancies are unplanned. Because of this, nutritional support during adolescent pregnancy is important and challenging, and the youngest adolescents are at the greatest risk. In particular, low pre-pregnancy BMI, poor gestational weight gain, impaired iron status, and poor calcium and vitamin D status can adversely affect pregnancy outcomes. Breastfeeding initiation rates and duration are lower in younger and unmarried mothers, although barriers to effective breastfeeding are thought to be more social and cultural than physical.

34.8.2 Dieting and anorexia nervosa

Western culture typically glorifies a thin body ideal and the media influences how adolescents view their body shape. Body dissatisfaction is rife in adolescent girls and it is not uncommon for teenagers to become preoccupied with their physical appearance. However, few adolescents actually go on to develop a diagnosed eating disorder (see Chapter 24), perhaps only 1%. Larger numbers of adolescents engage in unhealthy dieting behaviours which could place them at nutritional risk.

34.8.3 Alcohol

The independence of adolescents from their family is associated with an increased susceptibility to peer pressure, both positive and negative. In many countries, alcohol consumption commences during adolescence and intake is cause for concern. Although alcohol can be consumed safely and in moderation as part of an adolescent's dietary intake, many adolescents are exposed to a more negative side of alcohol and the dangers of alcohol intoxication. If consumed in excess, alcohol can replace more nutrient-dense foods from the diet. Adolescents who drink regularly tend to engage in other risky health behaviours, and careful campaigns are required in order to reach this target audience. It is unlikely that negative messages are well received, so that it may be better to focus on safe and legal drinking limits (rather than drinking and driving) and how to determine the alcohol content of drinks with which adolescents are unfamiliar.

34.8.4 Chronic disease

Chronic disease prevention should start early in life. Although the overt symptoms of most chronic disease may not be apparent until mid-adulthood, post-mortem studies have demonstrated that fatty streaks in the arteries are apparent in adolescents.

Although the majority of children and adolescents with diabetes have type 1 diabetes, up to 45% of new cases in some population groups now have type 2. This has been attributed to the escalating prevalence of obesity. Type 2 diabetes during growth occurs most often during the adolescent years and is more common in females. Thus there is considerable justification for encouraging adolescents to follow widely accepted dietary guidelines. However, it must be acknowledged that adolescence is a time of experimentation when young people inevitably experience the need to assert themselves and respond to peer pressure. This applies as much to food habits as to other aspects of their lifestyle. They generally, with their parents' help, manage to combine enough of the essential nutrients in their own individual way. If appropriate eating habits have been established in childhood, there is the expectation that food habits will improve when they have passed through this transitional stage.

Conclusion

Appropriate nutrition is essential for optimal growth and development in childhood and adolescence. Cognitive development is also influenced by nutritional factors. While one in four of children worldwide suffer from malnutrition, one in three in developed countries are overweight and, in some societies, undernutrition and obesity coexist. In childhood and adolescence overweight and obesity account for the emergence, in some population groups, of type 2 diabetes as a major health issue amongst young people, in addition to the well-recognized psychosocial consequences and risk of fractures. The conditions tend to continue into adult life, when the many comorbidities associated with excess body fat become apparent. Appropriate eating habits established in childhood will encourage healthier food choices in later life, even if in adolescence there is a tendency to adopt less conventional food habits. Thus implementation of dietary guidelines for young people should be regarded as a priority in families as well as in the context of public health.

Further Reading

1. **Cole, T.J., Bellizzi, M.C., Flegal, K.M., and Dietz, W.H.** (2000) Establishing a standard definition for child overweight and obesity worldwide: International survey. *BMJ*, **320**, 1240–43.
2. **De Onis, et al.** (2006) WHO Child Growth Standards. Length/height-for-age, weight-for-age, weight-for-length and body mass index-for-age. Methods and development. WHO, Geneva.
3. **Gordon R.C., Rose M.C., Skeaff S.A., Gray A.R., Morgan K.M.D., and Ruffman T.** (2009). Iodine supplementation improves cognition in mildly iodine-deficient children. *AmJ Clin Nutr* **90**,1264–71.
4. **Han, J.C., Lawlor, D.A., and Kimm, S.Y.S.** (2010) Childhood obesity. *Lancet*, **375**(9727), 1737–49.
5. **National Health and Medical Research Council** (2003) *Dietary guidelines for children and adolescents in Australia incorporating the infant feeding guidelines for health workers*. Canberra, National Health & Medical Research Council.
6. **Niinikoski, H., Lagström, H., Jokinen, J., Siltala, M., Rönnemaa, T., Viikari, J., Raitakari, O.T., Jula, A., Marniemi, J., Näntö-Salonen, K., and Simell, O.** (2007) Impact of repeated dietary counseling between infancy and 14 years of age on dietary intakes and serum lipids and lipoproteins. *Circulation*, **116**, 1032–40.
7. **Tanner, J. and Davis, P.S.W.** (1985) Clinical longitudinal standards for height and weight velocity for North American children. *J Pediatr*, **107**, 317–29.
8. A series of comprehensive international reports on maternal and child undernutrition appeared in consecutive issues of *The Lancet* starting on p. 243 of the issue of 19 January 2008.

Useful Websites

To see topical and scientifically robust updates on nutrition associated with this textbook and web links to many of the journals in the Further Reading sections, please see the dedicated Online Resource Centre at **http://www.oxfordtextbooks.co.uk/orc/mann4e/**

United States and Canada Dietary Reference Intakes:
http://www.nap.edu/
Growth references of the Centre for Disease Control:
http://www.cdc.gov/growthcharts/

More detailed growth charts for clinical use:
http://www.cdc.gov/growthcharts/clinical_charts.htm
Training module on the use of growth references:
http://www.cdc.gov/growthcharts/educational_materials.htm
Millennium Development Goals:
http://www.endpoverty2015.org/en/goals

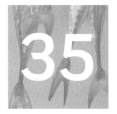

Nutrition and ageing

Wija van Staveren, Lisette de Groot, and Caroline Horwath

Nutrition interacts with the ageing process in numerous ways and the risk of nutrition-related health problems increases in later life. This chapter provides an overview of why nutrition is important in old age, what happens to our bodies as we age, the nutritional needs and status of older adults, and some special issues arising in nutrition–disease relationships.

35.1 Is nutrition one of the secrets to health and long life?

For thousands of years, the search for eternal life and youth has captured people's imagination. In about 1750 George Cheyne, physician to Samuel Johnson, David Hume, and Alexander Pope, wrote 'An Essay of Health and Long Life' in which he is emphatic that:

Nothing conduces more to Health and Long Life, than Abstinence and plain Food, with due Labour. Most chronical diseases proceed from Repletion ... Without due Labour and Exercise, the Juices will thicken, the Joints will stiffen, the Nerves will relax, and on these disorders, Chronical Distempers and a crazy old Age must ensue ... this [lessening the diet gradually with age] is a powerful means to make their old age Green and Indolent, and to preserve the remains of their Senses to the very last.

The similarities to recommendations derived from the latest research on ageing are remarkable. Still, it is questionable whether these recommendations have led to the currently continuing increase in life expectancy in many countries (UN 2007). This remarkable gain is not only observed in western Europe, North America, Australia, and New Zealand, with even larger gains in Japan and some southern European countries such as Spain

573

35.1 Is nutrition one of the secrets to health and long life?

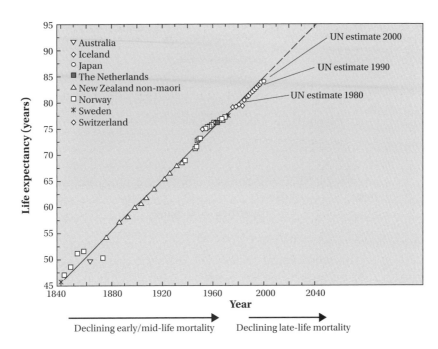

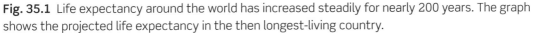

Fig. 35.1 Life expectancy around the world has increased steadily for nearly 200 years. The graph shows the projected life expectancy in the then longest-living country.

Source: Adapted by Kirkwood, T.B. (2008). A systematic look at an old problem. *Nature*, **451**, 644–7, from Oeppen, J., and Vaupel, J.W. (2002) Demography. Broken limits to life expectancy. *Science*, **296**, 1029–31.

and Italy, but also in some developing countries, although with differential speed. The segment of older adults is growing. Fig. 35.1 shows life expectancy from 1840 and projections to 2040 for the then longest-living country. It is generally accepted that these life expectancy improvements were not based on uniform reductions in mortality at all ages. During the nineteenth and early twentieth centuries, improvements in infant and childhood survival contributed most to the increase in record life expectancies. After successful combating of infectious diseases at young ages gains were caused by the decline in late-life mortality. This decline in mortality at age 80 years and over will continue, in some countries even at an accelerating pace.

The changes will lead to a very different population pyramid (Fig. 35.2). Rapidly growing older populations raise concern about whether or not a shrinking labour force will be able to support that part of the population who are commonly believed to be dependent on others, such as disabled and older adults. In order to delay or even prevent disabilities and chronic diseases, healthy ageing policies and programmes focusing on lifestyle are required.

But how can healthy ageing happen? Ageing is a multifactorial process. Genetic factors, for instance, may underlie the ageing process itself and aberrant gene expression is strongly involved in processes leading to the development of diseases that restrict lifespan. Consensus now exists that ageing is caused by the gradual, lifelong accumulation of a wide variation of molecular and cellular damage, eventually resulting in progressive loss of function, frailty, and disease. But if ageing is a matter of things falling apart, can research—and more specifically—can nutrition play a role in a 'healthy ageing' programme?

According to Kirkwood (2008) the answer is yes. How the ageing process plays out is—apart from chances or good luck—not only influenced by factors intrinsic to the individual but also by extrinsic factors such as environmental and lifestyle variables. There is plenty of mechanistic evidence that it is possible to intervene on the interplay

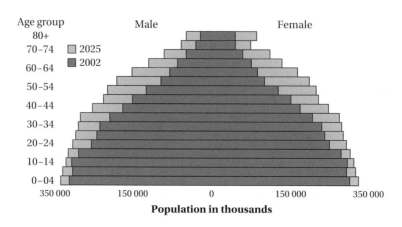

Fig. 35.2 Global population pyramids for 2002 and 2025. Note that as the proportion of children and young people declines and the proportion of people of 60 years and over increases, the triangular population pyramid of 2002 will be replaced with a more rounded structure in 2025.

Source: WHO (2002). *Ageing and life course program. Active ageing: A policy framework.* Geneva: World Health Organization.

between intrinsic factors and nutrition. Of the 20 leading risk factors for disability, chronic disease, and death, a number are nutrition-related and may lead, amongst others, to cardiovascular diseases, type 2 diabetes, Alzheimer's disease, and certain types of cancer. The global epidemiological data have motivated (WHO/FAO 2004, 2008) to update their dietary guidelines. These guidelines are evidence-based for younger adults, but may not have the same impact for elderly people. To get a better understanding of changing nutrient requirements in old age we first have to answer the question: 'What happens to our body as we age?'

35.2 What happens to our bodies as we age?

Changes in body composition, physical performance, and organ system function occur in all of us as we grow older. However, wide variation exists among people in the degree to which functions decline. As people become older, the more dissimilar they become from their contemporaries of the same chronological age. There can also be considerable variability in the rate at which different changes occur within the same person. Some of this variability in functional decline may reflect heterogeneity in true rates of ageing; however, lifestyle and other factors that can accompany ageing seem to be of importance. Changes in body composition and changes in the gastrointestinal tract have an impact on nutritional requirements. These changes will be further discussed here.

35.3 Changes in body composition and energy balance

Changes in body composition during ageing include loss of lean body mass (LBM), bone mass, body water, and a relative increase of fat mass. The latter is also redistributed from mainly subcutaneous to abdominal fat. The decrease in lean body mass is caused by a reduction in size and strength of skeletal muscle. On average the marked decline in LBM begins around the seventh decade, approaching as much as a 40% loss compared to young adulthood (Fig. 35.3).

A stable body weight in this process can be explained by a concomitant increase in body fat. This loss in lean body mass and change in fat mass is associated with sarcopenia, a term derived from the Greek words *sarx* (flesh) and *penia* (poverty). The term was introduced by Rosenberg (1997), who wanted the medical professionals to recognize this ageing condition in an early stage to diminish the negative impact on morbidity and mortality. Features of sarcopenia are, amongst others, loss of

muscle mass and strength (decrease of type 2 fibre number and strength, and less so of type 1 fibres). The pathophysiology is complex. The diagnosis of the medical condition is based on the combined presence of the two following criteria:

1 A low muscle mass, i.e. a percentage of muscle mass > 2 standard deviations below the mean measured in young adults of the same sex and ethnic background. This suggested T-score-based diagnosis is comparable with the diagnosis of osteoporosis; however, for sarcopenia there is a lack of suitable reference values in various populations.

2 Low gait speed, e.g. a walking speed below 0.8 m/s in the 4-minute walking test. This test can

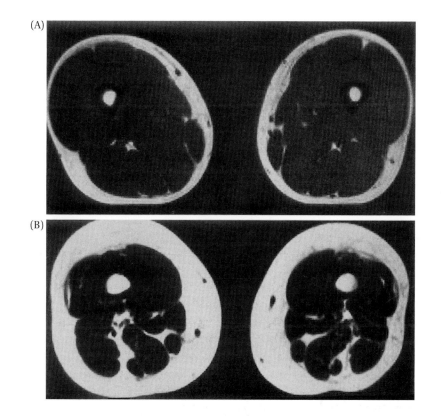

Fig. 35.3 Magnetic resonance images of the thigh showing differences in total muscle, intramuscular fat, subcutaneous fat, and bone between (A) a young woman athlete (age 20 years, body mass index 22.6 kg/m²) and (B) an elderly sedentary woman (age 64 years, body mass index 30.7 kg/m²).

Source: Evans, W.J., and Meredith, C.N. (1989) Exercise and nutrition in the elderly. In Munro, H.N., and Danford, D.E. (eds) *Nutrition, aging and the elderly*. New York, Plenum Press.

be replaced by another well-established functional test.

Effective prevention and treatment of sarcopenia is sought in physical activity programmes and the way nutrition and/or nutrition supplements and exercise regimens can be combined for the prevention or treatment of sarcopenia. Due to a lack of trials there is not yet a consensus on the management of sarcopenia.

Together with age-related metabolic diseases, as well as presence of individual handicaps, sarcopenia often coincides with decline of physical activity. Moreover, due to diminished maximum oxygen intake and muscle fibre atrophy, a greater physical effort for the same task is required in older people. As a consequence, older people will reduce physical activity further and have lower energy expenditure. Fig. 35.4 shows how the physical activity level (PAL) calculated as daily total energy expenditure

divided by the resting metabolic rate decreases with ageing.

Many nationwide food consumption studies have shown that older people respond to this lower activity with a smaller energy intake and may even over-respond, which results in a negative energy balance. This phenomenon is called anorexia of ageing and is common in people over 70 years of age. In contrast to younger adults, body weight tends to decrease at old age, even in healthy individuals. Weight loss in later life should be prevented, because it increases the risk of progressive malnutrition, micronutrient deficiency, nutrition-related diseases, and is associated with frailty and increased mortality (Fig. 35.5).

Bone mass and bone density may start to decrease already from the age of 35–40 years onwards (see Chapter 9) In women, bone loss accelerates during the menopause. They may lose half of their trabecular and about one-third of their cortical bone mass; in men, this loss is lower, only 50–70% of that of females. The decrease in bone mass density is associated with osteoporotic fractures. Osteoporosis is a multifactorial disease and inadequacies of the nutrients calcium and vitamin D are related to a decline in bone density and to fractures. Vitamin D deficiency is often observed in old age due to

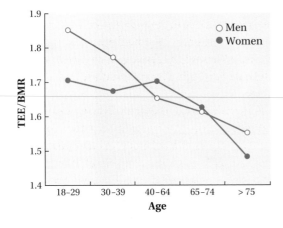

Fig. 35.4 Decrease of physical activity level (PAL) for men and women during ageing. PAL is derived as total energy expenditure (TEE, assessed by doubly labelled water method) and divided by basal metabolic rate (BMR, derived from proxy measures).

Source: Based on Black, A.E. (1996) Physical activity levels from a meta-analysis of doubly labeled water studies for validating energy intake by dietary assessment. *Nutr Rev*, **54**, 170–4; conclusion confirmed by Manini, T.M. (2010) Energy expenditure and aging. *Ageing Res Rev*, **9**, 1–11.

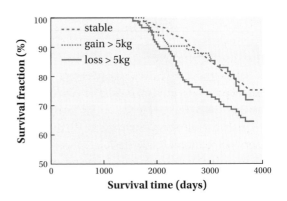

Fig. 35.5 Probability of survival for participants in the SENECA study with and without weight change.

Source: De Groot, C.P.G.M., and Van Staveren, W.A. (2002) Undernutrition in the European SENECA studies. *Clin Geriatr Med*, **18**, 699–708.

diminished synthesis in the skin (Fig. 35.6), as well as lack of sunlight exposure. Recommended intakes for the housebound elderly for vitamin D are 15 µg, which cannot be obtained from ordinary foods.

Dehydration is another problem often observed in elderly people. Due to less LBM, but also less interstitial fluid, the older adult contains less body water (<50% versus 70% of total body mass in younger adults). Further, decreased renal function, loss of thirst sensors, fear of incontinence, and increased arthritic pain resulting from numerous trips to the toilet may interfere with an adequate intake of fluid. Dehydration may result in constipation, faecal impaction, cognitive impairment, and even death. The recommended amount of fluid is about 1500 mL per day, which should be taken during and between meals.

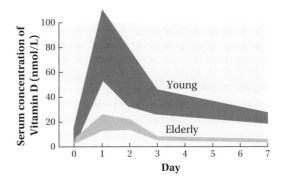

Fig. 35.6 Serum concentrations of vitamin D in healthy young and elderly adults in response to whole-body exposure to a dose of simulated sunlight on day 0.

Source: Holick, M. (1994) Vitamin D—new horizons for the 21st century. *Am J Clin Nutr*, **60**, 619–30.

35.4 Digestive function in old age

For many years it was thought that the efficiency of the digestive and absorptive functions of the gastrointestinal tract declines with age. This is now known to reflect also the effects of medications or disease states. Where malabsorption occurs in an older adult, investigation of possible pancreatic or small intestinal disease is required.

Diminished, altered, or lost taste perception with ageing may be caused by changes in the oral cavity (e.g. reduced taste bud numbers, saliva production, or dental problems) and/or changes in the neuronal fibres that are connected to the brain. Together with changes in the olfactory system (smell), the overall sensory perception of food declines. It is, however, difficult to distinguish between taste and smell dysfunctions that are directly related to ageing and those resulting from diseases and medication. Individuals are not able to discriminate between the loss of taste and smell. Many taste complaints are actually olfactory disorders. These complaints may cause malnutrition. Despite taste and smell losses, however, palatability is just as valuable in old age to promote food intake as it is in the young adults. This means that pleasantness might not decrease and

offering highly palatable foods in a stimulating ambiance increases food intake even in frail older adults. Difficulty in swallowing occurs in some older adults if neurological function is disturbed, e.g. after stroke.

Perhaps the most important change in gastrointestinal function with ageing is the reduction in gastric acid output in a subgroup of older people who have atrophic gastritis. Atrophy of the stomach mucosa becomes more common with ageing and appears to affect about one-third of those over 60 years. The result is lowered secretion of acid, intrinsic factor, and pepsin, which reduce the bioavailability of vitamin B_{12}, calcium, iron, and folate. The implications are most profound for vitamin B_{12} due both to the diminished dissociation of the vitamin from food proteins and binding of the small amount of freed vitamin B_{12} by the increased numbers of swallowed bacteria which are able to survive in the low-acid environment of the proximal small intestine. In recognition of this and the prevalence of atrophic gastritis in the older population, most of the current dietary reference intakes (DRIs) recommend that older adults meet their vitamin B_{12} needs from supplements or foods fortified with crystalline, free vitamin B_{12}. However, research is needed to determine whether functionality is improved by normalizing low vitamin B_{12} status and to determine the dose required (see Section 13.8.5).

Another change is reduced intestinal motility, which causes a slower clearance of the intestinal contents. The altered motility and additional dystrophy in the large intestine may lead to constipation or diarrhoea; both disorders occur in the elderly. Especially prevalence of constipation increases and contributes significantly to morbidity and affects the individual's feeling of wellbeing. Sufficient fluid and dietary fibre may at least partly prevent this disorder.

35.5 Do nutritional needs change as we age?

Since the late 1990s, many countries published nutrient recommendations with separate data for adults 51–70 years and ≥70 years. Until more specific information becomes available on the nutritional requirements of older adults, these broad age groupings will have to suffice for the entire heterogeneous older population (see Chapter 37 for a more extensive discussion on requirements and recommended intakes). How are the nutritional needs of older adults currently thought to differ from those of younger adults?

Older adults have reduced needs for energy and, as a result, presumably also for the B vitamins which are involved in energy metabolism, and postmenopausal women have lower needs for iron, as a result of cessation of menstrual blood losses. These differences are reflected in lower recommended nutrient intakes for older adults. The lower energy needs of older adults are the result of declines in metabolic rate (secondary to reduced lean muscle mass) and in activity levels. Neither of these changes are inevitable; indeed, it can be argued that morbidity and mortality could be lowered if LBM and physical activity were maintained at more youthful levels, rather than diminished in older persons. The greater food intake needed to balance higher energy expenditure is more likely to ensure adequate intakes of essential nutrients. If older adults consume low energy intakes, then it is important that the foods they eat are nutrient-dense, rather than low nutrient-density (high in sugars, fats, or alcohol).

The body's requirements for iron are lowest in old age; however, other factors in the lives of many older people can increase the risk of iron deficiency; chronic blood loss from ulcers or other disease conditions, poor iron absorption due to reduced stomach acid secretion, or medications like aspirin, which can cause blood loss.

Calcium needs are also higher in postmenopausal women (with low oestrogen levels) and this is reflected in increased recommendations for calcium intakes. An abundant calcium intake throughout life helps protect against osteoporosis, particularly in women (see Chapter 9). There is also evidence accumulating that older adults may have greater needs for vitamin D (see Section 35.3), riboflavin, and vitamin B_6, and need higher doses of vitamin B_{12} to correct poor status (see Section 35.4). The increase in vitamin B_6 requirement with age does not appear to be an absorptive problem, and subclinical deficiency of this vitamin may result in immune dysfunction. Furthermore vitamin B_6, along with folate and vitamin B_{12}, favourably affects serum homocysteine. Higher homocysteine levels might be an independent risk factor for cardiovascular disease and impaired cognitive functions. The high levels generally observed in older adults can be reduced by an increased intake of folate, vitamin B_{12}, and vitamin B_6 (in that order of effectiveness). Riboflavin requirements, which had previously been thought to be lower in older than in younger persons, are now recognized to be the same or slightly higher in older age categories. Since vitamin E is the only lipid-soluble, chain-breaking antioxidant found in biological membranes, this vitamin might play an important role in maintaining neuronal integrity and preventing cell loss. Thus it is logical to consider whether higher intakes may prove useful in neurological disorders where oxidative stress has been implicated. But three meta-analyses of randomized trials found that vitamin E supplementation did not reduce mortality.

Overall, compared with younger adults, most older adults need to obtain the same or even higher intakes of several micronutrients, but usually in substantially lower overall food intakes. Thus a nutrient-dense diet is a high priority in old age.

35.6 A look at the eating habits of older adults

A number of general conclusions can be drawn from studies of dietary intake conducted amongst older populations around the world. Contrary to the popular 'tea and toast' myth, it appears that most older adults outside institutions eat reasonably well. The dietary patterns of older adults have generally been found to be similar to those of younger adults, but vary within and between different cultures and regions. Energy intake decreases with ageing and only when the intake level falls below 1500 kcal or 6.3 MJ does it become

difficult to fulfil the recommended daily requirements (Table 35.1).

Since dietary intake of foods and nutrients are related and as people do not eat single nutrients or foods, evaluating dietary patterns in relation to health has attracted considerable interest. Strictly defined prospective studies found strong evidence for protective factors such as vegetables, nuts, monounsaturated fatty acids, and Mediterranean, prudent, basically plant-based and high-quality diets. Evidence was also found for harmful factors such as *trans*-fatty acids, foods with a high glycaemic index or load, and 'Western' dietary pattern. Adherence to a Mediterranean diet appears to be relevant even in old age. Reductions of 9% in overall mortality, mortality from cardiovascular diseases (9%), cancer (6%), and incidence of Alzheimer's disease (13%) followed from a meta-analysis of eight cohort studies.

Fig. 35.7 shows that, in addition to adherence to a healthy diet, other healthful practices are important, such as no smoking, moderate alcohol use, and physical activity. However, even with an apparently adequate food intake there are some nutrients for which there is a greater risk of inadequate supply. These nutrients are calcium, zinc, magnesium, vitamin B_6, folate, vitamin B_{12}, vitamin C, and vitamins D and E. The low calcium intakes and vitamin D supply of many older people, particularly women, have important implications for bone health. Vitamin C intake often seems to be adequate in older adults, but unfortunately vitamin C is readily lost from foods during storage and preparation. Low vitamin C intake in addition to low intakes of other antioxidants, e.g. vitamin E and carotenoids, has been associated—but not confirmed in trials—with

Table 35.1 Daily consumption of type of foods and number of portions suggested in this table supply about 6.3 MJ and recommended daily intakes of micronutrients for populations over 70 years of age as suggested in several countries.

• Sandwiches with filling	4 slices (margarine, cheese, meat, marmalade)
• Milk products	3 cups
• Fruit	1 to 2 pieces
• Potatoes	1 to 2 pieces
• Vegetables	4 serving spoons
• Meat	75–100 g
• Oil for preparation cooked meal	15 g
• Fluid	8 servings
• Vitamin D	10–20 µg

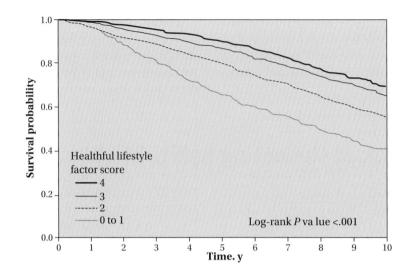

Fig. 35.7 Combined diet and lifestyle factors (smoking, alcohol consumption, and physical activity) for 10-year all-cause mortality in elderly Europeans. Note that individuals scored 1 or 0 points if they belonged to the low- or high-risk group, respectively, for diet or a particular lifestyle factor. For a maximum score, an individual could obtain 4 points: 1 point for the Mediterranean diet and 3 points for the lifestyle factors.

Source: Knoops, K.T., de Groot, L.C., and Kromhout, D. (2004) Mediterranean diet, lifestyle factors, and 10-year mortality in elderly European men and women: The HALE project. *JAMA*, **292**, 1433–9.

increased risk for senile cataract and coronary artery disease.

Daily intake of fruits, vegetables, whole grains, and dairy products as well as the inclusion in the diet of lean meat, fish, poultry, and legumes will ensure provision of those nutrients found to be most 'at risk' in the diets of older people. If elderly people eat these foods in amounts as suggested in Table 35.1, then about 6.3 MJ covers the daily recommended intake of most countries. However, with such a lower energy intake, there is no place for so-called social foods or snacks.

Inadequate nutritional intake is the predominant cause of undernutrition in older persons. The diagnosis of undernutrition is made with different methods and the prevalence depends on the methods and cut-off values applied. The literature describes a prevalence of 5–10% in community-dwelling persons above 70 years of age and up to 30–60% in institutionalized people of that age. It is crucial to identify older persons at risk and to make an early diagnosis for effective intervention. For a first screening, tools

have been developed from a number of parameters of the nutritional state. They are designed for self-assessment or for administering by healthcare professionals. Fig. 35.8 presents an example of a screening tool, that incorporates several domains including functionality, lifestyle, a few questions on diet, and subjective health and anthropometric indicators. The sensitivity and specificity of the tool validated against an extensive evaluation by clinicians were 96% and 98%, respectively.

Signs of poor nutrition in an older individual include recent weight loss, missing meals, infrequent grocery shopping, depression, loss of appetite, or declining food intake due to digestive problems, taste changes and chewing or swallowing difficulties. Table 35.2 shows other factors contributing to undernutrition in old age.

The three factors most consistently linked with poor dietary intake in old age are low socioeconomic status, depression, and, amongst older men, loneliness. Compared with men living with a spouse, older men living alone tend to have a poorer fruit

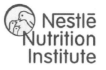 Nestlé
Nutrition
Institute

**Mini Nutritional Assessment
MNA®**

Last name: First name:

Sex: Age: Weight, kg: Height, cm: Date:

Complete the screen by filling in the boxes with the appropriate numbers. Total the numbers for the final screening score.

Screening

A Has food intake declined over the past 3 months due to loss of appetite, digestive problems, chewing or swallowing difficulties?
0 = severe decrease in food intake
1 = moderate decrease in food intake
2 = no decrease in food intake ☐

B Weight loss during the last 3 months
0 = weight loss greater than 3 kg (6.6 lbs)
1 = does not know
2 = weight loss between 1 and 3 kg (2.2 and 6.6 lbs)
3 = no weight loss ☐

C Mobility
0 = bed or chair bound
1 = able to get out of bed / chair but does not go out
2 = goes out ☐

D Has suffered psychological stress or acute disease in the past 3 months?
0 = yes   2 = no ☐

E Neuropsychological problems
0 = severe dementia or depression
1 = mild dementia
2 = no psychological problems ☐

F1 Body Mass Index (BMI) (weight in kg) / (height in m^2)
0 = BMI less than 19
1 = BMI 19 to less than 21
2 = BMI 21 to less than 23
3 = BMI 23 or greater ☐

IF BMI IS NOT AVAILABLE, REPLACE QUESTION F1 WITH QUESTION F2.
DO NOT ANSWER QUESTION F2 IF QUESTION F1 IS ALREADY COMPLETED.

F2 Calf circumference (CC) in cm
0 = CC less than 31
3 = CC 31 or greater ☐

Screening score ☐☐
(max. 14 points)

12-14 points: Normal nutritional status
8-11 points: At risk of malnutrition
0-7 points: Malnourished

For a more in-depth assessment, complete the full MNA® which is available at **www.mna-elderly.com**

Ref.   Vellas B, Villars H, Abellan G, *et al. Overview of the MNA®* — *Its History and Challenges.* J Nutr Health Aging 2006;**10**:456-65.
Rubenstein LZ, Harker JO, Salva A, Guigoz Y, Vellas B. Screening for Undernutrition in Geriatric Practice: Developing the Short-Form Mini Nutritional Assessment (MNA-SF) . J. Geront 2001;**56A**: M366-377.
Guigoz Y.The Mini-Nutritional Assessment (MNA®) Review of the Literature — What does it tell us? J Nutr Health Aging 2006; 10:466-487.
® Société des Produits Nestlé, S.A., Vevey, Switzerland, Trademark Owners Société des Produits Nestlé, S.A., Vevey, Switzerland, Trademark Owners
© Nestlé, 1994, Revision 2009. N67200 12/99 10M
For more information: www.mna-elderly.com

Fig. 35.8 Mini-nutritional assessment.

Source: Guigoz, Y. (2006) Mini-nutritional assessment (MNA) Review of the literature—what does it tell us? *J Nutr Health Aging*, **10**, 466–87.

Table 35.2 Potential contributors to nutritional problems in older people

Physical factors
Reduced total energy needs
Declining absorptive and metabolic capacities
Chronic diseases
Poor appetite
Changes in taste or odour perception
Poor dental health
Reduced salivary flow
Difficulty in swallowing
Lack of exercise
Physical disability (restricting the capacity to purchase, cook, or eat a varied diet)
Side effects of drugs (anorexia, nausea, altered taste, drug–nutrient interactions)
Restrictive diets
Alcoholism
Social and psychological factors
Depression
Loneliness
Social isolation
Bereavement
Loss of interest in food or cooking
Memory loss
Food avoidances
Socioeconomic factors
Low income
Inadequate cooking or storage facilities
Limited nutrition knowledge
Lack of transport
Shopping difficulties
Cooking practices that result in nutrient losses (e.g. soaking vegetables)
Inadequate cooking skills (particularly in men)

and vegetable intake, and more frequently choose less nutrient-dense, easy-to-prepare foods which also tend to be higher in fat and lower in fibre. Limited cooking skills and reduced motivation when cooking just for one are probably important contributors. Institutionalized older people and those living independently in the community but restricted in their mobility or depressed elderly, also tend to be at higher risk of poor dietary habits. Lack of social contact, loneliness, being less active socially and physically, and recent bereavement are also associated with poor dietary intake. On the other hand, a rich and varied lifestyle and maintenance of positive interests should lead to better dietary quality through an improvement in life satisfaction, a better social support network, and a lessening of the impact of some of the negative life events associated with growing older. In fact, participation in fewer activities outside the home is linked with higher mortality in old age.

35.7 Nutrition–disease relationships in old age

The role of diet in some chronic diseases is discussed elsewhere (see Chapters 18 and 21, for example). Outlined here are some special issues in older adults and differences in nutrition–disease relationships from those in younger adults.

It is often assumed that lifestyle changes to improve health are no longer worthwhile in old age, that the remaining years are not sufficient to reap the benefits of modifications which are often thought to lead to a reduction in enjoyment of food. Certainly very restrictive diets may impair the adequacy of dietary intake. However, benefits can be gained from nutrition education and lifestyle change in older people. In several studies, a high proportion of older men and women have been found to make dietary changes, often for health reasons, thus challenging the stereotyped view of older adults being 'set in their ways'.

The incidence and prevalence of coronary heart disease are highest in the older population. Smoking, hypertension, and diabetes continue to be strong risk factors for heart disease, and the prevalence of diabetes and impaired glucose tolerance rises steeply with age. Intervention trials clearly demonstrate that the health advantages of quitting smoking and managing hypertension remain in old age. The Dietary Approaches to Stop Hypertension, the so-called DASH diet, is high in fruits and vegetables, moderate in low-fat dairy products, and low in animal protein but with substantial amount of plant protein from legumes and nuts. Adherence to this diet, which is composed of almost the same items as the Mediterranean Diet, is associated with a lower risk of chronic heart disease and stroke, also in older adults.

The management of hypertension (i.e. weight reduction in the overweight, sodium restriction, limitation of alcohol) is particularly relevant for older adults who are more susceptible to severe adverse drug reactions and may be more responsive to sodium restriction. There appears to be further grounds for sodium restriction in older women from studies demonstrating increased obligatory urinary calcium loss and thus a higher dietary calcium requirement on high sodium intakes. Reducing salt intakes to 6g salt/day can lower dietary calcium needs by about a third. Non-insulin-dependent diabetes in older adults should be managed by weight reduction mainly by increased physical activity and hypoglycaemic agents. Even moderate weight reduction can have benefits for diabetic control in older people, when it occurs under professional guidance. The latter is important, because weight loss programmes may result in mainly loss of lean body mass instead of fat mass, which is detrimental for health. Other classic risk factors, such as serum cholesterol weaken in predicting cardiovascular risk. Cardiovascular disease is highly prevalent, even in older adults, even with low cholesterol levels, because those with the highest levels are more likely to have suffered early death. New biomarkers have been identified that are epidemiologically associated with cardiovascular diseases e.g. homocysteine, but they need to be validated more extensively.

We still have to consider the classic cardiovascular risk factors, because the absolute risk attributable to high cholesterol levels actually increases with age. Attributable risk infers the number of events or deaths that are avoided for people in the group with low exposure to the risk factor. All major risk factors, including elevated LDL cholesterol, show an increased attributable risk with advancing age. Evidence from clinical trials suggests that older adults are as responsive to drug and dietary treatment of high cholesterol levels as younger adults. It seems appropriate to consider functional rather than chronological age when deciding whether an individual should be given dietary advice to lower cholesterol levels. Someone who is generally healthy and appears likely to have a reasonable life expectancy should not be denied dietary advice. Still, more research is needed on the effects of cholesterol lowering particularly in those 70 years and older, though cholesterol lowering in people over 80 years would not seem worthwhile.

In Western societies the common pattern of weight gain up to the age of around 50–60 years would imply that overweight and obesity are common problems in old age. However, rather than being an inevitable part of growing older, this pattern is linked with sedentary lifestyles. The increase in abdominal or central obesity with advancing age is linked with greater risk of insulin resistance, hypertension, and dyslipidaemia. Overweight and obesity can also aggravate arthritis and impair physical mobility. Mortality too, among healthy adults who have never smoked, is greater in those with high body mass index (BMI) at least up until 75 years of age.

Surprisingly, systematic reviews conducted to determine the effect of an elevated BMI on all-cause mortality risk in men and women aged over 65 years concluded that those with overweight (25–29 kg/m^2) do not have increased risk of mortality. A BMI in the obese range is associated with only a modest increase in mortality, regardless of sex, disease status, and smoking. Of several explanations, the most important might be that BMI is not a good indicator of body composition. Kyphosis in old age makes it difficult to measure height reliably to estimate the BMI. Another suggestion is that an excess fat mass is less detrimental in old age. However, recent views on proinflammatory factors related to adiposity indicate that fat loss ameliorates some catabolic conditions of ageing since some cytokines may directly affect muscle

protein synthesis and breakdown. Moderate intentional weight loss may also ease mechanical burden on weak joints and muscle, and improve mobility. Therefore, in obese (not overweight) elderly weight-loss therapy is recommended, but on the condition that muscle and bone mass remain stable.

Another link between nutrition and disease in older people is that between the antioxidant nutrients and risk of cataracts (clouding of the lens of the eye resulting in diminished vision) and macular degeneration (for the latter, see Section 12.8.2). Cataracts afflict nearly half of the American population aged 75–85 years, and are a major cause of blindness worldwide. In the prevention of these eye diseases nutrients of interest may be the vitamins C and E, the carotenoids lutein and zeaxanthin, zinc, and ω-3 fatty acids. There is biological plausibility to support a role of these dietary components in the protection of the lens and the macula lutea from sunlight damage. Osmotic stress due to high glucose levels is believed to be why people with diabetes are particularly prone to cataracts.

Constipation and diverticular disease are common problems, and awareness of the need to increase fibre intake is high, as reflected in widespread use of unprocessed bran supplements in older populations. However, it is preferable for fibre intakes to be increased through the consumption of a variety of cereals and vegetables rather than relying on extensive use of bran supplements. These may have adverse effects on the bioavailability of zinc and calcium, which may be marginally supplied in the diets of many older adults.

Severe nutrient deficiencies clearly impair both brain and immune function, and researchers are exploring the possibility that long-term moderate (subclinical) nutrient deficiencies also produce memory impairments or declining immunity in older adults. On the other hand, dementia can also have nutritional consequences. Dementia may lead to difficulty in shopping or cooking, or an older person with dementia may forget to eat or experience changes in taste, and may even not recognize food or eat non-food items.

For older adults, probably the single most important health message is to achieve or maintain at least moderate levels of physical activity next to a balanced diet. There are numerous health benefits from exercise in old age: cardiovascular, musculoskeletal, and psychological benefits, improvements in fat and carbohydrate metabolism, and promotion of good bowel function. There are similarities between the deterioration accompanying ageing and that occurring with physical inactivity. Randomized controlled trials demonstrate that high-intensity strength-training exercises are effective and feasible means of preserving bone density while improving muscle mass, strength, and balance in old age.

35.8 Supplements for older adults

The use of supplements in the USA, Canada, Australia, and New Zealand is widespread amongst older men (35–60%) and women (45–79%). Advertisers often target older people, claiming their products prevent disease or promote longevity. Unfortunately, the nutrient supplements most commonly used are rarely those in shortest supply in the diet, and furthermore supplement users generally tend to have better dietary intakes than non-users. Particular concerns are the risk of supplement interference with drug absorption in an age group that heavily consumes both prescription and over-the-counter drugs.

There are, nevertheless, recommendations for specific supplement use by older adults: nutritional doses of vitamin D (15 μg per day) for all older adults, or general multivitamin including B vitamins and mineral supplements (at recommended intake levels) for those with very low food intakes (i.e. less than 6.3 MJ/day). The advice of vitamin B_{12} supplements is still under discussion (see Section 35.4). But a well-balanced diet will provide most healthy older people with the nutrients they need (except vitamin D), and for those whose food intakes are very low, the more important priority is to identify and try to correct any underlying physical or psychosocial reasons for eating problems or poor nutritional state (Table 35.2).

35.9 Drug–nutrient interactions

Drug–nutrient interactions should be considered as an issue of high clinical relevance for the older population first, because drugs may have different effects and side effects due to changes in body composition and functionality that occur with ageing. Second, dietary intake decreases and nutrient–nutrient interactions change as well as drug–nutrient interactions. Third, the use of (multi)medicinal preparations, including over-the-counter sold products and food supplement, is, on average, very high in this age segment. There are a number of means by which drugs can affect nutrition, usually increasing nutrient need. Many drugs can reduce appetite, produce nausea, gastrointestinal disturbances, or alter the senses of taste or smell and hence affect food intake; long-term laxative use can impair intestinal function; and laxatives and diuretics can lead to severe loss of potassium. As many as 30% of older adults complain that drugs change their sense of taste. It is very likely that undesirable drug–nutrient interactions are underdiagnosed, especially in frail, elderly people taking several drugs at a time and having low dietary intakes.

Conclusions

Logically, preventative measures to reduce diet-related disease should begin early in life; however, that is not to say that lifestyle modifications are worthless in old age. Improvements in diet and maintenance of exercise have been shown to benefit health, regardless of age. Behavioural risk factors (e.g. not regularly eating breakfast, lack of regular physical activity, unhealthy weight changes, smoking) remain predictors of 10-year mortality even at older ages (i.e. 70+). As the older population is more heterogeneous than any other age-group, individual judgement is critical in deciding on the advisability of dietary and lifestyle changes. Physiological, psychological, and sociological factors need to be considered. At one extreme are independent, vigorous, healthy people in their 70s, 80s, and even 90s. At the other extreme are patients who are dependent and have multiple diseases and limited reserves. For the latter, diet and lifestyle advice should focus on function and quality of life. It is, however, often overlooked that although average life expectancy at birth may only be to the late 70s, at age 65 men and women in developed countries still have a life expectancy of some 15 and 19 years, respectively. Furthermore, at age 75 these life expectancies are around 10 years, and recent studies have shown that a healthy diet and lifestyle may make these years healthier, more active, and independent.

Further Reading

1. **Black, A.E.** (1996) Physical activity levels from a meta-analysis of doubly labeled water studies for validating energy intake by dietary assessment. *Nutr Rev*, **54**, 170–4

2. **Bonjour, J.P., Guegen, L., Palacious, C., et al.** (2009) Minerals and vitamins in bone health: The potential value of dietary enhancement. *Br J Nutr*, **101**, 1591–6.

3. **Cruz-Jentoft, AJ., Balyens, J.P., Bauer, J.M., et al.** (2010) Sarcopenia: European consensus on definition and diagnosis. *Age Ageing*, **39**, 412–23.

4. **De Groot, C.P.G.M. and Van Staveren, W.A.** (2002) Undernutrition in the European SENECA studies. *Clin Geriatr Med*, 18, 699–708.

5. **De Groot, C.P.G.M., Van der Heijden, M., De Henauw, S., et al.** (2004) Lifestyle, nutritional status, health and mortality in elderly people across Europe: A review of the longitudinal results of the SENECA study. *J Gerontol Med Sci*, **59A**, 1277–84.

6. **Guigoz, Y.** (2006) Mini-nutritional assessment (MNA) Review of the literature—what does it tell us? *J Nutr Health Aging*, **10**, 466–87.

7. **Holick, M.** (1994) Vitamin D-new horizons for the 21st century. *Am J Clin Nutr*, **60**, 619–30.

8. **Houston, D.K., Nicklas, B.J., Ding, J., et al.** (2008) Dietary protein intake is associated with less lean body mass change in older, community-dwelling adults: The Health, Ageing and Body Composition (Health ABC) Study. *Am J Clin Nutr*, **87**, 150–5.

9. **Janssen, I. and Mark, A.E.** (2007) Elevated body mass index and mortality risk in the elderly. *Obes Rev*, **8**, 41–59.

10. **Kirkwood, T.B.** (2008). A systematic look at an old problem. *Nature*, **451**, 644–7.

11. **Knoops, K.T., de Groot, L.C., and Kromhout, D.** (2004) Mediterranean diet, lifestyle factors, and 10-year mortality in elderly European men and women: The HALE project. *JAMA*, **292**, 1433–9.

12. **Lairon, D., Defoort, C., Martin, J.C., et al.** (2009) Nutrigenetics: Links between genetic background and response to Mediterranean-type diets. *Publ Health Nutr*, **12**, 1601–6

13. **Manini, T.M.** (2010) Energy expenditure and aging. *Ageing Res Rev*, **9**, 1–11.

14. **Milne, A.C., Avenell, A., and Potter, J.** (2009) Meta-analysis: Protein and energy supplementation in older adults. *Ann Intern Med*, **144**, 37–48

15. **Morley, J.E., Perry, H.M., and Miller, D.K.** (2002) Something about frailty. *J Gerontol Med Sci*, **57A**, M698–704.

16. **Oeppen, J. and Vaupel, J.W.** (2002) Demography. Broken limits to life expectancy. *Science*, **296**, 1029–31.

17. **Raats, M., De Groot, L., and Van Staveren, W.** (eds) (2009) *Food for the ageing population.* Woodhead Publishing Limmited Cambridge pp 626.

18. **Rosenberg, I.H.** (1997) Sarcopenia: Origins and clinical relevance. *J Nutrition,* **127**, 990S–1S.

19. **Sofi, F., Cesari,F., Abbate, R.,** *et al.* (2008) Adherence to Mediterranean diet and health status: Meta analyses. BMJ, **337**, a1344,doi:10.1136/bmj.a1344.

20. **UN** (2007) *World Population Ageing.* New York, United Nations Department of Economic and Social Affairs.

21. **WHO** (2002). *Ageing and life course program. Active ageing: A policy framework.* Geneva: World Health Organization.

22. **WHO/FAO** (2004) *Vitamin and mineral requirements in human nutrition,* 2nd ed. Geneva and Rome, World Health Organization and Food and Agriculture Organization of the United Nations. http://whqlibdoc.who.int/publications/2004/9241546123.pdf (accessed 30 November 2008).

Useful Websites

To see topical and scientifically robust updates on nutrition associated with this textbook and web links to many of the journals in the Further Reading sections, please see the dedicated Online Resource Centre at **http://www.oxfordtextbooks.co.uk/orc/mann4e/**

Part 7

Changing food habits

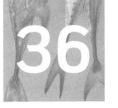

36 Food habits

Helen M. Leach

Many of the topics that form the chapters of this book represent specializations in the subject of human nutrition. Structurally speaking, they can be slotted into compartments within the overall framework of this scientific discipline. The study of food habits, however, might best be viewed as the exploration of a relatively unbounded field lying outside the construction of nutrition, but impinging on it at many points.

36.1 Studying food habits

A number of social scientists also locate their subject matter in this broad field of food habits: the American school of nutritional anthropology (e.g. Bryant, Fitzgerald, Jerome, Robson); a group of social anthropologists and sociologists interested in symbolism and structural order in food habits (e.g. Lévi-Strauss, Douglas, Nicod); anthropologists committed to more materialist explanations of food habits (e.g. Harris, Mintz); sociologists, economists, and social historians concerned with explaining change in food habits (e.g. Mennell, Burnett, Charsley); and social psychologists who have an interest in the interface between cultural beliefs and individual behaviour, as they affect food preference (e.g. Rozin).

Historically, the science of human nutrition developed in tandem with other medical sciences. At a clinical level, therefore, it has concentrated on the individual, and at a policy level, on the population, using epidemiological studies as a starting point. It has made by far the greatest progress with the biological aspects of human nutrition, and with the development of effective treatment of nutritional disorders in individuals. But in those aspects of human nutrition where individuals cease to behave as biological organisms or as members of biological populations, nutrition as an explanatory and applied science has had much less success. Of course, humans have to eat to survive, the environment constantly sets limits on food production, and populations will continue to show change in genetic factors affecting metabolism, but where humans exhibit any choice at all in what they eat, what they select is more likely to be socially influenced than the result of a biological craving, environmental determinism, or idiosyncratic whim.

In discussing food habits, therefore, a definition must be used that stresses the socially influenced food-related behaviour of humans as members of groups. Murcott's usage of the phrase 'food habits' as 'a provisional, convenient, and inclusive short-hand to cover the widest possible range of food choice, preferences, and meal patterns and cuisines' will be followed here.

36.2 Who chooses?

There can be no denying that in the course of a human lifetime, the decision whether to ingest a particular food item lies ultimately with the individual (except in cases of forced or tube feeding). Infants are particularly adept at exercising the right to reject food. But the power to decide what food items are made available for the selection process, and in what form, frequently lies beyond the individual. For the baby, the mother usually decides what should be offered, starting with the decision of either breast milk or formula. But her choice on behalf of the baby is usually influenced by advice from female relatives, or health professionals. In the case of the former, this permits a family tradition of infant feeding to be passed on, compatible with the beliefs of the family's ethnic group and with their religious affiliation. A nurse's or doctor's advice will normally reflect the society's prevailing scientific paradigm concerning infant nutrition, for example that solids should not be introduced until a certain age or that certain foods should be avoided.

The growing child has little control over the household menu, though at certain times (such as illness or the celebration of milestones in development), the person responsible for food acquisition and preparation will deliberately produce an item known to be the child's favourite. In some cultures, gender and position in the family may affect what is offered to each child in both quantity and variety. Similarly, the menu selected for the household may be strongly influenced by the preferences of a senior adult member. In societies where it is traditional for women to cook for their families, the desire to please their husbands may dictate the dishes they prepare for the whole household. Finally, in old age, any former control over the menu may be lost through institutionalization or displacement from the kitchen by a younger household member. Thus, for many humans, selection of food is subject to significant constraints for much of their lifetime, despite the apparent freedom of the individual to eat as they choose.

36.3 Social and cultural influences on food choice

It is not surprising then that the cook, food purchaser, housewife, or househusband, indeed any member of a group who makes food choices on behalf of that group, is sometimes referred to in research literature as the 'key kitchen person' (KKP), focal person, or gatekeeper, all terms that recognize a pivotal role in the diet and food habits of their group. What social factors influence their choice of food to prepare? The broad answer is that they select according to the unwritten rules or norms of the culture to which they belong. Even when they respond to the food preferences of a particular member of their group, they are choosing items, composing them into dishes, and combining the dishes into menus within particular culinary traditions.

Culinary traditions operate at many levels from small kin-based group traditions to the nearly global culinary styles of Western cultures. In some isolated Third World situations, only one culinary tradition may be relevant, but for most First World groups, food providers and KKPs choose to work within the tradition that they see as most appropriate for a particular eating situation. For many important social occasions, the family culinary tradition of the organizers and chief participants will be followed. The significance of the occasion (e.g. wedding breakfast, Christmas dinner, religious festival) and the desire for a successful outcome usually constrain the menu within the traditional family or community pattern.

Even at this lowest organizational level, the family pattern of eating may be distinctive from that of its neighbours, though both may belong to the same ethnic and religious group and occupy the same socio-economic position. Family food habits may be comparatively resistant to change in places where culinary knowledge and skills are learned primarily within the household and passed down between generations. Marriage residency practices, such as the wife joining her husband's extended family in a single household, may work to suppress, change, and reinforce the distinctiveness of the family tradition. Non-Western societies incorporate many different forms of household structure, depending on family lifecycle and kinship system. Each type will have a distinctive pattern of decision-making relating to food.

Urbanized communities also feature a wide range of household arrangements, from two-parent and two-generational families to groups of unrelated young adults. Food habits here are influenced by the background and social network of the group member who becomes the KKP for each main meal. If that person learned culinary skills in his or her own family setting, many of these will be transferred to the new household and applied according to the type of meal. However, in urbanized Western societies, such knowledge is frequently acquired outside the home (e.g. from the formal education system). For most of this century, cooking training in schools has been motivated by the goals of 'good nutrition' and has been responsible for reinterpreting Western culinary traditions within a scientific paradigm. There is ample evidence, however, that after schooling is complete, recipe repertoire is influenced by interaction with peers, within social networks, and by the media.

Magazines, newspapers, and television reflect an amalgam of culinary traditions depending on the contributing sources. A locally based food writer for a monthly newspaper column may work within a regional food tradition, combining new variants with well-established and familiar dishes. A national or internationally distributed magazine may offer more cosmopolitan fare, strongly influenced by international food fashion trends. However, there is little research on whether these fashions have a lasting impact on household food habits. For example, will the currently fashionable grain couscous become an important cereal in cosmopolitan cuisine, or will it be as short-lived as the fondue party?

The twentieth-century trend to a cosmopolitan culinary repertoire has probably been influenced by the range of dishes cooked in the commercial kitchens of restaurants and fast-food outlets, and sampled as part of the phenomenon of 'eating out'. For the household member who is not actively involved in food preparation, eating out means more choice is possible from an extended menu. For the KKP, the responsibility for selecting food for others is removed, along with control over the dishes on the menu and their composition. However, the characterization of restaurants and other food outlets into well-defined categories, such as vegetarian, wholefood, seafood, Italian, Thai, Cantonese, or other specified ethnic type suggests that consumers still prefer to choose their food from an identifiable culinary tradition, even if it is not that of their own birth culture.

Thus, for the purpose of food and menu selection, many Western households operate within multiple layers of culinary traditions, not simultaneously, but moving between them from meal to meal, through the weekly cycle and the annual calendar of festive occasions. Perhaps the unwritten rules for deciding which culinary tradition is appropriate are part of evolving culinary traditions in their own right.

36.4 Food habits in nutrition practice

From the viewpoint of the nutritionist offering clinical advice to an individual, it is clearly important to know how the patient relates to the KKP of the household where he or she normally resides.

Without the informed support of the KKP, long-term dietary modification is unlikely to occur. And even with that support, pressure from other members of the household or a high-status member might frustrate any change.

It is also valuable for the nutritionist to have some knowledge of the culinary tradition from which most of the patient's meals are derived. Any modification of intake must be compatible with that tradition. We tend to categorize other traditions by their starch staple and typical flavouring substances. But culinary traditions are more than just the combinations of dishes/recipes that characterize and distinguish the eating patterns of particular human groups. They also include the rules for selecting and preparing food for consumption (such as butchering practices and preservation techniques), rules for composing the menu according to an acceptable structure of courses, and the rules or norms concerning eating behaviour (e.g. time, location, participants). As with all human social behaviour, these rules or norms are culturally transmitted. They are not immutable, but variation and innovation tend to take place more frequently within the structure than radical alteration of the overall framework. Culinary traditions also include the nonnutrient-related meanings of food, including those that concern ethnic identity, values, and religious beliefs.

Within certain traditions, there is strong social pressure to prepare and serve more food on occasions than might be considered nutritionally desirable. In such instances, the food is satisfying more than biological needs, and the participants are well aware that it is carrying a coded message concerning social relationships and value systems. For example, the Oglala Sioux of Pine Ridge Reservation in South Dakota require participants at communal high feasts to eat beyond satiety, and to bring containers for the removal of leftovers. Since their culture values generosity as the most important of four cardinal virtues, overindulgence is a statement about the generosity of the host, and an affirmation that this virtue is more highly regarded by the Oglala than by Euro-Americans.

Similarly, on the Polynesian island, Tikopia, the anthropologist Raymond Firth observed that 'true hospitality consists in placing before a man more than he can possibly eat and then commanding him at intervals to continue when he shows signs of flagging'. In this Polynesian culture, which typically rates hospitality as an important virtue, the guest eats beyond satiety, regarding it as offensive to the host as well as shameful and embarrassing to confess to still being hungry. Food is used throughout Polynesia to confirm an agreement made between parties, and failure to partake could be interpreted as a sign that one party intends to break the contract.

Particular foods may encode metaphysical meanings that completely transcend any nutritional value. For the Christian taking communion, the wafer and the wine are clearly not food, but have been spiritually transformed. For modern Oglala Sioux Indians, ritual eating of dog involves equally complex rituals, reminding participants of the dog's role in Sioux cosmology and symbolizing all that is Indian in Oglala culture. The rejection of the dog as a food item by Euro-Americans adds to its symbolic importance for the Oglala, to the degree that the ceremonial stature of the dog feast has increased as Indian identity has been threatened. If dog consumption carried a health risk, a nutritionist who advised its avoidance would be threatening both group identity and religious belief.

Not all foods carry such complex spiritual meanings. However, under pressure, minority groups may encode particular items or dishes/recipes as markers of identity, when formerly they functioned simply as everyday food. Such is the case of 'soul food' in the USA. The pork and chicken products that provide the meat component of soul food, such as necks, backs, feet, and giblets, were originally eaten because they were rejected by wealthier white consumers and were therefore cheaper. In one Southern case study, it was found that black households of middle socioeconomic class described them as 'black people's food' and ate them not for their cheapness but as a marker of ethnic identity. Black families from lower socioeconomic classes and middle-class white families classified them as 'poor people's food'. Lower-class white people avoided them. These food items have acquired a

BOX 36.1 Food habits, modernization, and globalization

The Samoan archipelago in the South Pacific provides a powerful example of the effects of modernization on food habits. Modernization is usually associated with the adoption of a cash economy, urbanization, formal education, and increasing contact with the outside world. Globalization builds on those changes through the networks of multinational businesses and exposure to global media.

Although the recent arrival of fast-food outlets in the Samoan islands may be treated as a phenomenon of globalization, modernization began to affect Samoan people at least a century earlier. By the time that Paul Baker and his research team studied Samoan health in 1974–1983, modernization had already wrought significant changes.

Western Samoans and American Samoans share a Polynesian genetic heritage. Until the archipelago was partitioned in 1899, Samoans practised subsistence agriculture, obtaining most of their foodstuffs from fruit trees scattered through the landscape and from swidden gardens. Their staples (taro, breadfruit, and bananas) were supplemented with sea foods and occasionally pigs and chickens. In the traditional division of labour, young untitled men were responsible for the harvesting of crops and their preparation and cooking. At times, this was strenuous activity and the gardens might be located some distance from the village. Women were responsible for childcare, mat weaving, and village maintenance.

American Samoa was the first to begin the transition to a cash economy. Because Pago Pago Harbour on Tutuila Island was a strategic naval base, American Samoa was administered by the US Department of the Navy from 1900 to 1951. When the base closed, the territory was run by the US Department of the Interior. The naval base employed many Samoans and their wages allowed them to purchase imported foods, such as rice and canned meats. Improved health services and migration of relatives from Western Samoa fuelled a population boom. Fewer people engaged in gardening or fishing and Tutuila came to depend on food imports from Western Samoa, the USA, and Tonga. After 1951, the establishment of two canneries and creation of more public service jobs completed the economic modernization of American Samoa; a cash economy prevailed and population density built up around Pago Pago. Despite the US investment in health services, American Samoans suffered rising rates of obesity, cardiovascular diseases, and type 2 diabetes.

Were the same changes experienced in Western Samoa? After a short period as a German colony, it was administered by New Zealand, until it achieved independence in 1962. Until this time, most villagers practised subsistence agriculture, working unpaid with their extended families. There were only a few plantations employing wage labour, a small private sector, and some public servants in the capital, Apia. From 1920, a rapid rise in population occurred. As in American Samoa, migration provided an outlet for large numbers of young adults. While American Samoans migrated to Hawaii or California, Western Samoans travelled to New Zealand. Such was the strength of the extended family and concept of *tautua* (service to elders) that cash remittances from overseas relatives became significant sources of income and purchasing power for village Samoans.

Paul Baker's team found that modernization was less advanced in Western Samoa than in American Samoa. They obtained health data from isolated villages and urban centres in both Western and American Samoa, and extended the survey to Samoans resident in Hawaii and California. In weight, they found that adult men from Western Samoa averaged 76 kg and displayed a good level of physical fitness, especially those engaged in food production. American Samoan men living on more 'modern' Tutuila averaged 86.3 kg, while those in Hawaii averaged 89.8 kg and the Californian Samoans 98.8 kg. As weight increased, physical fitness measures declined. Modernization of the diet and increasingly sedentary lifestyles were identified as the main factors in the obesity epidemic affecting American Samoans. Instead of the men growing, transporting, and cooking their staple crops, waged workers (both women and men) increasingly purchased rice, mutton flaps, canned corn beef, chicken portions,

(Continued)

BOX 36.1 Food habits, modernization, and globalization (*Continued*)

bread, and soft drinks. Samoan women have taken on the role of cooking nontraditional foods, often with high fat and sugar content. Bottle-feeding has increased weight gains in infants as young women wean their babies in order to return to work.

Since the 1980s, globalization has accentuated the effects of modernization. With the arrival of fast-food outlets in American Samoa and recently Western Samoa, together with a dramatic increase in imported foods, traditional foods face greater competition than before, while imported four-wheel-drive vehicles now provide access to plantations formerly reached on foot.

status ranking and racial connotation that is perceived differently according to the socioeconomic status and ethnicity of the various groups in the case study. It would be difficult for a nutritionist to change the usage or nonusage of these foods by any of the groups concerned because of their acquired load of nonnutritional meanings.

For many societies, food choice is constrained by religious proscription. Many of these food taboos are of such antiquity that they are written into the formal teachings of the religion (such as the Jewish and Hindu dietary laws that proscribe pork or beef). However, more recent dietary regimens based on particular philosophical or ethical principles have evolved food taboos of equal force for their adherents. As a secular movement, vegetarianism has been important for nearly two centuries, throughout this period drawing for justification on the accumulating data from the science of nutrition. Not surprisingly, nutritionists faced with evidence of health benefits from vegetarian diets for adults have treated the movement with respect. However, the twentieth century has seen the development of far more restrictive dietary regimens allied to the 'health food' movement and the Western preoccupation with weight reduction. Food symbolism is highly developed in these regimens, with the polarization of 'natural' (= healthy) versus synthetic (= dangerous) constantly reworked and elaborated by those who benefit commercially from sales of diet books and the approved foods. For the clinical nutritionist, disentangling the pseudoscientific justifications and powerful symbolism of these restrictive and potentially damaging diets is a major challenge. Furthermore, the social networks into which adherents of 'fad' or extreme diets are drawn for mutual support are likely to counteract what is perceived as criticism by the health professionals.

36.5 Changing food habits in the modern world

So far, this introduction to food habits has stressed the inbuilt tendency to conservatism within a culinary tradition, the individual's lack of control over food choice at various periods in his or her life, and the symbolic loading on certain foods, which may exert powerful pressure against any change in usage or avoidance. Taken together, these factors explain why nutritional advice aimed at individual or group level may be listened to politely (because of the status of the health professional), but not subsequently acted upon.

At the same time, the success of multinational food companies provides ample evidence that throughout the world, even within highly conservative and symbol-rich culinary traditions, some substantial changes have occurred in diet during the twentieth century (Box 36.1). These have included the introduction of many new food items, and even new menus borrowed from other traditions. Food manufacturers have invested heavily in research on food acceptance and have realized that restrictive rules affecting food habits apply to meals rather than snacks. This observation, also made by Michael Nicod from his structuralist study of working-class food habits in Britain (1974), led to his definition of the meal as a structured food event and the snack as an unstructured event. Although meals have courses that must be served in a prescribed order and contain certain food categories, for snacks, consumers are free to eat the items in any order or combination, at any time, and with or without company. It is not surprising then that snack-food manufacturers have had a global impact, because their promotional advertising does not have to confront long-established culinary norms. The lack of structure in snacking behaviour has allowed it to become a global arena where multinationals compete with new products, or old ones, newly packaged.

Nutritionists have had some success in promoting snacks with lower fat and sodium content, but realize that because snacking is usually supplementary feeding, their long-term objectives can only be met by dietary reform of meals, the area in which the multinationals have made much less headway. It has taken several decades to achieve public acceptance of pizza- or burger-based main meals, when these items were originally conceived of more as snacks. Fast-food outlets have had to supply additional items such as potatoes, salads, and even desserts to meet the public's norms of what constitute 'proper' meals.

The key to effecting change in meal composition is to provide substitutions for existing elements without threatening the overall structure. Studies of dietary change in indigenous societies following contact with Europeans have shown that the way in which the new foods are slotted into existing native classification systems is a useful guide to their acceptability. The most rapidly accepted foodstuffs are those that are judged similar to existing foods, in attributes such as taste, appearance, style of preparation, or growth habit. In many Pacific Island cultures, plants closely related to species already grown were the most rapidly incorporated, for example the West Indian root crop *Xanthosoma* spp., which was predictably classified as a form of taro (*Colocasia esculenta*). South American cassava (also known as manioc) and solanum potatoes were similarly acceptable because they could be grown like traditional yams, arrowroot, and sweet potatoes. With no cereal precedent in Polynesia, maize took much longer to be slotted into local culinary and horticultural traditions. In most Pacific cultures, more than one starch staple was available, although they were seldom served at the same meal. This choice may have increased their readiness to accept the new staples introduced by Europeans. Monostaple cultures seem much more resistant to change. The depth of their attachment to their single staple may often be seen in the extension of the word used for the staple to mean food in general.

In some culture contact situations, foods that were initially disliked, but were essential to avoid starvation, eventually gained acceptance. This is reflected in the vernacular names, which give evidence of the crucial classification process. Faced by the loss of the symbolically and nutritionally important buffalo, the Oglala Sioux initially rejected government beef rations from cattle held in corrals as smelling offensive and no substitute for buffalo meat. Under pressure, they compromised by turning loose the cattle and then hunting, butchering, and ritually feasting on them as though they were buffalo. Cattle acquired buffalo terminology and became Indian.

The effects of globalization on developing countries constitute a special case of culture contact. The accompanying economic changes are of concern to nutritionists because they may lead to deleterious substitutions in traditional diets. These often involve replacement of higher-nutrient crops (such as millets in central Africa) with crops of lower nutritional value (such as cassava, which is more tolerant of drought and degraded soils). Studies have shown that given the local economic context, such diet shifts are based on rational choices designed to increase food security, even at the expense of optimal nutrition. Labour migration, pressure to produce cash crops, and increasing poverty produce adaptations in traditional food systems, which can transform adequate nutrition into chronic undernutrition or, in the most vulnerable groups, even malnutrition. In these cases, nutritional reform is unlikely to succeed unless poverty can first be reduced.

The message for nutritionists from such studies of culture contact is that the structural elements of culinary traditions are highly resistant to change. It is precisely these elements that, in giving stability and continuity, define the tradition. Where dietary change has occurred, it has involved substitution of new foods for old within the indigenous food system, using the classification process as a guide to how the new food is to be used. Judging from historical studies, actual structural changes involving things like course order and essential elements may take a century or longer. If thought nutritionally desirable, reform at such a fundamental level might be expected to add a new dimension to the notion of long-term planning! Ultimately, nutritionists must translate their findings into recommendations that will work within the culinary tradition, not against it.

Further Reading

1. **Baker, P.T., Hanna, J.M., and Baker, T.S.** (eds) (1986) *The changing Samoans: Behaviour and health in transition.* New York, Oxford University Press.
2. **Bryant, C.A., Courtney, A., Markesbery, B.A., and de Walt, K.M.** (1985) *The cultural feast: An introduction to food and society.* St Paul MN, West.
3. **Charsley, S.R.** (1992) *Wedding cakes and cultural history.* Routledge, London.
4. **Cox, D.N. and Anderson, A.S.** (2004) Food choice. In Gibney, M.J. *et al.* (eds) *Public Health Nutrition,* pp. 144–66. Oxford, Blackwell Science.
5. **Douglas, M.** (ed.) (1984) *Food in the social order: Studies of food and festivities in three American communites.* New York, Russell Sage Foundation.
6. **Douglas, M. and Nicod, M.** (1974) Taking the biscuit: The structure of British meals. *New Soc,* **30,** 744–7.
7. **Harris, M.** (1986) *Good to eat: Riddles of food and culture.* London, Allen and Unwin.
8. **Leach, H.M.** (1993) Changing diets—a cultural perspective. *Proc Nutr Soc NZ,* **18,** 1–8.
9. **Lentz, C.** (ed.) (1999) *Changing food habits: Case studies from Africa, South America and Europe.* Amsterdam, Harwood.
10. **Messer, E.** (1984) Anthropological perspectives on diet. *Annu Rev Anthropol,* **13,** 205–49.
11. **Murcott, A.** (1984) *The sociology of food and eating.* Aldershot, England, Gower.
12. **Murcott, A.** (1988) Sociological and social anthropological approaches to food and eating. *World Rev Nutr Diet,* **55,** 1–40.
13. **Robson, J.K.K.** (ed.) (1980) *Food, ecology and culture: Readings in the anthropology of dietary practices.* New York, Gordon and Breach.
14. **Sharman, A., Theophano, J., Curtis, K., and Messer, E.** (eds) (1991) *Diet and domestic life in society.* Philadelphia: Temple University.
15. **Truswell, A.S. and Wahlqvist, M.L.** (eds) (1988) *Food habits in Australia.* Richmond, Victoria, Australia, Heinemann.
16. **Visser, M.** (1988) Much depends on dinner. Toronto, McClelland and Stewart.

Useful Websites

 To see topical and scientifically robust updates on nutrition associated with this textbook and web links to many of the journals in the Further Reading sections, please see the dedicated Online Resource Centre at **http://www.oxfordtextbooks.co.uk/orc/mann4e/**

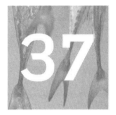

37 Nutritional recommendations for the general population

Katrine Baghurst

Nutrition research generates results that can often be translated by the media, or researchers themselves, into potentially confusing and conflicting messages. It is therefore critically important for governments, who develop food and nutrition policies, for those involved in health and nutrition education, and for consumers to have authoritative nutrition recommendations that represent consensus opinions of expert nutrition scientists. There are two major sets of recommendations: nutrient intake recommendations, and dietary guidelines and goals.

Nutrient intake recommendations were the earliest types of recommendations developed by governments and health authorities. They are based on authoritative quantitative estimates of human requirements for essential nutrients. The first set, which included only a few micronutrients, was issued by the nutrition committee of the old League of Nations in 1937. The best-known series of nutrient intake recommendations, the USA recommended dietary allowances, were first published in 1943 and have been revised 11 times since. Many other countries, groups of countries (e.g. Germany, Austria, and Switzerland; the European Community), or health authorities (e.g. FAO, WHO) have their own sets of recommended nutrient intakes.

More recently, there has been the recognition that in most relatively affluent societies, and indeed even in more affluent groups within many developing countries, inappropriate intakes of macronutrients are adversely affecting health status through increasing the prevalence of chronic degenerative diseases.

The distinction between chronic degenerative disease and deficiency disease is not always clear-cut. Some conditions, such as osteoporosis, can be considered both a deficiency disease and a chronic degenerative disease. One problem that arises in trying to set quantitative nutrient recommendations in relation to chronic disease prevention is the level of certainty surrounding the amount of a specific nutrient required for prevention of what is often a multicausal condition. Deficiency disease (e.g. scurvy, pellagra, beri-beri) is often, though not always (e.g. osteoporosis), related to a single nutrient, and quantification is sometimes more clear-cut.

In light of the increasing recognition of the role that diet plays in chronic disease aetiology, since the late 1960s many countries have developed *dietary goals*, which provide macronutrient targets aimed at achieving reductions of these diseases, and *dietary guidelines*, which help consumers to select, from the many available foods, a diet that will give them a better chance of long-term health. Dietary guidelines and goals should be based on knowledge about nutrient intake requirements. The guidelines generally address the balance of food groups required to attain a diet that will provide all the essential nutrients without the excesses that may increase chronic disease prevalence, or indeed overweight and obesity. The guidelines generally apply to total diet and not to the healthiness of particular foods. They are meant to be used as a framework for food choice at a time when the food supply in many affluent countries can be bewilderingly large and in some developing countries can be changing rapidly.

37.1 Nutrient intake recommendations

Most developed and developing countries have a set of average daily nutrient intake recommendations for various groups within their population. Recommendations are generally given by age category, by gender, and for pregnancy and lactation. Until recently, these recommendations focused on a single value per nutrient per age/gender/lifestage group, often called a recommended dietary allowance (RDA) or intake (RDI) or a reference or recommended nutrient intake (RNI) that would be sufficient to cover the needs of most people in that population group.

The original 1943 US National Research Council's RDAs were defined as a 'tentative goals towards which to aim in planning dietaries'. They were later described in the 1964 edition as 'designed to afford a margin of sufficiency above average physiological requirements to cover variations among practically all individuals in the general population'. Essentially the same definition continued in the 1989 edition: 'RDAs are the levels of intake of essential nutrients that, on the basis of scientific knowledge, are judged by the Food and Nutrition Board to be adequate to meet the known nutrient needs of practically all healthy persons'.

The latest revision of the nutrient intake recommendations for the USA was undertaken jointly with Canada and published in a series of reports from 1997 to 2005, as dietary reference intakes (DRIs). In contrast to their earlier publications, the DRIs incorporated several reference figures for each nutrient along the same lines as the UK dietary reference values for food and energy (DRVs) published in 1991. In November 2010, the USA–Canadian DRIs for calcium and vitamin D were revised. This new approach involves defining a set of values for each nutrient for each age/gender group and for pregnancy and lactation, which may include (in the case of the UK) a lower reference figure covering the needs of the 2–3% of the population with the lowest requirement; a figure assessed as being the average requirement for a particular age/gender and pregnancy/lactation group; a figure (equivalent to the traditional RDA) that would cover the needs of the majority of the population (e.g. 97–98%); an optimal range of intake; and an upper level that may indicate a regular daily intake level above which harm might result (Table 37.1).

Many different group names are used for these sets of nutrient intake recommendations such as dietary reference intakes (USA/Canada); dietary

Table 37.1 Different terms used for requirements of essential nutrients

R1	Lower diagnostic level of essential nutrient	EU: lowest threshold intake UK: lower reference nutrient intake (LRNI)
R2	Average nutrient requirement of a subgroup of an apparently healthy population	USA/Canada, Australia/New Zealand, UK, and FAO/WHO: estimated average requirement (EAR)
R3	Amount to cover most members of the apparently healthy population	USA/Canada: recommended dietary allowance (RDA) Austria/Germany/Switzerland: recommended intake (RI) Australia/New Zealand: recommended dietary intake (RDI) FAO/WHO: recommended nutrient intake (RNI) UK: reference nutrient intake (RNI)
R3B	Amount to cover most members of the apparently healthy population but where data is limited and certainty much less	USA/Canada, Australia/New Zealand: adequate intake (AI) UK: safe intake Germany/Austria/Switzerland: estimated values and guiding values (for certain nutrients)
R4	Suggested optimal range of intake	Intakes that give 'high-level' wellness or reduced risk of one, or more, degenerative diseases USA/Canada: acceptable macronutrient distribution ranges (AMDR) Australia/New Zealand: suggested dietary targets and acceptable macronutrient distribution ranges FAO/WHO: protective nutrient intake Germany/Austria/Switzerland: guiding values (for certain nutrients)
R5	Undesirably high intake or start of toxic level	USA/Canada, EU: tolerable upper intake level (UL) Australia/New Zealand: upper level (UL) UK: safe upper levels for vitamins and minerals

reference values for food and energy (UK); nutrient reference values (Australia/New Zealand), or reference values for nutrient intake (Germany/Austria/Switzerland). In addition, different names may be used for the individual values within each set (Table 37.1). For example, for estimates of the requirement to cover the needs of the majority of the population, terms used include recommended dietary allowance (USA/Canada); recommended dietary intake (Australia/New Zealand); recommended nutrient intake (FAO/WHO); recommended intake (Germany/Austria/Switzerland); or reference nutrient intake (UK).

There has also been an increasing recognition that for some nutrients data is so limited or con-

flicting that recommendations are made with less certainty than for other nutrients. In this case, some countries have used a different term such as adequate intake (USA/Canada and Australia/New Zealand); estimated or guiding values for adequate intake (Germany/Austria/Switzerland), or safe intake (UK). Table 37.2 shows some international comparisons.

Why does each country have a different set of these numbers? When the figures are compared, it will be seen that many are similar, if not the same, as those from other countries. Some countries simply adopt the figures from another country or authority. For example, many developing countries will use figures published by FAO/WHO and indeed take

Table 37.2 Nutrient intake recommendations (per day) from four national sets and FAO/WHO, for selected nutrients for men: RDA/RDI/RNI, R3s in Table 37.1

Nutrient	USA/Canada 1997–2004 RDA or AI (31–50 years)	Australia/New Zealand 2005 RDI or AI (19–50 years)	Germany/Austria/ Switzerland 2000 RI (25–51 years)	UK 1991 RNI (19–50 years)	FAO/WHO 2001 RNI (19–51 years)
Protein (g)	58	64	59	45	55[a]
Vitamin A (mg)	1.0	0.9	1.0	0.7	0.6
Vitamin D[d] (µg)	10	5.0	5.0	—	5.0
Vitamin E (mg)	15	10.0	12	(7)	—
Thiamin (mg)	1.2	1.2	1.2	1.0	1.2
Riboflavin (mg)	1.3	1.3	1.4	1.3	1.3
Niacin (mg)	16	16	16	17	16
Vitamin B$_6$ (mg)	1.7	1.3	1.5	1.4	1.3
Folate (µg)	400	400	400	200	400
Vitamin B$_{12}$ (µg)	2.4	2.4	3.0	1.5	2.4
Vitamin C (mg)	90	45	100	40	45
Calcium[d] (mg)	1000	1000	1000	700	1000
Iron (mg)	10	8	10	8.7	9[b]
Zinc (mg)	15	14	10	9.5	7
Iodine (µg)	150	150	200	140	140[c]
Selenium (µg)	55	70	30–70	75	34

[a]1985 figures for protein.

[b]For diets with 15% bioavailability.

[c]2 µg/kg body weight (assuming body weight of 70 kg).

[d]DRIs for calcium and vitamin D were revised in 2010. Calcium recommendation for this age remained the same; vitamin D was increased to 15 mg.

part in their initial development. Undertaking a major review of these figures is both time-consuming and expensive so many countries will use figures derived by another equivalent country (e.g. with a population with similar body size/culture/environment) but may vary their figures in the light of newer research data, a different philosophical approach, country-specific data, concerns about interpretation of the research data, or a perception that some key information was not considered. There may also be differences in the age groups used by different countries in relation to their own particular policy and assessment needs.

No matter what nomenclature is used, the purpose of the recommended figures in Table 37.2 is to set a standard for an adequate intake of each essential nutrient for individuals or groups in the population. They advise people how much, on the average, they should aim to eat each day of these nutrients. They have a prescriptive or health promotion role.

Table 37.3 Range of requirements for selected essential nutrients

Adult daily requirements (rounded)	Essential nutrients
2–5 µg	Vitamin B$_{12}$, vitamin D
30–40 µg	Chromium, molybdenum, biotin
70–100 µg	Selenium, vitamin K
~150 µg	Iodine
~400 µg	Folate
1–3 mg	Vitamin A, thiamin, riboflavin, vitamin B$_6$, fluoride, copper
5–15 mg	Pantothenate, manganese, vitamin E, niacin (equivalents), zinc, iron
50–100 mg	Vitamin C
400–500 mg	Magnesium, sodium
1–2 g	Calcium, phosphorus, essential fatty acids, potassium
~50 g	Protein
~2 kg (litres)	Water

They also serve as the reference unit for each essential nutrient. We need them because adult human requirements for individual nutrients range 1 billion-fold from just over 1 µg for vitamin B$_{12}$, through 1 mg for thiamin, to 1 g for calcium and greater than 1 kg for water (Table 37.3).

37.2 How should the various measures be used?

In the past, most countries published tables with only the single figure for population requirement (i.e. R3 in Table 37.1) variously known as the RDA, RDI or RNI, although an estimate of average requirement was generally necessary in order to derive the population figure. Since this 'population' figure is adequate to meet nutritional needs of practically all healthy people, it is more than most people need. It could not, therefore, be used directly to evaluate records of people's food intake for adequacy at the individual level, or if it was, there may be a misleading impression of inadequacy. Different approaches were used to define a diagnostic level for 'deficiency', with some people simply using two-thirds of the RDA, RDI, or RNI.

In recent publications, an estimated average requirement figure has received the same prominence as the population recommendation. Although the average requirement was often to be found in the text of earlier publications, it rarely appeared in the tabular form that nutrition and health practitioners and consumers regularly used. For micronutrients, it is prudent to encourage people to eat more than the estimated average requirement for the group. Those with higher requirements should then get enough, while those with low requirements will come to no harm from eating a little more than needed. However, for energy, it is important for people to match their intake with their needs by adjusting their dietary intake and/or physical activity. Having a little more calories than needed each day can only increase body weight in the long term.

The availability of published and tabulated estimated average requirements helps to make assessment at the individual level more accurate than in the past. Table 37.4 shows how the various types of values now made available can be used to assess adequacy of either individual or group intakes. As part of the process of review for the US/Canadian DRIs, a statistical probability method was developed by Beaton in Canada, to assess more accurately the probability that a selected nutrient intake would be adequate for a particular person or group of people. A statistical estimate of degree of risk of inadequacy can be made using Beaton's algorithms. The parameters used in Beaton's model are nutrient-specific, depending on the known variability in population needs for that particular nutrient (Beaton, 1994).

Publication of an upper level of intake in some sets of recommendations has occurred partly in response to increasing interest in and use of nutri-

tion supplements. It is difficult to overdose on vitamins and minerals from natural food sources; much easier if they are available as supplements. Consumers and pharmacists need guidance about a level that would be too much. It has long been known that vitamin A (retinol) and vitamin D can be toxic in some people at chronic intakes only 10 times the RDA/RDI. It used to be acknowledged that fat-soluble vitamins could be toxic but that water-soluble vitamins would simply be excreted. The finding that vitamin B_6 in excess could cause peripheral neuropathy and that other water-soluble vitamins could be harmful in people with compromised kidney function changed this. Table 37.5 shows a comparison of upper intake recommendations from a number of countries. The US/Canadian DRI review defines this level as the highest level of a nutrient that is likely to pose no risk of adverse health effects for almost all individuals in the general population. As intake increases above the upper level, the risk of adverse effects increases. While there is general agreement for many nutrients, for some, estimates can vary quite widely because of the limited data.

Table 37.4 Uses of the various values for assessing adequacy of intake in individuals and groups

Nutrient reference value	For individuals	For groups
Estimated average requirement (EAR)	Use to examine the probability that usual intake is inadequate	Use to estimate the prevalence of inadequate intakes within a group
Population recommendation (e.g. RDA, RDI, RNI)	Usual intake at or above this level has a low probability of inadequacy	Do not use to assess intakes of groups
Adequate intake (AI) or safe intake (population figure where data is limited or conflicting)	Usual intake at or above this level has a low probability of inadequacy. When the AI is based on median intakes of healthy populations, this assessment is made with less confidence	Mean usual intake at or above this level implies a low prevalence of inadequate intakes. When the AI is based on median intakes of healthy populations, this assessment is made with less confidence
Upper level of intake (UL)	Usual intake above this level may place an individual at risk of adverse effects from excessive nutrient intake	Use to estimate the percentage of the population at potential risk of adverse effects from excessive nutrient intake

Table 37.5 Proposed upper levels for essential nutrients for non-pregnant adults from three national sets of recommendations

	USA/Canada 1997–2000	Germany/Austria/ Switzerland 2000	Australia/New Zealand 2005
Vitamin A (mg)	3	3	3
Vitamin D[a] (µg)	50	50	80
Vitamin E (mg)	1000	800	300
Niacin (mg)	35	35	35
Vitamin B_6 (mg)	100	100	50
Folate (µg)	1000	1000	1000
Vitamin B_{12} (µg)	Not possible to set	5000	Not possible to set
Vitamin C (mg)	2000	1000	Not possible to set
Calcium (mg)	2500	2000	2500
Iron (mg)	45	—	45
Iodine (µg)	1100	500–1000	1100
Selenium (µg)	400	400	400

[a] In 2010, these were revised to 100 µg for vitamin D.

37.3 Optimal intakes for chronic disease prevention

Although the RDAs or RDIs are traditionally determined on the basis of needs for sustenance and avoidance of deficiency disease, it is obviously most beneficial if nutrient intakes are also compatible with intakes that may reduce chronic disease risk. There is an extensive and growing database related to diet and chronic disease risk in humans, but the population methodologies generally employed have a number of limitations in relation to identifying a specific level of intake that is optimal for reducing the risk of chronic disease. With that proviso in mind, there is some evidence that a range of nutrients could have benefits in chronic disease aetiology at levels above the RDI/RDA/RNIs.

The nutrients for which higher-than-recommended population intakes have been linked to benefits for chronic disease include the antioxidant vitamins such as vitamin C, vitamin E, and vitamin A (primarily its precursor, β-carotene), as well as selenium and nutrients such as folate, ω-3, fats and dietary fibre. For these nutrients, there is a reasonably large body of evidence of potential protective effects of higher than RDA/RDI levels for one or more chronic diseases such as coronary heart disease, certain cancers, degenerative eye diseases (such as cataract formation or macular degeneration) and conditions like Alzheimer's or cognitive decline. In the case of folate, higher than RDA/RDI levels may also further decrease the occurrence of neural tube defects. There is also a lesser volume of evidence for a number of other nutrients. The 'suggested dietary targets' for micronutrients for prevention of chronic disease from the Australian/New Zealand nutrient reference values (NRVs) are shown in Table 37.6. As it is difficult to identify accurately the levels of intake that confer optimal protection,

Table 37.6 Suggested dietary targets to reduce chronic disease risk—micronutrients, dietary fibre, and long-chain n-3 fats from the Australian and New Zealand nutrient reference values

Nutrient	Suggested dietary target (intake per day on average)[a]	Comments
Vitamin A	Vitamin A: — Men 1500 µg — Women 1220 µg Carotenes: — Men 5800 µg — Women 5000 µg	The suggested dietary target is equivalent to the 90th centile of intake in the Australian and New Zealand populations
Vitamin C	Men 220 mg Women 190 mg	Equivalent to the 90th centile of intake in the Australian/New Zealand populations
Vitamin E	Men 19 mg Women 14 mg	Equivalent to the 90th centile of intake in the Australian/New Zealand populations
Selenium	No specific figure can be set. There is some evidence of potential benefit for certain cancers but adverse effects for others	There are no available population intake data for Australia. New Zealand is a known low-selenium area; thus recommendations based on centiles of population intakes are inappropriate
Folate	An additional 100–400 µg DFE over current intakes (i.e. a total of about 300–600 µg DFE) may be required to optimize homocysteine levels and reduce overall chronic disease risk and DNA damage	Current population intakes are well below the new recommended intakes
Sodium/ potassium	Sodium: — Men 1600 mg, 70 mmol — Women 1600 mg, 70 mmol Potassium: — Men 4700 mg, 120 mmol — Women 4700 mg, 120 mmol	An upper level of 2300 mg (100 mmol)/day was set for the general population, but additional preventative health benefits (maintaining optimal blood pressure over the lifespan) may accrue if sodium intakes are further reduced to about 1600 mg (70 mmol)/day, in line with WHO recommendations. Reducing intakes to this level may also bring immediate benefit to older and overweight people with pre-existing hypertension. As potassium can blunt the effect of sodium on blood pressure, intakes at the 90th centile of current population intake may help to mitigate the effects of sodium on blood pressure until intakes of sodium can be lowered.
Dietary fibre	Men 38 g Women 28 g	Upper level at 90th centile of intake for reduction in CHD risk
Long-chain ω-3 fats (DHA, EPA, DPA)	Men 610 mg Women 430 mg	The suggested dietary target is equivalent to the 90th centile of intake in the Australian/New Zealand population

[a]For most nutrients, unless otherwise noted, this is based on the 90th centile of current population intake.

CHD, chronic heart disease; DFE, dietary folate equivalents; DHA, docosahexaenoic acid; DPA, docosapentaenoic acid; EPA, eicosapentaenoic acid.

these Australian/New Zealand targets were generally set at the 90th percentile of current population dietary intake, on the premise that many epidemiological findings are based on observational data comparing upper and lower quintiles of intake in the population under study and that this level of intake is unlikely to cause harm.

In addition to micronutrients, the role of the various types of carbohydrates (starches, sugars, high-glycaemic versus low-glycaemic carbohydrates, resistant starch, dietary fibres), fats (saturated, polyunsaturated, monounsaturated), and protein (animal, plant-based) have been variously assessed in relation to risk of conditions such as coronary heart disease, certain cancers, diabetes or insulin sensitivity, and risk of obesity. Unlike the micronutrients, the macronutrients (proteins, fats, and carbohydrates) all contribute to dietary energy intake.

For a given energy intake, increases in the proportion of one macronutrient necessarily involves a decrease in the proportion of one, or more, of the other macronutrients—a high-fat diet is usually relatively low in carbohydrate and vice versa. Imbalance in the proportions of macronutrients can increase risk of chronic disease and may adversely affect micronutrient intake. In addition, the form of fat (e.g. saturated, polyunsaturated, monounsaturated, or specific fatty acids) or carbohydrate (e.g. starches or sugars, high or low glycaemic index) has to be considered.

There appears to be quite a wide range of relative intakes of proteins, carbohydrates, and fats that are acceptable in terms of chronic disease risk. The risk of chronic disease (and of inadequate micronutrient intake) may increase outside these ranges, but data in free-living populations are limited at these extremes of intake. Much of the evidence is based on epidemiological studies with clinical endpoints but they generally show associations rather than causality and are often confounded by other factors that can affect chronic disease outcomes. The macronutrient recommendations from the US/Canadian DRIs and the Australian/New Zealand NRVs are shown in Table 37.7.

These acceptable macronutrient distribution ranges and the recommendations for micronutrient intakes for chronic disease prevention seem, on the surface, to resemble what are sometimes called 'dietary goals'. However, dietary goals are designed to direct national policy by outlining what nutrients or foods the nation should consume and provide, and are primarily addressed to bureaucrats and professionals. They are population targets, whereas the 'acceptable macronutrient distribution ranges' and 'suggested dietary targets' for chronic disease prevention are aimed at individuals in the population.

One recent example of population dietary goals was produced by the WHO in 2003, in a report called *Diet, nutrition and the prevention of chronic disease.* The suite of goals included some for percentage energy to be supplied by different macronutrients,

Table 37.7 Acceptable macronutrient distribution ranges for macronutrients to reduce chronic disease risk while still ensuring adequate micronutrient status

Nutrient	Australia/New Zealand 2005	USA/Canada 2005
Protein	15–25% of energy	10–35% of energy
Carbohydrate	45–65% of energy (predominantly from low-energy-density and/or low-glycaemic-index foods)	45–65% of energy
Fat	20–35% of energy	20–35% of energy
Linoleic acid (ω-6 fat)	From 4–5% to 10% of energy	5–10% of energy
α-Linolenic acid (ω-3 fat)	From 0.4–0.5% to 1% energy	0.6–1.2% of energy

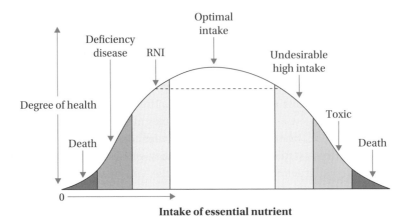

Fig. 37.1 The concept of optimal intake above the population recommended nutrient intake (i.e. RNI/RDA/RDI). Ingestion of the RNI/RDA/RDI should guarantee no deficiency disease, but beyond this there may still be additional health benefits (e.g. partial protection from a degenerative disease). The top of the dome beyond the RNI/RDA/RDI is then the optimal intake range.

and for cholesterol (less than 300 mg/day), sodium (less than 2 g/day) as well as for amounts of certain food groups (fruit and vegetable intake of 5400 g/day). When recommendations are made about nutrient intake for chronic disease prevention, it is thus important to be clear whether the cut-off numbers refer to populations or individuals. If the goal is set for the population, not every individual needs to conform for the population goal to be met.

Fig. 37.1 shows the general inter-relationships between the various levels of recommended intakes and health outcomes.

37.4 Reference numbers for nutrition labelling and food standards

In many countries, labels on food packaging carry information relating the content of that food to a daily reference figure for intake derived from the nutrient recommendations. Because of the limitations of size in most instances, a single reference figure for a given nutrient is derived from the range available across gender and age bands. In the USA, this kind of figure is called a daily value (DV) and the nutrient content of a food may be expressed as % DV per serving or per unit weight, based on their 1968 RDAs.

With adoption of the 1997–2004 DRVs in the USA/and Canada, it has been recommended that the concept of expressing nutrient content as % DV be retained and that the DV be based on the population-weighted estimated average requirement. Where no estimated average requirement (EAR) could be set, the AI would be used as the reference. In addition, it was recommended that the acceptable macronutrient distribution ranges should be the basis for the DVs for the macronutrients protein, total carbohydrate, and total fat; that 2000 calories should be used, when needed, as the basis for expressing energy intake when developing DVs; and finally that the DVs for saturated fatty acids, *trans*-fatty acids and cholesterol should be set at a level as low as possible in keeping with an achievable health-promoting diet. For infancy, toddlers aged 1–3 years, pregnancy, and lactation, different sets of DVs were recommended based on the EAR or AIs for those specific groups, as their needs vary markedly from the general population.

In Australia and New Zealand, before the 2005 revision of NRVs, the food law RDIs were based on the highest 1991 Australian/New Zealand RDIs for non-pregnant, non-lactating, younger adults. Thus, the RDI for younger adult men was generally used, with the exception of iron, for which the lower end of the range for younger women was used. This approach is likely to change with the advent of the new NRVs.

The wordings and the reference values used for food for labelling purposes are generally laid down by food law set by statutory bodies such as the Food and Drug Administration (FDA) in the USA or Food Standards Australia New Zealand (FSANZ) in Australia and New Zealand. The same reference value may be used in controlling permitted additions of micronutrients in food fortification (e.g. up to 50% DV may be added per reference quantity of food 'X').

37.5 Dietary guidelines

In contrast to dietary goals, 'dietary guidelines' are usually developed as advice to the general public about optimal food choices and consump-

tion behaviours, written in reader-friendly language for ordinary people, although they are often backed up by a technical explanation,

---

BOX 2.1 Comparison of nutrient intake recommendations (NIRs) and dietary goals and guidelines (DGGs)

- NIRs are primarily designed to ensure adequate intake of essential nutrients, while the focus of DGGs is promotion of general health as well as prevention of chronic disease. However, when developing dietary guidelines, this is done in such a way as to also ensure adequate essential nutrient intake. Some countries (e.g. the USA and Canada) now include consideration of chronic disease prevention in setting their NIRs.

- NIRs deal only with essential nutrients. DGGs deal more with the balance of macronutrients (although some chronic disease-related micronutrients such as sodium may be included). DGGs have a whole-diet approach with a focus on food groups and dietary behaviour for optimal health and wellbeing, avoidance of deficiency disease, and prevention of chronic disease.

- NIRs are expressed as weights (μg, mg, g) of nutrients required per day (and right now) for optimal physiological function and prevention of deficiency in a specified age, gender or lifestyle group (e.g. an estimated average requirement of 5 mg/day for women aged 19–51 years). NIRs have both diagnostic (EAR) and prespective (RDA/RDI/RNI) numbers. DGGs are traditionally population targets often expressed in relative terms (e.g. less than 10% energy as saturated fat). While appropriate for the here and now, they often have a time line attached for monitoring success of government initiatives to improve national dietary intake (e.g. a population mean intake of less than 10% saturated fat by the year 2010). DGGs are generally expressed qualitatively (e.g. 'eat plenty of fruits, vegetables, and legumes'; 'choose foods low in salt') but may be quantified in an accompanying food guide giving recommendations as specified 'serves' per day of various food groups (e.g. the US Dietary Pyramid).

- NRIs are relatively well established scientifically and usually depend on the results of short-term physiological experiments, DGGs are more provisional and are based on indirect evidence about the complex role of food components in multifactorial diseases with long incubation periods. They rely more on epidemiological evidence than NIRs.

Although there is never more than one NRI report in a country, there can be several sets of DGGs in a large country at any one time.

which may include quantitative expression of the guideline in the form of a food guide such as the US diet pyramid. Examples include statements such as 'enjoy a variety of nutritious food', 'eat plenty of vegetables, legumes and fruits', 'choose foods low in salt', 'care for your food, and prepare and store it safely', and 'encourage and support breastfeeding'. The dietary guidelines usually come as a set of recommendations that are meant to be adopted as a whole to produce an overall dietary pattern that will optimize health and wellbeing and prevent chronic disease, while providing all essential nutrients. Box 37.1 highlights some of the differences between dietary guidelines and goals, and nutrient intake recommendations.

In recent years, guidelines related to encouraging maintenance of desirable body weights and physical activity have been added to some countries' suite of guidelines, in recognition of the intimate relationship between dietary intake of energy and appropriate physical activity in maintenance of appropriate body weight.

Dietary guidelines have been published in at least 35 countries, starting with the Nordic countries in 1968. As an example, Table 37.8 shows the headings of the *Dietary guidelines for Australian adults* published in 2003 and Table 37.9 shows a comparison of key messages related to cereal consumption from various countries. In many countries, there have been several new editions or publications since the first appearance. In the USA, dietary guidelines are revised every 5 years.

Some countries produce a single set of recommendations for their population no matter what age or lifestyle; others (such as New Zealand and Australia (Tables 37.8 and 37.9)) have developed different sets of recommendations for various groups such as infants and toddlers, children, adults, the elderly, and, in the case of New Zealand, pregnant and lactating women. This latter approach was encouraged by the WHO at a 1993 symposium, which concluded that guidelines would be most effective if targeted to defined groups.

In May 2010, the US Dietary Guidelines Advisory Committee (DGAC) produced a report which formed

Table 37.8 Dietary guidelines for Australian adults

Enjoy a wide variety of nutritious foods
Eat plenty of vegetables, legumes, and fruits
Eat plenty of cereals (including breads, rice, pasta, and noodles)—preferably wholegrain
Include lean meat, fish, poultry, and/or alternatives
Include milks, yoghurts, cheeses, and/or alternatives—reduced-fat varieties should be chosen where possible
Drink plenty of water
Take care to:
Limit saturated fat and moderate fat intake
Choose foods low in salt
Limit your alcohol intake if you choose to drink
Consume only moderate amounts of sugars and foods containing added sugars
Prevent weight gain—be physically active and eat according to your energy needs
Care for your food—prepare and store it safely
Encourage and support breastfeeding

Table 37.9 Comparison of guidelines mentioning cereals from various countries

Country, year	Guideline
Australia 2003	Eat plenty of cereals (including breads, rice, pasta, and noodles)—preferably wholegrain
Denmark 1983	Eat more bread and corn products, potatoes, vegetables, and fruit
France 1981	For sufficient fibre, take wholemeal breads, vegetables, cereals, (dry) legumes, dried fruits, etc.
Hungary 1988	Always have wholegrain bread on the table; choose potatoes over rice
Japan 1985	Eat 30 (different) foodstuffs a day; take staple food (i.e. rice) main dish and side dish together
Singapore 1989	Increase intake of fruit and vegetables and wholegrain cereal products, thereby increasing vitamins A and C and fibre
UK 1990	Eat plenty of food rich in starch and fibre (examples given)
USA 2011	Consume at least half of all grains as wholegrains. Increase wholegrain intake by replacing refined grains with wholegrains.

the basis of the 2010 US Dietary Guidelines. In this revision, the DGAC has targeted a specific health issue namely obesity, including childhood obesity. There is a greater emphasis on a total diet approach, on the importance of physical activity, on ways to increase nutrient density, and on ways to overcome barriers to uptake of the recommendations both at the individual and societal level. Whilst the general food group recommendations do not differ markedly from earlier versions (e.g. increased consumption of plant-based food groups as well as fish and low-fat dairy, reduction of added sugars and solid fats and salt, etc.), there is a recognition that a range of different styles of diet can be accommodated within this general rubric. The report also acknowledges the need to address the needs of specific age groups such as children and the elderly, as well as the needs of pregnant and lactating women and infants.

In addition to the various national sets of dietary guidelines, organizations such as the WHO have been active in the development of food-based dietary guidelines, particularly aimed at assisting developing countries, and many health authorities such as heart, cancer, diabetes, or vegetarian foundations or societies have also produced guidelines for their constituencies.

Among the various sets of recommendations, there are some common themes shown in Box 37.2. Precise wording may vary.

Other guidelines that are more controversial and less widely recommended relate to issues such as polyunsaturated fats, dietary cholesterol and 'refined', 'extrinsic', 'added', or 'concentrated' sugars (i.e. not the natural sugars found in fruits and milk). On sugar, there is the widest range of opinions. Some countries recommend that less than 10% of

BOX 37.2 Dietary guidelines for which there is almost complete agreement across countries

- Eat a nutritionally adequate diet composed of a variety of foods
- Eat less fat (particularly saturated fat)
- Adjust energy balance for body weight control (less energy intake, more physical activity)
- Eat more wholegrain cereals, vegetables, and fruits
- Reduce salt intake
- Drink alcohol in moderation (if you drink at all)

energy comes from refined sugars (e.g. Nordic countries and Singapore); others do not mention sugar at all (e.g. Japan and South Korea). There are many different guidelines related to sugar including:

- Do not increase sugar consumption.
- Decrease sugar (not quantified).
- Consume only moderate amounts of sugars and foods containing added sugars.
- Cut down on sugary snacks and sweets between meals.
- Eat sweets seldom.
- Reduce sugary snacks.

A third group of recommendations appear only in a few sets of guidelines:

- Quench thirst with water.
- Drink fluoridated water (or fluoride tablets).
- Make sure you get enough calcium or milk.
- Preserve (by good food preparation) the nutritive value of foods.
- Keep food safe to eat.
- Eat three good meals a day.
- Do not eat too much protein.
- Eat foods containing iron.
- Reduced intake of salt-cured, preserved, and smoked foods.
- Limit caffeine intake.
- Eat happily for a happy family life.

37.6 How do the nutrient intake recommendations relate to the dietary goals and guidelines?

It should go without saying that a diet that may lower the incidence of chronic disease (e.g. one lower in dietary or saturated fat) will not bring optimal health and wellbeing in the community if, in lowering the intake of fat, it compromises attainment of intake of essential fat-soluble vitamins, essential fatty acids, or nutrients commonly found in foods also contributing to saturated fat intake (e.g. meats and milks). If goals aimed at reducing saturated fat result in people eating substantially less meat and milks, rather than choosing lower-fat versions, then intakes of certain nutrients that are borderline in the community, such as iron and zinc, which are primarily sourced from these food groups, may be compromised.

Thus, in order to develop goals and guidelines in such a way as to achieve the desired outcomes,

consideration of essential nutrient needs is a necessary first step (Fig. 37.2). It is a common misconception that dietary goals and guidelines are developed only from consideration of the evidence from chronic disease epidemiology. For example, in countries such as Australia and the USA, the more quantitative aspect of the guidelines are derived by a computerized modelling exercise linking nutrients to foods using national food databases to derive the amounts and types of various foods/food groups required to attain the nutrient needs of the various groups. Once basic requirements are met, this can then be refined and added to with reference to the evidence from chronic disease epidemiology.

37.7 Dietary goals and guidelines in developing countries

Dietary guidelines were originally introduced to address the nutrition problems of excess in affluent countries. In developing countries, the major nutri-

tional problem is that large sections of the population cannot afford or cannot grow enough food to meet all their family's requirements for essential nutrients.

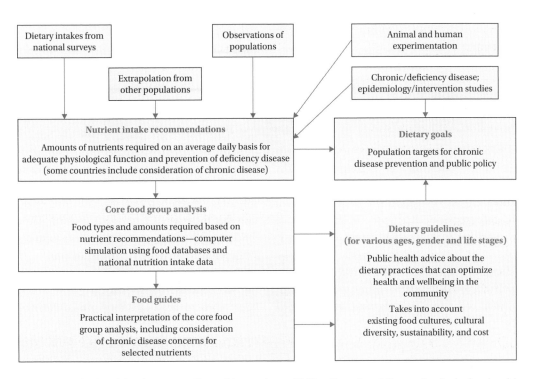

Fig. 37.2 Interrelationships between the evidence-based NIRs, Core Food Group Analysis food guides, dietary goals, and dietary guidelines.

There are, however, reasons why dietary goals and guidelines have a role in developing countries.

- Diet-related, non-communicable diseases in developing countries account for an increasing share of national mortality.
- Low-income countries cannot afford to add the burden of medical care of premature degenerative diseases to their already overstretched health budgets.
- Preparation and production of dietary guidelines is a low-cost measure.
- The affluent middle-class in a country such as India or Indonesia may only be 5% of the population, but this means many millions of people

(about 40 million in India—more than many whole nations). Many of these more affluent people in the community play a key role in the nation's development.

For India, Gopalan (1989) proposed two sets of guidelines. For the 'relatively poor' majority, diets should be least expensive and conform to tradition and cultural practice as far as possible. Some legumes (pulses) should be eaten along with the high-cereal diet, with some milk and leafy vegetable eaten each day. For affluent Indians, he recommends restriction of energy and of fat (especially ghee), sugar, and salt, with emphasis on unrefined cereals and green leafy vegetables in the diet.

37.8 Integrating nutrient recommendations and dietary guidelines in nutrition promotion

In most countries, for the general community, the 'public face' of the national recommendations relating to nutrient intake and dietary guidelines takes the form of a food choice guide, which can be summarized in a graphical form with some additional explanatory text.

Most countries base their guide on food groups, but the number of food groups varies widely from as few as three, in countries such as Fiji and a number of African countries, to seven or eight in countries such as the Caribbean. In industrialized countries, food guides generally contain between four and six food groups. Three-group systems often group foods under the headings of 'energy' foods (grains, tubers, etc. and sometimes fats and oils), 'protein' or 'growth' foods (meats, milks, legumes, etc.) and 'protective' foods to provide additional vitamins and minerals (fruits and vegetables, etc.). Groupings commonly used in the more complex guides include meat/fish/poultry and alternatives (including legumes), milk and milk products, fruits, vegetables, cereals, and fats and oils.

Because of the degree of commonality in their nutrient profile, fruits and vegetables often form a single group. Sometimes, because of the importance of a particular staple, such as potato in Finland, that particular food alone constitutes one of the categories. Sometimes the 'starchy' foods such as potato, rice, and other cereals are grouped together. Some countries also include an additional food group category of 'less healthy' extra or indulgence foods—generally these are energy-dense foods or drinks, high in fat, salt, sugar, or alcohol. They are addressed in recognition that these foods and drinks do form part of the food supply in many countries and can form part of a healthy diet if consumed in small amounts.

The graphic display of food group recommendations also varies from country to country (Fig. 37.3). In some countries, a pyramid form has been used.

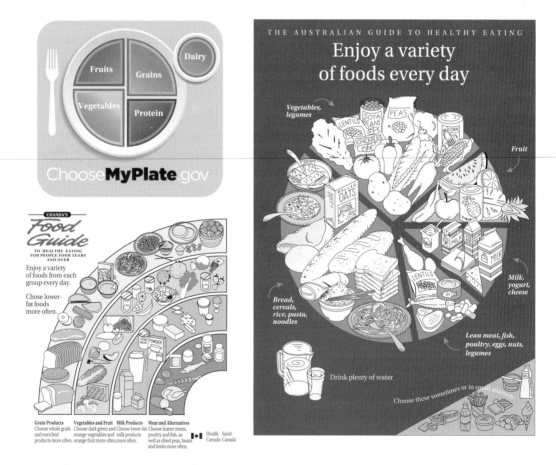

Fig. 37.3 Examples of three national food guides—the US updated 2011 MyPlate, the Canadian Rainbow, and the Australian Guide to Healthy Eating.

The 1990s US version showed breads and cereals at the base, with fruits and vegetables at the next level, followed by meat and alternatives and the milk group on the next level, and finally fats and sweets at the pinnacle. The 2005 revision aligned all food groups vertically in a pyramid with the groups represented by different-coloured segments, displayed in proportion to the recommended amounts. There were no representations of foods per se in the latest version of the Pyramid Guide graphic used until 2011. In 2011, the US changed from using a Pyramid Guide to a simpler Plate Guide (MyPlate). Some Nordic countries, together with health organizations in China, Australia and New Zealand, have also used pyramid or triangle designs. In the UK, Australia, many European countries, and the Caribbean, the national food guide is depicted as a plate or in a circular or semicircular design often divided up in proportion into the recommended amounts for the various food groups. Sometimes a food square is used in developing countries with each group equally represented (e.g. Iran). Other designs include a quarter-rainbow (Canada), steps (New Zealand), a wine glass (Israel), and a traffic light (UK Health Education Council), which is also often used in diabetic education materials.

Key points

There are several types of nutrition information and guidance based on expert opinion that governments provide for their population as a basis of nutrition education, to optimize health and address both deficiency and chronic disease prevalence.

Nutrient intake recommendations are primarily the amounts of the essential nutrients required to prevent deficiency in healthy people. Numbers differ for different age, gender, and physiological groups.

Dietary goals or guidelines assume adequate nutrient intake and advise on eating more or less of different foods to reduce the risk of chronic diseases. Uses of these two sets of recommendations include giving meaning to nutrient labelling of packaged foods and expression in user-friendly graphic food guides.

Further Reading

1. **Beaton, G.H.** (1994) Criteria of an adequate diet. In Shils, M.E., Olson, J.A. and Shike, M. (eds) *Modern nutrition in health and disease*, 8th edition, pp. 1491–505. Philadelphia, Lea & Febiger.
2. **Commonwealth Department of Health and Ageing, New Zealand Ministry of Health, NHMRC** (2005) *Nutrient reference values for Australia and New Zealand including recommended dietary intakes*. Canberra, National Health and Medical Research Council.
3. **Department of Health.** (1991) *Dietary reference values for food energy and nutrients for the United Kingdom*. Report of the panel on dietary reference values of the Committee on Medical Aspects of Food Policy. London, HMSO.
4. **Expert Group on Vitamins and Minerals** (2003) *Safe upper levels for vitamins and minerals*. London, Food Standards Agency.
5. **FAO/WHO** (1988) *Preparation and use of food-based dietary guidelines*. Report of a joint FAO/WHO Consultation. WHO Technical Report Series 880. Geneva, FAO/WHO.
6. **FAO/WHO** (2001) *Human vitamin and mineral requirements*. Report of a joint FAO/WHO Expert Consultation in Bangkok, Thailand. Rome, Food and Agricultural Organization.
7. **FAO/WHO/UN** (2004) *Human energy requirements*. Report of a joint FAO/WHO/UNU Expert Consultation. Food and Nutrition Technical Report Series 1. Rome, Food and Agricultural Organization of the United Nations.
8. **Food and Nutrition Board, Institute of Medicine** (1997) *Dietary reference intakes for calcium, phosphorus, magnesium, vitamin D and fluoride*. Washington, DC, National Academy Press.

9. **Food and Nutrition Board, Institute of Medicine** (1998) *Dietary reference intakes. A risk assessment model for establishing upper intake level for nutrients.* Washington, DC, National Academy Press.

10. **Food and Nutrition Board, Institute of Medicine** (1998) *Dietary reference intakes for thiamin, riboflavin, niacin, vitamin B$_6$, folate, vitamin B$_{12}$, pantothenic acid, biotin, and choline.* Washington, DC, National Academy Press.

11. **Food and Nutrition Board: Institute of Medicine** (2000) *Dietary reference intakes. Applications in dietary assessment.* Washington, DC, National Academy Press.

12. **Food and Nutrition Board: Institute of Medicine** (2000) *Dietary reference intakes for vitamin C, vitamin E, selenium and carotenoids.* Washington, DC, National Academy Press.

13. **Food and Nutrition Board: Institute of Medicine** (2001) *Dietary reference intakes for vitamin A, vitamin K, arsenic, boron, chromium, copper, iodine, iron, manganese, molybdenum, nickel, silicon, vanadium and zinc.* Washington, DC, National Academy Press.

14. **Food and Nutrition Board: Institute of Medicine** (2002) *Dietary reference intakes for energy, carbohydrate, fiber, fat, fatty acids, cholesterol, protein and amino acids (macronutrients).* Washington, DC, National Academy Press.

15. **Food and Nutrition Board: Institute of Medicine** (2003) *Dietary reference intakes: Guiding principles for nutrition labeling and fortification.* Washington, DC, National Academy Press.

16. **Food and Nutrition Board: Institute of Medicine** (2004) *Dietary reference intakes for water, potassium, sodium, chloride and sulfate.* Panel on the dietary reference intakes for electrolytes and water. Washington, DC, National Academy Press.

17. **German Nutrition Society/Austrian Nutrition Society/Swiss Society for Nutrition Research/Swiss Nutrition Association** (2001) *Reference values for nutrient intake.* Frankfurt, Main, Umschau, Braus, German Nutrition Society. Translated by S. Saupe and A.S. Truswell.

18. **Gopalan, C.** (1989) Dietary guidelines from the perspective of developing countries. In: Latham, M.C., and van Veen, M.S. (eds) *Dietary guidelines: Proceedings of an International Conference. International Monograph 21.* Ithaca, NY, Cornell.

19. **Hunt, P., Gatenby, S., and Rayner, M.** (1995) The format for the National Food Guide: Performance and preference studies. *J Hum Nutr Diet,* **8**, 335–51.

20. **Nordic Working Group on Diet and Nutrition** (1996) Nordic nutrition recommendations. *Scand J Nutr Naringsforskning,* **40**, 161–95.

21. **Truswell, A.S.** (1998) Dietary goals, and guidelines: National and international perspectives. In: Shils, M.E., Olson, J.A., Shike, M., and Ross, M.C. (eds) *Modern nutrition in health and disease,* 9th edition. Baltimore MD, Williams and Wilkins, pp. 1727–41.

22. **WHO** (2003) *Diet, nutrition and the prevention of chronic disease.* Report of a joint WHO/FAO Expert Consultation. WHO Technical Report Series 916. Geneva, World Health Organization.

Useful Websites

To see topical and scientifically robust updates on nutrition associated with this textbook and web links to many of the journals in the Further Reading sections, please see the dedicated Online Resource Centre at **http://www.oxfordtextbooks.co.uk/orc/mann4e/**

38 Dietary counselling: the effective dietary counsellor

Yasmin Mossavar-Rahmani

38.1 The case for client-centred counselling

Dietary counselling occurs in a rich context that employs all the senses. The effective dietary counsellor reads body language, seeks to understand the client's context, and responds to his/her emotional state while moving the conversation toward the ultimate goal—a healthier diet. To be effective, the counsellor needs to become a practitioner who is part psychologist, part anthropologist, part nutritionist. Dietary counselling occurs in a variety of places, from the counsellors' offices to clients' homes to the telephone or the web. It is also delivered in group sessions of related or unrelated individuals or in an individual session. The audience for nutrition services has also widened such that the socio-cultural background of the counsellor may be vastly different from that of the client. Given the need to deliver counselling in a time- and cost-effective manner for a diverse audience, effective counsellors are needed now more than ever.

In effective counselling, the practitioner empowers the client to resolve his/her challenges. Motivational interviewing (MI) or its abbreviated versions known as brief motivational interviewing (BMI) or motivational enhancement (ME) are approaches that can enable such an encounter (Miller and Rollnick, 2002; Resnicow et al., 2006; Mossavar-Rahmani, 2007; Schwartz et al., 2007; Rosengren, 2009). MI helps clients think thoughtfully about what matters most in their lives and to make decisions that are in consonance with their values and desires. The premise of this approach is that most people need help in accessing and bringing their values and life goals in front and centre. The practitioner accomplishes this goal through evoking desire, reason, ability, and need for change in the client.

In this chapter the essential skills for effective dietary counselling will be reviewed. In addition, narratives for interactions on commonly encountered themes will be used to illustrate these skills. These include: helping the client read food labels; changing a client's attitude about food preparation and large portions; helping a parent work with her overweight child.

38.2 Contexts for counselling: counselling diverse clients in varying contexts

The context within which counselling occurs presents great opportunities and challenges. When done on the web or in the office, which is the most common format, exposure to the client's context is limited. When done as a home visit, information about the client's environment is everywhere. This includes information about what foods the client consumes, where he or she stores and consumes it, and the neighbourhood in which the foods are likely purchased. What foods are stored in the refrigerator or in the cupboard can be elicited using a home inventory (Fulkerson *et al.*, 2008). If non-related individuals share the food in the fridge/cupboard, there may be issues with respect to the quality and quantity of foods purchased. Limited refrigerator space might explain why some families opt more for canned, rather than fresh or frozen produce. Limited incomes might mean that the cheapest foods that tend to also have the lowest nutrients are purchased. Other topics that can be investigated pertain to how meals are eaten. Eating alone in front of the television in the bedroom may be indicative of a dysfunctional family, as opposed to a family that eats together around a dining room table. The neighbourhood can provide additional information on the types of food available for purchase such as availability of low-fat milk. Some locales may not have any outlets for healthy foods such as fresh fruits or vegetables. Districts with limited or no availability of foods needed to maintain a healthy diet, but filled with fast food restaurants are known as 'food deserts'.

Additionally, the patient/client literacy level and learning disability may impact the delivery of nutritional counselling. Children with a learning disability need educational materials and counselling commensurate with their grade level for comprehension. Box 38.1 depicts the context of counselling from least to most removed from the client's life. Other issues point to the client's context: his/her family support, energy density of foods consumed and, if an immigrant, the level of acculturation. Box 38.2 illustrates these concepts.

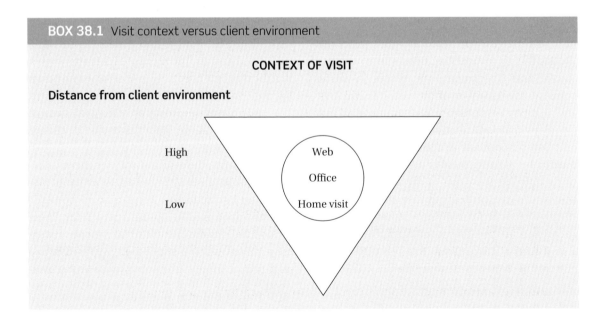

BOX 38.1 Visit context versus client environment

CONTEXT OF VISIT

Distance from client environment

High

Low

Web

Office

Home visit

38.3 Skills for client-centred counselling

MI, a directive, client-centred approach to counselling, is an effective approach to use in dietary counselling, as demonstrated in diverse populations and settings (Spahn *et al.*, 2010). Its effectiveness has been illustrated in numerous diet-related clinical trials and community studies (Bowen *et al.*, 2002; Newman *et al.*, 2005; Flattum *et al.*, 2009). The premise for using this approach is that a guided collaborative style is more effective in empowering clients to change behaviour than a style that is primarily of a directing nature. Miller and Rollnick identify 10 traits (see Box 38.3) for successful counselling integrating a MI approach.

38.4 The dietary counselling roadmap

38.4.1 Setting the stage

Setting the stage by engaging the client is an important component of the client–practitioner encounter. The dietary counsellor's tone and posture impact the exchange. Is the counsellor hurrying through the visit to see the next client? Does he/she appreciate the emotional state of the client? Asking about

BOX 38.3 Ten traits of motivational interviewing (MI)

1 The conversation focuses on change; not necessarily about behaviour change.

2 There is a purpose to the conversation to evoke and strengthen change.

3 It is collaborative, person-centred, and geared toward helpful change.

4 It honours autonomy and self-determination and is a conversation about choices.

5 It is evocative and evokes an individual's own motivation for change.

6 Specific skills are used: open-ended questions, affirmations, reflections, and summary.

7 It is goal orientated. MI moves toward a goal and is not merely for exploring ambivalence, although it will involve creating ambivalence.

8 It attends to specific speech and attends to client language.

9 It responds to specific change talk: elaborations, affirmations, reflections, summary.

10 It responds to resistance and sustains talk in specific ways. It is non-confrontational and is designed to avoid argument and does not resist resistance.

Source: Miller and Rollnick (2010), Second International Conference on Motivational Interviewing.

how things are going for the client before delving into the technical details of the encounter goes a long way in establishing a rapport (Box 38.4).

Next comes the *agenda-mapping* component, which involves asking on what the client would like to focus the discussion. The counsellor can present a host of topics that she/he may think are relevant. Is it diet, physical activity, or perhaps another matter that is more pressing at the moment that the counsellor may not have even thought of, but is of great importance to the client?

38.4.2 Assessing readiness to change

MI shifts the balance of the interaction into a guiding as opposed to a directing approach (Rollnick *et al.*, 2008). Through listening as indicated in reflections, confidence ruler, and clarifying values, the counsellor moves the client through change. Confidence rulers allow clients to think about how likely they might be able to see reason for or need or desire for change using a scale from 1–10. The counsellor queries the client about his/her choices on the confidence ruler to explore motivation for change. If the client places high importance in making a dietary change by selecting a 9, but only 2 for perceived ability to change, the counsellor needs to explore the reasons for this discrepancy. Does the client lack knowledge on how to make the change? Does he/she lack social support?

Values clarification allows clients to define what is important in their lives. For example, is it important to be healthy? To be spiritual? To reduce stress in the family?

The next step is working towards a goal. This step involves eliciting, responding to, and summarizing

---

BOX 38.4 The dietary counselling roadmap

1 **Setting the stage: (engaging, agenda mapping, exploring values)**

Looking to the future, what do you want to be doing differently about your diet?
What dietary changes would you most like to discuss today?
Where does that leave you?

2 **Assessing readiness to make a change (using open-ended questions, affirmations, reflections, summary (OARS), highlight motivational statements, use a confidence ruler)**

What concerns you? (open-ended question)
You have tried everything and nothing seems to work. (reflection)
Because you value your family's health, you are ready to do what it takes (affirmation)

Confidence ruler:

On a scale of 1–10 where 0 is 'not at all important' and 10 is 'very important': How important is it for you to make changes in your diet?
Why did you pick X as opposed to a lower number? What would have to be different for you to pick a higher number?
If ready, strengthen commitment; if unsure, explore ambivalence; if not ready, acknowledge client's decision.

3 **Planning and offering options to explore**

Would you like to keep track of your calories or increase your exercise?
What else would you like to try?

4 **Summarizing and planning for follow-up**

It sounds like your plan is to … and we will see you …

change talk in order to move the conversation towards the possibility of change.

38.4.3 Planning and offering options

This is the next part of the encounter and may consist of a negotiated plan. The plan could be action-oriented, such as self-monitoring calories or completing a food diary or it could be less action-

orientated by focusing on need for more information or for more time to contemplate choices and feelings of ambivalence.

38.4.4 Summarizing and planning for follow-up

Summarizing clarifies all the important points raised in the session and allows for strengthening commitment and plans for follow-up.

38.5 Examples of client-centred counselling

In each narrative *key phrases* that relate to the narrative's focus are *italicized*.

38.5.1 Narrative 1: Engaging phase in contrasting styles: directing (approach A) versus guiding (approach B)

Approach A

Dietary counsellor: 'Hi. Today I'd like to go over what you understand from nutrition labels.' (counsellor and not client maps the agenda).

Client: 'I know how to read nutrition labels.' (resistance)

Counsellor: 'But you indicated that you needed help with reading nutrition labels last time when we met?' (resistance from counsellor)

Client: 'I don't remember having said that plus I don't think I can do this. Reading labels is difficult for me. I am going to gain weight whether I read labels or not. Having a new baby is challenging.' (more resistance)

Counsellor: 'I will make it easy for you. All you need to do is look at the nutrition facts label; check the serving size and see how many calories you've eaten. So if you eat one serving of cereal—it says on this box—you've eaten 110 kcal (460 kJ). That's all. That wasn't too bad—was it?'

In this case the counsellor mapped the agenda and from the word go, the client showed resistance. The counsellor gave a lecture on reading the nutrition facts label without checking the client's knowledge and considered the work done.

Approach B

This session illustrates: engagement (agenda-mapping, information exchange by eliciting information and providing information)

Counsellor: 'Hi and congratulations on your new baby! That is wonderful news.' (engaging participant)

Client: 'Thanks. It has been both exciting and challenging. How have you been yourself?'

Counsellor: 'I am fine thanks. Being a new parent how exciting—you must be so proud. From our meeting last time you had indicated that you needed help with reading nutrition labels. Since we ran out of time, do you mind that we go over nutrition label reading now? Or is there something else that you'd rather we discuss today?' (engaging; asking permission; mapping the agenda)

Client: 'That is fine by me. I do want to talk about my weight too.'

Counsellor: 'OK. We will leave time to discuss both. Which would you rather do first?' (allows client to prioritize)

Client: 'Let's do the labels first. Maybe that will help me manage my weight better.'

Counsellor: Please tell me what you understand from this label.' (Counsellor points to the serving size section of the label for a cereal box—elicits client's understanding)

Client: 'That is the serving size. It is three-quarters of a cup (187 mL) and that is 110 kcal (460 kJ). It will tell me how much I am eating.'

Counsellor: 'Great. But *how can you tell* how much you are eating? Is there something you need to do first? (assesses client knowledge)

Client: 'I guess I need to figure out how much I eat. I usually guess, but I am not sure how to do that.'

Counsellor: 'That can be tricky. Would you like me to give you some tips?' (asking permission before providing information)

Client: 'Please do.'

Counsellor: 'You need to find out how the amount you eat compares to the amount listed on the box.' (provides information)

Client: 'Oh OK—but that is tough—I am not sure I know how much I am really eating.'

Counsellor: 'OK—let me show you different amounts of cereal so you can train your eye. Tell me how many cups each represent.' (Counsellor shows client 1/2 cup (125 mL), 1 cup (250 mL), 2 cups (500 mL) of cereals and asks client to tell her which is which.)

Counsellor: Great! So you are aware of the different steps you would need to go through before you realize the serving size you have actually eaten by checking the amount you eat from the box and how it measures up against the serving size on the nutrition label.' (summarizes and affirms client)

38.5.2 Narrative 2: Exchanging information: having a conversation with the client, a mother of an overweight child

Client: 'I pack a healthy lunch for my child every day. I include vegetables such as carrots and peas, but he eats very little of what I prepare for him. Most of the lunch comes straight back home with him. I found out today that he usually buys chips and cookies for lunches and may even trade the lunch I make for him for a friend's cookies.'

Counsellor: 'You are doing the best for your child, but he sabotages your efforts by eating an unhealthy lunch. *Tell me more.*' (reflection and asks for elaboration)

Client: 'Yes it is frustrating. I leave for work at 6 a.m. and need to be up earlier to prepare his lunch—after all that I do, nothing seems to work. He needs to lose weight, so I was hoping my lunches would do the trick.'

Counsellor: 'You are disappointed that the home-made lunches do not appeal to him. *Tell me* how your son is involved in helping you make lunch.' (elicits information)

Client: 'He is not involved at all. Maybe that is the problem. He doesn't like my choices. I could ask him to make his own lunch and pick fruits and vegetables he prefers. That way he may be more likely to eat a healthy lunch. I will also feel less rushed in the mornings.' (client comes up with a solution)

38.5.3 Narrative 3: Evoking: eliciting change talk: 'I'm used to eating "our" foods'

In this narrative, the client with diabetes who just moved from overseas feels that she can't prepare 'her' foods in this country and is having a hard time meeting her doctor's recommendation to eat healthily.

Counsellor: 'So *tell me* how are things going for you since you left India. What brings you here?'(elicits reason for visit)

Client: 'I am OK, but not too well since the doctor told me I need to lose weight. He told me to stop eating white rice and eat more vegetables. But I am used to eating white rice with every meal and cooking with ghee (clarified butter).' (client maps agenda)

Counsellor: 'So it is hard for you to stop eating white rice as often and change the way you cook.' (reflection)

Client: 'Yes. I love rice. Rice is part of our culture. I add ghee so the food has some taste.

Counsellor: 'Rice and cooking with ghee are important to you. *What then concerns you?*' (reflection and shift direction)

Client: 'Well, I have some concerns about my health. I am worried that I might get sick because of what I am eating.'

Counsellor: 'So you are here because you know that you need to change your diet, but you don't know how to do it. Would you like me to give you some ideas?' (elicits/asks permission)

Client: 'Yes.'

Counsellor: 'Changing foods you have eaten for so long is a challenging task; some people find it easier to make the change if they eat less of the food—so eating less rice—or substituting with something similar—maybe adding more vegetables and less rice and ghee—may be small steps you'd like to take. How does that sound to you?' (providing information)

Client: 'You just gave me an idea. Maybe I can use less ghee and add more vegetables and see how that goes. Maybe it will be more tolerable.'

Counsellor: 'Sounds like you have a plan.'

Summary

This chapter has introduced a general overview of client-centred dietary counselling illustrated through narratives. The skills and strategies outlined are essential in applying nutritional science to attain behaviour change in clients. Just as a pianist practises continuously to keep their skills honed, so too the effective dietary counsellor maintains skills through continuous practice.

Further Reading

1. **Bowen, D., Ehret, C., Pederson, M.,** *et al.* (2002) Results of an adjunct dietary intervention program in the Women's Health Initiative. *J Am Diet Assoc*, **102**, 1631–7.
2. **Flattum, C., Friend, S., Neumark-Sztainer, D.,** *et al.* (2009) Motivational interviewing as a component of a school-based obesity prevention program for adolescent girls. *J Am Diet Assoc*, **109**, 91–4.
3. **Fulkerson, J.A., Nelson, M.C., Lytle, L.,** *et al.* (2008) The validation of a household food inventory. *Int J Behav Nutr Phys Act*, **5**, 55.
4. **Miller, W.E. and Rollnick, S.** (2002) *Motivational interviewing: Preparing people to change addictive behavior.* London and New York, The Guilford Press.
5. **Mossavar-Rahmani, Y.** (2007) Applying motivational enhancement to diverse populations. *J Am Diet Assoc*, **107**, 918–21.
6. **Newman, V.A., Thomson, C.A., Rock, C.L.,** *et al.* (2005). Achieving substantial changes in eating behavior among women previously treated for breast cancer: An overview of the intervention. *J Am Diet Assoc*, **105**, 382–91.
7. **Resnicow, K., Davis, R., and Rollnick, S.** (2006) Motivational interviewing for pediatric obesity: Conceptual issues and evidence review. *J Am Diet Assoc*, **106**, 2024–33.
8. **Rollnick S., Miller W.R., and Butler, C.C.** (2008) *Motivational interviewing in health care: Helping patients change behavior.* New York, The Guilford Press.
9. **Rosengren, D.B.** (2009) *Building motivational interviewing skills: A practitioner workbook.* New York: The Guilford Press.
10. **Schwartz, R.P., Hamre, R., Dietz, W.H.,** *et al.* (2007) Office-based motivational interviewing to prevent childhood obesity. *Arch Pediatr Adoles Med*, **161**, 495–501.
11. **Spahn, J.M., Reeves, R.S., Keim, K.S.,** *et al.* (2010) State of the evidence regarding behavior change theories and strategies in nutrition counseling to facilitate health and food behavior change. *J Am Diet Assoc*, **110**, 879–91.

Useful Websites

 To see topical and scientifically robust updates on nutrition associated with this textbook and web links to many of the journals in the Further Reading sections, please see the dedicated Online Resource Centre at **http://www.oxfordtextbooks.co.uk/orc/mann4e/**

Part 8

Applications

39 Sports nutrition

Louise M. Burke

Enhancements in research technology and methods over the past decade have opened up new areas of understanding and practice in sports nutrition. In particular, our increased ability to measure intracellular events has increased appreciation of training and nutrient interactions, and the importance of timing of nutritional interventions in relation to exercise. New sports nutrition strategies have been shown to enhance the preparation and performance of athletes. They also offer potential benefits to those wishing to use the combination of exercise and nutrition to prevent or treat health problems such as obesity and the metabolic syndrome, or the sarcopenia of ageing.

This chapter focuses on outcomes related to exercise performance, particularly for competitive sport, in particular new areas of knowledge since the last edition of this book, with emphasis on the outcomes of the third Consensus on Nutrition for Sport held in 2010 by the International Olympic Committee (http://www.olympic.org/Documents/Reports/EN/CONSENSUS-FINAL-v8-en.pdf). Since the goals of sports nutrition are typically related to basic principles of body function rather than the calibre of the person who is exercising, they apply both to elite performers and the much larger number of highly motivated recreational athletes.

39.1 Goals for the everyday or training diet

Although exact nutritional needs vary among athletes, there are common goals for the everyday diet eaten in training (Table 39.1). The achievement of most goals is underpinned by an adequate energy intake and a well-chosen variety of foods. Energy requirements are determined by several factors including gender, age, size, and the volume, intensity, and frequency of the training programme. Athletes undertaking prolonged sessions of moderate–high intensity exercise generally have high energy requirements. Energy intake may be manipulated to increase body size, for example during periods of growth or when attempting to achieve a gain in muscle mass or a decrease in body mass (BM) and body fat levels. Difficulties arise when athletes face practical challenges in meeting the high energy cost of intensive training/competition or growth, or when they reduce energy intake too drastically in order to achieve or maintain low BM/fat goals.

Energy availability is a new concept in sports nutrition which can be applied to assess the suitability of an athlete's energy intake. It provides a rough assessment of the amount of energy that the body can utilize for everyday activities required for good health and is defined operationally as energy

Table 39.1 Sports nutrition goals for the athlete in training

The athlete should aim to:
• Meet energy and fuel requirements needed to support their training programme
• Achieve and maintain an ideal physique for their event; manipulate training and nutrition to achieve a level of body mass, body fat, and muscle mass that is consistent with good health and good performance
• Refuel and rehydrate well for key training sessions where it is important to perform at their best
• Practise any intended competition nutrition strategies so that beneficial practices can be identified and fine-tuned
• Enhance adaptation and recovery between training sessions by providing all the nutrients associated with these processes
• Maintain optimal health and function, especially by achieving the increased needs for some nutrients resulting from a heavy training programme
• Reduce risk of sickness during heavy training periods by maintaining healthy physique and energy balance and by supplying nutrients believed to assist immune function (e.g. consume carbohydrates during prolonged exercise sessions)
• Make use of supplements and specialized sports foods that have been shown to enhance training performance or meet training nutrition needs after considering the potential risks associated with their use
• Eat for long-term health by paying attention to community nutrition guidelines
• Continue to enjoy food and the pleasure of sharing meals

intake minus the energy cost of the training programme. Studies have shown that when energy availability drops below about 30 kcal (125 kJ) per kg of the athlete's fat-free mass, there is inadequate energy to fuel all activities required for good health, including hormone function and bone function. Table 39.2 summarizes various levels of energy availability with examples of situations in which it has been reduced to less than optimal levels to achieve weight loss.

39.1.1 Achieving optimal physique

Physique plays a role in the performance of many sports, and elite competitors typically display the optimal physical characteristics for their event. This results from genetic factors that have helped to determine the athlete's pursuits combined with the conditioning effects of nutrition and training. Some athletes achieve an ideal physique easily, others need to manipulate their training and dietary programmes to achieve their desired size and shape.

In some sports, including combative events (e.g. boxing, wrestling, judo), weight-lifting, and lightweight rowing, athletes compete in weight divisions, which attempt to match competitors based on size. Competition classification is decided at 'weigh-ins', just before competition. 'Making weight' is a common activity whereby athletes, many of whom are already lean, shed kilograms in the hours or days prior to the weigh-in to qualify for a division lighter than their normal BM. Although this strategy is used to gain advantage in strength or reach over a smaller opponent, it must be balanced against the problems of dehydration or suboptimal nutritional status resulting from rapid weight-loss techniques.

Table 39.2 Examples of different levels of energy availability

Situation	Energy availability (energy intake—energy cost of exercise)	Case studies
Weight gain, growth, hypertrophy, etc.	>45 kcal (189 kJ) per kg fat-free mass (FFM)	
Weight/physique maintenance	~45 kcal (189 kJ) per kg FFM	
Healthy weight loss (or weight maintenance at reduced metabolic rate)	30–45 kcal (125–189 kJ) per kg FFM	Runner A: 55 kg (20% body fat = 80% FFM); Weekly training = 5600 kcal (23.5 MJ); Daily energy intake = 2520 kcal (10.6 MJ) Energy availability = $(2520-800)/(0.8 \times 55)$ = 39 kcal/kg FFM (164 kJ)
Low energy availability, health implications	<30 kcal (125 kJ) per kg fat-free mass	Runner B: 55 kg (25% body fat = 75% FFM) Weekly training = 5600 kcal (2.35 MJ) Daily energy intake = 1980 kcal (8.3 MJ) Energy availability = $(1980-800)/(0.75 \times 55)$ = 29 kcal/kg FFM (120 kJ)

Medical committees and governing organizations have issued guidelines warning against extreme 'making weight' activities.

Low BM and body fat levels offer biomechanical and physical (power to weight) advantages in a range of other sports including distance running, uphill cycling, diving, and gymnastics. Aesthetic considerations are important in gymnastics, figure skating, and bodybuilding. Many athletes embark on extreme weight-loss schemes, often involving excessive training, chronic low energy and nutrient intake, and psychological distress. Problems arising from these activities include fatigue, inadequate intake of protein and micronutrients (especially iron and calcium), reduced immune status, altered hormonal balance, disordered eating, and poor body image.

Targets for 'ideal' BM and body fat should be set in terms of ranges and should consider measures of long-term health and performance, rather than short-term benefits alone. Athletes should be encouraged to set individual targets within these ranges, and where it is warranted, loss of body fat should be achieved by a gradual programme of

sustained and moderate energy deficit. Each athlete should be able to achieve targets while eating a diet adequate in energy and nutrients, and free of unreasonable food-related stress. Most importantly, low body fat levels of elite athletes should not be considered natural or necessary for recreational and subelite performers. Even then, most elite athletes periodize their BM and body fat levels, achieving their 'race weight' only for times they are at their competition peak.

At the other end of the spectrum are athletes who are interested in gaining muscle mass and strength. These athletes often focus dietary interests on excessive protein intake and special supplements that claim to enhance the gain of lean BM. However, emerging evidence suggests that the key nutritional support for a resistance-training programme is well-timed intake of nutrition. Modest amounts (15–25 g) of high-quality protein (particularly from dairy, eggs, or animal sources) consumed close to the workout promote maximal protein synthesis during the immediate recovery period. Total protein requirements are generally easily met within the high energy intakes typical of athletes undertaking heavy training. Meanwhile, carbohydrate is the nutrient needed to fuel training sessions and recovery, and an energy surplus may be needed to promote optimal gain in BM or general growth.

39.1.2 Achieving fuel and fluid needs for training

Carbohydrate Energy for muscle contraction is provided by breakdown of adenosine triphosphate (ATP). Since muscle ATP stores would be consumed in only a few seconds of high-intensity exercise, the body uses a range of energy pathways to regenerate ATP. In most situations of exercise or sport, the integration of the energy systems (non-oxidative pathways involving creatine phosphate and carbohydrate, and the oxidative pathways involving fat and carbohydrate) means that ATP replenishment matches ATP demand. A major advantage of the provision of ATP via anaerobic pathways is that the rate of ATP synthesis is five or six times higher than that from aerobic pathways; such pathways are turned on rapidly at the onset of exercise. However, oxidative metabolism of fat and carbohydrate provides the majority of the energy supply for longer-duration exercise of lower intensity. Several interrelated factors influence selection of muscle fuel during exercise; these include availability of endogenous substrates (muscle glycogen and triglyceride stores), training status of an individual, intensity and duration of exercise, environmental conditions, and nutrient intake during exercise, especially carbohydrate.

Of these factors, the availability of muscle glycogen is an important determinant of the performance of many types of sport and exercise activities. Depletion of body carbohydrate stores causes fatigue or impaired performance during prolonged sessions of submaximal or intermittent high-intensity activity. Unfortunately, total body carbohydrate stores are limited, and are often substantially less than the fuel requirements of the training and competition sessions undertaken by many athletes. Therefore, sports nutrition guidelines provide targets for adequate daily carbohydrate intake to support the needs of training and recovery. The principles and terminology of guidelines have changed over the past two decades.

The first guidelines recommended ideal carbohydrate intake in terms of 'percentage of dietary energy intake'. However, when energy intakes are very high (growing athletes) or restricted (weight-loss diets), the same percentage of energy will translate into very different amounts of carbohydrate that may be unrelated to the muscle's fuel needs for exercise. Thus modern guidelines for carbohydrate intake are scaled to the size of the athlete and the fuel cost of their training.

As for energy, carbohydrate intake should be recommended in terms of 'carbohydrate availability' to ensure that total daily intake, and timing of its consumption in relation to exercise maintains an adequate supply of carbohydrate substrate for the muscle and central nervous system. The evidence is sound, at least in the competition setting where the primary goal is optimal performance, that high carbohydrate availability is desirable. Table 39.3 provides suggestions for ballpark figures that should be fine-tuned with individual consideration of total energy needs, specific training needs, and feedback from training performance. This approach acknowledges that the athlete's needs are not static, but move between categories according to changes in daily, weekly, or seasonal goals and exercise commitments in a periodized training programme. Furthermore, a useful way in which an athlete can be guided to adjust their carbohydrate intakes is to adopt eating patterns in which meals/snacks providing carbohydrate and other important nutrients are placed strategically around exercise sessions. This permits nutrient and energy intake to track with fuel needs of the athlete's exercise commitments, as well as specifically enhance carbohydrate availability and its potential to enhance performance and recovery for key exercise sessions.

Fluid Fluid needs are also increased in response to training, with additional fluid losses from sweating being determined by factors such as intensity and duration of exercise, environmental conditions (heat and altitude), and degree of acclimatization of the athlete. Athletes must make a conscious plan to increase fluid intake to balance sudden increases in sweat losses, which may occur when moving to hot climates or undertaking substantial increases in training load. Thirst does not provide an adequate guide to acute dehydration or sudden changes in fluid need in the short term. The drinking plan should consider total fluid needs over the day, as

Table 39.3 Summary of guidelines for carbohydrate intake by athletes

	Situation	Carbohydrate targets	Comments on type and timing of carbohydrate intake
DAILY NEEDS FOR FUEL AND RECOVERY—these general recommendations should be fine-tuned with individual consideration of total energy needs, specific training needs, and feedback from training performance			
Light	• Low-intensity or skill-based activities	3–5 g/kg of athlete's body mass (BM)/day	• Timing of intake may be chosen to promote speedy refuelling or to provide fuel intake around training sessions in the day. Otherwise, as long as total fuel needs are provided, the pattern of intake may simply be guided by convenience and individual choice
Moderate	• Moderate exercise programme (i.e. ~1 hours per day)	5–7 g/kg/day	
High	• Endurance programme (e.g. 1–3 hours/day moderate–high-intensity exercise)	6–10 g/kg/day	• Protein- and nutrient-rich carbohydrate foods or meal combinations will allow the athlete to meet other acute or chronic sports nutrition goals
Very high	• Extreme commitment (i.e., >4–5 hours/day moderate–high intensity exercise	8–12 g/kg/day	
ACUTE FUELLING STRATEGIES—these guidelines promote high carbohydrate availability to promote optimal performance in competition or key training sessions			
General fuelling up	• Preparation for events <90 min exercise	7–12 g/kg per 24 hours as for daily fuel needs	• Athletes may choose compact carbohydrate-rich sources that are low in fibre/residue and easily consumed to ensure that fuel targets are met and to meet goals for gut comfort or lighter 'racing weight'
Carbohydrate loading	• Preparation for events >90 min of sustained/ intermittent exercise	36–48 hours of 10–12 g/kg BM per 24 hours	
Speedy refuelling	• <8 hours recovery between 2 fuel-demanding sessions	1–1.2 g/kg/hour for first 4 hours, then resume daily fuel needs	• There may be benefits in consuming small, regular snacks • Compact, carbohydrate-rich foods and drink may help to ensure that fuel targets are met

(Continued)

Table 39.3 Summary of guidelines for carbohydrate intake by athletes (*Continued*)

Pre-event fuelling	• Before exercise >60 min	1–4 g/kg consumed 1–4 hours before exercise	• Timing, amount, and type of carbohydrate foods and drinks should be chosen to suit the practical needs of the event and individual preferences/experiences • Choices high in fat/protein/fibre may need to be avoided to reduce risk of gastrointestinal issues during the event • Low glycaemic index choices may provide a more sustained source of fuel for situations where carbohydrate cannot be consumed during exercise
During brief exercise	• < 45 min	Not needed	
During sustained high-intensity exercise	• 45–75 min	Small amounts, including mouth rinse	• A range of drinks and sports products can provide easily consumed carbohydrate • Beneficial effects are generally seen when exercise is undertaken in fasted state or several hours post meal
During endurance exercise including 'stop and start' sports	• 1–2.5 hours	30–60 g/hour	• Opportunities to consume foods and drinks vary according to the rules and nature of each sport • A range of everyday dietary choices and specialized sports products ranging in form from liquid to solid may be useful • The athlete should practise to find a refuelling plan that suits their individual goals, including hydration needs and gut comfort
During ultra-endurance exercise	• >2.5–3 hours	Up to 90 g/hour	• As above • Higher intakes of carbohydrate are associated with better performance • Products providing multiple transportable carbohydrates (glucose/fructose mixtures) are necessary to achieve high rates of oxidation of carbohydrate consumed during exercise

Source: Burke, L. M., Hawley, J. A., Wong, S. H., *et al.* (2011) Carbohydrates for training and competition. *J Sports Sci* **8**, 1–11.

well as specific intake before, during, and after each workout. Strategies for fluid and carbohydrate replacement before, during, and after exercise will be further examined in the context of the competition diet.

39.1.3 Achieving protein needs

Prolonged daily training may increase protein requirements, to meet the small contribution of protein oxidation to fuel requirements of prolonged exercise, as well as the protein needed to support muscle gain and repair of damaged body tissues. Athletes undertaking recreational or light training activities will meet protein needs within population protein RDIs. However, the need for an increased protein intake for heavy endurance and strength training has been a highly debated issue. The 2010 International Olympic Committee consensus suggests that athletes engaged in intensive exercise are likely to need more protein than the RDIs for sedentary people (perhaps 1–1.5 g/kg BM per day. Generally, total intakes of protein by athletes are within or above these goals because of the increased energy allowances that accompany a regular exercise programme. Those who restrict energy to lose weight are at risk of protein intakes below this range.

The key issue related to protein needs is the timing of intake of high-quality protein around training and competition sessions. Early intake of protein after exercise (and perhaps, in some cases before and during the session) has been shown to enhance protein synthesis and net protein balance. The consumption of quality protein provides a source of amino acids to act as substrate for the building of new proteins, and in the case of the amino acid leucine, to act as a trigger to activate protein synthesis. Recent studies suggest that maximal rates of protein synthesis are achieved during the early recovery phase by the intake of 15–25 g of protein. Protein consumed in excess of these amounts may increase protein oxidation rates. Although the value of protein synthesis is recognized by resistance athletes, stimulation of protein synthesis is part of

the recovery from all modes of exercise by trained individuals, with the type of exercise coding for specific types of muscle protein that are preferentially involved (e.g. mitochondrial, myofibrillar, sarcolemmal). New techniques which distinguish rates of synthesis of muscle protein subfractions provide evidence that endurance exercise and repeated high-intensity sprints (i.e. team sport activities) also stimulate protein synthesis. Therefore, recovery meals and snacks following key training sessions should include high-quality protein to promote optimal adaptation to the training session, e.g. increase in muscle mass, formation of new enzymes and signalling proteins, and repair of muscle damage.

39.1.4 Micronutrient needs

The key factors ensuring adequacy of vitamin and mineral intakes in athletes are a moderate-to-high energy intake and a varied diet based on nutrient-rich foods, so typically reported intakes of vitamins and minerals are well in excess of RDIs and likely to meet any increases in micronutrient demand caused by training. Thus routine supplementation with vitamins is not justified, and research has failed to show evidence of an increase in performance following vitamin supplementation except in the case where a pre-existing deficiency was corrected. However, not all athletes eat varied diets of adequate energy intake, with energy restriction, fad diets, and disordered eating being typical causes of reduced micronutrient intake. Food range may also be restricted by poor practical nutrition skills, inadequate finances, and an overcommitted lifestyle that limits access to food and causes erratic meal schedules. Athletes require education about the quality and quantity of food intake, but a low-dose, broad-range multivitamin/mineral supplement may be useful when an athlete is unwilling or unable to make dietary changes or when travelling to places with uncertain food supplies or eating schedules.

Minerals are the micronutrients at most risk of inadequate intake in the diets of athletes. Inadequate *iron status* can reduce exercise performance via suboptimal levels of haemoglobin and perhaps iron-related muscle enzymes. However, it may be difficult to distinguish true iron deficiency from alterations in iron status measures that are caused by exercise itself (e.g. changes in plasma volume, acute-phase responses to training). Reduction of blood haemoglobin concentrations due to plasma expansion, often termed 'sports anaemia', does not impair exercise performance.

Nevertheless, some athletes are at true risk of becoming iron-deficient. Iron requirements may be increased in some athletes because of growth, or to increased gastrointestinal or haemolytic iron losses. However, the most common risk factor among athletes, as in all young people, is a low-energy diet or low intake of available iron. Females, athletes who restrict dietary energy intake or variety, vegetarians, and athletes eating high-carbohydrate/low-meat diets are most at risk. Evaluation and management of iron status may need assessment by a sports medicine expert. Low iron status (serum ferritin levels lower than 20 ng/mL), should be considered for further assessment and treatment. Prevention and treatment of iron deficiency may include iron supplementation. However, long-term management should be based on dietary counselling to increase intake of bioavailable iron (increasing intake of haem iron sources and complementary intake of vitamin C or meat foods with non-haem iron foods). These strategies can be integrated with the athlete's other dietary goals.

Previously, it was considered that low iron status without anaemia did not reduce exercise performance. However, many athletes with low iron stores, or a sudden drop in iron status, complain of fatigue and inability to recover after heavy training. Many of these respond to strategies that improve iron status or prevent a further decrease in iron stores.

Some athletes are at risk of problems with *calcium status* and bone health. Reduced bone density in athletes seems contradictory, since exercise is considered to be an important protector of bone health. However, a serious consequence of low energy availability and menstrual disturbances frequently observed in female athletes is the high risk of either direct loss of bone density or failure to optimize the gaining of peak bone mass that should occur during the 10–15 years after the onset of puberty. Calcium requirements may be increased to 1200 mg/day in female athletes with impaired menstrual function. Where adequate calcium intake cannot be met through dietary means, usually through use of low-fat dairy foods or calcium-enriched soy alternatives, a calcium supplement may be considered. Low bone density is also seen in male athletes, with high-risk groups including elite cyclists; this presumably results from the low energy availability associated with heavy energy expenditure and a desire for low body fat levels, but may be exacerbated by the lack of bone loading during cycling activities.

Vitamin D deficiency or insufficiency is now recognized as a potential problem in some at-risk sections of the population at large. Some athletes should be considered as such a group with risk factors including indoor training (e.g. gymnasts, swimmers), residing at latitudes greater than 35 degrees, training in the early morning or late evening, thus avoiding sunlight exposure, wearing protective clothing or sunscreen, and consuming a diet low in vitamin D. Athletes with these characteristics should seek professional advice and have their vitamin D status monitored. Although there is dispute over optimal vitamin D status, prevention or treatment of vitamin D insufficiency may require supplementation.

39.2 The competition diet

The nutritional challenges of competition vary according to length and intensity of the event, the environment, and factors that influence the recovery between events or the opportunity to eat during the event itself. To achieve optimal performance, the athlete should identify potentially preventable factors that contribute to fatigue during the event and undertake nutritional strategies before, during, and after the event that minimize or delay the onset of this fatigue. In most cases, dehydration and/or depletion of body carbohydrate stores present the major nutritional challenges. Various goals of competition nutrition are summarized in Table 39.4.

Dehydration is a likely outcome in most sports events, with most athletes drinking fluid at a rate that is lower than their rate of sweat loss. The effects of dehydration on exercise performance vary according to degree of fluid deficit, environment, type of exercise, and characteristics of the individual. Dehydration of as little as 2% of BM (1.5–2 L for most athletes) is sufficient to cause detectable changes to work output, and perception of effort, especially when exercise is carried out in a hot environment or at altitude. Other penalties of fluid deficits include impairment of thermoregulation, reductions in skill and decision-making abilities, and increased risk of gastrointestinal problems. Carbohydrate depletion can manifest as central fatigue (low blood glucose

concentrations) and/or peripheral fatigue (glycogen depletion in the working muscle). When nutrition strategies enhance or maintain carbohydrate status during exercise, they can be demonstrated to enhance endurance. The effect on exercise *performance* is more difficult to assess but a number of studies have shown benefits following various strategies to enhance carbohydrate availability.

39.2.1 Fuelling up before an event

Optimizing carbohydrate stores in muscle and liver is a primary goal of pre-exercise preparation. The key factors in glycogen storage are dietary carbohydrate intake and, in the case of muscle stores, tapered exercise or rest. In the absence of muscle damage, muscle glycogen stores can be normalized by 24–36 hours of rest and an adequate carbohydrate intake

Table 39.4 Sports nutrition goals for the athlete in competition

The athlete should aim to:

- In weight-division sports, achieve the competition weight division with minimal harm to health or performance

- 'Fuel up' adequately prior to an event; consume carbohydrate and achieve exercise taper during the day(s) prior to the event according to the importance and duration of the event; and utilize carbohydrate-loading strategies when appropriate before events of greater than 90 minutes' duration

- Use opportunities to drink before and during the event to minimize dehydration by replacing most of the sweat losses, but without drinking in excess of sweat losses

- Consume carbohydrates during events >1 hour in duration with a sliding scale of intake according to the need to prime the brain or to provide an additional source of muscle fuel.

- Achieve pre-event and during-event eating/drinking strategies without causing gastrointestinal discomfort or upsets

- Promote recovery after the event, particularly during multiday competitions such as tournaments and stage races

- During a prolonged competition programme, achieve these goals without compromising overall energy and nutrient intake goals

- Make use of supplements and specialized sports foods that have been shown to enhance race performance or meet race nutrition goals after first considering the risk of side effects from their use

(7–12 g/kg BM/day). Such stores appear adequate for the fuel needs of events of less than 60–90 minutes in duration.

Carbohydrate loading refers to practices that aim to supercompensate muscle glycogen stores; such protocols may elevate muscle glycogen stores by 125–200%. Pioneering studies undertaken in the late 1960s by Scandinavian sports scientists produced the 'classical' 7-day model of carbohydrate loading, involving a 3–4-day 'depletion' phase of hard training and low carbohydrate intake and finishing with a 3–4-day 'loading' phase of high carbohydrate eating and exercise taper. Early field studies of prolonged running events showed that carbohydrate loading can enhance sports performance, not by allowing the athlete to run faster, but by prolonging the time that race pace can be maintained.

Studies extended to trained subjects have produced a 'modified' carbohydrate loading in which the depletion or 'glycogen stripping' phase is omitted. For well-trained athletes at least, carbohydrate loading may be seen as an extension of 'fuelling up' (rest and high carbohydrate intake) over 3–4 days. In fact, a recent study has shown that in well-trained subjects, glycogen supercompensation may be achieved in as little as 30–48 hours of such preparation. The modified carbohydrate-loading protocol (Table 39.3) offers a more practical strategy for competition preparation, by avoiding the fatigue and complexity of the extreme diet and training protocols associated with the previous depletion phase. Carbohydrate loading is useful for events of greater than 90 minutes' duration and will typically postpone fatigue and extend the duration of steady-state exercise by about 20%, or improve performance over a set distance or workload by 2–3%.

39.2.2 Pre-event meal

Food and fluids consumed in the 4 hours prior to an event may continue to fuel muscle glycogen stores if they have not been fully restored since the last exercise session, restore liver glycogen content after an overnight fast, and ensure that the athlete is well hydrated. Gastric comfort issues must be balanced to prevent hunger, yet must avoid the gastrointestinal discomfort and upset often experienced during exercise. From the psychological viewpoint, the pre-event meal should include foods and practices that are important to the athlete's superstitions or feelings of wellbeing.

A carbohydrate-rich, low-fat meal is generally recommended as the ideal pre-event meal. Some experts have speculated, however, that the elevation of plasma insulin concentrations following pre-exercise carbohydrate feedings could potentially disadvantage exercise metabolism and performance. A rise in insulin suppresses lipolysis and fat utilization, accelerating carbohydrate oxidation, and perhaps causing premature fatigue. This situation is at most risk of occurring when small amounts of carbohydrate (e.g. <1 g/kg BM) are consumed in the hour prior to exercise. One safeguard is to ensure that the amount of carbohydrate in the pre-event meal is substantial rather than minor (Table 39.3); thus, any increase in carbohydrate utilization during exercise will be more than offset by the large increase in carbohydrate availability. Others have argued that low-glycaemic-index (GI) carbohydrate foods provide a superior pre-event meal choice, since they provide a reduced insulinaemic response. In general, however, studies have failed to show that a low-GI pre-event meal produces a superior performance outcome. In fact, when carbohydrate is consumed during the event to maintain carbohydrate availability, the type of carbohydrate consumed before exercise may be largely irrelevant. However, a low-GI pre-exercise meal may be useful for some situations or individual athletes where a sustained release of carbohydrate is desirable during exercise but carbohydrate cannot be consumed during the session.

The type, timing, and amount of food chosen for the pre-event meal will be determined by individual situations and experience. In general, meals that are low in fat and moderate in fibre and protein are recommended, especially for athletes who are at risk of gastrointestinal problems during their event. Fluid should be consumed in the hours prior to exercise to ensure that the athlete is well hydrated at the onset of the event. Above all, the athlete should experiment with their intended pre-event meal strategies to fine tune the plan that suits their individual needs.

39.2.3 Fluid and carbohydrate during the event

In events of greater than 30 minutes, there is likely to be both a need and opportunity for fluid replacement. Ideally, an athlete should drink at a rate that replaces most of their sweat loss; however, this is impractical and uncomfortable when sweat rates exceed 1 L/hour. There have been some recent changes in the education messages provided to athletes about fluid replacement during sports and exercise activities. Instead of receiving prescriptive advice (e.g. drink 150–250 mL of fluid every 15–20 minutes), athletes are advised to be aware of their own sweat losses and use opportunities that exist within their activities to drink as often and as much as is practical to replace *most* of these losses. Since studies find that athletes typically replace only 30–60% of fluid losses across a range of sporting activities, most athletes can aim for an improvement in their fluid intake. However, recent observations from sporting events attracting large numbers of recreational participants have shown that there is a need specifically to warn against drinking excessively before and during exercise. Slower participants in running, cycling, and triathlon races have been observed to consume fluids at rates that greatly exceed their sweat losses—combining low sweat rates with aggressive use of aid stations during the event. Such drinking patterns, which can lead to a weight gain over the race, are a major risk factor for the development of hyponatraemia (low plasma sodium concentrations). Several athletes have died in marathons as a result of severe hyponatraemia.

The literature clearly shows that intake of carbohydrate during prolonged sessions of moderate-intensity or intermittent high-intensity exercise can improve work capacity and performance. Even when there is no significant positive effect of carbohydrate ingestion on exercise capacity, performance is not adversely affected by increasing the availability of carbohydrates. The major mechanisms to explain the benefits of carbohydrate feedings during prolonged exercise are maintenance of plasma glucose concentration and high rates of carbohydrate oxidation when muscle carbohydrate stores become depleted. Recently, a number of studies have shown that carbohydrate intake may benefit shorter-duration, high-intensity sports (of about 1 hour duration), even when carbohydrate stores are not thought to be limiting. This is may be a result of effects on the brain and central nervous system that promote enhanced pacing strategies. In fact, the effect can be achieved simply by swilling carbohydrate-containing fluid in the mouth; apparently, receptors in the oral cavity communicate with reward centres in the brain.

In practice, athletes consume carbohydrates during exercise using a variety of foods and drinks, and a variety of feeding schedules. In general, a carbohydrate intake of 30–60 g/hour is recommended, with carbohydrate feedings starting well in advance of fatigue or depletion of body carbohydrate stores and being achieved according to the practical opportunities provided in each sport or exercise (Table 39.3). The value of sports drinks (commercial solutions providing 4–8% carbohydrates, electrolytes, and palatable flavours) is recognized, since these allow carbohydrates to be delivered while attending to needs for fluid replacement. Such drinks have been shown to increase voluntary fluid intake during exercise, thus enhancing fluid balance as well as providing an additional source of fuel.

More recently there has been growing evidence of a dose–response relationship between carbohydrate intake during exercise and the performance of sustained exercise lasting longer than 2–3 hours. In these events, rates of carbohydrate intake of up to 80–90 g appear optimal (Table 39.3). However, such an intake exceeds the rate of intestinal absorption of carbohydrate from a single carbohydrate source; the ceiling for uptake of glucose in its various forms (e.g. maltodextrin, glucose polymers) appears to be ~60 g/hour. Fortunately, the mixture of two carbohydrate sources which use different intestinal absorption routes ('multiple transportable carbohydrates') allows a higher rate of carbohydrate delivery to the muscle during exercise. This has been shown to enhance performance of prolonged exercise and to reduce the risk of gastrointestinal discomfort when high rates of carbohydrate are consumed. Formulas providing glucose to fructose in a ratio of 2:1 are now becoming available in sports products aimed at endurance and ultra-endurance events, and seem well tolerated as sports gels or solid bars. Athletes who are intending to use such products should practise in training, since there is some evidence that this can increase their tolerance and capacity to absorb carbohydrate consumed during exercise; at least it will allow the athlete to fine-tune successful competition strategies.

39.3 Post-exercise recovery

The main dietary factor in post-event refuelling is the amount of carbohydrate consumed, with a threshold for muscle glycogen storage being within the range of 7–12 g/kg BM/day (Table 39.3). There is some evidence that moderate-GI and high-GI carbohydrate-rich foods and drinks may be more favourable for glycogen storage than some low-GI food choices. Since glycogen storage may occur at a slightly faster rate during the first couple of hours after exercise, athletes are often advised to begin refuelling immediately after exercise. However, the main reason for promoting carbohydrate-rich meals or snacks soon after exercise is that effective refuelling does not start until a substantial amount of carbohydrate (about 1 g/kg BM) is consumed (Table 93.3). Rapid refuelling strategies are important when there is less than 8 hours between exercise sessions but when recovery time is longer, immediate intake of carbohydrate after exercise is unnecessary and the athletes should choose their preferred meal/snack schedule for achieving total carbohydrate intake goals. The co-ingestion of protein with carbohydrate-rich recovery meals and snacks may enhance glycogen synthesis when the total intake of carbohydrate is below optimal targets. Nevertheless, the main reason to consume high-quality protein after exercise is to promote protein synthesis during the recovery phase.

Rehydration is another issue in post-event recovery, since athletes can expect to be at least mildly dehydrated at the end of their session. In essence, the success of post-exercise rehydration is dependent on how much the athlete drinks, and then how much of this is retained and re-equilibrated within body fluid compartments. It may take 6–24 hours for complete rehydration following fluid losses of 2–5% of BM.

When it is important to encourage voluntary fluid intake, flavoured drinks have been shown to encourage greater intake than plain water. Urine losses appear to be minimized by the simultaneous replacement of lost electrolytes, particularly sodium. The inclusion of sodium in a rehydration drink is an important strategy in the rapid recovery of moderate-to-high fluid deficits. However, the optimal sodium level is about 50–80 mmol/L, as found in oral rehydration solutions used in the treatment of diarrhoea. This is considerably higher than the concentrations found in commercial sports drinks and may be unpalatable to many athletes. Alternatively, sodium can be consumed in recovery meals in the form of sodium-rich foods (e.g. bread, cheese, breakfast cereals) or by adding salt to cooking or food preparation. Creatively planned meals and snacks may be able to simultaneously provide the athlete's needs for carbohydrate, protein, fluid, and electrolytes.

Since alcohol promotes diuresis, consumption of large amounts of alcoholic drinks may interfere with speedy restoration of fluid balance. However, the most important problem with excessive intake of alcohol is indirect: it is likely to interfere with the athlete's commitment or interest in undertaking sound recovery practices. Caffeine has also been identified as a compound that causes diuresis. However, this effect has recently been reviewed, with the finding that it is overstated when consumed in small to moderate doses by habitual caffeine users. The value of the voluntary intake of well-liked beverages should not be forgotten. It is likely that athletes who are prevented from consuming their normal pattern of tea, coffee, and cola drinks may not replace these fluids with an equivalent amount of another beverage.

39.4 Supplements and sports foods

The sports world is filled with supplements and sports foods that claim to make the athlete faster, stronger, leaner, better recovered, healthier, with greater endurance, or whatever other factors are important to performance. The ever-growing range of products can be divided into two separate categories: sports supplements and nutritional ergogenic aids. Sports supplements may be considered as products that address the special nutritional needs of athletes. This category includes sports drinks, sports bars, liquid meal supplements, and micronutrient supplements that are part of a prescribed dietary plan. Many of these products are specially designed to help an athlete meet specific needs for energy and nutrients, including fluid and carbohydrates, in situations where everyday foods are not practical to eat. This is particularly relevant for intake immediately before, during, or after exercise. These supplements can be shown to improve performance when they allow the athlete to achieve their sports nutrition goals. However, they are more expensive than normal food, a consideration that must be balanced against the convenience they provide.

Nutritional ergogenic aids—products that promise a direct and 'supraphysiological' benefit to sports performance—are the supplements that seem most appealing to athletes. These products, which continually change in popularity, include megadoses of vitamins and some minerals, free-form amino acids, ginseng and other herbal compounds, bee pollen, coenzyme Q10, and inosine. In general, these supplements have been poorly tested or have failed to live up to their claims when rigorous testing has been undertaken. Exceptions to this are creatine (Box 39.1), caffeine (Box 39.2), and the buffering agents bicarbonate and beta-alanine (Box 39.3), each of which may enhance the performance of certain athletes under specific conditions. Athletes should seek expert advice about such supplements to see if their sport/exercise warrants experimentation with these products, and to ensure that a correct protocol is tried. The Sports Supplement Program of the Australian Institute of Sport provides information

---

BOX 39.1 Evidence for use of creatine by some athletes

Dose and mode of action

- Loading: 20–30 g taken in multiple doses (e.g. 4×5 g) for 5 days
- Maintenance dose 2–5 g/day

Creatine loading can significantly increase muscle creatine and phosphocreatine levels to reach the muscle storage threshold for these compounds. There is some variability in response to creatine loading, perhaps due to initial creatine stores (i.e. people with pre-existing high levels fail to respond, while those with low levels show the greatest response). Weight gain of about 1 kg occurs with loading because of fluid retention. New studies also show that prior creatine loading may assist the muscle to store glycogen or carbohydrate load more effectively.

Phosphocreatine serves a number of important roles in exercise metabolism: the most well-known role is the rapid regeneration of ATP by the phosphagen power system. The long-term effects of creatine supplementation are not known; however, studies to date have not shown an increased prevalence of problems that are anecdotally linked to creatine use (e.g. muscle strains and tears, thermoregulatory problems). Even so, creatine supplementation is not recommended to young athletes, and athletes are reminded to adhere to the well-proven supplementation protocols. In real life, there have been anecdotal reports that some athletes take creatine in doses that far exceed the amounts that are shown to saturate muscle creatine stores.

(Continued)

BOX 39.1 Evidence for use of creatine by some athletes (*Continued*)

Supported uses

Studies show that creatine loading enhances the performance of exercise involving repeated high-intensity bouts with short recovery intervals (<2 minutes recovery). Performance benefits are seen only in subjects who experience significant increases in creatine stores following loading. Most studies have been undertaken in the laboratory and more research is needed to confirm the benefits of creatine loading by well-trained and elite athletes in sports-specific situations. No benefits to aerobic endurance have been reported, although protocols that involve the effectiveness of carbohydrate loading have not been undertaken. Creatine loading may enhance competition performance involving repeated short sprints (e.g. team games and racquet sports). It is also likely to assist interval and resistance training programmes, thus enhancing training adaptations and the gain of muscle mass and strength.

---

about many products and rates supplements and sports foods into four categories based on the amount of scientific support for the claims made about the use of the product and whether it is considered a banned substance (see http://www.ausport.gov.au/ais/nutrition).

One risk that should be considered in contemplating the use of supplements is the potential for a product to contain impurities and contaminants. Since the mid-1990s it has become apparent that some supplements contain prohormones and stimulants that are banned under antidoping

---

BOX 39.2 Evidence for use of caffeine by some athletes

Dose and mode of action

- Traditional protocol: 5–6 mg/kg BM taken about 1 hour prior to exercise
- New protocols: 2–3 mg/kg BM taken before exercise or during prolonged exercise prior to the onset of fatigue

Caffeine affects numerous body tissues in a variety of ways, causing difficulty in isolating a specific mechanism for any observed changes in exercise performance and endurance. Possible effects include stimulation of the central nervous system and reduction in perception of effort or fatigue, an increase in adrenaline release and activity, and direct effects on muscle recruitment and contractility. New research shows that these effects occur at much lower levels of caffeine intake than previously suggested and the benefits to performance of endurance exercise do not increase with increasing caffeine doses. Therefore, athletes may gain maximum benefit with a reduced risk of side effects such as sleep disturbances from using the low to moderate doses of caffeine found in a range of everyday foods, drinks, and special sports foods. Previous beliefs that the intake of caffeine impairs hydration status, or that it achieves its effects by stimulating lipolysis leading to enhanced fat oxidation and glycogen sparing during prolonged exercise, are now discredited.

Supported uses

Studies show that caffeine intake is associated with performance enhancements in prolonged moderate-intensity exercise (>90 minutes), prolonged intermittent events (e.g. team games), high-intensity events of around 20 minutes' duration and short very-high-intensity exercise of about 5 minutes' duration. Additional studies using sports-specific protocols and well-trained athletes are required, particularly using strategically timed intake of small to moderate doses of caffeine. Individual variability in beneficial response and side effects also warrants further research.

Caffeine was removed from the banned list of the World Anti-Doping Agency in January 2004.

BOX 39.3 Evidence for use of buffering agents by some athletes

Background

During sustained or intermittent activities at high-intensity in which non-oxidative glycolytic pathways contribute significantly to fuel needs, there is a build-up of H^+ which gradually impairs muscle function, causing fatigue. Strategies that enhance the capacity to buffer this drop in muscle pH can delay the onset of such fatigue. These include the old and well-supported strategy of acutely increasing blood (extracellular) buffering capacity via supplementation with bicarbonate and the new strategy of chronically increasing muscle (intracellular) content of the buffering dipeptide carnosine via supplementation with the amino acid beta-alanine.

Dose and mode of action

Bicarbonate

- Acute protocol: 300 mg/kg BM taken 1–2 hours prior to exercise acutely increases buffering capacity for a single exercise session.
- Some research also suggests that a multiday protocol may be effective for repeated days of exercise: 500 mg/kg BM daily, split into four doses. Effects of buffering may be maintained for at least 24 hours after the last dose with this protocol.
- Increases blood bicarbonate levels and pH to provide additional extracellular buffering capacity. Theoretically can mop up excessive levels of H^+ which efflux from muscle cell following high levels of anaerobic glycolytic activity.
- Gastrointestinal upsets are often reported and may be reduced by the intake of large volumes of fluid (1–2 L) or a meal/snack with the bicarbonate dose.

Beta (β)-alanine

- Recent studies have shown that supplementation with 3–5 g/day beta-alanine can increase muscle carnosine content by 80% after 10 weeks of supplementation
- It is unclear how long supplementation needs to continue to maximize muscle carnosine concentrations, or how long muscle carnosine remains elevated if supplementation is stopped; however, the rise and fall of muscle carnosine may take several months to occur.
- Some beta-alanine preparations cause a side effect of paresthesia—an uncomfortable prickling or 'pins and needles' sensation—occurring for ~60 minutes about 15–20 minutes following a dose. This side effect is greatly reduced or eliminated with controlled-release beta-alanine products.

Supported uses

Meta-analysis of bicarbonate studies confirms that bicarbonate supplementation enhances the capacity for high-intensity exercise, which results in the production of high blood levels of lactate and H^+ ions. Events that are likely to benefit from bicarbonate loading are high-intensity events lasting 1–7 minutes and perhaps prolonged events involving intermittent high-intensity bursts. Further study is needed to investigate buffering protocols for events in which a series of heats and finals are undertaken over a day or days to decide the final outcome. The research on performance benefits associated with beta-alanine supplementation is only just appearing, but there are early signs that it also offers advantages for these same sports. Since beta-alanine supplementation involves a chronic increase in intracellular buffering capacity, it is likely that it will also offer benefits to the athlete's ability to undertake high-intensity training. There is a potential for an additive effect of bicarbonate and beta-alanine supplementation protocols through the interaction of enhancements of extra- and intracellular buffering capacity.

codes. While these products should be declared as ingredients on supplement labels, there is evidence that this does not always occur. In fact, a study by an IOC-accredited laboratory found that 15% of supplements contained detectable levels of undeclared banned prohormones. Situations of 'contamination' can include products containing therapeutic doses of banned stimulants or steroids, not identified on the ingredients list, presumably to ensure that the supplement 'works'. More frequently, however, the contamination occurs in trace amounts. These impurities may be sufficient to cause an inadvertent doping outcome in drug testing. Athletes face a code of strict liability under antidoping laws and they will be held responsible for any failed drug test even when it can be proved that they unwittingly ingested a supplement containing banned ingredients.

The decision to use a supplement or sports food should include consideration of the likely benefits and disadvantages (Fig. 39.1). At best, most purported nutritional ergogenic aids offer a placebo to athletes, and at worst, they represent a waste of

considerable amounts of money. Athletes will be better rewarded by investing their resources and interest in a more credible area of sports performance, such as better equipment, improved training techniques, or advice about nutrition or psychological preparation, before directing them to the majority of supplements on the market. Another disadvantage of the use of supplements is the possibility of contamination of products with substances that are illegal in sport, leading to a 'positive' doping offence for the athlete.

Summary

The goals of sports nutrition vary according to the athlete and their event (see Box 39.4). However, these can be divided into issues of training and issues for optimal competition outcomes. Acute nutrition strategies can directly enhance performance by reducing or delaying the onset of factors that would otherwise cause fatigue. Competition performance also benefits when everyday eating strategies assist the athlete to stay healthy and in

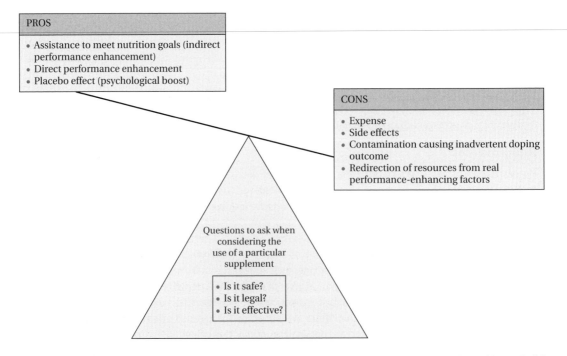

Fig. 39.1 Considerations for using a supplement or sports food *Source*: Burke, L., and Deakin, V. (eds) (2010) *Clinical sports nutrition*, 4th edition. Sydney, McGraw-Hill. p. 488.

BOX 39.4 Case study

Jack is a 26-year-old triathlete who has recently undertaken his first 70.3 event (1.2-mile swim, 56-mile cycle and half-marathon). He is disappointed with his performance, struggling to complete the run leg after 'hitting the wall' just after the half-way point. It was a hot day at the beginning of the summer season and Jack realized that he had sweated more heavily during the cycling leg than he had been prepared for. His bike only carried one drink cage and Jack hadn't liked to slow down too much at the aid stations to take new drink bottles. However, he had tried to drink plenty of fluid during the half-marathon to make up for it—or at least as much as he could stomach without feeling ill. His previous experiences in Olympic distance triathlons hadn't required too much nutrition during the event, so he admitted to being unpractised at the skills required to grab supplies at the aid stations or consume them. He had made sure to drink only water during the run, since his previous attempts at drinking a sports drink during a marathon many years previously had left him feeling queasy. After this experience he had read somewhere that sports drinks were too concentrated to empty from the stomach and should be drunk at a very dilute concentration, if at all. Realizing that he might need some expert advice on how to hydrate during his next attempt at the 70.3 event, he consulted a sports dietitian.

The sports dietitian explained the importance of meeting fuel and fluid needs during an event of this duration (Jack's goal time = 4.45 hours). She corrected the 'hearsay' regarding the concentration of sports drinks, advising him that they were well formulated to contribute to effective delivery of water and carbohydrate to the muscle during exercise. She noted that new sports nutrition research showed that fuelling during ultra-endurance events of this type favoured even higher rates of carbohydrate replacement than previously thought. Whereas a target of 60 g/hour had been the previous benchmark for endurance events (perhaps up to 2–3 hours), intakes of up to 90 g/hour were likely to be even better during lengthier sustained events. She agreed that tolerating this intake would require a number of strategies. The first was to choose a range of newer sports products containing a carbohydrate blend of 2:1 glucose to fructose. These products allowed a greater absorption from the intestine when consumed at those high intakes, enhancing fuel strategies and reducing the likelihood of gut discomfort from unabsorbed contents. The second was to start practising to use these during some training sessions—particularly those mimicking race pace or other race characteristics. It appeared that the gut, like the muscle, was a trainable body part and could learn to tolerate and better absorb/utilize the fuel consumed during exercise. The third strategy was to develop a race plan that allowed for early and regular intake of carbohydrate intake as well as fluid. Jack needed to have a proactive plan, rather than wait until dehydration or fuel depletion had occurred and to overturn it.

Jack practised with a range of products including sports drinks, gels, and some bananas during the month of training leading up to his next race. He found that he was able to tolerate an intake of about 50 g/hour: while not totally reaching his intended target, this was a major improvement on his total lack of intake in the first race. He settled on a brand of sports products and flavours that he liked and found that some occasional solid food in the form of the banana helped to avoid the hunger that he had previously diagnosed as queasiness. At such intakes he wouldn't take specific advantage of the increased absorption of the carbohydrate blends in the new-generation sports products, but at least he seemed to have found a formula that he could quickly learn to be comfortable with. He implemented this menu on race day and was overjoyed to find that he felt 'fuelled' right to the finish line this time. All had gone to plan, although he had found himself reaching for some defizzed Cola at the last feed zones in the run, looking forward to a new taste other than the fruity flavours of his sports products. Between the sports drinks at some feed zones and the flask of gels he carried on his bike, he had easy access to the fuel supplies he needed. He was able to swallow some additional water to rinse out his mouth or add to his fluid needs at times, but otherwise tried to refuel as well as hydrate. After finishing so well, Jack is now reading up on Ironman races (2.4 miles, 112-mile cycling, marathon) to consider his next challenge. He realizes that this will be a true test of a good nutrition plan, but feels he now has the confidence to build this into his training programme.

shape and to optimize the adaptations from their training programme. The various strategies that make up these training and nutrition goals are summarized in Tables 39.1 and 39.4. The athlete can be assisted by the advice of a sports dietitian to adopt eating practices that achieve these goals, often integrating a number of goals into the same menu choices.

Further Reading

1. **Burke L.** (2007). Practical sports nutrition. Champaign, Illinois, Human Kinetics Publishers.
2. **Burke, L. and Deakin, V.** (eds) (2010) *Clinical sports nutrition*, 4th edition. Sydney, McGraw-Hill.
3. **Maughan, R.J.** (ed.) (in press) *Foods, nutrition and sports performance III*. Supplement to *Journal of Sports Science*.

Useful Websites

To see topical and scientifically robust updates on nutrition associated with this textbook and web links to many of the journals in the Further Reading sections, please see the dedicated Online Resource Centre at **http://www.oxfordtextbooks.co.uk/orc/mann4e/**

Sports Nutrition, Australian Institute of Sport http://www.ausport.gov.au/ais/nutrition/
Sports Dietitians Australia http://www.sportsdietitians.com.au

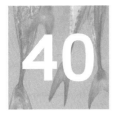

40

Nutritional consequences of poverty and food insecurity in developed countries

Winsome R. Parnell

'It upsets me that I'm not feeding the kids the food I want to and they want to eat.'

Traditionally, the many nutritional consequences of poverty have been identified and discussed in the context of developing countries. However, developed countries, particularly those with changes in their economic environments, have begun to identify an increasing prevalence of poverty-related health issues. Nutritionists recognize the overriding effects of the economic, social, and educational factors, which together can influence nutritional status. Research in this area has therefore had to encompass new definitions and methodologies to assess the magnitude of the problem and the multifaceted causes in order to develop strategies to alleviate them. Specific definitions of poverty and deprivation are always made in relative terms (between the haves and have-nots) and therefore only apply to the society or group under discussion. Poverty is defined in terms of money and equivalent income; deprivation refers to the lack of certain material items regarded as essential in that society. Different degrees of deprivation can occur over a range of income levels with low monetary income (below a defined poverty level) not necessarily being associated with severe deprivation.

Social and material circumstances are known to affect health outcomes. However, it is more difficult to ascertain whether food and nutrient intakes have actually been impaired by socioeconomic disadvantage and can therefore be viewed as a cause of poorer health. Research focus has mostly been to link socioeconomic factors with health outcome, and, to a limited extent, to link food and nutrient intake with poverty.

The major areas of nutritional concern, specifically found to be related to poverty in developed countries, include:

- energy intake—both undernutrition and overnutrition;

- insufficient intake of some micronutrients, such as iron;

- more babies with low birth weight and fewer babies being breastfed;

- lower intakes of vegetables and fruits.

40.1 Methodology

The selection of appropriate methodologies to study the nutritional consequences of poverty is not easy. First, a definition of poverty needs to be developed that is appropriate to the specific population group under consideration. Many researchers have used purely economic definitions; for example, a percentage of mean equivalent disposable household income. Others recognize that deprivation criteria should be part of the definition of poverty, such as a lack of adequate housing, transport, or clothing. The length of time a group or individual experiences deprivation will be a determining factor in the effects of poverty.

Second, in developed countries with adequate food supplies, it has been difficult to define the concept of hunger. It is not an isolated outcome, but one consequence of the larger problem of poverty. Hunger can be cyclical, short term, or long term; it is not just physiological need. From the debate has emerged the term *food insecurity*. Food insecurity may be said to exist when the availability of nutritionally adequate and safe foods or the ability to acquire adequate supplies of culturally acceptable foods in socially acceptable ways is limited or uncertain.

Whereas most people living in poverty, defined in economic terms, are at risk of food insecurity, not all are food insecure. Also, some households will experience food insecurity in the face of events such as sudden ill heath, job loss, or unexpected expenses, even though income *per se* might place them well above a poverty line. National food and nutrition surveys often now include specific measures of food insecurity at household or individual level, which can potentially be correlated with food- and nutrient-intake data. Studies targeted at subgroups that

are at risk require special consideration of their particular circumstances when developing the methodology and establishing sampling procedures. Participation may be affected by poor access to transport and telephones and language and literacy problems, along with a variety of other social stresses. Sensitivity to these issues, including those of confidentiality and privacy, must be taken into account.

A landmark study among an at-risk population was carried out in London, UK, by Dowler and Calvert. Their report *Nutrition and diet in lone-parent families in London* describes the socioeconomic circumstances, food-intake patterns, and nutrient intakes of 200 lone-parent families, with the aim of identifying the most important factors that differentiate diets of those at higher or lower risk for long-term ill health. Data collected included 3-day weighed intake records for each lone parent and at least one child, a food-frequency questionnaire, and a taped, semi-structured interview. The main conclusion from this work was 'that poor material circumstances combined with severe constraints on disposable income are the main factors characterising nutritional deprivation in lone parents, and sometimes their children'. The diets of parents (predominantly mothers) were affected more than children's diets, and patterns of food shopping and food-management skills had little effect on nutritional outcome. 'These mothers are not bad managers who do not know how to look after their children. They face impossible odds in making ends meet, and the aim of policy should be to help them, not to blame them'. This study encapsulates the root causes of food insecurity: inadequate financial resources and constraints on those resources that result in money not being available for food.

Further examples of studies of at-risk population groups have been carried out in Canada and New Zealand. In New Zealand, a convenience sample of 40 families receiving government benefits responded to a questionnaire developed to assess the aspects of food security relevant to them. Nutritional status was measured by means of weights and heights; nutrient intakes were measured by multiple 24-hour dietary recalls. Women in these families were the most nutritionally disadvantaged. A further study in New Zealand examined the food-purchasing habits and behaviours surrounding food acquisition among families with children from a range of socioeconomic backgrounds. Although behaviours were found to be similar across the socioeconomic spec-

trum, financial constraints impacted greatly on low income families' ability to obtain a nutritious diet. There was a lower expenditure on food overall, and in particular a lower expenditure on vegetables compared to medium- and high-income families.

In Canada, a study of women receiving emergency food assistance included assessment of dietary intake by three repeated 24-hour dietary recalls and examination of dietary adequacy across levels of self-reported household-level hunger. The prevalences of inadequacy of nutrient intake of those reporting the most food insecurity were 'in a range that could put women at risk of nutrient deficiencies'.

Studies such as these have provided a step forward in the development of useful methods in this area. The surveillance of diets of people living on low incomes is important in developed countries.

40.2 Undernutrition and obesity

Studies of the growth rates and weight/height relationships of children in the 5–12-year age range, of varying socioeconomic circumstances, generally conclude that disadvantaged children have lower height-for-age and are more likely to have lower weight-for-height. This suggests that overt undernutrition (insufficient energy intake) over a period of time does have a negative effect on children's growth in developed countries.

However, it is clear that obesity also occurs in socioeconomically disadvantaged children, although to a lesser extent than among those of wealthier backgrounds. Evidence is emerging that food insecurity may contribute to overweight, particularly among girls. Further research is necessary and must include measures of dietary intake, along with measures of growth patterns and income, in order to determine the role of nutrition in growth in developed countries.

Few studies on adults in developed countries have linked poor socioeconomic status with frank under-nutrition. Undoubtedly some extremely deprived men and women—for example, the homeless—exhibit clinical signs of undernutrition.

Prevalence studies do not appear to have been conducted among these groups. In contrast, extensive work has documented the inverse relationship between socioeconomic status and obesity among women; this relationship has not been shown in men. Whereas poverty has long been held to be a cause of obesity among women, recently the inverse has been suggested, that obesity will result in lower socioeconomic status, mediated through unequal work and partnership opportunities.

Although the relationship between obesity and lower socioeconomic status clearly exists, there is little evidence from food and nutrient data that excess energy intake is the main influencing factor.

Criticisms of the existing studies on the energy intakes of obese women focus on the fact that they are more likely than non-obese women to under-report food intake and to eat less than their habitual intake during study periods. Until the problem of accurately determining energy intake among obese women is solved, no conclusions can be made about the primary cause of obesity in socioeconomically disadvantaged women. The applicability of standard cut-off values for the ratio of energy intake to estimated basal metabolic rate for estimating under-reporting has been questioned, as they were not developed for population sub-groups so different from the populations on which the approach was developed. It seems also that the notion of habitual intake is less applicable to socio-economically disadvantaged women than wealth-ier women, because their economic resource base is not stable and they experience times of feast and famine. Food insecurity is associated with over-weight, particularly among women. Given that food insecurity is characterized by an uncertain supply of food, this lends support to the point of view that fluctuations in energy intake and in body weight can contribute ultimately to accumulation of excess body fat. Whether obese women of low socioeconomic status are less physically active than obese women of wealthier backgrounds is not

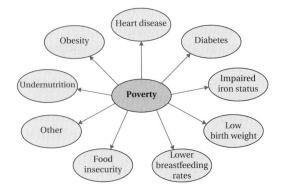

Fig. 40.1 Nutritional consequences of poverty.

known. Economic deprivation is, however, known to affect motivation and self-esteem and it limits opportunities for many forms of recreational exer-cise (Fig. 40.1).

40.3 Heart disease and diabetes

Research has shown that the prevalence of coronary heart disease and accompanying changes in risk and mortality rates appear to be influenced greatly by socioeconomic factors. Although coronary heart disease is more common in more affluent countries, it appears to have a higher incidence in less affluent subgroups of these countries. Overall, declining mortality rates have been largely at the higher end of the socioeconomic spectrum, and in some regions mortality has risen among lower socioeco-nomic groups of men and women. These differences have in part been attributed to differences in rates of blood pressure and obesity. Blood pressure, within average community levels, is influenced by sodium intake. Lower socioeconomic conditions in child-hood have also been linked to increased risk of cor-onary heart disease in adulthood, in both women and men. This association has not been fully explained, but several studies provide some evi-dence to link nutritional status in childhood to sub-sequent coronary heart disease.

There is no obvious link between socioeconomic status and either quality or quantity of fat in the diets of men or women. However, there is clear evidence across all socioeconomic groups that fat intake, par-ticularly intake of saturated fat, is a significant die-tary factor associated with the incidence of coronary heart disease (see Section 21.3). Many studies in developed countries document distinctive differ-ences in eating habits and food choices between high and low socioeconomic groups, but this seldom has a profound effect on the contribution to energy intake from macronutrients, including fat. Indeed, some authors conclude that there is a general uni-formity of nutrient-density consumption patterns across different socioeconomic groups. Evidence that the consumption of fresh vegetables and fruits is inversely related to socioeconomic indices is undis-puted. Foods that are perishable and not nutrient-dense are less likely to be consumed in the context of food insecurity. If diets high in fruits and vegetables decrease degenerative diseases (e.g. by means of the antioxidative properties in these foods), then it may well be that their lack contributes to the burden of coronary heart disease and diabetes, as well as some cancers, among the poor.

Whereas obesity is one identified risk factor for coronary heart disease, it is also a major predictor in the onset of type 2 diabetes mellitus, with both the duration and magnitude of obesity increasing the risk of development of type 2 diabetes. Since obesity is associated with lower socioeconomic status, it would be expected that type 2 diabetes will occur more frequently in groups of lower socioeconomic status. The incidence of type 2 diabetes and impaired glucose tolerance was found to be inversely related to annual gross household income but not to an occupation-based index of socioeconomic status (the Elley–Irving Index) in a multiracial workforce study in New Zealand. The prevalence of type 1 diabetes mellitus in children has been noted to be associated with material deprivation, but it has not been possible to link this with any particular nutrient. Recent research suggests that early exposure to cow's milk or diminished breastfeeding may be an important determinant of subsequent type 1 diabetes.

40.4 Iron deficiency

The aetiology of iron deficiency can be viewed as a negative balance between iron intake and iron loss. During the periods of rapid growth, iron balance is difficult to maintain; that is, during infancy, early childhood, adolescence, and pregnancy.

In infancy, lower iron status is associated with lower socioeconomic status, although iron deficiency occurs in all strata of society. Low iron status among adolescent girls of all socioeconomic groups is largely attributable to their increased dietary requirement of iron to balance the needs of growth and menstruation. Studies have not shown any difference in iron intakes among adolescent girls in low socioeconomic groups when compared with those from more affluent backgrounds.

Women of childbearing potential in the USA have lower intakes of some nutrients, including iron, if they are of lower socioeconomic status. This can contribute to low iron status during pregnancy. Iron-deficiency anaemia has been shown to be associated with poverty and to be linked with an increased risk of preterm delivery and low birth weight.

40.5 Low birth weight

Low socioeconomic status is predictive of low birth weight in most developed countries. A number of factors have been found to increase the incidence of low birth weight: cigarette smoking, low maternal weight gain during pregnancy, low pre-pregnancy weight, iron-deficiency anaemia, alcohol intake, and possibly caffeine. Some of these factors are more prevalent in lower socioeconomic groups and others are not. For example, cigarette smoking, which has a direct effect on the flow of nutrients across the placenta, is higher among low socioeconomic groups. Smokers have also been shown to eat less than non-smokers. Alcohol intake, however, has in some studies been higher among the wealthy.

Women in whom birth outcome is most at risk from a nutritional cause enter pregnancy with a low body mass index and do not gain sufficient weight during their pregnancy. Poor socioeconomic circumstances could contribute to this scenario, but no studies show that it is confined to such groups. Future studies may be able to discern whether poverty has a significant influence on low birth weight because maternal nutrition has been impaired, rather than because, for example, smoking rates are higher or other lifestyle factors, such as prenatal health care, are less than optimal.

40.6 Breastfeeding

Social class is an important marker of breastfeeding success, which is more common in mothers of high socioeconomic status. Solo mothers, who are over-represented in the lower socioeconomic groups and obese mothers are less likely to initiate or continue breastfeeding. The reasons for this are complex, but it is generally acknowledged that women need adequate support and encouragement to breastfeed successfully, and this help may be most limited among solo mothers. Infants who are not breastfed are at greater risk of respiratory illness and infections and are more likely to be subject to feeding practices that do not enhance iron status and are at greater risk of childhood obesity.

40.7 Behaviour

The issue of whether inadequate nutrient intake and particularly hunger affect behaviour has been most studied among school children. After World War II, policy-makers in the UK and USA felt that food programmes for lunches and/or breakfasts in schools would have a significant impact on school performance, including alertness, intelligence, educational attainment, and general behaviour patterns. These programmes were made available regardless of socioeconomic circumstances, although those in higher socioeconomic groups were expected to pay. Fifty years on, when many such programmes have been reduced or dropped, hunger is again considered a problem among school children and the reasons given are inadequate family income and lifestyle factors, such as time for food preparation and food habits. Thus, socioeconomic status is still believed to impact negatively on children's behaviour patterns. Whereas many believe that nutrition is a significant issue, it is very difficult to disentangle the effects of the many disadvantageous factors of low socioeconomic status and how they impact on children's behaviour. Nutrition may well be one of these but few studies adequately address the issue in totality. For example, a study of 'perceived hunger' in schools in New Zealand found that the prevalence was higher in inner-city areas and where ethnic diversity was greatest. No measures of behaviour at school were made, or of nutritional status. Reviews of school feeding programmes in the USA conclude that they have positive nutritional impact, but have not adequately evaluated such programmes in terms of their effect on academic performance. Data from the USA have examined the ongoing effects of household food insecurity on children's academic performance and social skills and found that they are associated with developmental consequences. The fact that so many outcomes of poverty, in both the home and school environment, have the potential to influence behaviour of children means that adverse food patterns and nutrition will always be a part of the spectrum to a varying degree.

40.8 Food insecurity

From the above sections it can be concluded that it is difficult, in developed countries, to quantify the effect of poverty on nutritional status, both for methodological reasons and possibly because nutritional status is seldom profoundly affected, particularly in the short term. In addition, poor nutritional status is not confined to low socioeconomic groups.

Food security, however, is clearly difficult to achieve when economic status drops suddenly or when it is inadequate and remains so for long periods of time. To be food secure, individuals need more than adequate disposable income. They may need to overcome obstacles such as lack of transport, inadequate cooking or storage facilities, and access to food that is culturally acceptable (Fig. 40.2).

'I don't buy 5 kg of potatoes as I can't carry it.'
'I hope my husband will agree to give us the car.'

What is measurable is the growth of the many and varied programmes to alleviate shortage of food for groups of economically disadvantaged people. Food banks or pantries set up by charitable organizations continue to increase in number and size of operation in most developed countries. Their aim is to provide free food to the needy in an emergency or on a short-term basis. In some countries, government purchasing assistance such as food stamps serve as a permanent or semi-permanent source of food income. The efficacy of surplus-food redistribution is fiercely debated. Many consider that it perpetuates food poverty and provides no long-term solutions.

'It's hard to ask people for help. I don't want to be a burden.'

There is little dispute that the underlying causes of food insecurity are socioeconomic and political. These must be addressed by economists and politicians. What can nutritionists do? Many have attempted an educational approach, on the premise that budgeting and food-preparation skills should be improved. In some instances, this is helpful. But many communities of people in constrained circumstances vocalize their need to find

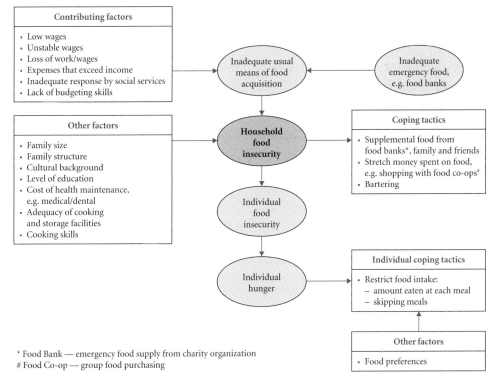

Fig. 40.2 Household food insecurity.

Source: Adapted from Williams, C., and Dowler, E.A. (1994) *A working paper for the Nutrition Task Force Low Income Project Team*. London, Department of Health.

solutions and coping strategies using their own skills and resources, alongside appropriate professional input.

'People are the experts on their own lives.'

Public health policy in many developed countries states that the effects of socioeconomic disadvantage on nutritional wellbeing is a public health priority. Australia's 1992 *Food and Nutrition Policy* document opens: 'The Government's food and nutrition policy is to facilitate and support action through the entire food and nutrition system, in order to achieve better nutrition for Australians, especially for those most disadvantaged'. New Zealand's National Plan of Action for Nutrition listed 'Improving household food security' as a first priority, noting the need to establish baseline information on the current situation with respect to accessibility, acceptability, and affordability of food.

It is apparent that developed countries cannot assume that all segments of their population are food-secure. There is an emerging body of research demonstrating associations with, or consequences of, food insecurity which include psychological issues and socio-familial disturbances. Several countries are developing tools to document the prevalence of food insecurity and monitor the nutritional outcomes. An example is in New Zealand, where eight indices of household food security were developed and ranked in order of severity. Categories of food security (fully/almost fully

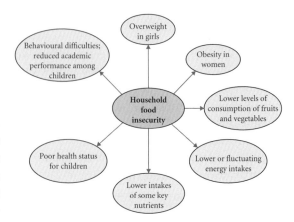

Fig. 40.3 Consequences of household food insecurity—emerging evidence.

secure, moderately secure, and low security) have been shown to be associated with nutritional outcomes in the population. For adults, those with the lowest household food-security status have the highest intake of fats and the lowest intakes of glucose, fructose, and vitamin C. For New Zealand children, those in households with lower food security have lower intakes of lactose, calcium, vitamin A and β-carotene. Such data confirm the hypothesis that without ready access to affordable and appropriate food, nutritional status will be compromised (Fig. 40.3). They also assist efforts to develop and coordinate economic policies, educational strategies, and social action to alleviate the consequences of poverty, among which poor nutritional status is undoubtedly one.

40.9 Case study

Mary Smith is a 40-year-old solo mother (sole parent) with two sons aged 14 and 8 years. She has been co-owner/operator of a lunchtime cafe in a small town for a little over 1 year. She entered this venture after receiving money from a relative's estate, all of which was invested in the business. The cafe is making no profit. The local district Health Board scheduled gall-bladder surgery without warning, which was necessitated by an acute attack of

gall stones 6 months before. This obliges her to leave her partner to cope alone without arrangements for adequate cover. The surgery is followed by complications that delay her recovery and she is away from work for a month, so that the partner demands the business be sold. Debts have been incurred for intercity ambulance transport to enable urgent hospital readmission in relation to the surgical complications and early discharge. Childcare costs for 2 months' 'board' for her two sons have accrued.

Mary leaves the business with no assets and 2 months' rent in her bank account. Her car requires repairs if it is to be roadworthy. She is not well enough to seek new paid employment for the foreseeable future and anticipates eligibility for a government benefit in 2 months' time.

How should she provision her household until then? There are staple foods in the pantry: rice, pasta, some canned goods, and condiments. Normally her garden would be a source of fresh vegetables but this has been neglected since she began to work in the cafe for 12 hours each day.

Once the government benefit payments begin, they will need to stretch to service debts for her sons' school uniforms, in addition to paying the debts for the ambulance and car repairs. Her immediate recourse is to the local food bank, which provides dried and canned foods. Neighbours supply some fresh vegetables. There is no money available to pay for fresh milk and fruit.

Further Reading

1. **Bailey, V.F. and Sherriff, J.** (1992) Reasons for the early cessation of breast-feeding in women from lower socio-economic groups in Perth, Western Australia. *Aust J Nutr Diet*, **49**, 40–3.

2. **Dowler, E. and Calvert, C.** (1995) *Nutrition and diet in lone-parent families in London.* London, Family Policy Studies Centre.

3. **James, W.P.T., Nelson, M., Ralph, A., and Leather, S.** (1997) The contributions of nutrition to inequalities in health. *BMJ*, **341**, 1545–9.

4. **Jyoti, D.F., Frongillo, E.A., and Jones, S.J.** (2005) Food insecurity affects school children's academic performance, weight gain and social skills. *J Nutr*, **135**, 2831–9.

5. **Miller, J.E. and Korenman, S.** (1994) Poverty and children's nutritional status in the United States. *Am J Epidemiol*, **140**, 233–43.

6. **Nelson, M.** (2000) Childhood nutrition and poverty. *Proc Nutr Soc*, **59**, 307–15.

7. **Nutrition Taskforce Low Income Project Team** (1996) *Health of the nation. Low income, food, nutrition and health: Strategies for improvement.* Wetherby, Department of Health.

8. **Position of the American Dietetic Association** (2010): Food insecurity in the United States. *J Am Diet Assoc*, **110**, 1368–76.

9. **Sobal, J. and Stunkard, A.J.** (1989) Socioeconomic status and obesity: A review of the literature. *Psychol Bull*, **105**, 260–75.

10. **Tarasuk, V.S. and Beaton, G.H.** (1999) Women's dietary intakes in the context of household food insecurity. *J Nutr*, **129**, 672–9.

11. **Williams, C. and Dowler, E.A.** (1994) *A working paper for the Nutrition Task Force Low Income Project Team.* London, Department of Health.

Useful Websites

To see topical and scientifically robust updates on nutrition associated with this textbook and web links to many of the journals in the Further Reading sections, please see the dedicated Online Resource Centre at **http://www.oxfordtextbooks.co.uk/orc/mann4e/**

41

Nutrition and HIV and AIDS

Hester Vorster

The global pandemic as a result of infection with the human immunodeficiency virus (HIV) and consequent development of acquired immunodeficiency syndrome (AIDS) has been described as 'the first postmodern pandemic', 'a human tragedy', 'one of the greatest calamities ever to befall humankind', one of the 'most devastating events in human history', and 'a threat to development, security and economic growth'.

The Joint United Nations Programme on HIV/ AIDS (UNAIDS) reported in 2009 that globally, an estimated 33.4 million people were living with HIV infection, of whom more than 30 million were from low- and middle-income countries. South Africa has the largest population living with the infection (about 5 million in 2008). Nigeria is second with 2.6 million, and India third with about 2.5 million in 2008. Countries such as the USA and China have low prevalence rates (0.6 and 0.2%, respectively), but at least 1.2 and 0.7 million people in these countries are living with the disease. An estimated 25 million people have already died from HIV/ AIDS. In 2007 alone, 2.5 million people were newly infected and 2.1 million died because of HIV/AIDS-related causes.

The consequences and impact of the pandemic are devastating. Life expectancy at birth in Southern Africa has already plummeted to levels last recorded in the 1950s (to 47 years) and infant mortality rates are severely affected in developing countries. It is a disease with a profound social impact in the developing world. It turns grandparents into parents, and orphaned children into main breadwinners and heads of households, because it is usually young, sexually active adults in their reproductive years that are victims of the disease.

Kallings, the founding president of the international AIDS society, pointed out in 2008 that the scientific and public health response to the infection were relatively successful: 'we have identified and described the aetiology, pathogenesis, and transmission routes and developed diagnostic tests and antiretroviral drugs'. The World Health Organization reported in 2009 that global scaling up of treatment had resulted in 4 of the 9 million people needing antiretroviral drugs in developing countries in 2008 gaining access to these drugs. However, despite this progress, the unique characteristics of the virus have prevented the development of a vaccine, and there is little hope that one will become available in the near future.

This chapter focuses on the role of nutrition in the prevention, progression, care, and treatment of HIV and AIDS. Optimizing nutritional status is often the only option to assist infected people in resource-limited countries. To understand how nutrition influences the disease and management of patients with HIV and AIDS, the viral aetiology of the infection, clinical features, and pharmacological therapy are briefly summarized in Section 41.1 and

Boxes 41.1 and 41.2. The discussion of metabolic abnormalities associated with HIV and AIDS in Section 41.2 leads into the discussion of the role of nutrition in HIV and AIDS in Section 41.3.

41.1 HIV and AIDS

41.1.1 Human immunodeficiency virus characteristics

HIV is a member of the lentivirus family of retroviruses and was first isolated in 1983. Currently, six subtypes are known, with two major subtypes, HIV-1 and HIV-2, the principal cause of the pandemic. Human beings are not the natural hosts of the virus. These viruses probably entered the human population as a result of cross-species transmission from chimpanzee species (HIV-1) and sooty mangabeys (HIV-2), possibly around 1930.

After HIV entry into the human body, it binds to the CD4$^+$ receptor on the surface of CD4$^+$ cells of

---

BOX 41.1 Stages of HIV infection

Stage 1: Acute infection (seroconversion)

- rapid viral replication
- symptoms: fever, malaise, headache, myalgia, skin rashes, lymphadenopathy syndrome
- duration: 1 week to several months

Stage 2: Asymptomatic HIV infection

- none or only a few symptoms
- subclinical loss of lean body mass
- vitamin B$_{12}$ deficiency
- changes in blood lipids and liver enzymes
- susceptibility to pathogens in food and water
- duration: 10 years or longer (depending on nutritional status and drug treatment)

Stage 3: Symptomatic HIV infection

- CD4$^+$ counts between 200 and 500 cells/μL
- symptoms: loss of appetite, white plaques in mouth, skin lesions, fever, night sweats, tuberculosis, shingles, other infections
- wasting: involuntary weight loss > 10% baseline body weight, caused by reduced food intake, chronic incurable diarrhoea, malabsorption, nutrient losses, and increased energy needs ('slim disease'); nutrition interventions may help to preserve lean body mass and strengthen the immune system

Stage 4: AIDS

- CD4$^+$ cell counts below 200 cells/μL
- final, fatal stage if not treated by antiretroviral (ARV) drugs
- immunosuppression leads to opportunistic (secondary) infections with fungi, protozoa, bacteria, and other viruses
- malignant diseases and dementia may develop

BOX 41.2 Pharmacological (ARV drug) therapy of HIV and AIDS

Treatment of primary infection

- HAART: highly active ARV therapy, with at least three drugs (protease inhibitors such as amprenavir, indinavir, etc. and reverse transcriptase inhibitors such as abacavir, nevirapine, etc.) There are now more than 20 different ARVs available

- slow progression of HIV to AIDS, restore immunofunction partially, decrease morbidity and mortality

- start drug treatment with onset of symptoms or when $CD4^+$ counts are below 200 cells/μL

- individualize and monitor treatment to prevent drug resistance, interactions, and side effects

- daily, lifelong adherence required

- World Health Organization's '3 × 5' programme showed that drug treatment in developing countries is possible, affordable, and sustainable

Treatment of wasting

- megestrol acetate, testosterone, other metabolic steroids, growth hormone, or thalidomide may be useful to use in adjunction to diet therapy and increased activity

Treatment of secondary (opportunistic) infections

- individualized therapy of specific fungi, protozoa, bacteria, or other virus infections, using appropriate drugs

the immune system. This allows the virus to penetrate the $CD4^+$ cells and replicate, using reverse transcriptase to produce viral DNA. The new viral particles are secreted into the circulation and the $CD4^+$ host cells are destroyed. The body produces new $CD4^+$ cells to fight the HIV infection, but eventually the $CD4^+$ cell counts drop, the immune system loses its ability to resist other infections, and signs of immune failure appear, namely mucocutaneous conditions, persistent generalized lymphadenopathy, and high risk of infections and malignancies. At this stage, patients have developed AIDS and, without effective antiretroviral therapy (see Boxes 41.1 and 41.2), will die within a few years. The persistency of the infection, the ability of the virus to mutate, and its destruction of the immune system are some reasons why no vaccine is available as yet.

41.1.2 HIV transmission

The virus is transmitted via certain body fluids: blood, semen, pre-seminal fluid, vaginal secretions, and breast milk. Previously, and today in most developed countries, the principal modes of transmission were and are unprotected sexual contact between men and sharing of needles by intravenous drug abusers. The majority of infections globally, are because of unprotected heterosexual contact and vertical transmission from an infected mother to her child: antenatally, during labour, or by breastfeeding. A small number have been infected by transfusion of contaminated blood or blood products. Extreme care when working with body fluids and the use of condoms reduces the risk of infection.

41.1.3 Stages of HIV infection and progression to AIDS

The destruction by the virus of the ability of the immune system to fight infections results in four stages of the disease (Box 41.1), which form the basis of clinical classifications.

41.2 Metabolic and endocrine abnormalities during HIV infection

The changes in metabolism and endocrine function during HIV infection, resulting from both the primary and several possible secondary infections, and the pharmacological therapy of the disease influence its nutritional management.

41.2.1 Changes in energy metabolism

Wasting associated with HIV and treated or untreated AIDS is an independent predictor of mortality. Wasting results from inadequate macronutrient and energy intake, malabsorption, increased losses, and increased energy expenditure or needs. Studies in adults show that resting metabolic rate (RMR) is about 10% higher in HIV-infected adults compared with healthy adults, especially when secondary infections occur. However, total energy expenditure is usually not raised, probably because of decreased physical activity. In asymptomatic HIV, energy intake is normal or slightly increased (15%), probably to compensate for malabsorption or increased RMR. Later, secondary infections lead to decreased intake. Antiretroviral drugs also cause anorexia, which disappears when clinical symptoms improve and drug therapy is established. HIV damages intestinal villi, causing malabsorption. Gut infections further exacerbate malabsorption through diarrhoea, all contributing to wasting. Energy needs during convalescence following severe infection may increase by an additional 20–50%.

41.2.2 Changes in protein metabolism and turnover

Potential changes in protein metabolism and turnover are of importance to determine whether HIV and AIDS patients require higher-than-usual protein intakes. Some studies suggest that this may be the case. There is evidence of increased protein turnover

(possibly explaining the increased RMR) and that, on energy-deficient diets, protein rather than fat stores may be preferentially metabolized. Definitive recommendations regarding protein intake are not possible at this stage, but it does seem that additional protein and amino acids are not utilized adequately until secondary infections have been treated.

41.2.3 Changes in lipid metabolism and development of the lipodystrophy syndrome

HIV increases lipid oxidation, while carbohydrate oxidation in AIDS decreases. Fasting triglyceride and sometimes cholesterol levels increase, lipoprotein lipase activity and triglyceride clearance decrease, and hepatic *de novo* lipogenesis increases. Severe hyperlipidaemia may occur in patients treated with antiretroviral drugs. The most striking abnormality of lipid metabolism is the development of the lipodystrophy syndrome seen in some patients treated with antiretroviral drugs. Body composition, fat distribution, and shape changes include the development of a 'spider body' and 'buffalo hump' (extra fat deposits in the dorsocervical fat pad), increased intra-abdominal fat deposition and loss of subcutaneous fat in the cheeks, arms, and legs, leading to prominent veins and muscles. Some patients on HAART (see Box 41.2) develop insulin resistance and type 2 diabetes mellitus. Conventional dietary and drug treatments are recommended for the hyperlipidaemia and abnormalities of glucose metabolism.

41.2.4 Other metabolic and endocrine abnormalities

Raised levels of cytokines and disturbed levels of adiponectin, growth hormone, leptin, insulin-like growth factor, and glycerol have all been observed in AIDS patients. Increased venous lactate levels (>2.0 mmol/L) and low arterial pH (<7.3) are potential consequences of antiretroviral therapy, especially in the presence of liver damage. Lactic acidosis is accompanied by nausea, abdominal pain, shortness of breath, fatigue, and weight loss, and can be fatal. Hypogonadism occurs in 30–50% of men with AIDS, and the resultant male steroid hormone deficiency may play a role in HIV wasting.

41.3 Nutrition and HIV and AIDS

Appropriate nutrition cannot cure HIV and AIDS. However, based on the established relationship between nutrition and the immune system, it could enhance immune function and reduce the risk and severity of infections. Furthermore, there is evidence that improved nutritional status can reduce the risk of transmission, reduce HIV-associated wasting, slow the progression of HIV to AIDS, and optimize drug treatment of both the primary and secondary infections. Nutrition interventions can, therefore, help to improve the quality of life of infected people, promote a sense of wellbeing, and keep them mobile and working. Unfortunately, HIV-infected persons are often exposed to inappropriate, untested, and unproven advice regarding benefits of specific foods and supplements. This advice exploits ignorance and fear and raises false hope. In the following section, only nutrition interventions that have been proven and with a sound scientific basis are considered.

41.3.1 Specific nutrient requirements

Deficiencies of several nutrients including protein, essential fatty acids, vitamins A, B_6, folate, C and E, iron, zinc, copper, and selenium, as well as an energy deficit, are associated with impaired immune function. This has led to speculation that some of these nutrients may have specific beneficial effects in HIV and AIDS. Attempts to definitively establish their roles have been hampered by a multitude of methodological problems and ethical considerations. Further studies are underway but in the light of existing knowledge, the following nutrients deserve attention.

Protein While there is no definitive evidence (see Section 41.2.2) that the presence of HIV or AIDS *per se* warrants additional protein, there are some situations in which protein intake should be at the upper end of the recommended range (1.5–2.0 g/kg): presence of infection, catch-up growth in children, and wasting in adults. In such situations it is essential to optimize, as far as possible, conditions for the utilization of protein, e.g. by the treatment of infections. For most others, protein intake should be 1.0–1.4 g/kg body weight. Those with severe hepatic or renal disease should be recommended reduced protein intakes.

Fat Fat has a high energy density and is a useful nutrient to include in small frequent meals of individuals with anorexia and others requiring increased energy intake. However, reduced fat diets are indicated for those with a decreased fat tolerance, fat malabsorption, and diarrhoea. Medium-chain fatty acid oils may be better tolerated and absorbed than long-chain ones by HIV-infected people. Supplementation with fish oils (ω-3 fatty acids) may be useful because they are less inflammation-promoting than ω-6 fatty acids. Saturated fatty acids should be reduced in those with hyperlipidaemia as a consequence of antiretroviral treatment.

Fluids and electrolytes Fluid and electrolyte requirements of HIV-infected and uninfected individuals are similar: 30–35 mL/kg or 1.5 L/day for adults. However, additional fluids and electrolytes are often required because of losses during diarrhoea, vomiting, and night sweats. These should be replaced by oral rehydration solutions, which may be prepared at home (e.g. 1 L boiled, cooled water plus half a teaspoon of salt (sodium chloride) and 8 teaspoons of sugar or cooked cereal).

Vitamins HIV infection is associated with low serum vitamin A levels and low maternal serum vitamin A is associated with increased perinatal transmission of the virus. There is evidence that in HIV-infected children vitamin A supplementation will decrease morbidity and mortality. Vitamin A is necessary for maintaining epithelial integrity and is suspected to help prevent transmission of the virus. However, there is no convincing evidence that vitamin A supplementation decreases risk of transmission of HIV or slows the progression of the disease in adults. Several large studies have indicated that vitamin A supplementation of pregnant women actually increases mother-to-child transmission and vitamin A supplementation of pregnant women is not recommended. There is consistent evidence that several of the B vitamins may decrease transmission of the virus and that the antioxidant vitamins (C and E) may decrease progression of the infection and improve birth outcomes. Therefore, except for vitamin A in pregnant women, multivitamin supplementation to a level not more than twice the daily needs, are strongly recommended for HIV-infected people.

Minerals Iron stores decrease during the asymptomatic stages (1–3) of HIV infection, probably because of decreased absorption. In the later stages of AIDS, iron accumulates in macrophages and other cells. Iron supplements are recommended in pregnancy and anaemia. However, iron may increase the risk of opportunistic infections. Moreover, the effects of iron on viral replication and load are not clear. Zinc deficiency is prevalent in many developing country populations, and supplementation with zinc is known to decrease the risk of diarrhoea and respiratory tract infections. It is also known that zinc is essential for the normal function of the immune system. However, in high doses, zinc has been shown to be immunosuppressive. There are conflicting results about the role of zinc in the progression and morbidity of HIV and AIDS. Selenium is another micronutrient (antioxidant)

suspected to play a role in HIV. It seems that a selenium deficiency is associated with an increased virulence of the virus, but there is no evidence on the effects of selenium supplementation on the course of HIV and AIDS.

Supplements There are gaps in our knowledge about the primary effect of HIV on micronutrient status and requirements and about the effects of supplementation with specific micronutrients on the course of HIV infection. Thus, at present the recommendations are that intakes of infected individuals should reach levels of intake that will prevent clinical and biochemical signs of any deficiency. A food-based approach with diversified diets is always the most appropriate. However, many infected individuals are food insecure. Furthermore, HIV infection lowers food intake and absorption and leads to loss of micronutrients. Therefore, the distribution and the use of fortified foods and micronutrient supplements may be necessary. As in the case with antiretroviral treatment, the distribution of micronutrient supplements should be health-facility based and accompanied with detailed explanations on how to use them to prevent overdosage.

41.3.2 Public health versus therapeutic nutrition interventions

Fig. 41.1 gives a conceptual framework to help understand how targeted nutrition interventions leading to improved nutrition status can influence the outcomes of HIV and AIDS. The figure illustrates two important concepts: first, that poverty, underdevelopment and malnutrition, and the social dimensions of the disease create ideal circumstances for the propagation of the HIV epidemic, which should be addressed by public health nutrition interventions. Second, the diagram illustrates that the biological dimensions of HIV infection call for individualized therapeutic nutrition interventions.

The top of Fig. 41.1 shows how the vicious circle of underdevelopment, food and nutrition insecurity,

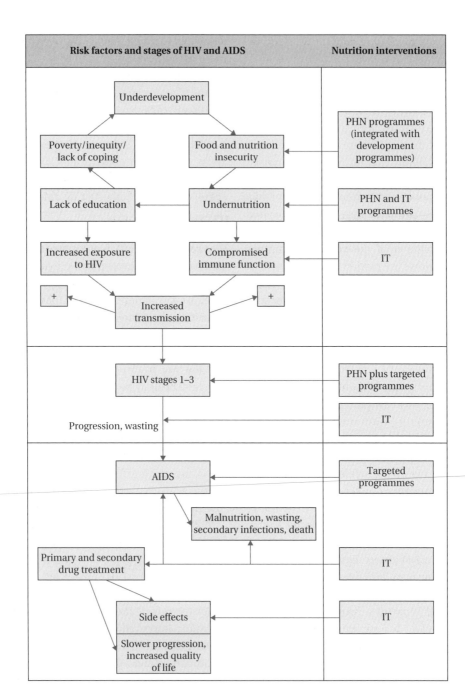

Fig. 41.1 A conceptual framework to show the role of public health nutrition (PHN) and individualized therapeutic (IT) nutrition interventions in HIV and AIDS. The top left section shows that increased transmission of HIV has a positive (+) feedback effect, exacerbating undernutrition and compromised immune function, as well as worsening the factors leading to increased exposure to HIV.

undernutrition, lack of education, poverty, inequity, and lack of coping skills can lead to a lack of knowledge about HIV and AIDS, high-risk behaviours, and increased exposure to the virus. At the same time, undernutrition will lead to a compromised immune system, damage to epithelial barriers, increased susceptibility, and decreased resistance to infections. Collectively, these factors will all increase risk of transmission. The development of HIV will exacerbate the vicious cycle by further worsening nutritional status and impact on all factors contributing to poverty in developing communities. The public health nutrition interventions needed should form part of other health, education, and development programmes. The aims should be to: educate people about AIDS; optimize nutritional status, immunity, and resistance to infections; and promote preventive behaviours, collectively to decrease transmission of the virus. Programmes should be targeted at specific risk groups. The approach, focus, and programme content in the developed and developing worlds will differ and should be tailored to fit specific needs.

The middle of Fig. 41.1 shows the outcome of transmission, namely infection with HIV. The public health nutrition interventions needed during the progression of the infection should include specific nutrition guidelines to all people living with HIV and AIDS and food-aid programmes to assist people living with hunger and food insecurity. The deterioration of immune function, the effect of the virus on reduced food intake and absorption, and increased nutrient requirements and losses all lead to wasting, which requires individualized therapeutic nutrition interventions. The aims are to provide the needy with appropriate foods and supplements and to increase food intake by treating anorexia and wasting, in order to strengthen the immune system and slow the progression of HIV to AIDS.

The bottom of Fig. 41.1 shows that if stages 1–3 are not adequately managed, AIDS develops. If untreated, AIDS will lead to further malnutrition, wasting, secondary infections, and death. If treated with a combination of antiretroviral drugs and appropriate individualized nutrition therapy, further progression of the disease, decreases in viral loads (and therefore less risk of transmission), improved immune function, and an improved quality of life will result. The aims of nutrition therapy during AIDS are to address wasting and side effects of the treatment of primary (HIV) and secondary (opportunistic) infections and to improve immune function. All AIDS patients should have written dietary and lifestyle guidelines and should be educated on how to avoid foodborne and waterborne pathogens, how to ensure nutrient adequacy by diet diversification, and how to use fortified foods and nutrient supplements.

41.3.3 Individualized, therapeutic nutrition interventions

The progression of HIV is associated with changes in nutritional status that require individualized, therapeutic nutrition interventions. The aims of these interventions should be to treat wasting (preserve and restore lean body mass), prevent nutritional deficiencies or excesses that may compromise immune function, minimize complications that interfere with food intake and nutrient absorption, and support antiretroviral and other drug therapies. The standard components of nutrition therapy should be followed: screening, referral, assessment, intervention, outcomes evaluation, and communication. Algorithms for the nutritional support, care, and management of wasting and other symptoms are available in dietetic or clinical nutrition texts (see Box 41.3). Principles of nutrient–drug interactions should be applied. In addition to the general knowledge of food and nutrient effects on absorption and metabolism of drugs, some information is available on how antiretroviral treatment can be optimized. Table 41.1 summarizes practical dietary advice that can be followed to disguise the taste of these drugs, avoid nausea and other symptoms, and ensure optimal absorption. Patients should be counselled and issued with dietary guidelines and recommendations to help them cope with all the side effects and symptoms of both the primary and secondary infection drug therapies. The dietary advice should be based on the known effects of foods to alleviate these problems, but adapted and individualized to fit in with the patient's usual eating pattern. There are indications that some traditional herbal supplements and also garlic- and caffeine-rich foods and drinks may inhibit antiretroviral drug absorption.

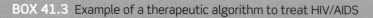

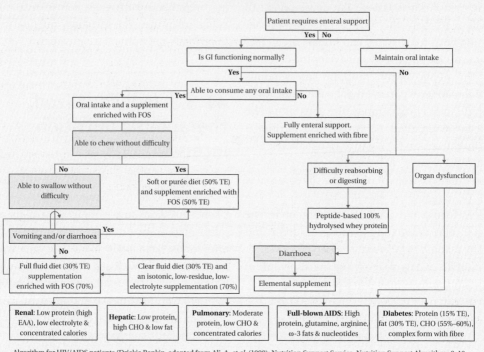

BOX 41.3 Example of a therapeutic algorithm to treat HIV/AIDS

Patient requires enteral support
Yes | No

Is GI functioning normally?

Maintain oral intake

Yes

Able to consume any oral intake
Yes | No

Oral intake and a supplement enriched with FOS

Fully enteral support. Supplement enriched with fibre

Able to chew without difficulty

Difficulty reabsorbing or digesting

Organ dysfunction

No | Yes

Able to swallow without difficulty

Soft or purée diet (50% TE) and supplement enriched with FOS (50% TE)

Peptide-based 100% hydrolysed whey protein

Vomiting and/or diarrhoea
Yes

Diarrhoea

No

Full fluid diet (30% TE) supplementation enriched with FOS (70%)

Clear fluid diet (30% TE) and an isotonic, low-residue, low-electrolyte supplementation (70%)

Elemental supplement

Renal: Low protein (high EAA), low electrolyte & concentrated calories

Hepatic: Low protein, high CHO & low fat

Pulmonary: Moderate protein, low CHO & concentrated calories

Full-blown AIDS: High protein, glutamine, arginine, ω-3 fats & nucleotides

Diabetes: Protein (15% TE), fat (30% TE), CHO (55%–60%), complex form with fibre

Algorithm for HIV/AIDS patients (Driekie Rankin, adapted from Ali, A. *et al.* (1998): Nutrition Support Service, Nutrition Support Algorithms 8, 13
EAA, essential amino acids, FOS = fructo-oligosaccharides, CHO = carbohydrate, GI = gastrointestinal tract, TE = total energy.

These supplements and foods should be avoided until more scientific information on putative beneficial effects are available.

41.3.4 Public health nutrition interventions

Two main types of public health nutrition interventions are needed to address the nutrition problems associated with HIV and AIDS. The first are integrated programmes aimed at optimizing nutrition status of whole populations, communities, and groups of people. The second are targeted programmes that address specific needs of people living with HIV and AIDS.

Integrated nutrition programmes These general programmes form part of policies, strategies, and services within countries aimed at improving the nutrition status of all, and are based on existing nutrition problems in these countries. Examples are programmes to address food and nutrition insecurity, poverty, and undernutrition, but also childhood and adult obesity and programmes to decrease risk factors of non-communicable diseases, as well as efforts to increase fruit and vegetable consumption.

Targeted public health nutrition programmes These are programmes and efforts that address specific nutrition problems associated with HIV and AIDS in groups of infected people. An essential element of these programmes is education of people living with HIV and AIDS to understand the disease, its influence on nutritional status, and how to choose appropriate foods to manage its complications. The World Health Organization has developed a set of user-friendly, practical guidelines for people living with HIV and AIDS. They can be adapted to local circumstances, basing advice on

Table 41.1 Dietary advice to optimize drug treatment of HIV and AIDS

Drug	Objectives	Dietary advice
All drugs	Disguise taste Minimize side effects	Take drug with small quantities of honey, jelly, ice cream, yoghurt, milk shake, fruit juice, fruit ice, or fruit purée
Nevirapine	Avoid aggravating sore mouth	Can be taken with food or on empty stomach Use smooth and moist foods
Indinavir	Avoid nausea, vomiting, change in taste, diarrhoea Optimize absorption	Take on an empty stomach or with a low-fat snack, supplemented with fruit juice or other fluids taken in small, regular amounts
Ritonavir	Avoid nausea, vomiting, diarrhoea, abdominal pain, burning and prickling sensations in mouth	Take with food
Nelfinavir	Avoid loose stools and diarrhoea Optimize absorption	Take with food
Saquinavir (contains lactose)	Avoid nausea, diarrhoea Optimize absorption	Take after a high-energy, high-fat meal
Etavirenze	Optimize absorption	Take with or after meals

existing food-based dietary guidelines within countries. Such guidelines should also include advice on food safety, food preparation, and healthy lifestyles. In countries where hunger and food insecurity are problems, the best advice can only be followed when recommended foods and supplements are available and affordable. Part of these programmes, therefore, could be food aid, providing energy-dense fortified products that are compatible with local culture and eating patterns.

41.4 HIV and AIDS during pregnancy, lactation, and infancy

Without pharmaceutical intervention, the risk of vertical transmission of HIV from pregnant mothers to infants is between 15% and 20%, and during breastfeeding between 20% and 45%. *In utero* and *postpartum* transmission can be reduced to less than 10% by treating pregnant women with oral ARV drugs from 14 to 34 weeks of gestation, and with intravenous ARVs during labour to reduce the viral load in blood and vaginal secretions. Ideally, infants born to infected mothers should also be treated for 6 weeks after birth. There are indications that poor nutritional status of pregnant women increases the risk of transmission.

Human milk can transmit the virus. The rate of HIV infection in breastfed infants increases with the duration of breastfeeding. The risk depends on the viral load and is increased during mastitis, nipple disease, and when breast and bottle feedings are alternated. To reduce risk of transmission, HIV-infected mothers are advised to avoid breastfeeding. In the developing world, this may be difficult because replacement feeding is not always acceptable, feasible, affordable, sustainable, or safe. A lack of clean water and unhygienic practices during replacement feeding are known causes of high rates of infant mortality. In these instances, exclusive breastfeeding is recommended for a few months, to be replaced by alternative feeding when it is available, affordable, and safe. To assist mothers in this difficult choice between breast and replacement feeding, mothers from resource-poor developing countries should be supported with counselling and education regarding the risks to the infant.

Children born to HIV-infected mothers are mostly below the 50th percentile for weight and height. Uninfected, but not infected, children show catchup growth. The poor growth in infected children not receiving antiretroviral therapy is reflected in their reduced survival rates. Energy and protein needs of infected children may be double that of uninfected infants. Increases in energy intake without antiretroviral treatment increase the weight but not the height of infected children. Antiretroviral treatment improves weight, height (growth), development, and survival, provided that secondary infections are prevented or adequately managed. Infected babies, therefore, should be assessed at baseline and nutritionally supported as necessary. All micronutrient intakes should reach dietary recommendations. There is some evidence that megadoses of vitamin A in children under 5 years decrease diarrhoea-related morbidity as well as all-cause and AIDS mortality. For further information and references, see Fawzi *et al.* (1999) and Mehta and Fawzi (2007).

Concluding key points

- The experience with HIV/AIDS in the developed world has shown that although there is no cure or vaccination at present, it is a preventable and manageable disease in which optimum nutrition can help to improve quality of life.

- Unfortunately, in most low- and middle-income countries, underdevelopment, poverty, malnutrition, a lack of education, lack of sufficient health infrastructures and services, and lack of informed, concerned, and committed politicians, as well as the social stigmata associated with the disease, have resulted in the epidemic continuing unabated.

- International cooperation has resulted in scaling up of access to HIV/AIDS prevention and treatment. In 2008, 4 of the 9 million people needing treatment received antiretroviral drugs.

- There are gaps in our knowledge about the effects of HIV/AIDS on nutritional status and the benefits of specific nutrients in the management of the infection.

- At present, the most responsible approach is to optimize nutritional status by diet diversification and the use of fortified foods and micronutrient supplements where indicated to prevent signs and symptoms of nutrient deficiencies. However, pregnant women should not receive vitamin A supplements.

- Hopefully, the gaps in knowledge will motivate further research in this area, providing results and nutrition tools to ensure better outcomes in the management as well as prevention of transmission of HIV infection.

Further Reading

1. **Anon.** (1999) *The demographic impact of HIV/AIDS.* New York, Population Division, Department of Economic and Social Affairs and the Joint UN Programme on HIV/AIDS (UNAIDS).
2. **Fawzi, W.W., Mbise, R., Hertzmark, E., et al.** (1999) A randomized trial of vitamin A supplements in relation to mortality among human immunodeficiency virusinfected and uninfected children in Tanzania. *Paed Infect Dis J,* **18**, 12–13.

3. **Fenton, M. and Silverman, E.** (2000) Medical nutrition therapy for human immunodeficiency virus (HIV) infection and acquired immunodeficiency syndrome (AIDS). In: Mahan, L.K., and Escott-Stump, S. (eds) *Krause's food, nutrition, and diet therapy*. Philadelphia, W. B. Saunders. pp. 889–911.

4. **Kallings, LO.** (2008) The first postmodern pandemic: 25 years of HIV/AIDS. *J Int Med*, **236**, 218–43.

5. **Mehta, S. and Fawzi, W.** (2007) Effects of vitamins, including vitamin A, on HIV/AIDS patients. *Vitam Horm*, **75**, 355–83.

6. **WHO** (2009) *Towards universal access: Scaling up priority HIV/AIDS interventions in the health sector*. Progress report 2009. Geneva, World Health Organization.

7. **WHO/FAO** (2002) *Living well with HIV/AIDS. A manual on nutritional care and support for people living with HIV/AIDS*. Rome, Food and Agriculture Organization.

8. **Zhu, T., Korber, B.T., Nahmias, A.J., Hooper, E., Sharp, P.M., and Ho, D.D.** (1998) An African HIV-1 sequence from 1959 and implications for the origin of the epidemic. *Nature*, **391**, 594.

Useful Websites

To see topical and scientifically robust updates on nutrition associated with this textbook and web links to many of the journals in the Further Reading sections, please see the dedicated Online Resource Centre at **http://www.oxfordtextbooks.co.uk/orc/mann4e/**

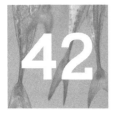

42 Nutritional support for hospital patients

Ross C. Smith

42.1 Enteral nutrition

Surgical staff in the 1960s and 1970s would provide puréed food directly through a large-bore gastrostomy tube into the stomach of patients who were unable to eat. The concept of 'enteral nutrition' is much more refined than this and has developed as a specialized form of nutrition therapy out of the space programme, where a balanced nutrition that resulted in minimal excretion was a distinct advantage (Box 42.1). It is interesting that in the late 1960s the concept of parenteral nutrition was also at a phase of rapid development in the era of early space exploration, and this probably helped to evolve the use of 'space diets' as a type of complete nutrition in a liquid form that could be delivered by a tube directly into the gastrointestinal tract for the treatment of hospitalized patients. The first such product was an elemental formula, but there are benefits for polymeric products because of cost and more efficient metabolism. Following on from the success of enteral nutrition for complex hospitalized patients, the concept has been successfully evolved for nutritional treatment for nursing-home patients and outpatients who are otherwise unable to eat.

Currently, patients entering hospital are screened for nutritional status by admitting doctors, nurses, and dietitians. The at-risk patient is referred to the ward dietitian, who undertakes a more detailed nutritional assessment and considers the best method of treatment: specialized oral diet, enteral nutrition, or parenteral nutrition. Nutritional support becomes indicated for all patients who are unable to nourish themselves with oral intake for more than 5 days, or sooner if they are malnourished on admission and when it is predicted that the time to oral intake will be more than 5 days. Enteral nutrition should always be used in preference to parenteral nutrition when it can be administered safely because it is cheaper, more physiological, and less complicated than parenteral nutrition. It is important to understand the safety issues when deciding on a patient's suitability for treatment.

> **BOX 42.1** Enteral nutrition
>
> Feeding by tube directly into the stomach or upper small intestine by using a formula that is a mixture of nutrient sources that can be passed in water emulsion through a fine tube.

42.1.1 Indications for enteral nutrition

Enteral nutrition is indicated as a means of nutritional support for patients who are unable to sustain themselves with an oral diet and who have a sufficient normal intestine available for absorption of enteral formula. The frequently quoted statement 'If the gut works, use it!' should be remembered in all patients who are referred for nutritional therapy. There are many different clinical situations where enteral nutrition becomes the preferred method of feeding (Table 42.1).

Patients with a stroke or other neurological deficit who are unable to swallow satisfactorily are a good example of a situation where enteral nutrition

Table 42.1 Indications for enteral nutrition

Indication	Examples
Anorexia due to illness	Eating disorders
	Weakness due to illness or surgery
	Cancer
Swallowing disorders	Cerebrovascular disease
	Motor neurone disease
	Oesophageal stricture
Gastric stasis (gastroparesis)	Postoperative, intensive-care patients
Inability to take sufficient oral nutrition	Burns Pancreatitis
	Open, infected wounds
	Trauma
	Inflammatory bowel disease
	Some patients with sepsis

has been found to be invaluable. Critically ill patients who have a functioning gut are also suitable, but there may be an initial period when the gut is not functioning and parenteral nutrition should be considered.

42.1.2 Contraindications to enteral nutrition

The main contraindication to the use of enteral nutrition is poor functioning of the gastrointestinal tract. In general in this circumstance, the enteral nutrition causes vomiting, gastrointestinal distension, or severe diarrhoea. Patients who are frail and have loss of sensation in the pharynx are at great risk of aspiration of enteral nutrition into the lung; an example of such a patient in this circumstance would be following a stroke involving the muscles of the pharynx. Aspiration should be particularly considered when patients are vomiting or have a respiratory disorder. This is a most important issue and needs to be emphasized.

Another important contraindication to the use of enteral nutrition is the presence of inadequate circulation to the gut, which occurs during conditions such as septic shock and the use of high doses of vasopressor agents. Other extreme conditions, such as mesenteric artery thrombosis and abdominal compartment syndrome, cause gross impairment of absorption.

Ethical issues are also important when considering the need for enteral nutrition. Because enteral nutrition allows complete nutritional therapy, withholding such treatment can be seen as denying a patient their normal and natural requirements. Withholding nutritional support from a patient who is unable to eat is an emotionally charged ethical problem. It is inappropriate to withhold treatment from a patient who has reasonable potential for extended quality of life. Alternatively, it is unreasonable to extend a patient's life when there is no hope of relief from pain and suffering. Unfortunately these decisions are not always black and white and there are frequently discrepancies between the expectations of some relatives and of medical and nursing staff. Mostly these issues can be settled by discussion and by helping all parties understand the potential outcomes of the patient's condition. Funding issues are also an important consideration. In some communities, enteral nutrition is funded by government bodies, while in other communities, the patients' families have to pay.

42.1.3 Access to the gastrointestinal tract

Enteral nutrition can be given by mouth as a bolus but, because it is unpalatable and uninteresting when repeated over a number of days, this is not frequently successful. It is therefore mostly given through a tube into the stomach or intestine (Fig. 42.1). The tube can be small and placed as a nasogastric tube. Because it is small and made of soft material, it is quite acceptable for many patients. Although these tubes are fine and can be used for bolus feeding to allow for disconnection and mobility of the patient free from the infusion, they are best tolerated as a continuous infusion over a 24-hour cycle. In some situations nutritional requirements are achieved as an overnight infusion to provide supplementation. Such a programme would require daily insertion of the tube, which would present difficulties.

A gastrostomy tube can be safely inserted through the abdominal skin into the stomach to allow for direct delivery of the nutrition. Gastrostomy tubes are most frequently placed with the aid of the endoscope. Under vision with an endoscope in the stomach, a needle is passed through the skin into the stomach and a guide is passed through the needle. This guide is pulled back into the mouth and attached to the tube. The tube is then pulled in through the mouth and pulled out of the stomach along the needle, leaving a bulbar portion of the tube in the stomach to anchor it in position. These tubes are designed to lie comfortably in the stomach and to be fixed to the skin. Such tubes are more easily used for intermittent feeding and can be disconnected from the nutrition infusion to allow mobility.

Jejunostomy tubes can be placed to lie in the small bowel for conditions that result in poor gastric emptying. Again they can be inserted via the nose, via a gastrostomy, or directly into the small intestine. When the tube is placed into the jejunum, it is best used for continuous infusion.

42.1.4 Enteral formulations

In each class of enteral nutrition formulation, there are numerous commercial products. The reason for choosing one over the other often depends on the presentation or method of delivery. Some formulae are presented as dry powder, while others are presented already prepared in a sterile container with easily connected delivery tubing. Therefore, the choice of solution is frequently not directly related to whether one formula has more or less than another of a particular nutrient. In early formulations, milk was a predominant protein source and with this, lactose was a significant carbohydrate; intolerance to lactose leads to diarrhoea in many patients. In general, lactose has been replaced by corn starch.

The majority of popular formulae use casein hydrolysates for protein and a mixture of different oils for the provision of lipid. They provide 1 kcal/mL

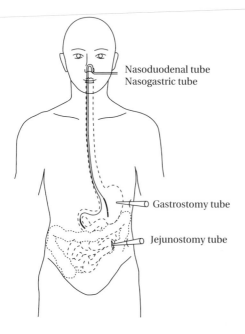

Nasoduodenal tube
Nasogastric tube

Gastrostomy tube

Jejunostomy tube

Fig. 42.1 Routes of enteral (tube) feeding.

of a solution containing about 110 kcal/g N (nitrogen) and have a balance of vitamins, trace elements, and electrolytes with an osmolality of from 300 to 700 mosm/kg.

Polymeric diets These are more commonly used because they are well utilized and are cheap to manufacture. They contain maltodextrins, milk protein, and vegetable oils. They provide recommended dietary intakes (RDIs) of vitamins and minerals and are presented in various manners for ease of clinical use.

Elemental diets Elemental diets were developed for space travel to have low residue. They mainly use amino acids as nitrogen source and are enriched with glutamine. They have a low fat content but provide essential fatty acids along with the RDI of vitamins, trace elements, and electrolytes. Although the amino acids are free, they are not necessarily absorbed more easily because the peptidases in the brush border improve the uptake of amino acids.

Added fibre Some enteral nutrition solutions contain a suitable form of added dietary fibre, which is important for some patients with diarrhoea. The fibre is also an important nutrient for the colonic mucosa and may be useful in patients with colitis.

Prebiotics, probiotics, and synbiotics Some ill patients who are on long-term antibiotics have an alteration of the bowel flora that causes diarrhoea and may lead to endotoxaemia. Strains of lactobacilli, which are normal commensal organisms in the small bowel and may help with digestion of fibre, are able to compete with and reduce the effect of the pathogenic organisms. Different strains of lactobacilli have been recommended. A recent study indicated that these products are dangerous in acutely ill and immune-compromised patients, where they increased the risk of bowel perforation.

Special formulations

- *Immunonutrition*: these solutions contain added amounts of different nutrients considered to be useful in promoting the immune system. They include: ω-3 fatty acids and medium-chain triglycerides, L-arginine and L-glutamine, and dietary nucleotides. These solutions have been shown to reduce postoperative wound infections.
- *Hepatic failure with encephalopathy*: these patients require solutions containing added branched-chain amino acids.
- *Renal failure*: it is important in these patients to reduce solute load to reduce the need for dialysis. The past concept of limiting protein is considered to lead to malnutrition, but there may be improvement in outcome by using a greater proportion of essential amino acids.
- *Acutely stressed patients*: these patients may need high-protein enteral nutrition.

42.1.5 Initiating enteral nutrition

Once the tube is in place, the enteral nutrition is commenced slowly to ensure that there is good tolerance. It is recommended to reduce the rate rather than the concentration of the solution. This author's preference is for continuous feeding because bolus feeding can induce vomiting and dumping with diarrhoea. Regular monitoring of blood glucose, urea and electrolytes, and liver function is important. After 12–24 hours, the rate can generally be increased to provide daily calorie and protein requirements. Frequent assessment of the patients for respiratory distress or abdominal distension should be part of routine care in these patients. Continuous enteral nutrition was not found to reduce the appetite in patients recovering from surgery.

42.1.6 Monitoring for efficacy

Monitoring of patients undergoing enteral nutrition therapy is not an exact science. It is important to monitor the amount that the patient receives and whether or not the patient has nausea, vomiting, or diarrhoea. Patients should have serum urea, electrolytes, albumin, and liver function monitored. By following weight each week, a judgement can be made as to whether more or less nutrition should be provided.

42.1.7 Complications and toxicity

Major complications include aspiration pneumonia, which is a particular threat in patients with weakness and reduced pharyngeal reflexes. It is particularly risky in patients with poor gastric emptying, who may aspirate when vomiting. Other possible major complications are:

- acute intestinal distension and ischaemic damage to the intestine causing intestinal necrosis and disruption;

- dislodgement of the catheter into the peritoneal cavity with spillage of nutrient solution into the peritoneal cavity;

- severe diarrhoea causing electrolyte disturbances.

Moderate to minor complications include:

- diarrhoea;
- metabolic complications;
- glucose intolerance;
- low serum sodium;
- low serum potassium;
- low serum phosphate;
- low serum magnesium;
- essential fatty acid deficiency;
- low serum zinc.

Mechanical issues include:

- blocked feeding tubes;
- dislodged feeding tubes;
- bacterial contamination.

42.2 Parenteral feeding

Parenteral feeding is indicated when patients cannot be nourished with oral nutrition or enteral feeding for more than 5 days. Although the desire to feed directly into the vein had tempted doctors over the centuries, it was not until the development of pyrogen-free fluids in the 1920s and the development of protein hydrolysates and lipid emulsions by Arvid Wretland in the 1940s that this became possible. The technique of complete feeding was further advanced in 1968 by Stanley Dudrick and colleagues with central vein (line) placement and care, so that hypertonic glucose and amino acid solutions could be delivered. They neatly demonstrated that beagle puppies could grow with parenteral nutrition, and subsequently that human infants could develop at a similar rate to breastfed infants. The system of

Dudrick was termed 'hyperalimentation' because it allowed the delivery of large amounts of nutrition that sometimes caused problems of overfeeding. There were fears about the use of lipid emulsions for many years but their safety with admixtures of amino acids and glucose in a three-in-one solution was demonstrated by French workers, and this has gradually become a most common presentation. Three-in-one solutions allow the provision of the daily nutrient requirements in a 3 L bag with an osmolality of about 1000 mosm/L. These solutions can be delivered into peripheral veins, particularly if a fine catheter is used in a larger vein such as the basilic vein. Parenteral nutrition also needs to provide all necessary electrolytes, trace elements, and vitamins in balanced amounts.

42.2.1 Constituents of parenteral nutrition

The glucose concentration ranges from 10% to 50%, which is much higher then the usual 5% of replacement intravenous fluids. One gram of glucose provides approximately 4 kcal (16.8 kJ), so 1 L of 25% glucose will provide about 1000 kcal (4200 kJ).

Lipid emulsions are presented as 10%, 20%, and 30% solutions and provide about 8 kcal/g lipid so 500 mL of 20% solution provides about 1000 kcal (4200 kJ). They have traditionally been composed of soy bean oil with lecithin as emulsifying agent. Some also contain medium-chain triglyceride or safflower oil. They provide the requirement for essential fatty acids (see Section 4.4.2). It is generally considered that 'lipid burns in a carbohydrate fire' and therefore it is usual that no more than 50% of non-protein calories are given as lipid.

Amino acids are provided as crystalline *laevo* form in solutions providing from 5.5 to 11.4 g amino acid per 100 mL. This value needs to be divided by 6.25 to derive grams of nitrogen. The amino acid pattern corresponds to that of high-quality dietary protein.

The glucose, lipid, and amino acid solutions are combined to provide between 110 and 150 non-protein calories to 1 g N in the final solution. Electrolytes, vitamins, and trace elements are also necessary. It is particularly important to provide a balance of the intracellular electrolytes potassium, magnesium, and phosphate because with the provision of nutrition the intracellular compartment expands. If one nutrient is deficient, the response to nutrition is impaired.

An example of an adult formula is given in Table 42.2. This solution is run to provide about 0.25–0.3 g N/kg/day to the acute patient. Long-term patients may require less than this when they are not stressed. The maximum nutritional input that stressed hypermetabolic patients can metabolize is up to twice their basal metabolic rate, but there has been a tendency to be conservative to prevent the complications of overfeeding in these patients.

Table 42.2 Parenteral nutrition, per day

Nitrogen	1 litre 18 g/L (114 g protein)
Glucose	1 litre 25% (1000 kcal)
Lipid emulsion	500 mL 20% (1000 kcal)
Sodium	70–100 mmol
Potassium	60–80 mmol
Magnesium	10–15 mmol
Phosphate	10–20 mmol
Balanced water-soluble and lipid-soluble vitamins	
Balanced trace element solution (zinc, selenium, copper)	
Water	2500 mL

42.2.2 Methods of venous access

When solutions of glucose and amino acids are given, they have an osmolality of about 2000 mosm and a pH approaching 5. This is therefore very irritating to the endothelium in veins and leads to *thrombophlebitis* in a short period of time if such solutions are delivered into small peripheral veins. However, when delivered into a large pool of blood it can be buffered and diluted. It therefore has to be delivered through a catheter placed in a large central vein like the superior vena cava (Fig. 42.2). Central lines require special care to prevent sepsis, and the catheter used for parenteral nutrition should be dedicated to this purpose. Antibiotics and other drugs should be delivered through a separate line. Apart from the risks of insertion of central lines, there is a constant risk of major sepsis either around or through a central line and it needs to be dressed and monitored carefully to prevent overwhelming sepsis. One always needs to be alert to the possibility of sepsis.

The combination of lipid emulsion with the glucose and amino acids results in a complex three-in-one solution. Three-in-one solution allows the buffering of the solution and a marked reduction of osmolarity. When this is at or below 1000 mosm/kg, it can be delivered into peripheral veins using normal cannulae, but these need to be rotated regularly to prevent thrombophlebitis. An improved thrombophlebitis rate can be achieved with a mid-line placed about 15 cm into the basilic vein (Fig. 42.2). There are a number of advantages to midlines because they can be placed without radiological guidance and can be monitored clinically for any tenderness over the vein. These lines need to be 2–3 Fr in size and can only be used for continuous infusion for rates up to 120 mL/hour. They cannot be used for resuscitation. Studies have demonstrated a reduced risk of sepsis with the use of midlines. Another advantage for these lines is that they can be safely managed by nursing staff without the need for referral to the radiology department.

A peripherally inserted central catheter (PICC) line is a further choice because it is safer to insert. Again, it has to be managed very carefully to ensure that sepsis is not introduced around or through the catheter.

42.2.3 Monitoring when on parenteral nutrition

Monitoring of electrolytes in patients treated with parenteral nutrition is required more frequently in the acute setting because the introduction of nutrition can induce severe acute depression of blood values of many nutrients that are marginally deficient. The *refeeding syndrome* (Box 42.2) is prevented by the slow introduction of the parenteral nutrition and the provision of increased amounts of phosphate, potassium, and magnesium. Patients at risk of refeeding syndrome may need to have their electrolytes checked twice daily until they are stable.

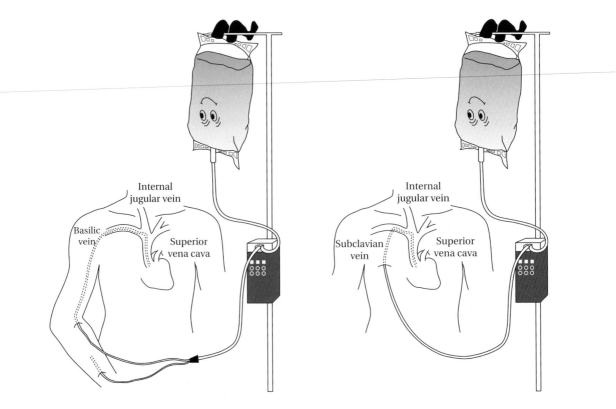

Fig. 42.2 Routes of parenteral feeding.

This occurs in very malnourished patients who are refed too fast. The starved body adapts to use less carbohydrate and more fat. The introduction of artificial nutrition stimulates insulin secretion. There is enhanced uptake into the cells of glucose, water, phosphate, potassium, and magnesium with consequent subnormal extracellular fluid and plasma levels of these electrolytes. This can lead to cardiac arrhythmia. Thiamin deficiency is also a risk.

Monitoring of vitamins and trace elements needs to be undertaken at weekly intervals in the acute setting and 3-monthly in the long-term patients. The vitamins and trace elements most frequently depressed during parenteral nutrition are folate, vitamin C and D, vitamin B_6, zinc, selenium, and copper. Essential fatty acid deficiency occasionally occurred in patients who had glucose as the only nonprotein calorie source and was prevented by twice-weekly lipid infusions. However, one needs to be aware that there may be depression of any nutrient that is not included in the parenteral nutrition formula.

Protein-calorie nutritional status is monitored with blood values that reflect protein metabolism, such as plasma proteins, albumin, transferrin, and C-reactive protein. Serum creatinine and urea are depressed in patients with malnutrition and it is important to observe these return to the normal range. Measures of body composition can be simple, by anthropometric measures of skin folds and arm muscle circumference. There are a number of techniques for estimating muscle and fat mass, including electrical bioimpedence, DEXA, CT assessment, and neutron activation analysis (see Chapter 31).

Blood glucose is also important to monitor to prevent hyperglycaemia. In intensive-care patients, this requires a 4-hourly finger-prick for blood glucose. In the more stable ward patient, a urinalysis is undertaken twice daily and followed by blood glucose measures if urine glucose is elevated.

Acid–base balance should be measured on arterial blood samples if the patient's condition suggests a metabolic disturbance. After the patient has reached goal amounts of parenteral nutrition infusion, the frequency of blood electrolyte measures can be reduced to every other day if the patient is stable. Home parenteral nutrition patients are frequently sufficiently stable that electrolytes only need to be measured at monthly intervals.

42.2.4 Complications

Complications of parenteral nutrition include:

- Complications of venous catheter insertion. These are greatest when a central venous catheter is used; there is a risk of significant injury to the subclavian and related vessels or a pneumothorax can occur.

- Sepsis is a constant risk for patients with parenteral nutrition. Again, this is greater with central venous access than with peripheral venous access, and any spike in fever or persistent fever has to alert the medical team to the possibility of line sepsis. Such events should be treated with removal of the line and blood culture.

- Metabolic complications are mostly related to hyperglycaemia. The many possible nutrient deficiencies are discussed in the monitoring section (see Section 42.2.3).

Requirements of several *vitamins* given parenterally are approximately 2 × the RDI (i.e. food by mouth): thiamin, riboflavin, niacin, pantothenate, vitamin B_{12}, and vitamin C. This is because of oxidation in the bag or faster urinary excretion when they go into a peripheral vein rather than the portal system. On the other hand, requirements are lower for several *inorganic* elements that are poorly absorbed when taken by mouth: about half or a third of the RDI for calcium, phosphorus, zinc, and copper, and about a tenth for iron.

42.3 Nutritional support teams

Many studies have demonstrated the benefit of nutritional support teams. With complex medical treatment for patients in intensive care, gastroenterology, surgical, oncology, and renal failure wards, many patients have poor nutritional status, and the prevention of significant nutritional deficiency has been shown to improve outcome. Multidisciplinary teams help make this process happen in a complex tertiary hospital but all medical and paramedical staff need to be aware of the importance of good nutritional care.

42.3.1 Decision path for nutritional therapy

When a patient is at risk of developing malnutrition, Fig. 42.3 may help in considering nutritional therapy. Clearly it is unacceptable to allow patients to become malnourished in hospital when there are well-designed therapies that have proven efficacy for preventing this. There is a large body of evidence that malnutrition increases the risk of complications and death. Nutritional assessment of patients entering hospital is important, and there should be a greater stress on recording body weight and weight loss, plasma proteins, lymphocyte count, and haemoglobin values on a nutritional assessment form.

Enteral nutrition should be used if the gut is available and functioning. Enteral nutrition is most commonly delivered through a fine-bore nasogastric tube. In complex patients in intensive care, it may be important to pass the tube into the jejunum. Long-term access may require the placement of a feeding gastrostomy or jejunostomy tube. Enteral nutrition

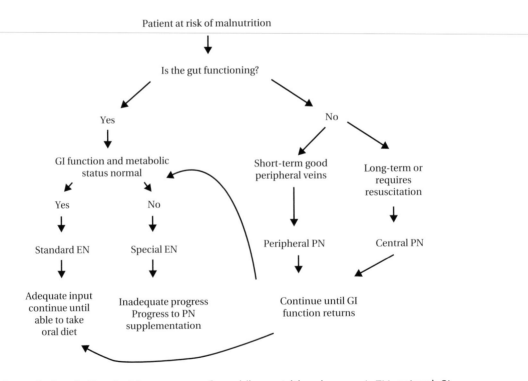

Fig. 42.3 Some factors in the decision process of providing nutritional support. EN, enteral; GI, glycaemic index; PN, parenteral.

is frequently prescribed to provide 20–25 kcal/kg/day, while the infusion rate for parenteral nutrition is frequently 25–35 kcal/kg/day. The decision to use either peripheral or central parenteral nutrition depends on the presence of suitable peripheral veins. Peripheral parenteral nutrition is preferred because the nutrient composition is satisfactory for repletion when given peripherally, and sepsis and complications of venous access are reduced. Infusion rates need to be individualized, depending on tolerance and complication and whether there is a positive response to treatment.

Useful Websites

To see topical and scientifically robust updates on nutrition associated with this textbook and web links to many of the journals in the Further Reading sections, please see the dedicated Online Resource Centre at **http://www.oxfordtextbooks.co.uk/orc/mann4e/**

Index